PARASITOLOGY

PROTOZOOLOGY AND HELMINTHOLOGY

IN RELATION TO CLINICAL MEDICINE

With two hundred fourteen illustrations

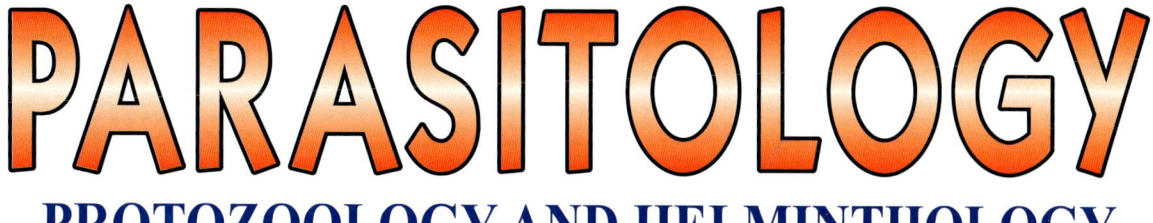

By

K.D. CHATTERJEE M.D. (CAL)

Professor of Medicine

THIRTEENTH EDITION

Dr. D. CHATTERJEE M.D. (CAL)

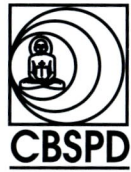

CBSPD

CBS Publishers & Distributors Pvt Ltd

New Delhi • Bengaluru • Chennai • Kochi • Kolkata • Lucknow • Mumbai
Hyderabad • Jharkhand • Nagpur • Patna • Pune • Uttarakhand

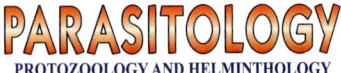

PROTOZOOLOGY AND HELMINTHOLOGY

IN RELATION TO CLINICAL MEDICINE
With two hundred fourteen illustrations

ISBN : 978-81-239-1810-5

First Edition: August 1957
Twelfth Edition: April 1980
Reprinted: January 1981
Reprinted: January 1982

Thirteenth Edition: September 2009
Reprinted: February 2011
Revised and Reprinted: February 2012
Reprinted: January 2014
Reprinted: January 2015
Reprinted: January 2017
Reprinted: January 2019
Reprinted: 2022, 2023, 2024, **2025**

Copyright © by Dr. D. Chatterjee M.D. (Cal)
6, Amrita Banerjee Road, Kolkata - 700 026

Published by Satish Kumar Jain and produced by Varun Jain for
CBS Publishers & Distributors Pvt Ltd
4819/XI Prahlad Street, 24 Ansari Road, Daryaganj, New Delhi 110 002, India.
Ph: 011-23289259, 23266861   Website: www.cbspd.com
e-mail: delhi@cbspd.com

Corporate Office: 204 FIE, Industrial Area, Patparganj, Delhi 110 092
Ph: 011-4934 4934   Fax: 011-4934 4935   e-mail: publishing@cbspd.com;
publicity@cbspd.com

Branches

• **Bengaluru:** Seema House 2975, 17th Cross, KR Road, Banasankari 2nd Stage, Bengaluru 560 070, Karnataka, India
Ph: +91-80-26771678/79   Fax: +91-80-26771680   e-mail: bangalore@cbspd.com
• **Chennai:** 18/8B, Subbarayan Street, Shenoy Nagar, Chennai 600 030, Tamil Nadu, India
Ph: +91-44-42032115, 26681266   e-mail: chennai@cbspd.com
• **Kochi:** 42/1325, 1326, Power House Road, Opp KSEB, Power House, Ernakulum Kochi 682 018, Kerala, India
Ph: +91-484-4059061-65,67   Fax: +91-484-4059065   e-mail: kochi@cbspd.com
• **Kolkata:** 147, Hind Ceramics Compound, 1st Floor, Nilgunj Road, Belghoria, Kolkata-700056, West Bengal, India
Ph: +033-25633055, 033-25633056   e-mail: kolkata@cbspd.com
• **Lucknow:** Basement, Khushnuma Complex, 7 Meerabai Marg (Behind Jawahar Bhawan),Lucknow-226001, UP, India
Ph: +0522-4000032   e-mail: tiwari.lucknow@cbspd.com
• **Mumbai:** PWD Shed, Gala no 25/26, Ramchandra Bhatt Marg, Next to JJ Hospital Gate no. 2, Opp. Union Bank of India,
Noorbaug, Mumbai-400009, Maharashtra, India
Ph: 022-66661880/89   e-mail: mumbai@cbspd.com

Representatives

• Hyderabad	0-9885175004	• Jharkhand	0-9811541605	• Nagpur	0-8692091830
• Patna	0-9334159340	• Pune	0-9664372571	• Uttarakhand	0-9716462459

Printed at Nutech Print Services, Faridabad, Haryana, India

PREFACE TO THE THIRTEENTH EDITION

The text has been revised and brought up to date by adding new informations wherever necessary. The volume of the book however has been appreciably enlarged, maintaining the original purpose, namely, to provide a book of handy size.

The book was out of print for a considerable period. The inconvenience caused thereby is regretted.

I am sincerely thankful to Mrs. N. Chatterjee, Miss S. Chatterjee and Mr. S. Nath for their efforts to bring out this edition.

Calcutta   Dr. D. Chatterjee M.D. (Cal)
28th September 2009
Revised and Reprinted: February 2012

ACKNOWLEDGEMENTS

Prof. K.D. Chatterjee acknowledged the help which he had received in the past from the following persons:

Dr. D.R. Seaton of Liverpool School of Tropical Medicine.

Dr. T. Clive Backhouse, Hony. Consultant Parasitologist to the Tropical Section of St. Vincent's Hospital, Sydney; formerly Senior Lecturer in Parasitology, School of Public Health and Tropical Medicine, University of Sydney.

Dr. Leroy J. Olson, Assistant Professor, Department of Microbiology and Dr. Howard C. Hopps, Professor and Chairman, Department of Pathology, University of Texas.

Dr. John W. Orr, Professor of Pathology, University of Birmingham.

Dr. J.J.C. Buckley, Professor of Helminthology, London School of Hygiene and Tropical Medicine.

Dr. W. Peters, Professor of Parasitology, Liverpool School of Tropical Medicine.

Dr. H. Spencer, Professor of Pathology, St. Thomas's Hospital Medical School, London.

Dr. George S. Nelson, Professor of Helminthology, London School of Hygiene and Tropical Medicine.

Dr. D. Chatterjee acknowledges the help which he received for this edition from the following persons:

Dr. A.K. Bandyopadhyay, Retd. Associate Prof. & Head, Dept. of Helminthology, School of Tropical Medicine, Calcutta.

Dr. N.K. Jana, Reader, Dept. of Zoology, Charuchandra College, Calcutta.

Dr. B.B. Bandyopadhyay, Head, Dept. of Physiology, R.P.M. College, Hoogly, West Bengal.

Mr. U. Hazra, Reader & Head, Dept. of Zoology, R.P.M. College, Hoogly, West Bengal.

PREFACE TO THE FIRST EDITION

This book has been developed from the author's previous book entitled *Human Parasites and Parasitic Diseases* which, according to many, was considered to be a comprehensive treatise—a reference book—though not so appealing to the undergraduates on account of its large size.

This present volume has therefore been reduced to a handy size, in which elaborate discussions have been avoided, but all basic facts with which a medical student should be familiar, have been dealt with. In short, it should serve as a book of ready reference on Parasitology, dealing with the essential characters of parasites infecting man, as also the pathogenic effects and methods of diagnosis.

The book has been divided into four sections. The first is an introductory section describing the terminology and general principles of parasitological studies. Then there are two sections: Protozoology and Helminthology. In each section the parasites of man have been classified and described under the following headings: Geographical distribution, habitat, morphology and life cycle, pathogenicity and clinical features, diagnosis, treatment and prophylaxis. The concluding section is by way of an appendix, detailing various techniques adopted for parasitological diagnosis. (Treatment of parasitic infections has been added in the appendix from the 4th Edition.)

This book is adequately illustrated with the line diagrams and coloured plates and there are also specially compiled tables to assist the reader in readily grasping the essential points discussed in the text. In fact, no pains have been spared to make the book as attractive and appealing to the students as possible and the author hopes that he has been able to provide a complete guide to the students reading Medical Parasitology, which will not only be of help in their class-work but will also give them a better understanding of the subject. If the book should be equally useful to teachers, laboratory workers and practitioners, the author would feel amply rewarded for his efforts.

The author desires to record his appreciation of the valuable services rendered by Sree Saraswaty Press Ltd., in the printing of the book.

Calcutta
21st August 1957

K.D. Chatterjee

CONTENTS

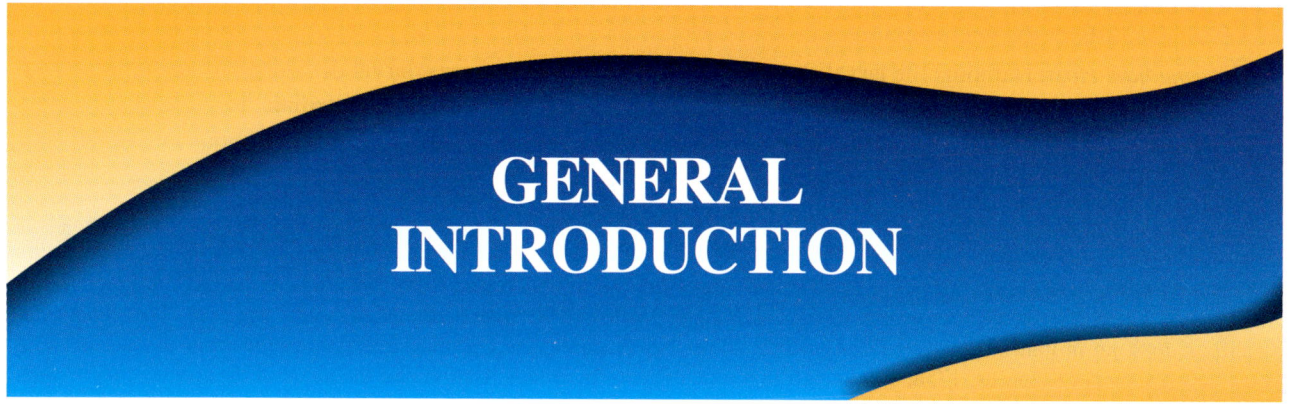

GENERAL INTRODUCTION

Terms Employed in Parasitology

Parasite. A living organism* which receives nourishment and shelter from another organism where it lives.

Host. An organism which harbours the parasite.

Association of living things which live together: An association which is formed between animals of different species may be divided into three categories:

Symbiosis. An association in which both are so dependent upon each other that one cannot live without the help of the other. None of the partners suffers any harm from the association.

Commensalism. An association in which the parasite only is deriving benefit without causing injury to its host. A *commensal* is capable of leading an independent life.

Parasitism. An association in which the parasite derives benefit and the host gets nothing in return but always suffers some injury, however slight the injury may be. The host, at the same time, offers some resistance to the injury done by the parasite and there may be some adaptation (*tolerance*) between the parasite and the host. A *parasite* has lost its power of independent life.

Zoonosis. Evolution of a human disease naturally acquired from an infection primarily confined to vertebrate animals. Literally, the term "zoonosis" means a disease of animals. Leishmaniasis, trypanosomiasis (Chagas' disease and "Rhodesian" sleeping sickness), trichinelliasis and echinococcosis are typical examples of zoonotic diseases.

Classes of Parasites

Ecto-parasite (Ectozoa): Lives outside on the surface of the body of the host.

Endo-parasite (Entozoa): Lives inside the body of the host: in the blood, tissues, body cavities, digestive tract and other organs.

Temporary Parasite: Visits its host for a short period.

Permanent Parasite: Leads a parasitic life throughout the whole period of its life.

Facultative Parasite: Lives a parasitic life when opportunity arises.

Obligatory Parasite: Cannot exist without a parasitic life.

Occasional or Accidental Parasite: Attacks an unusual host.

Wandering or Aberrant Parasite: Happens to reach a place where it cannot live.

---

*The living organisms may be animals, plants (bacteria) or viruses but this book is concerned only with animals that are parasitic in man.

Classes of Hosts

Definitive Host: Either harbours the adult stage of the parasite or where the parasite utilises the sexual method of reproduction. In the majority of human parasitic infections, man is the definitive host; in malaria and hydatid disease, however, man acts as the intermediate host.

Intermediate Host: Harbours the larval stages of the parasite. In some cases, larval developments are completed in two different intermediate hosts, which are being referred to as *first* and *second* intermediate hosts, respectively.

Paratenic Host (A carrier or transport host): A host, where the parasite remains viable without further development.

Nomenclature of Parasites

Each parasite possesses two names, a generic and a specific; the former begins with an initial capital and the latter with an initial small letter, after which comes the designator's name, followed by punctuation and finally the year. The generic and specific names are in italics but not the designator's name. For example, the common intestinal roundworm of man is named *Ascaris lumbricoides* Linnaeus, 1758. This means that it belongs to the Genus *Ascaris* and the name of the species *lumbricoides* was given by Linnaeus in the year 1758. When the name assigned to the parasite is later transferred, the correct name is written as usual followed by the original name with the year in parenthesis.

The animal parasites which medical men have to deal with are divided into three main groups:

   I. Phylum Protozoa—*Medical Protozoology.*

  II. Phylum Platyhelminthes and Phylum Nemathelminthes—*Medical Helminthology.*

 III. Phylum Arthropoda—*Medical Entomology.*

While describing animal parasites certain rules of zoological nomenclature are followed and each phylum may be further subdivided as follows:

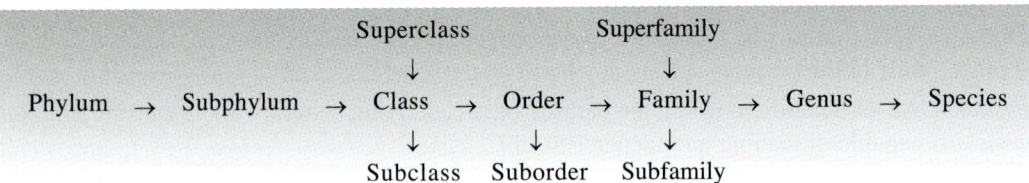

SCHEME FOLLOWED IN PARASITOLOGICAL STUDIES

The study of animal parasites infecting man and producing clinical manifestations should include the following:

1. History of the discovery of the parasite.
2. Geographical distribution.
3. Habitat inside the human host.
4. Morphology and life cycle (staining methods and cultivation).
5. Modes of infection: Reservoir host, sources of infection, portal of entry, vehicle of transmission.
6. Effect of the parasite: Pathogenic lesions, Clinical manifestations.
7. Immunological responses.
8. Methods for specific diagnosis.
9. Approved therapy for eradication of the parasitic infection.
10. Prophylactic measures for the prevention of parasitic infection of the individual as well as of the community.

History. The date and the year in which the parasite was first identified and any important discovery and knowledge regarding it.

Geographical Distribution. Environmental factors, social customs and habits of person greatly influence the distribution of parasites and accordingly each parasite has got a specific distribution.

Habitat. Each parasite, according to the mode of its existence, selects a particular place of abode in the host. The parasite, after entering into the body, may directly establish itself in the place where it is introduced or the parasite, on entering the body through a particular route, may travel through various organs till it reaches its normal abode for its growth to sexual maturity. In some cases, the larval form of the parasite, after getting into its normal habitat, does not develop directly into adult worm, but takes a circumroutous path and on arrival for the second time, at the same place starts growing to maturity, as in the case of *Ascaris lumbricoides*. The parasite, in some cases, may grow to maturity at its normal site of localisation and then may migrate to a suitable site to enable its progeny to be transferred to a second host, as in Schistosoma; or it may discharge its larvae which are carried to some distant places either to be taken up by an intermediate host, as in Wuchereria, or remain encysted in the striped muscle, as in Trichinella. The sites of such localisation (Figs. 1 & 2) will no doubt give an idea about the pathogenic effects and the channels through which the progeny may come out of the human host.

Immunology. There are two main types of immunity: Innate and Acquired. *Innate immunity* is not dependent upon previous exposure to infection and is not the result of specific responses of immunocompetent cells. It is probably related to the genetic constitution of the host. The example of genetic innate immunity of man to "human" parasitic infection is seen amongst west Africans who are more resistant than white Americans to hookworm infection and vivax malaria. It is also known that African children carrying the sickle-cell trait (HbS heterozygotes) are relatively resistant to *P. falciparum* infection. *Acquired immunity* may be gradually built up after a natural infection or may be induced artificially, as in cutaneous leishmaniasis (Oriental sore). This is known as *active immunity*. Immune bodies (IgG fraction or 7S immunoglobulin) may be passively transferred to a newborn infant *via* placenta and milk of an immune pregnant woman which is known as *passive immunity*. In hyperendemic malarious area, infants born from immune mothers are thus protected for the first 6 months of life against *P. falciparum* infection. Thereafter, the child suffers from malarial attack for 2-5 years, when the acquired immunity is gradually built up and as the child grows up becomes tolerant to re-infection, i.e., a balance is achieved between infection and resistance.

ACQUIRED ACTIVE IMMUNITY: UNDERLYING MECHANISM

Immune reactions in acquired active immunity are mediated by cellular or humoral mechanism or both.

I. Humoral mechanism: *Synthesis of specific immunoglobulins.* In this case, the antigens are first taken up by macrophages before passing them on to the immuno-competent cells — "thymus-dependent" lymphocytes and plasma cells. The antibody producing plasma cells are derived from bone marrow stem cells and are not dependent on thymus. Of the five major classes of immunoglobulins, IgA, IgD, IgE, IgG and IgM, the last two are important. A high level of specific immunoglobulins is found in many protozoal and helminthic infections. They may be protective and help recovery from infections, whereas others are precipitating and may be utilised for various serological tests for the immuno-diagnosis of parasitic infections. The concentration of IgG and IgM are both increased in malaria, the former has an antiplasmodial effect, whereas the latter helps phagocytosis. In trypanosomiasis, the concentration of IgM fraction of serum immunoglobulin is greatly increased but it has no affinity for the infecting organism and is non-specific. Serum antibodies are demonstrable in kala-azar, but they do not help recovery from infection. Protective antibodies also develop in helminthic infections, such as strongyloidiasis, ancylostomiasis and ascariasis, which lower the worm burden.

II. Cellular mechanism: *(a) Development of cell-mediated immunity.* "Thymus-derived" lymphocytes seeded out to spleen and lymph nodes are required for cell-mediated immunity. They become sensitised and play the dominant role in eliminating the parasites. Such immunity can be transferred by lymphoid cells and inhibited by immuno-suppressive agents. They also participate in formation of certain types of antibody, which remains firmly bound to the cells and not readily released, thereby acting as a specific antigen-recognising mechanism of these sensitised cells. A marked cell-mediated immunity develops in self-curing cutaneous leishmaniasis, like Oriental sore and chiclero's ulcer which can be demonstrated by a delayed type of hypersensitivity skin reaction. A cell-mediated immunity also develops in trichinosis and schistosomiasis.

II. Cellular mechanism: *(b) Development of non-specific cellular response.* Antigenic stimulus provokes cells of the reticulo-endothelial system (macrophage system) to proliferate and actively phagocytose the antigen. This is particularly seen in African trypanosomiasis, where the macrophages play the dominant role of the defensive mechanism in clearing the trypomastigotes. In malaria, the main agent in immunity is serum antibodies but their effectiveness may depend upon a synergic action with the macrophage system.

OTHER TYPES OF IMMUNE REACTIONS

Autoimmune reaction. This is an immune reaction in which antibodies develop against some constituents of body's own tissues, e.g., autoimmune antibody developing against erythrocytes and causing anaemia in kala-azar and malaria.

Hypersensitivity reaction. Immune reactions not only protect but on access to the antigen for a second time can produce an abnormally exaggerated response which may themselves be injurious or may be responsible for various pathological reactions in tissues. These reactions may be of two types:

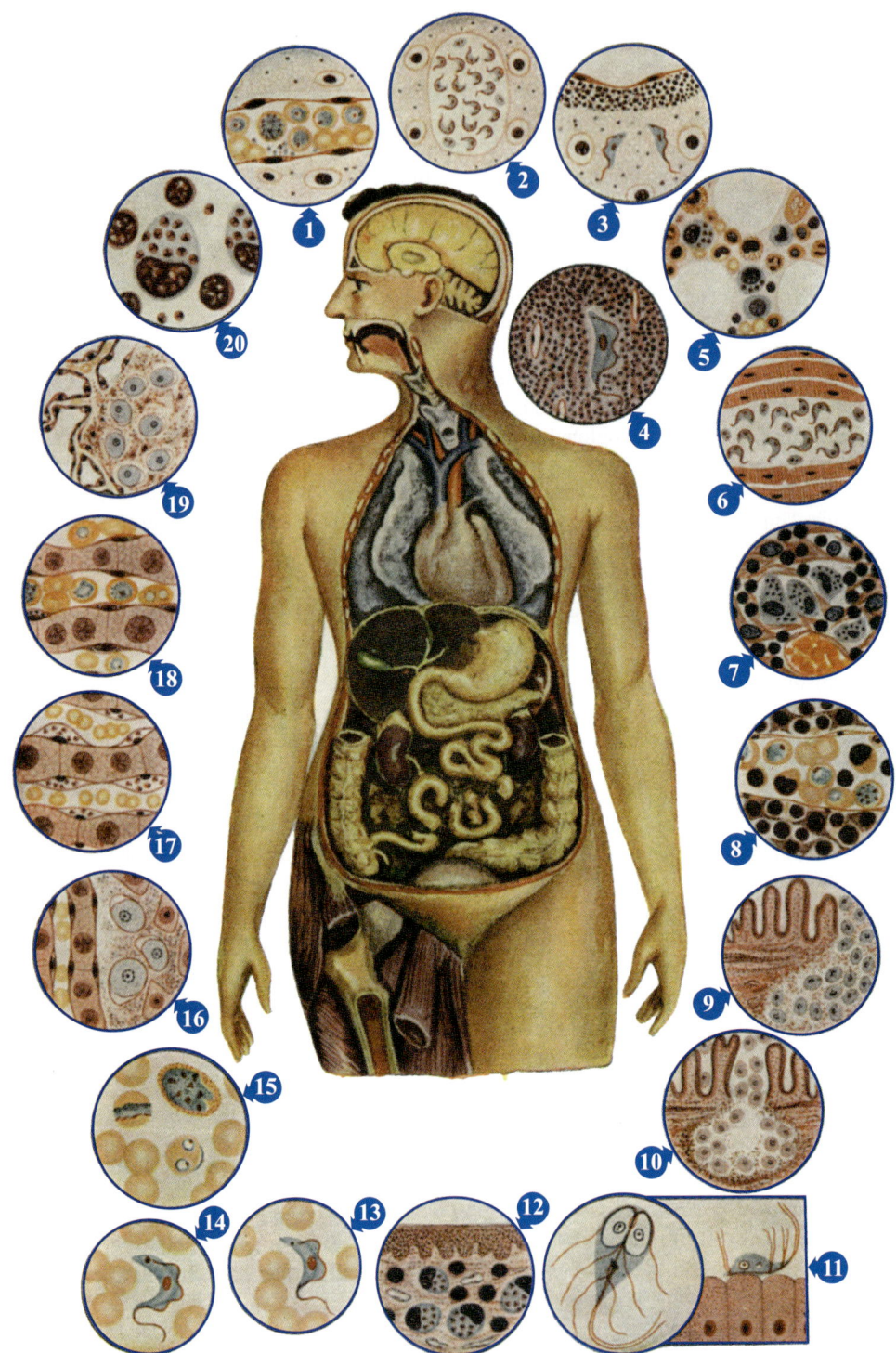

Fig. 1—Distribution and localisation of protozoal parasites inside the human body.

BRAIN: 1, *P. falciparum*; 2, *T. cruzi*; 3, *T. brucei* subgroup. LYMPH NODE: 4, *T. brucei* ("gambiense" strain). BONE MARROW: 5, *L. donovani*. HEART MUSCLE: 6, *T. cruzi*. SPLEEN: 7, *L. donovani*; 8, *P. falciparum*. LARGE INTESTINE: 9, *B. coli*; 10, *E. histolytica*. SMALL INTESTINE: 11, *G. intestinalis*. SKIN: 12, *L. donovani* and *L. tropica*. BLOOD: 13, *T. brucei* subgroup; 14, *T. cruzi*; 15, *P. vivax*, *P. malariae* and *P. falciparum*. LIVER: 16, *E. histolytica*; 17, *L. donovani*; 18, *P. falciparum*. LUNG: 19, *E. histolytica*. ORO-NASAL MUCOUS MEMBRANE: 20, *L. brasiliensis*.

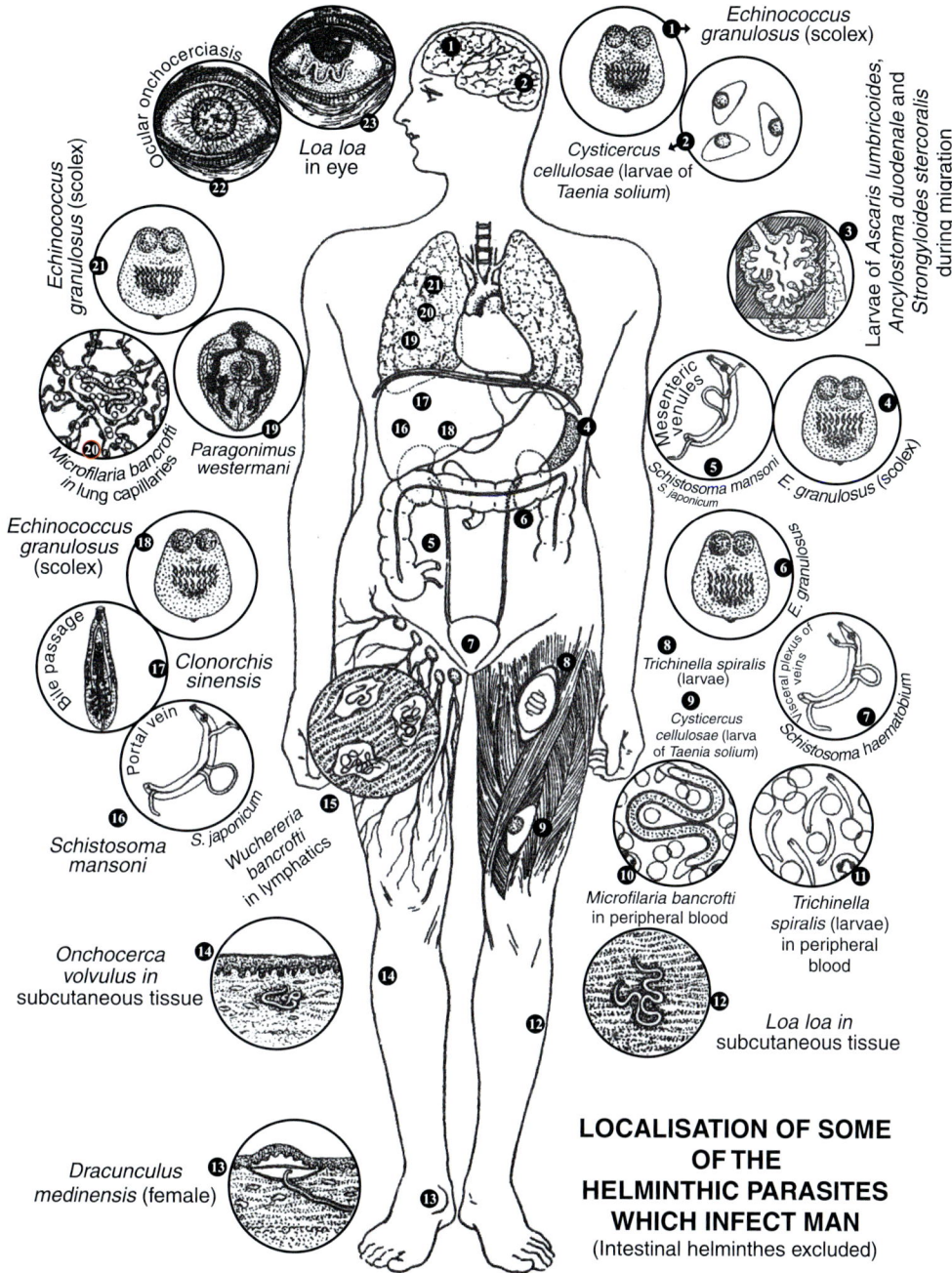

Fig. 2—Somatic helminthiasis.
Forms of helminthic parasites encountered in tissues or organs are inserted within the
circle with their names outside. The numbers of the circles correspond to those
in the human body and represent the areas of localisation.

(a) An immediate type of hypersensitivity reaction resulting from antibody-mediated immunity. This may occur from contact of antigen with antibody fixed to the cells, as in anaphylactic reaction, or the antigen-antibody complexes may induce pathological changes, as in nephrotic syndrome in quartan malaria.

(b) A delayed type of hypersensitivity reaction resulting from a cell-mediated immunity. This is often used as an intradermal test for parasitological diagnosis as in Montenegro reaction in leishmaniasis and is also responsible for the granulomatous reaction provoked by Schistosome eggs.

Premunition. This is a concomitant immunity or infection immunity in which there is a relative resistance to reinfection of host still carrying the infecting organism. It disappears with the cure of parasitic infection. It is seen in many parasitic infections, particularly in malaria and schistosomiasis. In malaria, as long as, the erythrocytic parasites survive the "premunition" persists but with total destruction of parasites it disappears. In schistosomiasis, the adult worms resist immunological attacks and persist in the host for long periods. It has been attributed to the acquisition of a coating of host antigen, which prevents their destruction by the immune responses excited by the adult worms themselves.

Tolerance. This term is applied to an infection immunity where there is a host-parasite adjustment, so that the infection is allowed to continue without producing adverse effect on the host and the individual becomes resistant to reinfection. This explains why resistance to infection tends to increase as the age advances.

Note: Prophylactic immunisation has not been successful or practical against human parasitic diseases, except in a few protozoal infections, e.g., Oriental sore.

Morphology and Life Cycle. Under this heading, the general structure of the parasite and the various stages through which it passes, are studied. The parasite may pass its life cycle in one and the same host or it may change its host.

Modes of Infection. Transmission of the parasite from one host to another is effected by certain forms which are known as infective stages. The means by which different infecting agents are transferred from one host to another and the avenues through which they enter the human host require careful consideration. In an endemic area, a parasitic infection is continually kept up by the presence of hosts acting as reservoirs of infection; such hosts may be either animals or man. Where an insect intermediate host (vector) plays the part in dissemination of the disease, its bionomics should also be carefully studied.

Reservoirs of Infection. In a majority of cases, man is the main reservoir. In such cases, the parasite does not produce any manifest symptoms but remains in the host and keeps up the infection, thus helping to maintain a "carrier state". During this "carrier state", the parasite evolves certain resistant forms which help in the dissemination of the disease, *e.g.,* cysts of *E. histolytica*, gametocytes of malarial parasite. In certain species of parasites, both men and lower animals are infected, the latter serving as reservoirs of infection: examples are "Rhodesian" trypanosomiasis (antelope), Oriental sore (dog), kala-azar occurring in China and Mediterranean areas (dog), balantidiasis (pig), trichinelliasis (pig and rat) and hydatid disease (sheep and cattle).

Sources of Infection and Portal of Entry. Infective stage of the parasite may reach the human body in the following ways (Fig. 3 and *vide* table below).

1. BY CONTAMINATION OF FOOD OR DRINK. The pathogenic species under this group gain entrance into the digestive tract. Some of the examples are:
    (a) Cysts of *E. histolytica* and eggs of *A. lumbricoides* which contaminate the food or drink.
    (b) The infective forms may remain in the flesh of some intermediate hosts, which are taken as food, such as: *(i)* Beef containing the larval stages of *T. saginata (Cysticercus bovis); (ii)* Pork containing the larval forms of *T. solium (Cysticercus cellulosae)* and the larval forms of *T. spiralis; (iii)* Fish containing the plerocercoid larvae of *D. latum* and metacercarial forms of *C. sinensis; (iv)* Crab or crayfish containing metacercarial forms of *P. westermani.*
    (c) Sometimes the intermediate host harbouring the infective form may be taken up as a whole, *e.g.,* cyclops infected with the larval forms of *D. medinensis* are ingested with water.
    (d) The infective forms may come out of its intermediate host and encyst in aquatic plants, eaten as food by man, *e.g.,* metacercarial forms of *F. buski* and *F. hepatica.*

2. BY CONTAMINATION OF THE SKIN OR MUCOUS MEMBRANE. Examples are:
    (a) The filariform larvae of *A. duodenale, N. americanus* and *S. stercoralis* which abound in damp soil, may penetrate the unbroken skin of an individual walking over such places bare-footed.
    (b) The cercarial forms of *S. haematobium, S. mansoni* and *S. japonicum* in infected water, may penetrate the skin of a person coming in contact with such water.

3. BY THE AGENCY OF INSECT HOST. An infected blood-sucking arthropod may introduce the organism directly into the blood or into the skin or into the skin layers at the time of obtaining a blood-meal, *e.g.,* Plasmodia (malarial parasites) by Anopheline mosquitoes, Trypanosoma by Glossina (tsetse flies), Leishmania by Phlebotomus (sandflies) and Wuchereria by Culicine mosquitoes. In this group, the parasites undergo a biological development for a certain period before becoming infective to man.

4. BY SEXUAL CONTRACT: Trophozoites of *T. vaginalis* can be transmitted by sexual contract.

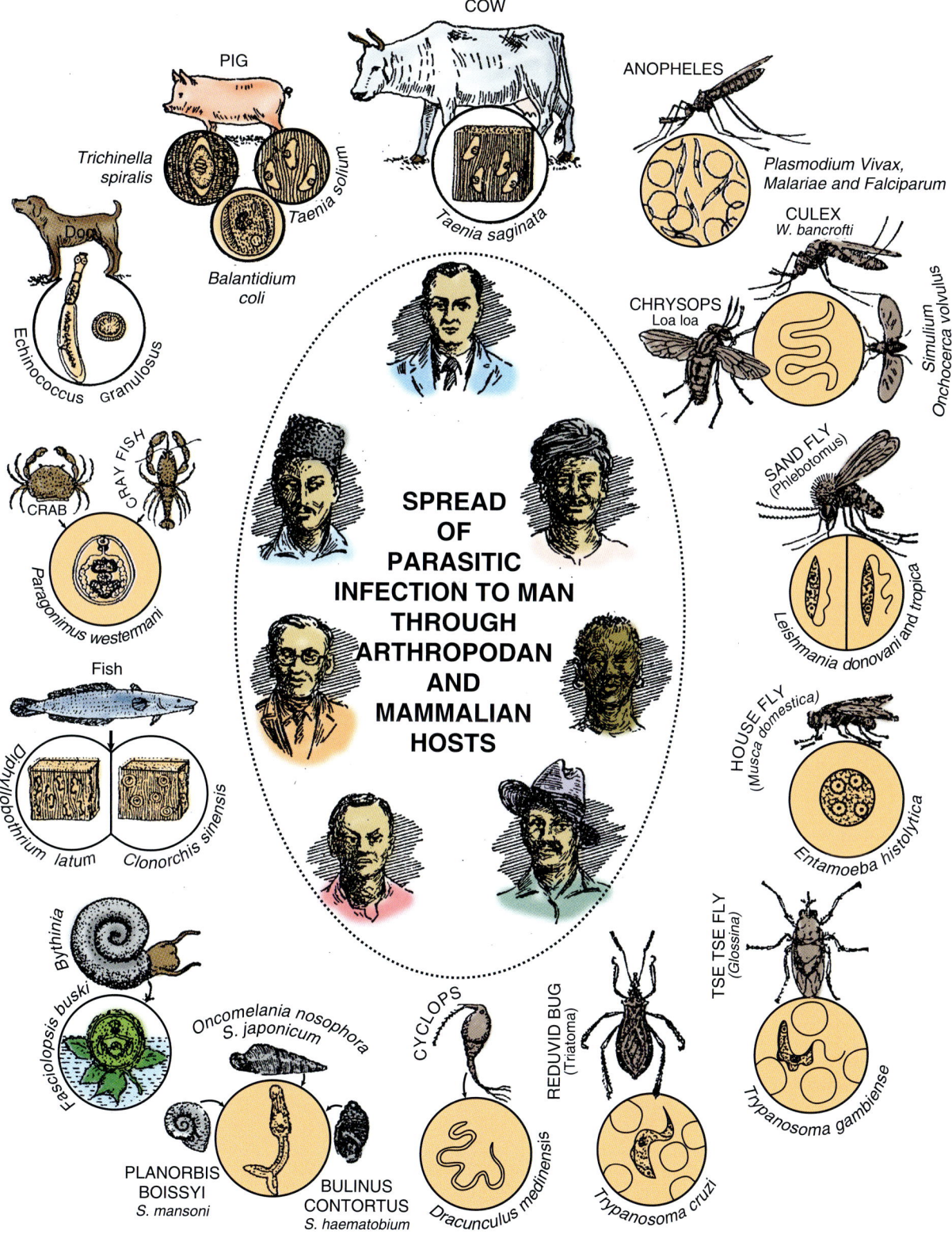

COW

PIG

ANOPHELES

Trichinella spiralis

Taenia solium

Balantidium coli

Taenia saginata

Dog

Plasmodium Vivax, Malariae and Falciparum

CULEX
W. bancrofti

CHRYSOPS
Loa loa

Echinococcus   Granulosus

Simulium Onchocerca volvulus

CRAY FISH

CRAB

SAND FLY
(Phlebotomus)

Paragonimus westermani

Leishmania donovani and tropica

Fish

SPREAD OF PARASITIC INFECTION TO MAN THROUGH ARTHROPODAN AND MAMMALIAN HOSTS

HOUSE FLY
(Musca domestica)

Diphyllobothrium latum   *Clonorchis sinensis*

Entamoeba histolytica

Bythinia

TSE TSE FLY
(Glossina)

Fasciolopsis buski

Oncomelania nosophora S. japonicum

CYCLOPS

REDUVID BUG
(Triatoma)

PLANORBIS BOISSYI
S. mansoni

BULINUS CONTORTUS
S. haematobium

Dracunculus medinensis

Trypanosoma cruzi

Trypanosoma gambiense

Fig. 3—The infective forms of the parasite are depicted within the circle under each host. In *Echinococcus granulosus*, the egg is the infective form. Dog and anopheles represent the definitive hosts of the parasite shown in the diagram, all other animals are intermediate hosts.

TABLE SHOWING THE SPREAD OF PARASITIC INFECTIONS

Sources of Infection	Infective forms, where found	Portal of Entry	Infection of Parasite
THROUGH MAMMALIAN HOST			
COW	C. bovis in muscles	Ingestion, Al. tract*	T. saginata
PIG	(a) C. cellulosae in muscles	Ingestion, Al. tract	T. solium
	(b) Encysted larvae in muscles	Ingestion, Al. tract	T. spiralis
	(c) Plerocercoid larvae in muscles	Ingestion, Al. tract	Spirometra larval stage
	(d) Cysts of B. coli in faeces	Ingestion, Al. tract	B. coli
DOG	Eggs of E. granulosus and T. canis in faeces, contamination of food	Ingestion, Al. tract	E. granulosus
			Larva migrans (Visceral)
CAT	Oöcysts in faeces	Ingestion, Al. tract	T. gondii
THROUGH PISCINE HOST			
FRESH-WATER FISH	Plerocercoid larvae in fish flesh	Ingestion, Al. tract	D. latum
	Metacercariae in fish flesh	Ingestion, Al. tract	C. sinensis
	Metacercariae in fish flesh	Ingestion, Al. tract	H. heterophyes
	Metacercariae in fish flesh	Ingestion, Al. tract	M. yokogawai
THROUGH MOLLUSC (SNAIL)	Cercariae encysted in aquatic vegetation	Ingestion, Al. tract	F. buski
			F. hepatica
	Cercariae liberated in water	Penetration, Skin	Schistosomes
THROUGH ARTHROPOD			
CRAB OR CRAYFISH	Metacercariae in fish	Ingestion, Al. tract	P. westermani
CYCLOPS	(a) Larvae inside the body cavity	Ingestion, Al. tract	D. medinensis
	(b) Procercoid larvae inside the body	Ingestion, Al. tract	Plerocercoid larvae Spirometra
REDUVIID BUG	Metacyclic forms in hind-gut	Contamination, Skin	T. cruzi
TSETSE FLY (Glossina)	Metacyclic forms of trypomastigotes in salivary gland	Inoculation, Skin	T. brucei subgroup
SANDFLY (Phlebotomus and Lutzomyia)	Promastigotes in pharynx and buccal cavity	Inoculation, Skin	L. donovani
			L. tropica
			L. brasiliensis
MOSQUITOES			
Anopheles	Sporozoites in salivary glands	Inoculation, Skin	Malaria parasites
Culex	Larvae in proboscis	Dropped on Skin	W. bancrofti
Mansonioides	Larvae in proboscis	Dropped on Skin	B. malayi
CHRYSOPS	Larvae in proboscis	Dropped on Skin	L. loa
SIMULIUM	Larvae in proboscis	Dropped on Skin	O. volvulus
HOUSE-FLY	Cysts in Al. canal, contamination of food	Ingestion, Al. tract	E. histolytica
THROUGH HUMAN FAECES			
Contamination of food	(a) Eggs of Enterobius, Hymenolepis nana, T. solium	Ingestion, Al. tract	E. vermicularis
			H. nana
			C. cellulosae
	(b) Cysts of E. histolytica and B. coli	Ingestion, Al. tract	E. histolytica
			B. coli
THROUGH SOIL			
Polluted with human faeces	(a) Embryonated eggs of Ascaris, Trichuris	Ingestion, Al. tract	A. lumbricoides
			T. trichiura
	(b) Filariform larvae of Hookworm and Strongyloides	Direct penetration, Skin	A. duodenale
			N. americanus
			S. stercoralis
Polluted with faeces of dogs and cats	(a) Embryonated egg of Toxocara canis and T. catis	Ingestion, Al. tract	Larva migrans (Visceral)
	(b) Filariform larvae of A. caninum and A. braziliense	Direct penetration, Skin	Larva migrans (Cutaneous)
THROUGH WATER**			
Infective forms liberated from snail	Cercariae of Schistosoma free in water	Direct penetration, Skin	S. haematobium
			S. mansoni
			S. japonicum
Infected cyclops	Dracunculus larvae in cyclops	Ingestion, Al. tract	D. medinensis

*Al. tract—Alimentary tract   **Also mentioned under snail and cyclops.

Pathogenic Effects. These vary with the nature of parasitic infections:

In protozoal infections, the lesions are greatly influenced by proliferation, multiplication and metastasis to distant organs. In *E. histolytica*, the trophic form secretes a powerful histolytic toxin, causing destruction of the tissues. In plasmodia the parasite, while undergoing erythrocytic schizogony, causes destruction of erythrocytes (R.B.C.).

In the majority of helminthic infections, the adult parasites are found inside the human body and *no multiplication occurs* except in cases of strongyloidiasis and hymenolepiasis. It is the number of invading organisms gaining entrance during primary infection and re-infection that constitutes the most important problem in the development of clinical manifestations in helminthiasis. The effects produced therefore depend upon their habitat, i.e., the sites where the parasites attack the tissues and also on the pattern of laying eggs or larvae. In certain helminthic infections, the normal secretions and excretions of the growing larvae and the products liberated from dead parasites behave like foreign proteins and give rise to various *allergic manifestations*. Allergic state of various helminthic infections may be recognised by skin tests (intradermal) with specific antigens (*vide infra*).

Other pathogenic effects

Some parasitic infections produce an immunosuppressive state, thereby allowing the pathogenic bacteria to invade the tissues which the patient is unable to resist, as in trypanosomiasis, kala-azar and malaria. Immunosuppressive states or agents may help parasitic multiplication, resulting in fulminant parasitaemia, as in falciparum malaria or may favour massive invasion of the tissue, as in strongyloidiasis or may help "opportunist infection", as in toxoplasmosis.

The parasitic infection may contribute to the development of neoplastic growth. Examples are (*i*) adenocarcinoma of the bile duct and primary liver cell carcinoma in fascioliasis and clonorchiasis, (*ii*) colonic, rectal, hepatic and vesical carcinoma in schistosomiasis and (*iii*) Burkitt's lymphoma in malarial infection.

In some helminthic infections, the migrating larvae may carry viruses and Gram negative bacteria from the intestine to the blood and tissues, as in strongyloidiasis, trichinosis and ascariasis.

The pathological changes induced by the parasite may be the result of immunological responses. The following are some examples: (a) Nephrotic syndrome and idiopathic tropical splenomegaly in malaria, (b) Autoimmune haemolytic anaemia observed in malaria and kala-azar, (c) Granuloma formation with consequent fibrosis in schistosomiasis, the result of a cell-mediated immunity, (d) Manifestations of occult filariasis.

Laboratory Diagnosis. Depending on the nature of the parasitic infections, the following materials should be collected for specific diagnosis:

1. *Blood*. In those parasitic infections, where the parasite itself, or in any stage of its development, circulates in the blood stream, examination of blood film forms one of the main procedures for specific diagnosis. Examples are:

In malaria, the parasites are found inside the erythrocytes (R.B.C.).

In kala-azar, *L. donovani* are found inside the monocytes of blood.

In African sleeping sickness and Chagas' disease, trypomastigotes are found in the blood plasma.

In Bancroftian and Malayan filariasis, microfilariae are found in the blood plasma.

In case of leishmaniasis and trypanosomiasis blood culture and animal inoculation are helpful, but not used now as routine procedure.

2. *Stool*. Examination of the stool forms an important part in the diagnosis of intestinal parasitic infections and also for those helminthic parasites, which localise in the biliary tract and discharge their eggs into the intestine.

In protozoal infections, either trophozoites or cystic forms may be detected; the former, during the active phase and the latter, during the chronic phase. Examples are amoebiasis, giardiasis and balantidiasis.

In the case of helminthic infections, either the adult worms or their eggs are found in the stool. Examples are:

  (i) Eggs are found in intestinal helminthiasis (ascariasis, hookworm infection, trichuriasis, fasciolopsiasis, intestinal schistosomiasis, taeniasis, diphyllobothriasis, hymenolepiasis and dipylidiasis) and also where the adult worms inhabit the biliary tract (fascioliasis and clonorchiasis).

  (ii) In enterobiasis, eggs are *rarely found* in the stool, because they are deposited on the perianal skin and hence *anal swabs* are to be taken for the diagnosis.

  (iii) In strongyloidiasis, larvae, not *eggs*, are commonly present in freshly-passed stool.

  (iv) Adult worms are found in ascariasis and after a vermifuge in hookworm infection and enterobiasis. Segments of adult worms are found in taeniasis, diphyllobothriasis and other intestinal tapeworm infections.

3. *Urine.* When the parasite localises in the urinary tract, examination of the urine will be of help in establishing the parasitological diagnosis. Examples are:

(i) In vesical schistosomiasis, terminal-spined eggs of *S. haematobium* are found.

(ii) In cases of chyluria caused by *W. bancrofti*, microfilariae are found (very very rarely).

4. *Sputum.* Examination of the sputum is useful in the following:

(i) In cases, where the habitat of the parasite is in the respiratory tract, as in paragonimiasis, the eggs of *P. westermani* are found.

(ii) In amoebic abscess of lung or in the case of amoebic liver abscess bursting into the lungs, the trophozoites of *E. histolytica* are detected.

(iii) In cases of rupture of hydatid cyst of the lung, scolices and hooklets of *E. granulosus* are obtained.

5. *Other Body Fluids.* Examination of vaginal and uretheral discharge may demonstrate *T. vaginalis.* Trophozoites of *G. intestinalis* and larvae of *S. stercoralis* may be found duodenal aspirates.

6. *Biopsy Material.* It varies with different parasitic infections. As for example:

(i) Spleen puncture in cases of kala-azar.

(ii) Bone marrow puncture in cases of kala-azar and African trypanosomiasis.

(iii) Lymph node puncture in cases of African sleeping sickness and filariasis; also in cases of kala-azar occurring in China and Mediterranean areas.

(iv) Skin biopsy in cases of dermal leishmanoid, espundia and onchocerciasis.

(v) Muscle biopsy in cases of cysticercosis, trichinelliasis and Chagas' disease.

(vi) Rectal biopsy in cases of intestinal schistosomiasis.

(vii) Liver biopsy in cases of visceral schistosomiasis.

(viii) Aspiration of (a) hydatid fluid, (b) material from amoebic liver abscess and (c) fluid from hydrocele for revealing scolex of *E. granulosus*, trophozoite of *E. histolytica* and microfilaria of *W. bancrofti* respectively. Tropozoites of *G. lamblia* may be demonstrated in duodenal aspirates.

(ix) Lumbar puncture. Cerebrospinal fluid may be collected for the diagnosis of African trypanosomiasis (sleeping sickness). Tropozoites of *N. fowleri* and *acanthemeba* may be detected in the CSF.

7. X-ray, ultrasound, CT scan and MRI are also useful in diagnosis of various parasitic diseases.

8. *Indirect Evidences.* Changes indicative of internal parasitic infection are:

(i) *Cytological Changes in the Blood.* Eosinophilia* often gives an indication of tissue invasion by a helminth, leucopenia is a feature of kala-azar and neutrophilic leucocytosis is observed in amoebic liver abscess. Anaemia (a reduction of erythrocytes) is a feature of hookworm infection and malaria.

(ii) *Biochemical Alteration of the Blood.* Hypergammaglobulinaemia in cases of kala-azar, African trypanosomiasis, schistosomiasis and visceral larva migrans. This is detected as a formol-gel test (aldehyde test of Napier) or as a precipitation reaction (Brahmachari's or Sia's test, antimony test of Chopra *et al.*).

(iii) *Serological Tests* are used to detect antigens or antibodies in the patient's serum and other clinical specimens. In some parasitic infections such as toxoplasmosis and hydatidosis, where parasites are seldom detected, serological tests are most helpful.

(a) Specific complement fixation test is used in many protozoal and helminthic infections, such as Chagas' disease, amoebiasis, toxoplasmosis, filariasis, trichinelliasis, hydatid disease, schistosomiasis and clonorchiasis.

Non-specific complement fixation test, as in kala-azar.

(b) Specific precipitin test, as in schistosomiasis, hydatid disease and amoebiasis. Specific precipitin antibody may also be demonstrated by flocculation test, such as bentonite flocculation test in trichinelliasis and hydatid disease.

(c) Specific agglutination test, as in leishmaniasis.

(d) Specific dye test of Sabin and Feldman, as in toxoplasmosis.

(e) Immobilisation test, as in amoebiasis.

(f) Reaction of the parasite with fluorescein-tagged homologous antibody, as in *E. histolytica* and Toxoplasma. The fluorescent antibody technique has also been employed for the serological diagnosis of certain helminthic infections (schistosomiasis, trichinelliasis and onchocerciasis), and also in malaria and visceral leishmaniasis.

---

* Eosinophilia is not found when helminths have settled at their sites of election. Helminths, not adapted to man, when gain access to man's tissues often provoke a marked eosinophilia.

(g) ELISA test, (Enzyme linked immunosorbent assay), RIA (Radioimmunoassay), IEP (Immunoelectrophoresis), CIEP (Countercurrent immunoelectrophoresis) and double diffusion tests are now available for diagnosis of the disease.

(h) Molecular method—Use of PCR, DNA probes hold better scope for diagnosis of many parasitic infection.

(iv) *Intradermal Reaction (Skin Test).* This is positive in many helminthic infections, such as hydatid disease (Casoni's test), schistosomiasis (Fairley's test), filariasis, trichinelliasis, ascariasis and strongyloidiasis; it is positive in certain protozoal infections, such as Chagas' disease, espundia, Oriental sore, amoebiasis and toxoplasmosis.

Note: Most of the immunological tests mentioned above can be carried out only in laboratories where special antigens are available.

Treatment. Many of the parasitic infections can be cured by specific chemotherapy and the greatest advance has been made in the treatment of protozoal diseases (*vide* respective chapters).

For the treatment of intestinal helminthiasis, drugs are given orally for direct action on the helminths. To obtain maximum parasiticidal effect, it is desirable that the drugs administered should not be absorbed and the drugs should also have minimum toxic effect on the host.

In the treatment of somatic helminthiasis, drugs administered by mouth should be readily absorbable and they should have marked parasitotropic and the least organotropic action. When administered by parenteral injections, the drugs must reach the various tissues of the body, where the helminths are located. Although effective remedies have not yet been discovered for somatic helminthiasis, some advances have recently been made regarding the treatment of paragonimiasis, clonorchiasis, schistosomiasis, fascioliasis and wuchereriasis.

Prophylaxis. Prophylactic measures that may be adopted in parasitic infections include the following:

1. *Therapeutic Prophylaxis.* The parasite is attacked within the host, thereby preventing the dissemination of the infecting agent.

2. *Drug Prophylaxis.* Measures are adopted not to prevent the infection but to abort the clinical manifestations by specific drug therapy, hence this method is also known as *clinical prophylaxis* or *suppressive therapy.*

3. Eradication of the infection in the reservoir hosts and destruction of intermediary hosts. The infective agents may also be destroyed while they exist free outside the human host.

4. Personal prophylaxis may further be ensured by preventing the susceptible individuals coming in contact with infecting agents.

5. Avoidance of consumption of raw and under-cooked flesh of beef or pork, non-cooked fish, crab, cray fishes, cyclops and watercress.

SECTION I

PROTOZOOLOGY

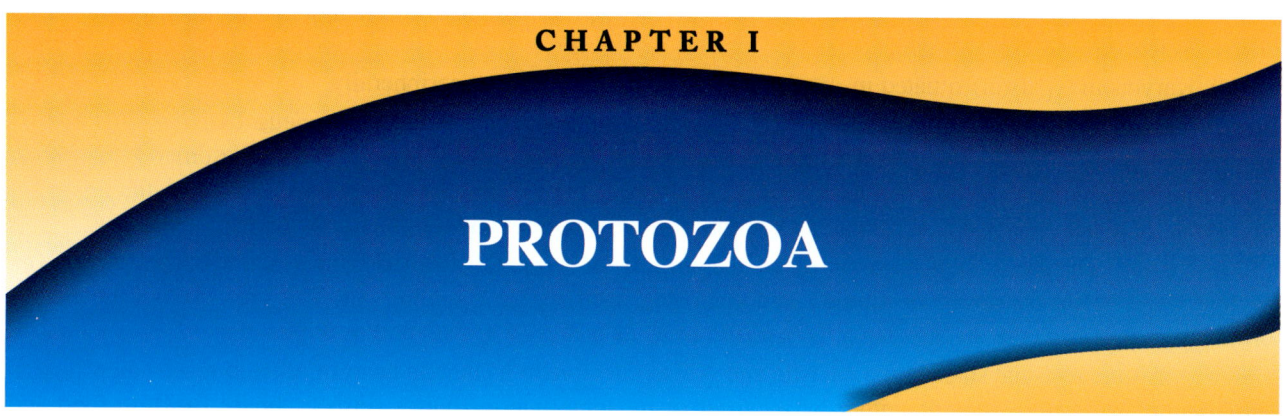

CHAPTER I

PROTOZOA

Definition. Protozoal parasite consists of a single "cell-like unit", which is morphologically and functionally complete. The differences between protozoa and metazoa are as follows:

	Protozoa	Metazoa
Morphology:	Unicellular. A single "cell-like unit".	Multicellular. A number of cells, making up a complex individual.
Physiology:	A single cell performs all the functions: reproduction, digestion, respiration, excretion etc.	Each special cell performs a particular function.

Morphology. The structure of a protozoal "cell" is composed of (1) a cytoplasmic body and (2) a nucleus.

CYTOPLASM. It may be divisible into two portions:

(a) *Ectoplasm.* The external hyaline portion; its function is protective, locomotive and sensory.

(b) *Endoplasm.* The internal granular portion; its function is nutritive and reproductive.

STRUCTURES DEVELOPED FROM ECTOPLASM

(i) *Organelles of Locomotion*

    (a) PSEUDOPODIA. Prolongation of temporary ectoplasmic process, seen in Rhizopodea.

    (b) FLAGELLA. Long delicate thread-like filaments, seen in Zoomastigophorea.

    (c) CILIA. Fine needle-like filaments covering the entire surface of the body, seen in Ciliatea.

        Speed of Locomotion:

            Amoeba—0.2 to 3 micrometres (μm) per second.

            Flagellates—15 to 30 micrometres (μm) per second.

            Ciliatea—400 to 2,000 micrometres (μm) per second.

                1 micrometre (μm) = 0.001 millimetre (mm).

(ii) *Contractile Vacuoles.* Situated inside the endoplasm; excretory function.

(iii) *Rudimentary digestive organ*, such as cytostome ("cell mouth") and cytopharynx, seen in *Balantidium coli*.

(iv) *Cyst-wall.* A thickened resistant wall, seen in the cystic stage.

NUCLEUS. It is the most important structure, as it controls the various functions and regulates reproduction. It is situated inside the endoplasm and its structure is often of great help in the differentiation of genera and species. Its structure comprises of the following:

(i) Bounded externally by a well-defined nuclear membrane.

(ii) Made up of a network of linin, enclosing within it the nuclear sap.

(iii) Chromatin granules, lining the inner side of the nuclear membrane or appearing as condensation on linin threads.

(iv) Karyosome (palstin) situated inside the nucleus either centrally or peripherally.

Kinetoplast, Micronucleus and Macronucleus. In most of the protozoa there is one nucleus. In Ciliatea two nuclei are present—a small micronucleus and a large macronucleus. Certain protozoa, such as trypanosomatid flagellates, show in addition to the nucleus, a non-nuclear DNA-containing body called the *kinetoplast*, near which the flagellum originates; there is a small body at the point of origin of the flagellum known as the *basal body*.

ENCYSTMENT. The protozoal parasite possesses the property of being transformed from an active (trophozoite) to an inactive stage, losing its power of motility and enclosing itself within a tough wall. The protoplasmic body thus formed is known as a cyst. At this stage, the parasite loses its power of growth and multiplication.

The *cyst* is the resistant stage of the parasite and is also infective to its human host. In order to reach a new host, it must be transferred mechanically, either by a carrier or by some intermediaries (insect—house-flies), to food and drink which become contaminated with the cysts of protozoa.

Reproduction. The protozoal parasites may exist in two stages: trophozoite and cyst, as in intestinal flagellates and amoebae. In such cases, the parasite multiplies only in the trophic stage. The methods of reproduction or multiplication among the parasitic protozoa are of the following types:

1. *Asexual Multiplications:*

   (i) BY SIMPLE BINARY FISSION. In this process, the individual parasite divides either longitudinally or transversely into two more or less equal parts. Before division all the structures are duplicated.

   (ii) BY MULTIPLE FISSION OR SCHIZOGONY. In this process, more than two individuals are produced, as in Plasmodia. The nucleus of the parent cell at first undergoes repeated divisions which are then surrounded by the cytoplasm. When the multiplication is completed, the parasitic body or the schizont ruptures and liberates these daughter individuals which in their turn repeat their life cycle.

2. *Sexual Reproduction:*

   (i) BY CONJUGATION. In this process, a temporary union of two individuals occurs during which time interchange of nuclear material takes place. Later on, the two individuals separate, each being rejuvenated by the process, as in Ciliatea.

   (ii) BY SYNGAMY. In this process, sexually differentiated cells, called gametes, unite permanently and a complete fusion of the nuclear material takes place. The resulting product is then known as a zygote, as in Plasmodia.

Life Cycle. A protozoal parasite may multiply vigorously by asexual method for a long time, and later by a change of process, it either has recourse to sexual method of reproduction or undergoes encystment for a change of its host. The sexual method of reproduction often occurs in a different host other than the one utilised for asexual multiplication; the process is known, as alternation of generation accompanied by alternation of host, as seen in Plasmodia. A protozoal parasite may pass its life cycle in one or two hosts.

Second Host Not Required. Examples are Rhizopodea, intestinal flagellates and Ciliatea. The parasites in this group adapt themselves for passive transfer from one host to another by encystment. The species multiplies asexually in its trophic stage and in circumstances unfavourable for its existence, secretes a resistant cyst-wall, transforming itself into a cyst. When the condition becomes favourable again, the organism leaves the cyst (excystment) and continues its life in the trophozoite stage. Thus, encystment is not a reproductive process, but a means of protection of the species from extinction. In amoeba, however, multiplication may take place within the cyst where the nucleus divides into 2, 4 or 8 daughter nuclei. Later, when the organism leaves the cyst, complete division of the cell occurs and a number of individual organisms are liberated. Both the processes, encystment and excystment, occur in one and the same host, but after encystment, a transference to another new host is required for further development.

Second Host Required. Examples are Trypanosoma, Leishmania and Plasmodia. In Trypanosoma and Leishmania, the second host is required for the development of a special cycle, which is essential for the continuation of the species from one host to another. In Plasmodia, the asexual method of multiplication is carried out in one host and the sexual method of reproduction in another host.

Classification of Protozoa

A. *Systematic Classification*

(1) Based on the recommendation of the Committee on Systematics and Evolution of the Society of Protozoologists consisting of Levine *et al.* (1980), the protozoal parasites of man are classified as follows:

Phylum	Subphylum	Superclass	Class	Subclass	Order	Suborder	Genus
KINGDOM PROTISTA **SUBKINGDOM PROTOZOA**							
Sarcomastigophora	Mastigophora		Zoomastigophorea		Kinetoplastida	Trypanosomatina	Leishmania Trypanosoma
					Retortamonadida		Chilomastix Retortamonas
					Diplomonodida	Diplomonadina Enteromonadina	Giardia Enteromonas
					Trichomonadida		Trichomonas Pentatrichomonas Dientamoeba
	Sarcodina	Rhizopoda	Lobosea	Gymnamoebia	Amoebida	Tubulina	Entamoeba Amoebae Endolimax Iodamoeba
						Acanthopodina	Acanthamoeba
					Schizopyrenida		Naegleria
*Apicomplexa			Sporozoea	Coccidia	Eucoccidiida	Eimeriina	Eimeria Isospora Toxoplasma Sarcocystis
						Haemosporina	Plasmodium
				Piroplasmia	Piroplasmida		Babesia
Microspora			Microsporea		Microsporida	Apansporoblastina	Enterocytozoon Encephalitozoon Nosema
Ciliophora			Kinetofragminophorea	Vestibuliferia	Trichostomatida	Trichostomatina	Balantidium

* Some workers place *Pneumocystis* under phylum Apicomplexa whereas others consider it as protozoa of uncertain classification. Other Apicomplexa parasites under the subclass Coccidia include *Cryptosporidium* and *Cyclospora*.

(2) A revised scheme of classification of protozoa replacing the scheme conventionally in use has been proposed by Honigberg *et al.** (1964) and is given below:

The phylum PROTOZOA has been divided into 4 subphyla: Subphylum I Sarcomastigophora, Subphylum II Sporozoa, Subphylum III Cnidospora (no human representative) and Subphylum IV Ciliophora.

Phylum PROTOZOA Goldfuss 1918, emend, von Siebold, 1845.

Subphylum I **Sarcomastigophora** Honigberg & Balamuth, 1963. It is divided into 3 superclasses.

Superclass I MASTIGOPHORA Diesing, 1866. It has 2 classes.

Class 1 PHYTOMASTIGOPHOREA Calkins, 1909 (no human representative).

Class 2 ZOOMASTIGOPHOREA Calkins, 1909. It has 9 orders.

Order 4 KINETOPLASTIDA Honigberg, 1963. It has 2 suborders.

Suborder 1 *Bodonina* Hollande, 1952.

Suborder 2 *Trypanosomatina* Kent, 1880.

*B. M. Honigberg *et al. J. Protozoology*, **11**, 7-20, 1964.

Order 5 RETORTAMONADIDA Grassé, 1952.

Order 6 DIPLOMONADIDA Wenyon, 1926.

Order 8 TRICHOMONADIDA Kirby, 1947.

Order 9 HYPERMASTIGIDA Grassi & Foâ, 1911.

Superclass II OPALINATA Corliss & Balamuth, 1963 (no human representative).

Superclass III SARCODINA Hertwig & Lesser, 1874. It is divided into 3 classes.

Class 1 RHIZOPODEA von Siebold, 1845. It has 5 subclasses.

Subclass 1 LOBOSIA Carpenter, 1861. It has 2 orders.

Order 1 AMOEBIDA Kent, 1880.

Class 2 PIROPLASMEA Levine, 1961.

Class 3 ACTINOPODEA Calkins, 1909 (no human representative).

Subphylum II **Sporozoa** Leuckart, 1879. It is divided into 3 classes.

Class 1 TELOSPOREA Schaudinn, 1900. It has 2 subclasses.

Subclass 1 GREGARINIA Dufour, 1828 (no human representative).

Sublcass 2 COCCIDIA Leuckart, 1879. It has 2 orders.

Order 1 PROTOCOCCIDA Cheissin, 1956 (no human representative).

Order 2 EUCOCCIDA Léger & Duboseq, 1910. It has 3 suborders.

Suborder 1 *Adeleina* Léger, 1911 (no human representative).

Suborder 2 *Eimeriina* Léger, 1911.

Suborder 3 *Haemosporina* Danilewsky, 1885.

Class 2 TOXOPLASMEA Biocca, 1957. It has one order.

Order 1 TOXOPLASMIDA Biocca, 1957.

Class 3 HAPLOSPOREA Caullery, 1953 (no human representative).

Subphylum III **Cnidospora** Doflein, 1901 (no human representative).

Subphylum IV **Ciliophora** Doflein, 1901. It has one class.

Class 1 CILIATEA Perty, 1852. It is subdivided into 4 subclasses.

Subclass 4 SPIROTRICHIA Bütschli, 1889. It has 6 orders.

Order 1 HETEROTRICHIDA Stein, 1859.

It is to be noted that the suffixes have also been altered as will be seen from the following:

A system of uniform endings has been adopted for the names of the higher taxa Phyla, Subphyla and Superclasses which end in "-a". Classes end in "-ea", Subclasses end in "-ia", Orders end in "-ida" and Suborders end in "-ina".

B. *Classification Based on Pathogenicity*

According to the degree of pathogenicity, the protozoal parasites are divided into two main groups: (i) Pathogenic and (ii) Non-pathogenic.

Protozoal Parasites Pathogenic to Man				
PHYLUM	GENUS	SPECIES	HABITAT	PATHOGENIC EFFECTS
Sarcomastigophora	Entamoeba	*E. histolytica*	Large intestine	Dysentery, Liver abscess
Intestinal flagellate	Giardia	*G. intestinalis*	Small intestine	Diarrhoea
Genital flagellate	Trichomonas	*T. vaginalis*	Vagina	Vaginitis
Blood and tissue flagellates	Trypanosoma	*T. brucei*	Blood, Lymph node, C.N.S.	African trypanosomiasis (Sleeping sickness)
		T. cruzi	Heart, Nervous system	South American trypanosomiasis (Chagas' disease)
	Leishmania	*L. donovani*	R. E. system	Kala-azar and Dermal leishmanoid
		L. tropica	Skin	Oriental sore
		L. brasiliensis	Oro-nasal mucous membrane	Espundia

PHYLUM	GENUS	SPECIES	HABITAT	PATHOGENIC EFFECTS
Apicomplexa	Plasmodium	*P. vivax*	R.B.C.	Benign tertian malaria
		P. falciparum	R.B.C.	Malignant tertian malaria and pernicious malaria
		P. malatiae	R.B.C.	Quartan malaria
		P. ovale	R.B.C.	Ovale tertian malaria
	Isospora	*I. belli*	Ep. cells of intestine	Diarrhoea
	Toxoplasma	*T. gondii*	R. E. system, parenchyma cell	Encephalomyelitis, choroidoretinitis, etc.
	Sarcocystis	*S. hominis*	Large intestine	Sarcocystosis
		S. suihominis	Large intestine	Sarcocystosis
	Cyclospora	*C. cayentanensis*	Ep. cells of intestine	Cyclosporiasis
	Cryptosporidium	*C. parvum*	Large intestine	Cryptosporidiosis
	Babesia	*B. bovis*	RBC	Babesiosis
		B. divergens	RBC	Babesiosis
		B. Microti	RBC	Babesiosis
Ciliophora	Balantidium	*B. coli*	Large intestine	Dysentery
Microspora	Enterocytozoon	*E. bieneusi*	Ep. cells of intestine	Microsporidiasis
	Encephalitozoon	*E. intestinalis*	Ep. cells of intestine	Microsporidiasis

Protozoal Parasites Non-pathogenic to Man				
SUBPHYLUM	SUPERCLASS	GENUS	SPECIES	HABITAT
Sarcodina	Rhizopodea	Entamoeba	*E. dispar*	Large intestine
			E. hartmani	Large intestine
			E, gingivalis	Mouth
			E. coli	Large intestine
		Endolimax	*E. nana*	Large intestine
		Iodamoeba	*I. bütschlii*	Large intestine
Mastigophora		Dientamoeba	*D. fragilis**	Large intestine
		Chilomastix	*C. mesnili*	Caecum
		Trichomonas	*T. hominis*	Ileocaecal region
			T. tenax	Teeth and gum
		Enteromonas	*E. hominis*	Large intestine
		Embadomonas	*E. intestinalis*	Large intestine
		Trypanosoma	*T. rangeli*	Blood

* Formerly believed to be non-pathogenic but it is now found to cause various abdominal symptoms and signs and now has been reclassified as an aberrant trichomonad flagellate.

CHAPTER II

PHYLUM SARCOMASTIGOPHORA

Subphylum: SARCODINA Superclass: RHIZOPODA
Class: LOBOSEA Subclass: GYMNAMOEBIA Order: AMOEBIDA

The protozoal parasites belonging to this group, while in motion, throw out cytoplasms called pseudopodia which represent the organs of locomotion. The genera included in the order Amoebida are:

1. Genus Entamoeba: *E. histolytica, E. coli* and *E. gingivalis.*
2. Genus Endolimax: *E. nana.*
3. Genus Iodamoeba: *I. bütschlii.*

The three genera are distinguished by the structure of the nucleus (Fig. 4) as follows:

In *Entamoeba*—The nuclear membrane is lined by chromatin granules and the compact karyosome is either centrally or eccentrically placed.

In *Endolimax*—The karyosome is a large irregular mass situated peripherally; it may be connected with another small mass.

In *Iodamoeba*—The karyosome is a large circular mass surrounded by refractile globules.

The amoeba infecting man may be classified according to their pathogenicity and habitat as follows:

A. PATHOGENIC
   Intestinal Amoeba: *E. histolytica.*
B. NON-PATHOGENIC (HARMLESS COMMENSALS)
   1. Mouth Amoeba: *E. gingivalis.*
   2. Intestinal Amoebae: *E. coli, E. nana, I. bütschlii* and *D. fragilis.*

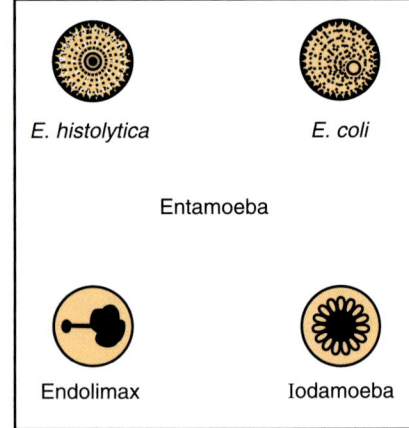

Fig. 4—**Nuclear character of various genera under Amoebida.**

Genus: Entamoeba

Entamoeba histolytica Schaudinn, 1903

The parasite causing diarrhoea, dysentery and liver abscess in man.

Lambl (1859) first discovered the parasite, Lösch (1875) proved its pathogenic nature, while Schaudinn (1903) differentiated pathogenic and non-pathogenic types of amoebae.

Geographical Distribution. World-wide. More common in the tropics and sub tropics than in the temperate zone.

Habitat. Trophozoites of *E. histolytica* (the "large race" or the tissue-invading forms) live in the mucous and submucous layers of the large intestine of man.

Morphology. The structural character of the parasite can be studied both in unstained and stained preparations (iodine and iron-haematoxylin). The morphology of the three phases (Fig. 5) in the life cycle of *E. histolytica* is described.

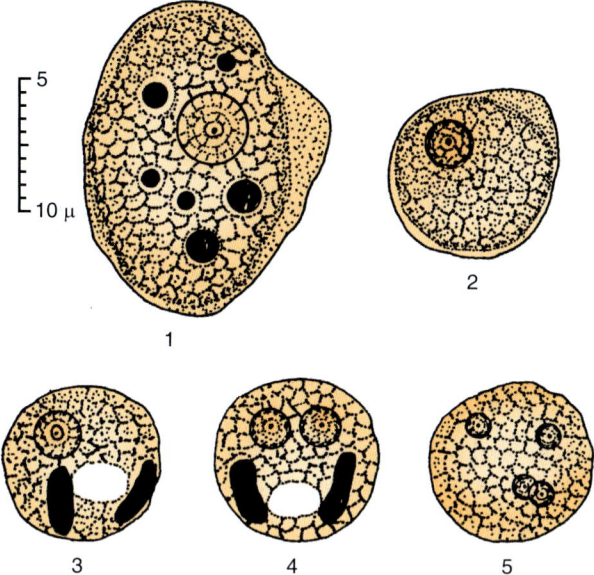

Fig. 5—**Three stages of** *Entamoeba histolytica.*
1, Trophozoite; 2, Pre-cystic stage; 3, 4, 5, Uninucleate, binucleate and quadrinucleate cysts.

1. *Trophozoite* (The Growing or Feeding Stage). Under the microscope, the living parasite, in a warm stage, is seen to exhibit slow gliding movement. The clear hyaline ectoplasm (pseudopodium) has a jerky movement, as if it were ejected under high pressure, followed by flowing in of the whole granular endoplasm. The morphological characteristics (Fig. 6) are as follows:

SHAPE: Not fixed because of constantly changing position.

SIZE: Ranges from 18 to 40 µm, average being 20 to 30 µm.

CYTOPLASM: Divisible into two portions—a clear translucent *ectoplasm* and a granular *endoplasm*. Red blood cells, occasionally leucocytes and tissue debris, are found inside the endoplasm.

NUCLEUS: Spherical in shape and varying in size from 4 to 6 µm. In fresh preparations due to rapid movement, the nucleus is not visible but with the decrease of motility a faint outline of the nucleus occupying an eccentric position inside the body of the parasite may be observed. In stained preparations, the nuclear structure shows: (i) *karyosome*, small dot-like, central in position and surrounded by a clear halo, (ii) *nuclear membrane*, delicate and lined with a single layer of uniformly distributed fine chromatin granules, and (iii) the space between the karyosome and the nuclear membrane is traversed by a fine thread of *linin network* having a spoke-like radial arrangement.

2. *Pre-cystic Stage.* It is smaller in size, varying from 10 to 20 µm. It is round or slightly ovoid with a blunt pseudopodium projecting from the periphery. The endoplasm is free of red blood cells and other ingested food particles. The relatively larger nuclear structure retains the characteristics of the trophozoite.

3. *Cystic Stage.* During encystment, the parasite becomes rounded and is surrounded by a highly refractile membrane, called the cyst-wall. A mature cyst is a quadrinucleate spherical body, its cytoplasm is clear and hyaline, and the nuclear structure retaining the characters of the trophozoite. The cyst varies greatly in size—the "small race" being 6 to 9 µm and the "large race" 12 to 15 µm.

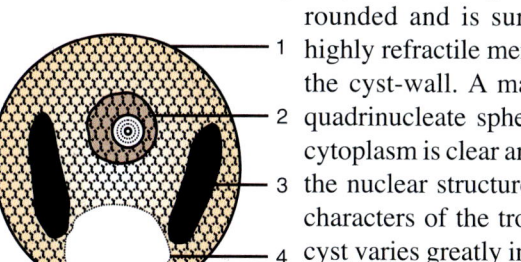

Fig. 7—**Cyst of** *E. histolytica.*
1, Cyst wall; 2, Nucleus;
3, Chromatoid bodies;
4, Glycogen vacuole.

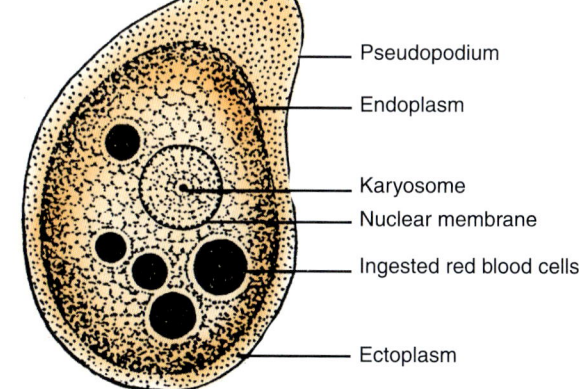

Fig. 6—**Trophozoite of** *E. histolytica.*

- Pseudopodium
- Endoplasm
- Karyosome
- Nuclear membrane
- Ingested red blood cells
- Ectoplasm

The cyst begins as a uninucleate body but soon divides by binary fission and develops into binucleate and quadrinucleate bodies. The single nucleus multiplies by two successive divisions into 2 and ultimately to 4 daughter nuclei. During the process of division, the nuclei undergo gradual reduction in size, becoming 2 µm in diameter.

The cytoplasm of the cyst (Fig. 7) shows, in early stage of development, the following:

(i) CHROMATOID OR CHROMIDIAL BARS: These do not stain with iodine but are seen as refractile oblong bars with rounded ends in preparations with normal saline and as black when stained with iron-haematoxylin; the number varying from 1 to 4 and the size varying from one-half to two-thirds the diameter of the cyst.

(ii) A GLYCOGEN MASS: This stains brown with iodine.

As the cyst matures (passing from the uninucleate to the quadrinucleate stage), both the glycogen mass and the chromidial bars gradually disappear. Immature cysts passed in the faeces may however complete their development outside.

Resistance of Cysts. The mature quadrinucleate cysts, passed in the stool, do not undergo any further development and remain alive for a few days, if they are not dried or heated. As moisture is essential for the long continued existence of the cysts, they may live up to 10 days in moist stool. Although covered by a resistant cyst-wall, the cysts are very susceptible to desiccation. The thermal death point of cysts is 50°C. In the strengths used for bacteriological sterilisation of public water supply by chlorination, the cysts are not destroyed. The capacity for taking up eosin stain is the generally accepted method of determining the vitality of cysts. It is observed that dead cysts are stained with weak eosin solution but the living cysts do not take up the stain.

SALINE (FRESH) AND STAINED PREPARATIONS:

In saline preparations, the trophozoite of *E. histolytica* is identified by the motility and the presence of red blood cells, which appear yellowish-green inside the endoplasm. The nucleus is not visible but a faint outline may be detected. The endoplasm shows a bluish or ground glass appearance. In the cystic form, the chromatoid bodies are seen as round refractile bars and the cyst-wall, smooth and thin. The glycogen mass is not visible but the outlines of nuclei may be visible.

In preparations stained with iodine, the body of the parasite stains yellow to light brown, and the nucleus is clearly seen with a central karyosome. The cytoplasm of the cyst shows a smooth and hyaline appearance. Chromatoid bodies are not stained but the glycogen mass stains brown.

In fixed and stained preparations (with iron-haematoxylin), the chromatoid bodies and the nucleus stain jet black. The cytoplasm appears bluish or greyish and the glycogen mass (dissolved in the process of staining) remains un-stained as a vacuole.

Formal ether concentration method and zinc sulphate centrifugal floatation method may be used to decect cyst in the faeces.

For the technique of making a saline preparation and staining with iodine solution and iron-haematoxylin, *see Appendix I.*

Methods of Reproduction: Excystation, Encystation & Multiplication (Fig. 8).

Excystation. This is the process of transformation of cysts to trophozoites and occurs only when the cysts enter into the alimentary canal of man (a susceptible host). During excystation a quadrinucleate cyst gives rise to eight amoebulae, each one of which is being capable of developing into a trophozoite.

Encystation. This is the process of transformation of trophozoites to cysts and occurs inside the lumen of the intestine of an infected individual. The whole process of encystation takes place within a few hours and the life span of a mature cyst inside the lumen of the bowel of the original host is only two days. It is to be noted that the cysts are not developed inside the tissues of man, neither in the intestinal wall nor in the areas of metastatic invasion (liver, lungs or other organs). The mature cyst is a quadrinucleate body, because during encystment the nucleus has under-gone multiplication and given rise to four daughter nuclei.

Note: Both the processes of *excystation* and *encystation* may occur in one and the same host but after the formation of cysts, a transference to another new host is required for the continuation of species.

Multiplication. This occurs only in the trophozoite phase. The trophic forms of *E. histolytica* are exclusively parasitic in their habit, growing at the expense of living tissues and multiplying in large numbers. Reproduction of trophozoites occurs by simple binary fission, first of the nucleus which divides by a modified type of mitosis and then, of the cytoplasmic body of the organism.

Note: As already stated, encystment is not a reproductive process but a means of protection of species from extinction. In *E. histolytica* however the nucleus of the cyst multiplies into 4 daughter nuclei from which ultimately 8 amoebulae are developed.

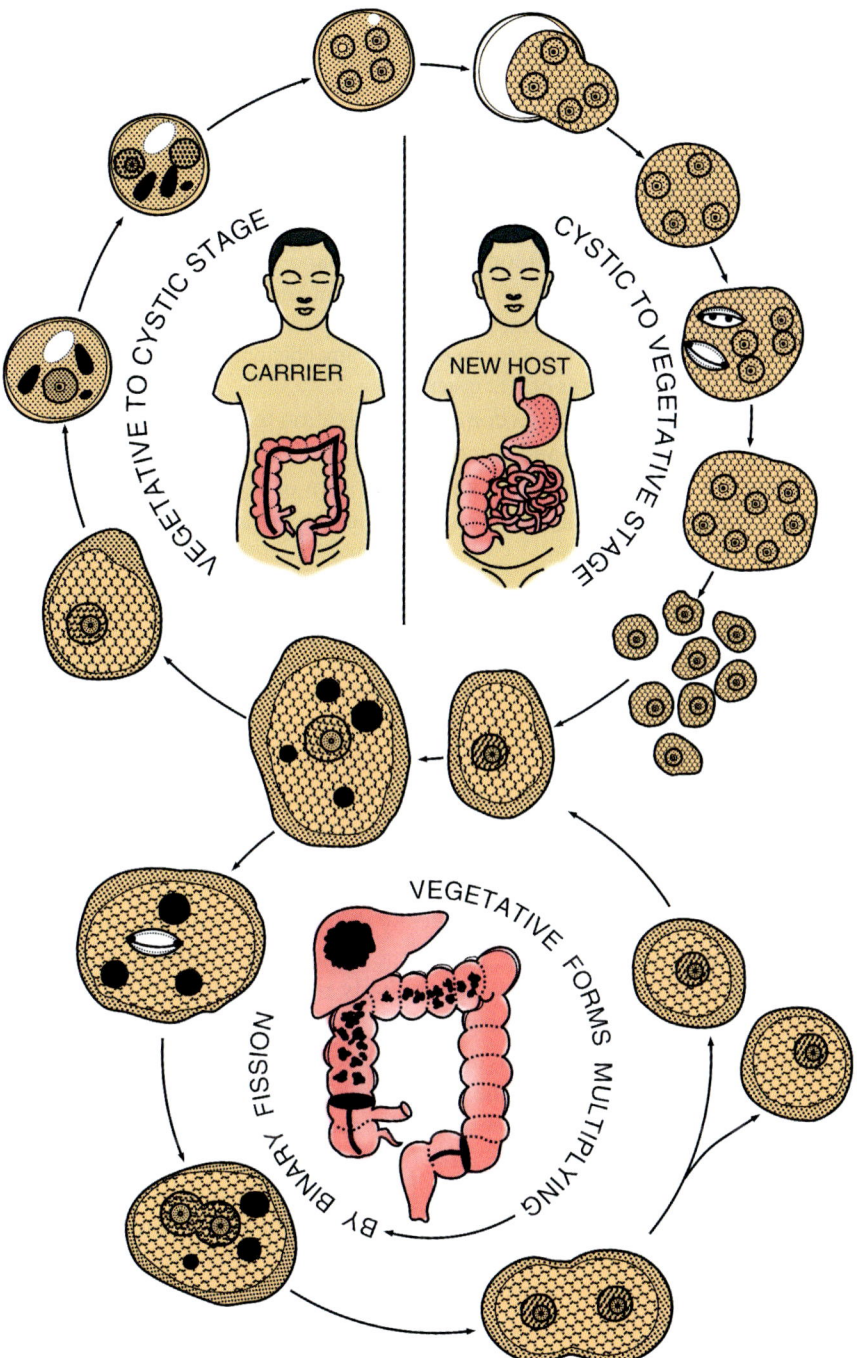

Fig. 8—Methods of reproduction of *Entamoeba histolytica*.
Showing excystation and encystation at the top and multiplication of trophozoites below.

Cultivation. A successful culture of *E. histolytica* was first made by Boeck and Drbohlav (1925) using solidified blood agar or solidified egg slopes covered with Locke's solution. The growth of *E. histolytica* requires in cultures the presence of starch or rice flour and some metabolic associates, such as enteric bacteria, organism t (a non-pathogenic bacterium) or the parasitic flagellate *T. cruzi*, living or dead. Micro-cultures are made from a single washed amoeba in micro-tubes (4 × 50 mm) containing a medium of thioglycollate preparation, horse serum and an overlay of a rich culture of *T. cruzi* (Philips' medium). *E. histolytica* has also been grown in a serum medium containing thioglycollate and penicillin-inhibited streptobacilli which are living but not multiplying (Shaffer and Frye's medium). Robinson's culture media & NIH polyxenic culture media are now available for culture of the stool for isolation of amoeba. Diamond in 1961 developed axenix cultivation, which does not require the presence of other microorganisms and produces pure growth of the amoeba. Culture is not a routine diagnostic procedure.

Susceptible Animals. Amoebic lesions may be experimentally reproduced in cats, dogs and monkeys. In *kittens* an extensive sloughing and ulceration of the colonic mucosa occur and the infection is invariably fatal within a period of 2 to 3 days. Encystment does not occur in kittens. In *dogs* (pups), the intestinal lesions are similar in morphology to those found in man and the animals live much longer than kittens.

Lesions in other experimental animals. Hepatitis has been produced in hamsters. Intracaecal inoculation in white rats produced caecal ulceration and intra-ileal injection in guinea pigs also produced ulceration of the colon. Experimental amoebiasis helps not only to study the progress of infection but also the effect of amoebicidal drugs; pathogenic property of an attenuated strain may be restored by passage through the liver of a hamster.

Immunology. Certain serological tests, such as complement fixation test, precipitin test, immobilisation test of *E. histolytica* with hyper-immune sera of rabbits and reaction of *E. histolytica* with fluorescein-tagged homologus antibody suggest the development of specific immune bodies in the sera of individuals suffering from amoebiasis, particularly invasive (hepatic) amoebiasis. Such humoral antibodies however do not protect the individual who has recovered from amoebiasis against re-infection.

Life Cycle. *E. histolytica* passes its life cycle (Fig. 9) only in one host, the man. There are mainly two phases of development, *trophozoite* and cyst with a transitory stage of *pre-cystic form.*

The mature quadrinucleate cysts are the infective forms of the parasite. When these cysts are swallowed along with the contaminated food and drink by a susceptible person, they are capable of further development inside his gut. The fully developed cysts, thus gaining entrance into the alimentary canal, pass unaltered through the stomach. The cyst-wall is resistant to the action of the gastric juice but is digested by the action of trypsin in the intestine. The *excystation* occurs when the cyst reaches the caecum or the lower part of the ileum (neutral or slightly alkaline medium). During the process, the cytoplasmic body retracts and loosens itself from the cyst-wall. Vigorous amoeboid movements cause a rent to appear in the cyst-wall through which at first a small mass of cytoplasm and then ultimately the whole body comes out. Each cyst liberates a single amoeba with four nuclei, a *tetranucleate amoeba* which eventually forms eight amoebulae (*metacystic trophozoites*) by the division of nuclei with successive fission of cytoplasm. The young amoebulae being actively motile, invade the tissues and ultimately lodge in the submucous tissue of the large gut, their normal habitat. Here they grow and multiply by binary fission. It is to be noted that the trophozoite phase of the parasite is responsible for producing the characteristic lesion of amoebiasis.

During growth, *E. histolytica* secretes a proteolytic enzymes of the nature of histolysin which brings about destruction and necrosis of tissues and thereby helps the parasite in obtaining nourishment through absorption of these dissolved tissue juices. The tissue-invading amoebae gradually recede from the dead tissues towards the margin of healthy ones and in this way the trophozoites of *E. histolytica* often wander about in the tissues of the gut-wall, entering into deeper layers and may sometimes actually find their way into the radicles of the portal vein to be carried away to the liver where their further progress may be arrested. In the liver the trophic forms may for a time grow and multiply but encystation does not occur. Hence such an invasion is always to be looked upon as an accident on the part of the parasite because so far as its biological aspect is concerned it has reached a dead end.

Those parasites that remain in the intestinal wall may cause an attack of acute dysentery (ulcerative colitis) in which a large number of trophozoites are discharged along with the slough. This again is a loss to the species itself because by causing acute dysentery it may completely exterminate its own race. It is not the ultimate design of the parasite to cause such a destructive lesion but to live in a comparative peace with the host, establishing a mutual adjustment between them so that it can produce strains which are capable of giving rise to cysts. A high degree of pathogenicity of the parasite is obviously a disadvantage to itself.

After sometime, when the effect of the parasite on the host is gradually toned down together with the concomitant increase in the tolerance of the host, the lesions become quiescent and commence to heal. The parasite now finds it difficult to continue its life cycle solely in the trophozoite stage and therefore, prepares itself to produce strains which will save the race from extinction. A certain number of these trophozoites are discharged into the lumen of the bowel and are transformed into small pre-cystic forms from which the cysts are developed.

LIFE CYCLE OF *ENTAMOEBA HISTOLYTICA*

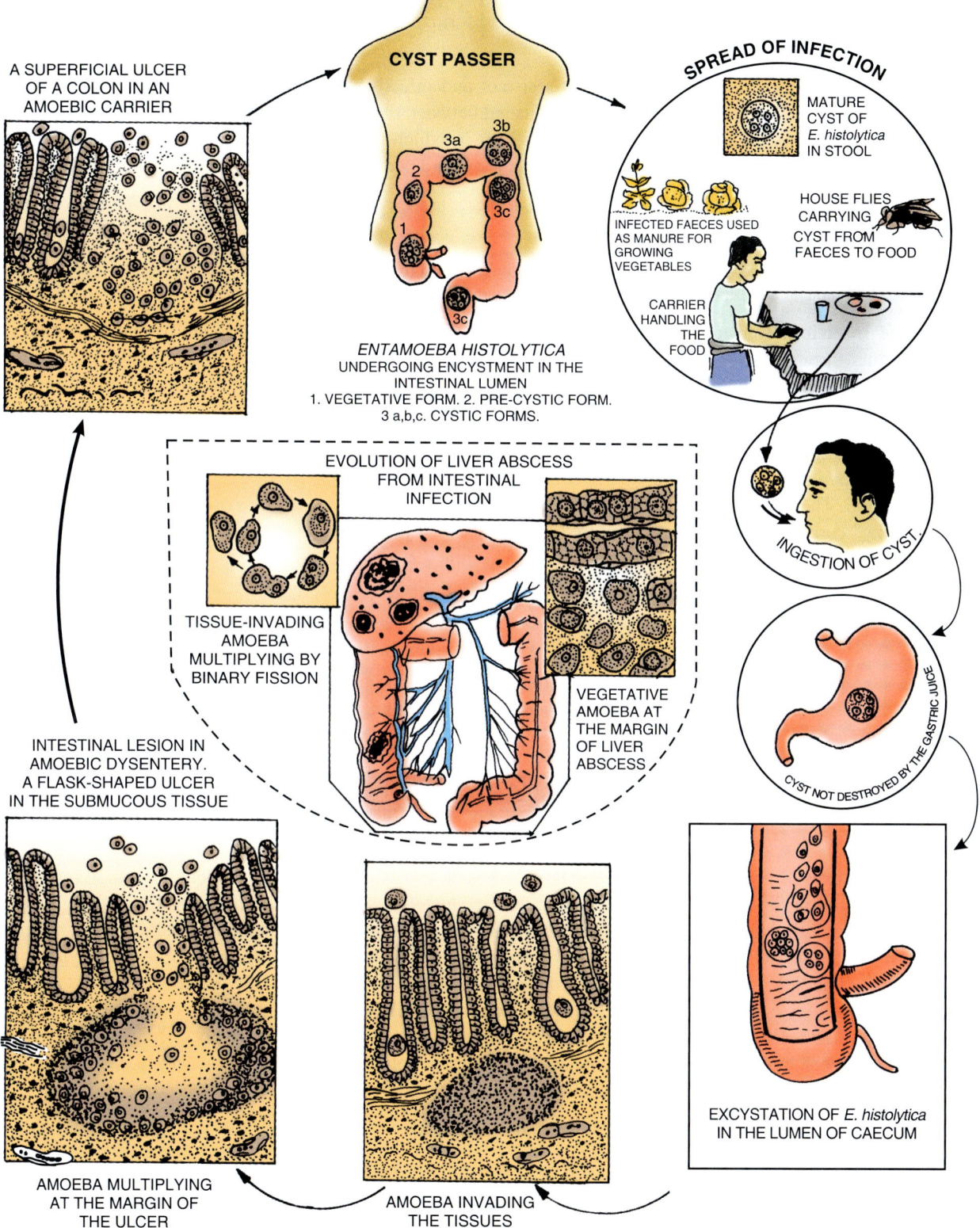

A SUPERFICIAL ULCER OF A COLON IN AN AMOEBIC CARRIER

CYST PASSER

SPREAD OF INFECTION

MATURE CYST OF *E. histolytica* IN STOOL

INFECTED FAECES USED AS MANURE FOR GROWING VEGETABLES

HOUSE FLIES CARRYING CYST FROM FAECES TO FOOD

CARRIER HANDLING THE FOOD

ENTAMOEBA HISTOLYTICA UNDERGOING ENCYSTMENT IN THE INTESTINAL LUMEN
1. VEGETATIVE FORM. 2. PRE-CYSTIC FORM.
3 a,b,c. CYSTIC FORMS.

INGESTION OF CYST.

EVOLUTION OF LIVER ABSCESS FROM INTESTINAL INFECTION

TISSUE-INVADING AMOEBA MULTIPLYING BY BINARY FISSION

VEGETATIVE AMOEBA AT THE MARGIN OF LIVER ABSCESS

CYST NOT DESTROYED BY THE GASTRIC JUICE

INTESTINAL LESION IN AMOEBIC DYSENTERY. A FLASK-SHAPED ULCER IN THE SUBMUCOUS TISSUE

EXCYSTATION OF *E. histolytica* IN THE LUMEN OF CAECUM

AMOEBA MULTIPLYING AT THE MARGIN OF THE ULCER

AMOEBA INVADING THE TISSUES

Fig. 9—Showing the mode of infection, evolution of intestinal and hepatic lesions and development of carrier state.

If the parasite happens to enter a resistant host, the injuries produced are minimal (superficial ulcers only). In such a host, *E. histolytica* not only remains in the trophozoite stage and multiplies at the margin of these superficial ulcers, but also discharges from time to time pre-cystic and cystic forms to propagate its species. These persons are thus a constant source of infection to others.

The mature quadrinucleate cysts are the most resistant and infective forms of the parasite and are particularly developed when a state of equilibrium has been established between the host and the parasite. But the cysts produced in an infected individual are unable to develop in the host in which they are produced and therefore necessitate a transference to another susceptible host, where they can grow and continue their life cycle as stated above.

Reservoirs of Infection. Natural infection of *E. histolytica* is seen only among men and monkeys. Hence, man is the commonest source of infection.

In China, dogs are supposed to be the possible source of infection to man. It has been shown that wild rats, although not an important factor in the spread of the disease to man, may be regarded as reservoirs of *E. histolytica*.

Modes of Infection. Transmission of *E. histolytica* from man to man is effected through its encysted stage and infection occurs through the ingestion of these cysts. Mature quadrinucleate cysts are the infective forms of this parasite. Faecal contamination of drinking water, vegetables and food are the primary causes. Eating of uncooked vegetables and fruits which have been fertilised with infected human faeces has often led to the occurrence of the disease. Occasionally, drinking water supply contaminated with infected faeces gives rise to epidemics.

Role of Carriers. Handling of food by infected individuals (cyst-passers or cyst-carriers) appears to be a very common method. There are two types of carriers: "contact" and "convalescent". The former are supposed to be so-called "healthy" carriers who have never suffered from amoebic dysentery and whose health appears to remain un-impaired. The latter are those who have recovered from a clinical attack of acute amoebic dysentery.

The trophozoites which pass out with the evacuation (blood and mucus) of a patient suffering from an attack of amoebic dysentery cannot survive for more than a couple of hours and so are an unlikely source of infection. Even if they are ingested during this short period of existence, they are digested by the action of the gastric juice.

House-flies may transmit cysts while passing from faeces to unprotected food-stuff, but seem usually to be of relatively little importance. The cysts of *E. histolytica* have been found in the droppings of cockroaches which also serve as a source of infection.

Pathogenicity of *Entamoeba histolytica*

Incubation Period. In man, the incubation period varies a great deal but is generally four or five days.

Clinical Features or Symptomatology. The term "*amoebiasis*" is used clinically to denote all those conditions which are produced in the human host by infection with *E. histolytica* at different areas of its invasion. The term "*amoebic dysentery*" signifies a condition in which the infection is confined to the intestinal canal and is characterised by the passage of blood and mucus in the stool. It is to be noted that "*amoebic dysentery*" is not a synonym of "*amoebiasis*" and neither does the term "*amoebic dysentery*" give the full picture of the manifestations of "*intestinal amoebiasis*". Dysentery is a symptom characteristic of extensive intestinal ulcerations representing only a part of the clinical picture of intestinal amoebiasis, but there are a large number of cases which are not accompanied by dysenteric symptom. Clinical features vary from acute colitis to chronic colitis and asymptomatic carrier state. Asymptomatic carrier can pass cysts of both non-pathogenic and pathogenic strains of *E. histolytica*.

Pathogenic Lesions. These may be considered under two heads:

1. *Primary or Intestinal Lesions*. The infection is limited entirely to the large intestine, the initial site of location of the parasite.

2. *Secondary or Metastatic Lesions*. The extra-colonic areas where the trophozoites of *E. histolytica* can migrate and produce lesions include (a) liver, (b) lungs and (c) brain.

INTESTINAL LESIONS

Genesis of Intestinal Lesions. The metacystic trophozoites* liberated after excystation enter through the crypts of Lieberkühn and penetrate directly through the columnar epithelium of the mucous membrane by their amoeboid activity and by also dissolving the intestinal epithelial cells with a proteolytic ferment they secrete. They then burrow their way deeper and deeper by continuous lysis of tissue cells till they reach the submucous coat (Figs. 10 & 11). Here the amoebae rapidly multiply and increase in number, form colonies, destroy the tissues in their vicinity and utilise the cytolysed material as their food. The amoebae then begin to pass in various directions, dissolving all surrounding tissues, till ultimately, a considerable area of the submucosa is destroyed, undermining the mucous membrane above. The invasion of the tissues by this protozoal parasite brings in its train coagulative necrosis and the formation of abscess which finally breaks down, leading to the development of ulcers.

Intestinal Lesions in Acute Amoebic Dysentery

MACROSCOPIC PATHOLOGY (MORBID ANATOMY)

Distribution of Ulcers. Amoebic ulcerations are strictly confined to the large gut. The lesions may be generalised or localised.

  (i) Generalised—The whole length of the large gut as far down as the internal anal sphincter is involved.

 (ii) Localised—There are two levels of involvement:

    (a) Ileo-caecal region—Here the caecum, ascending colon, ileo-caecal valve and appendix are involved.

    (b) Sigmoido-rectal region—Here the sigmoid colon and rectum are involved.

  As a rule, the preponderance of lesion in the region (a) is found to be about twice as that in the region (b).

Character of Ulcers. The sites of amoebic ulcers are not easily detected externally (from the peritoneal surface) unless they are deep and extensive. The characteristic appearance of the ulcers is best seen from the mucous surface. The ulcers are discrete and a healthy mucous membrane always intervenes between the ulcers even when they are

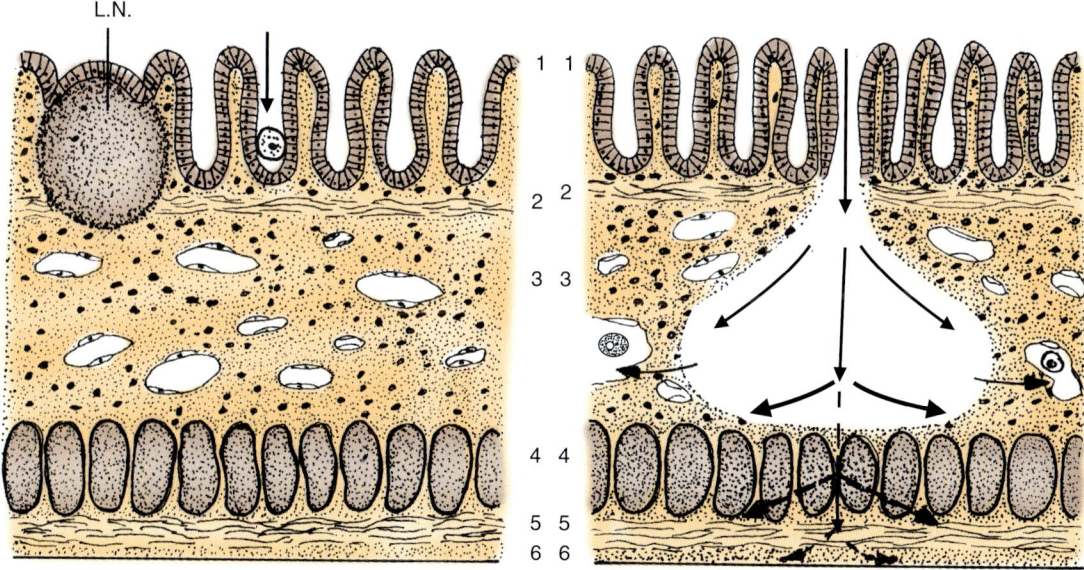

Fig. 10—Microscopic anatomy of the large intestine.
1, crypts of Lieberkühn; 2, muscularis mucosae; 3, submucosa; 4, circular muscles; 5, longitudinal muscles; 6, peritoneum. L.N., solitary lymph node.

Fig. 11—Invasion of *E. histolytica* **through the intestinal wall.** Flask-shaped clear area represents the process of tissue necrosis. Continuous lines indicate the usual progress and dotted lines, the occasional approach.

---

*There are certain strains of *E. histolytica* which may live superficially in the crypts of Lieberkühn's glands of the large intestine, eroding the mucous surface and utilising the mucous secretion as food. At this stage, it metabolises anaerobically and lives in association with certain intestinal bacteria (symbiotic associates) but not feeding upon them. These strains have a low pathogenic index.

extensive. The *earliest lesion* is characterised by the formation of scattered areas of small nodular elevations (Fig. 12), having an opening at the centre with hyperaemia and oedema of the marginal tissues. When the nodules are incised, brownish-yellow material of necrotic tissue comes out in which amoebic trophozoites may be found. With the liberation of cytolysed tissues from these nodular areas, small superficial ulcers are produced.

A typical *amoebic ulcer* has the following peculiarities:

Size—Varying from a pin's head to one inch or more in diameter.

Shape—Round or oval; transverse in large coalescing ulcers.

Margin—Ragged and undermined, being formed by the overhanging mucous membrane. Such an ulcer, on vertical section, has the appearance of a flask (flask-shaped ulcer).

Base—Generally formed by the muscular coat and filled up by the necrotic material, yellowish or blackish slough (Fig. 13).

Extension of Ulcers. Superficial ulcers do not extend beyond the muscularis mucosae. Deep ulcers are limited to the submucous coat and may extend laterally to communicate with adjacent ulcers. When the destruction is not limited to the submucosa but extends deeper into the muscular and even the serous layers, the following complications may arise—local peritonitis, haemorrhage, perforation and generalised peritonitis, pericaecal or pericolic abscess, sloughing and gangrene of the large gut.

Healing of Ulcers. After the separation of slough, granulation tissue begins to form on the floor of the ulcerated area. *In small superficial ulcers*, scar tissue is not formed and the mucous membrane is completely restored over the area. In these cases, regeneration is so effective that the sites of the healed ulcers can hardly be recognised later. In *large and deep ulcers*, healing is associated with the formation of scar tissue over which the epithelium of the mucous membrane does not grow and these areas can later be detected as smooth depressed scars, the centres of which may or may not be pigmented. Excessive formation of scar tissue may lead to strictures and partial obstruction to the passage of the faecal matter, or it may produce a generalised thickening of the intestinal wall.

MICROSCOPIC PATHOLOGY (HISTOPATHOLOGY). In an early ulcer, the lesion will be found to be limited above the muscularis mucosae (Fig. 14) and the amoebae may be seen marching along the interglandular spaces causing cytolysis. At this stage, the epithelial cells of the crypts of Lieberkühn will show varying degrees of necrosis and with the destruction of its basement membrane, the amoebae will be found to penetrate deeper (Fig. 15). If a section is made through the middle of an early ulcer, one would find the following:

1. In the *centre*, an area of necrosed tissue in which the cells are in various stages, of degeneration. Hardly any amoeba can be seen in this central degenerated area.

2. Towards the *periphery*, amoebae (trophozoite forms) are to be found in large numbers lying singly or in groups, with no cellular infiltration.

In a fairly advanced lesion, the trophozoites of *E. histolytica* may be seen migrating a considerable distance away from the actual ulcer and invading the intermuscular spaces to reach the peritoneal coat. The parasites may also be observed burrowing into the small venules or lying within the lumina of dilated venous radicles as free cells alongside the red blood cells and leucocytes. Hyperplasia of the endothelial cells of many small blood vessels causing their thrombosis may also be seen. In these thrombi, the trophic forms of *E. histolytica* have often been detected.

Intestinal Lesions in Chronic Intestinal Amoebiasis. The pathological picture of individuals suffering from chronic intestinal amoebiasis and those suffering from acute dysentery varies only in degree. The course and progress of such lesions are entirely guided by the resisting power of the host. The lesions which are observed in this group of cases are characterised by ulcerations and regenerative tissue changes and hence, a combination of the following is observed:

1. Small ulcers involving only the mucosa.
2. Extensive superficial ulcers with hyperaemia.
3. Marked scarring of intestinal wall with thinning, dilatation and sacculation.
4. Extensive adhesions with the neighbouring viscera.
5. Localised thickening of the intestinal wall leading to a narrowing of the lumen of the bowel.

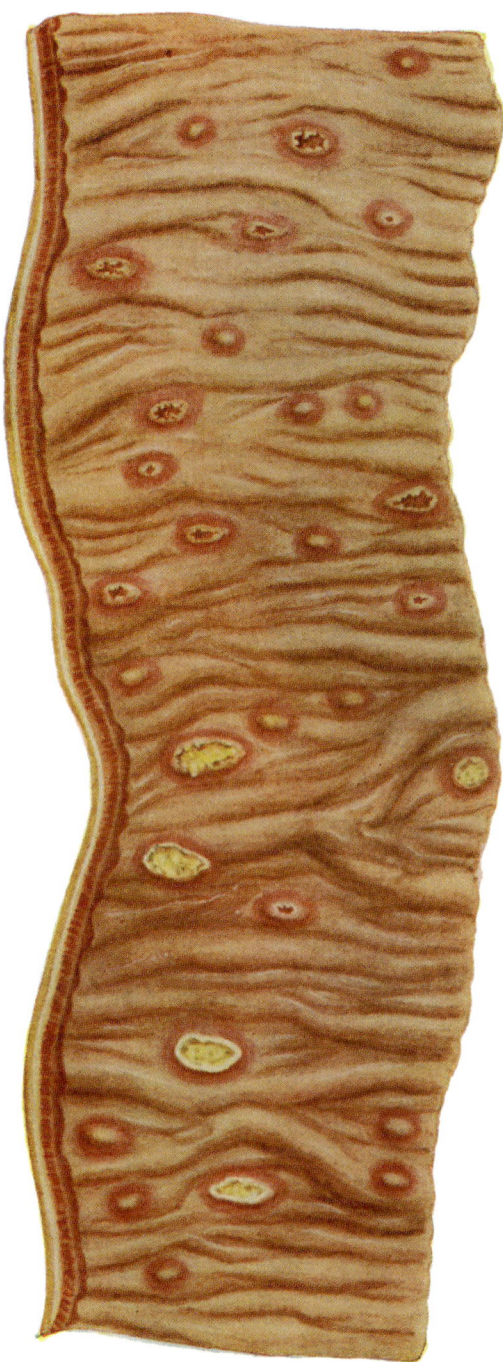

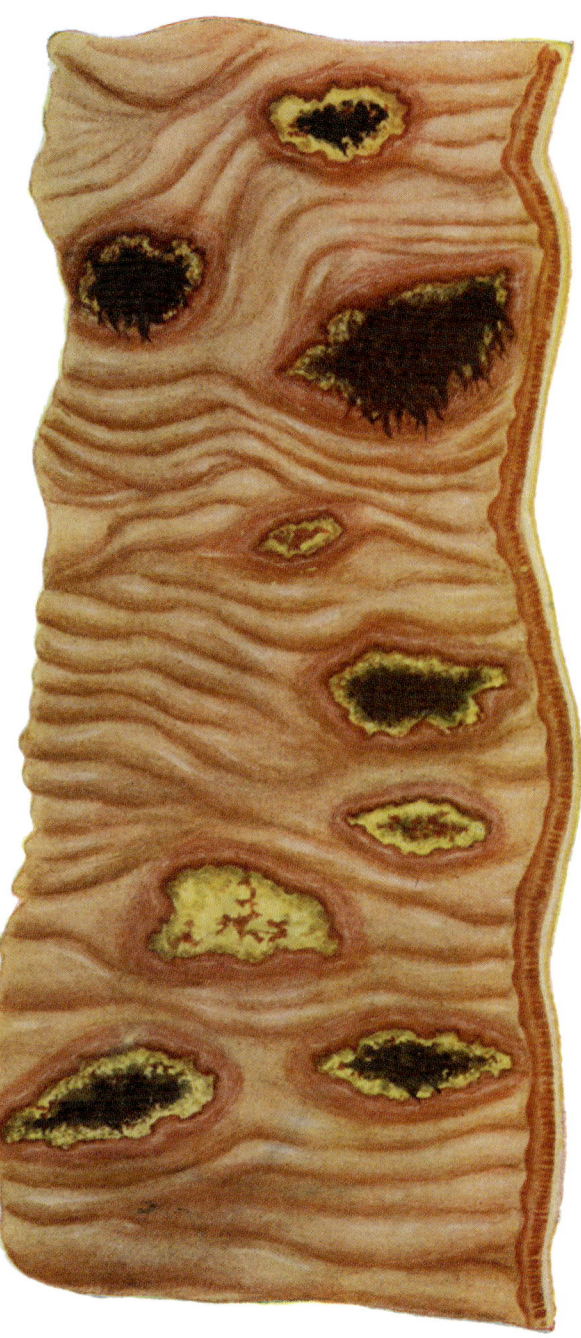

Fig. 12—Early intestinal lesions in acute amoebic dysentery.

Showing the nodular elevations and ulcerations.

Fig. 13—Intestine of acute amoebic dysentery.

Showing advanced lesions. The base of most of the ulcers is filled with blackish slough and a hyperaemic zone surrounds each of these ulcers.

6. Generalised thickening of the bowel wall rendering it palpable. In emaciated patients the course of the entire thickened colon may become easily visible and palpable.

7. Formation of tumour-like masses of granulation tissue (amoebic granuloma or *amoeboma*). Clinically it is difficult to differentiate amoeboma from carcinoma and the diagnosis rests upon the demonstration of trophozoites of *E. histolytica* in sections of tissues, obtained by biopsy or at autopsy.

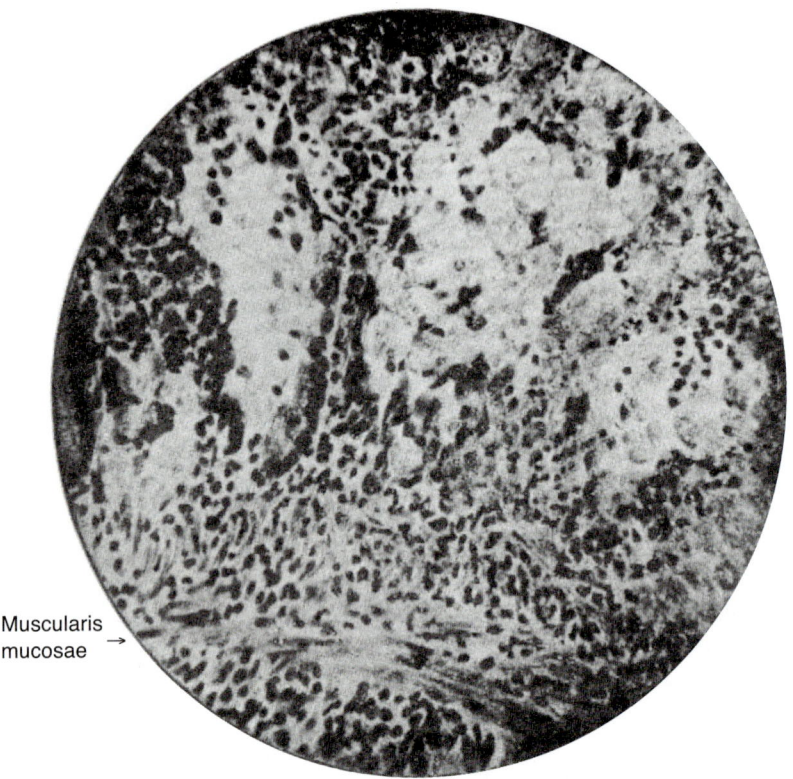

Muscularis mucosae →

Fig. 14—Section from the margin of an amoebic ulcer of the caecum.
Showing a collection of *E. histolytica* (trophozoite forms) lying along the interglandular spaces.

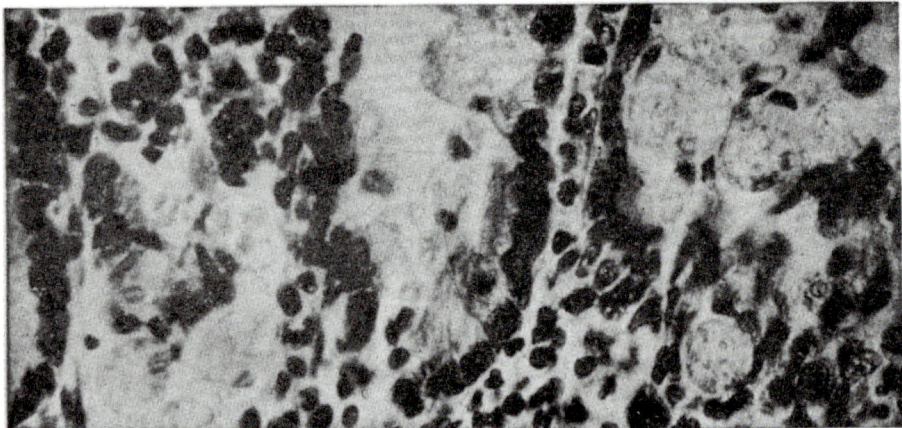

Fig. 15—Photomicrograph from an early amoebic ulcer of the caecum.
Trophozoites of *E. histolytica* are seen marching along the crypts of Lieberkühn (4 of them are shown—2 intact and 2 destroyed), eroding the basement membrane of the epithelial lining and penetrating deeper into the tissues (one trophozoite can be seen passing the barrier).

Definite ulcers involving the muscular coat or even extending up to the peritoneal coat may be seen in cases where acute exacerbation has occurred.

Stool in Intestinal Amoebiasis. The general character of the stool will vary with the inestinal condition. It may be fluid (diarrhoeic), semi-fluid or even formed, with or without adherent traces of mucus and/or blood. Examination of the stool, both macroscopically and microscopically, helps not only to establish the diagnosis of intestinal amoebiasis but to differentiate from other dysenteric conditions. Although the demonstration of *E. histolytica* in the stool of infected persons forms one of the conclusive evidences, the importance of making a cytological study of the dysenteric stool has been greatly emphasised. It has been observed that the cellular character of the stool in amoebic and bacillary dysentery is so specific that a diagnosis can be based on this point alone. A table is appended below to show the macroscopic and microscopic differences between the stools of amoebic and bacillary dysentery.

	AMOEBIC DYSENTERY	BACILLARY DYSENTERY
Macroscopic:		
NUMBER:	6 to 8 motions a day.	Over 10 motions a day.
AMOUNT:	Relatively copious.	Small.
ODOUR:	Offensive.	Odourless.
COLOUR:	Dark red.	Bright red.
NATURE:	Blood and mucus mixed with faeces.	Blood and mucus; no faeces.
REACTION:	Acid.	Alkaline.
CONSISTENCY:	Fluid mucus not adherent to the container.	Viscid mucus adherent to the bottom of the container.
Microscopic (Figs. 16 & 17):		
R.B.C.	In clumps; reddish-yellow in colour.	Discrete or in rouleaux; bright red in colour.
PUS CELLS:	Scanty.	Numerous.
MACROPHAGES:	Very few.	Large and numerous; many of them contain R.B.C.; hence mistaken for *E. histolytica*.
EOSINOPHILS:	Present.	Scarce.
PYKNOTIC BODIES:	Very common.	Nil.
GHOST CELLS:	Nil.	Numerous.
PARASITE:	Trophozoites of *E. histolytica*.	Nil.
BACTERIA:	Many motile bacteria.	Nil.
C.L. CRYSTALS:	Present.	Nil.

METASTATIC LESIONS IN LIVER

Hepatic Amoebiasis (Amoebic Liver Abscess)

Incidence of Liver Abscess. In the tropics about 2 to 10 per cent (average 5 per cent) of the individuals infected with *E. histolytica* suffer from hepatic complications. The incidence of liver abscess is less common in women and is rare in children under ten years. History of amoebic dysentery may not be obtained in more than 50 per cent of cases.

Hepatic complication may develop at any time during intestinal infection and generally appears when the intestinal symptoms have subsided. In the majority of cases, the hepatic complication appears after about one to three months of the disappearance of the dysenteric attack. Cases have been reported where liver abscesses have developed after a lapse of months or even years. It is rather a peculiar feature that patients suffering from acute dysenteric symptoms do rarely present hepatic complications. Only in a small number of cases both the intestine and the liver are involved at the same time, and these cases are invariably fatal.

Genesis of Hepatic Lesions. The trophozoites of *E. histolytica* are carried as emboli by the radicles of the portal vein from the base of an amoebic ulcer in the large intestine, usually from the caecum and the ascending colon. The capillary system (Fig. 18) of the liver acts as an efficient filter and holds these parasites. Once established, they multiply in large numbers and proceed to carry on their cytolytic action. In course of time, a local accumulation of the amoebae will cause obstruction to the circulation and produce thrombosis of the portal venules (sinusoids) resulting in anaemic necrosis of the surrounding liver cells. The primary lesion thus appears to be a focal necrosis of the liver cells which forms the starting point of a liver abscess and the process of destruction then continues in concentric layers (Fig. 19). At first the necrotic material consists of a solid slough and later the centre liquefies by cytolytic action of amoebae and the liquefaction extends radially. A fairly big-sized abscess is formed by coalescence of these miliary abscesses.

Diffuse Amoebic Hepatitis. The syndrome of slightly enlarged and tender liver, right upper quadrant pain, intermittent fever and leucocytosis in patients with amoebic dysentery is sometimes referred to as *"diffuse amoebic hepatitis"*. *The existence of such a condition is doubted*, because careful postmortem and biopsy studies of material obtained from liver do neither reveal any

Microscopic appearances of cellular exudate in amoebic and bacillary dysentery
(Fresh preparations)

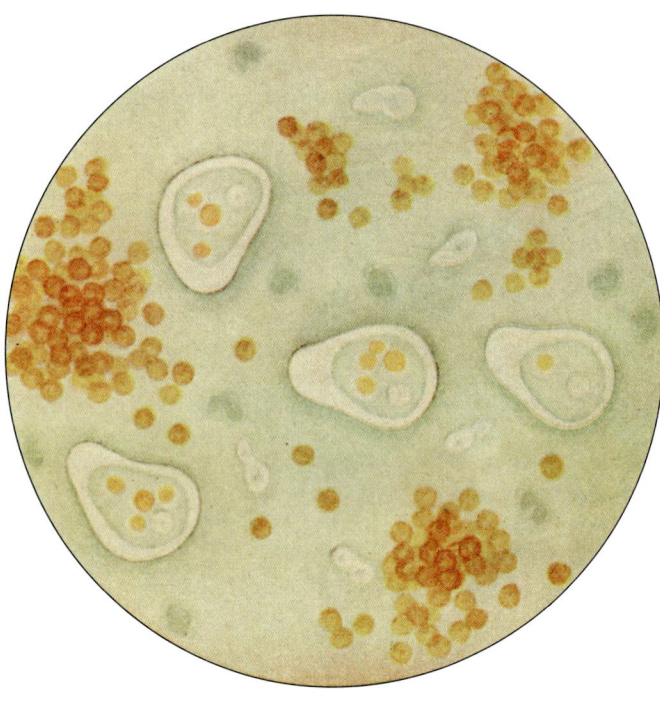

Fig. 16—Stool in acute amoebic dysentery. Note the scanty cellular exudate, clumped red blood cells, pyknotic bodies and trophozoites of *E. histolytica* with ingested red blood cells.

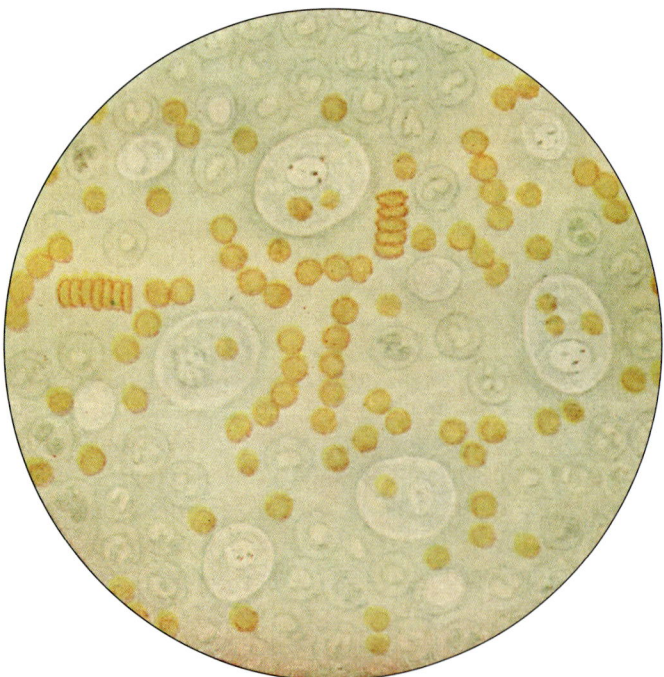

Fig. 17—Stool in acute bacillary dysentery. Note the abundant cellular exudate containing pus cells, macrophages with phagocytosed red blood cells, ghost cells and discrete red blood cells with occasional rouleaux formation.

pathological evidence of diffuse amoebic hepatitis nor the presence of *E. histolytica* in the hepatic tissues. Hence it is now considered to be a non-specific hepatomegaly, the result of periportal inflammation (a general congestion and enlargement of the organ) due to substances or bacteria carried to the liver by the blood stream from an ulcerated gut and not a prelude to amoebic liver abscess. Moreover the control of intestinal amoebiasis by tetracycline, a drug having no action on *E. histolytica* in the liver, causes disappearance of this tender hepatomegaly.

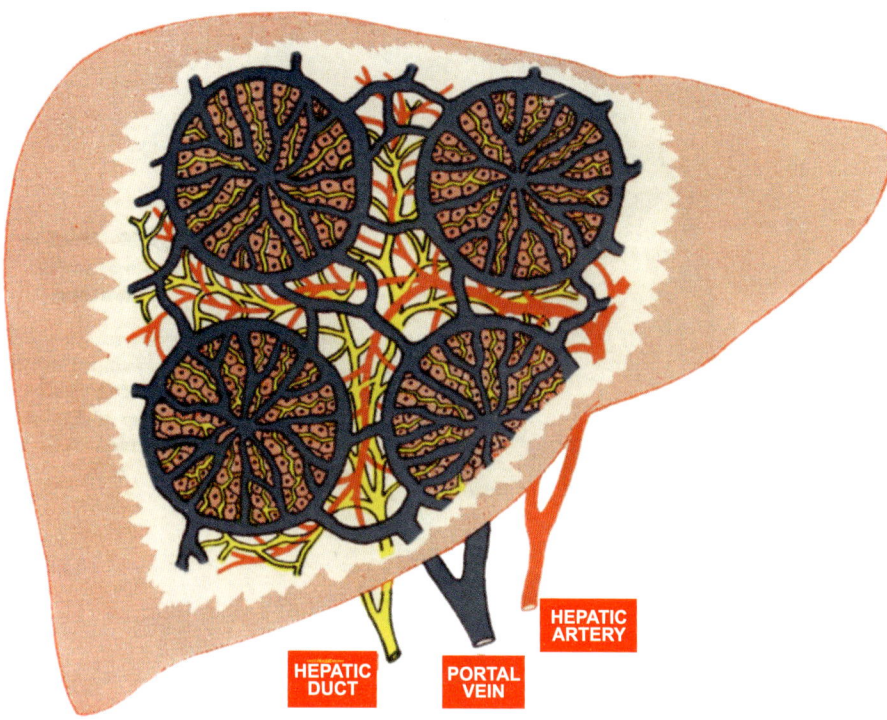

Fig. 18—Anatomy of the vascular supply of the liver.

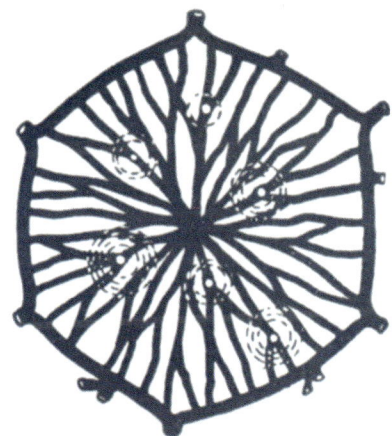

Fig. 19—Portal venous system of a liver lobule.
Showing the genesis of liver abscess. Note the focal necrosis (miliary abscess)
and extension in concentric circles.

Macroscopic Pathology. Amoebic liver abscess varies greatly in size. It may occur in any part of the liver but is generally confined to the postero-superior surface of the right lobe. Ordinarily only one large solitary abscess is found. To the *naked eye*, the appearance of the abscess area is reddish brown in colour with a semi-fluid or grumous consistency (Fig. 20). If the cytolysed liver tissue is completely destroyed or is washed out in running water, shreds of connective tissue may be seen running across the abscess cavity. The wall of the abscess cavity is ragged and shaggy in appearance and is formed by the necrotic liver tissues which gradually merge into the healthy zones with an intervening zone of hyperaemia. In an old abscess, the wall is smooth and is formed by dense connective tissues.

Cases have been observed where the whole liver has been transformed into a huge abscess sac, holding litres of pus, the wall being formed by a narrow strip of liver tissue.

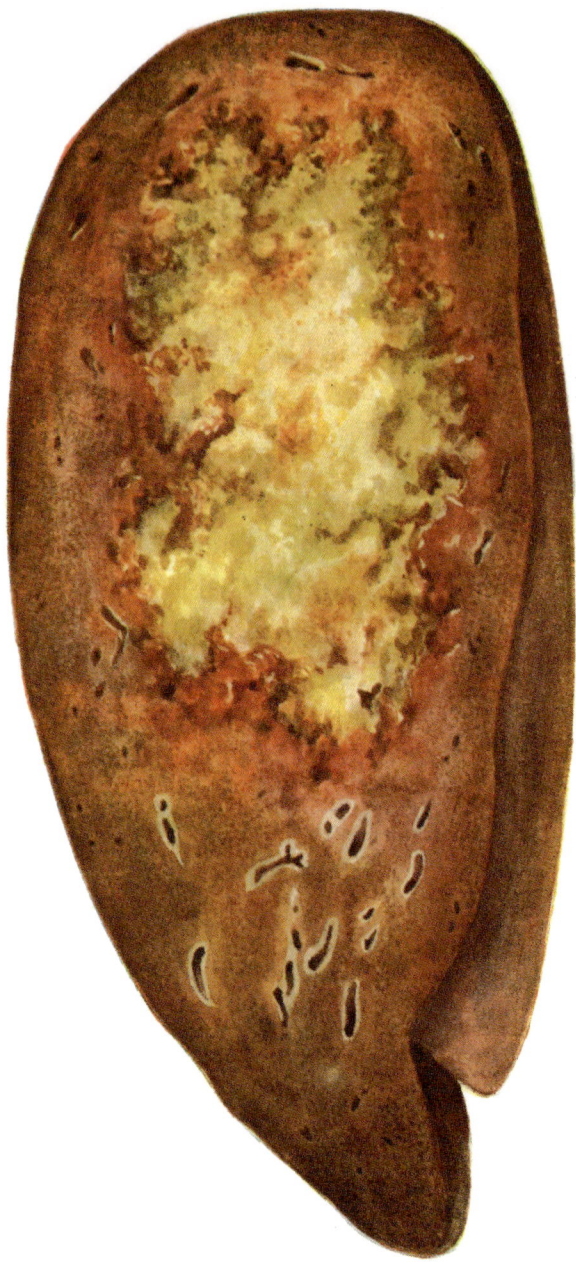

Fig. 20—Macroscopic pathology of amoebic liver abscess.
Note the characteristic coagulative necrosis caused by *Entamoeba histolytica*.

Multiple small abscesses in which the whole organ becomes riddled with scattered foci of necrosis, are probably more common than is usually supposed.

Microscopic Pathology. If a section is made through the margin of a liver abscess, three zones can be differentiated from the centre to the periphery (Fig. 21):

1. A central zone of cytolysed granular material with no amoebae.
2. An intermediate zone consisting of degenerated liver cells, a few leucocytes, connective tissue cells, red blood cells and an occasional trophozoite of *E. histolytica*.
3. A peripheral zone consisting of congested capillaries with varying degrees of necrosis of liver cells. The amoebae can be seen to be multiplying in this area and invading the adjoining healthy liver tissue.

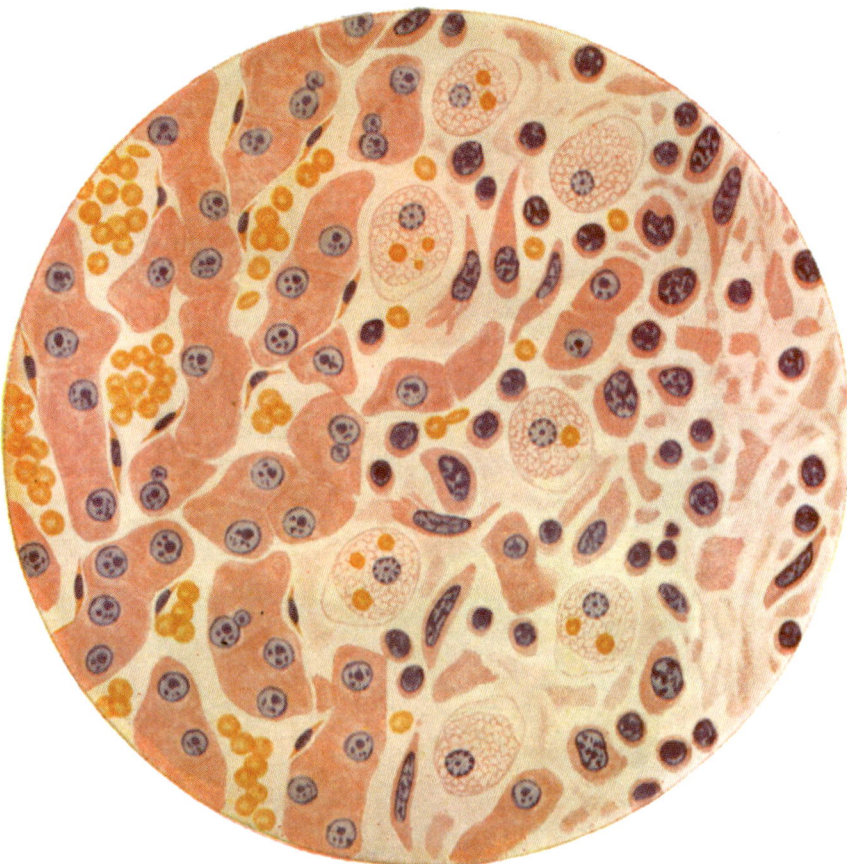

Fig. 21—Microscopic pathology of amoebic liver abscess.
Note the trophozoites of *Entamoeba histolytica* at the margin.

In a long-standing abscess, the third zone may consist of actively proliferating connective tissue cells, lympho-cytes, to wall of the abscess cavity.

Note: For the demonstration of trophozoites of *E. histolytica*, the material should be taken from the tissues of the abscess-wall by scraping, and not from the abscess contents.

Pus of Liver Abscess. The "pus" is not of suppuration but is a mixture of sloughed liver tissue and blood. It is chocolate brown in colour and thick in consistency (the so-called "anchovy-sauce pus"). The smell is rarely offensive. The "pus" is bacteriologically sterile. *Microscopical* examination of the "pus" reveals degenerated liver cells, a few red blood cells and occasional leucocytes. The trophozoites of *E. histolytica* are not generally found in freshly aspi-rated liver pus.

Intestinal Lesions in Amoebic Liver Abscess. In all cases of hepatic amoebiasis as also in other metastatic amoebiasis, the primary lesion is in the large gut. The changes in the intestine observed at autopsy may be any one of the following:

1. Small superficial ulcers with thickening of the colon.
2. A single latent ulcer, located most commonly in the caecum.
3. Pigmented or non-pigmented scars in the large intestine, representing the sites of previous ulcers.
4. No change in the large gut. This is due to the fact that while the amoebae are causing damage to the liver, the intestinal ulcers have been completely healed up.
5. Extensive ulcers scattered throughout the large intestine are not at all common.

Clinical Features of Amoebic Liver Abscess (Fig. 22)

(Located in the postero-superior surface of the right lobe of the liver.)

Onset is insidious.

Pain and *tenderness* in the right hypochondrium are the earliest manifestations and this is due to the stretching of the capsule of the liver. Pain is sometimes referred to the right acromial region (shoulder pain) due to the irritation of

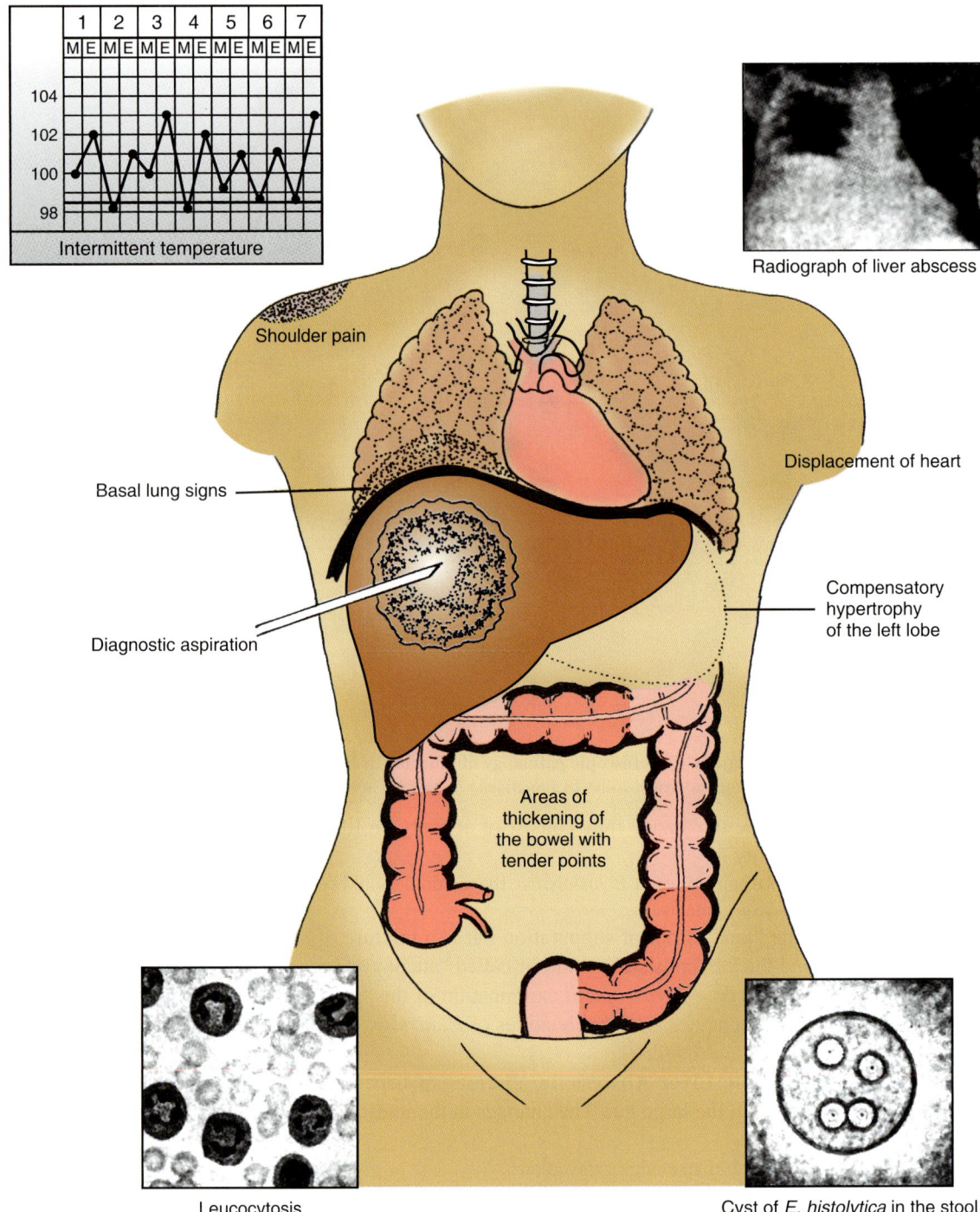

Intermittent temperature

Radiograph of liver abscess

Shoulder pain

Basal lung signs

Diagnostic aspiration

Displacement of heart

Compensatory hypertrophy of the left lobe

Areas of thickening of the bowel with tender points

Leucocytosis

Cyst of *E. histolytica* in the stool

Fig. 22—Clinical, laboratory and radiological findings in a case of amoebic liver abscess.

the phrenic nerve which supplies the undersurface of the diaphragm; a dry cough may often be associated with it for similar reason. Occasionally, the pain is referred to the lower abdomen or the right iliac region.

Fever. A slight rise of temperature in the evening or a low remitten temperature which later becomes quotidian and takes on a hectic character. This is due to the pyrogenic effect of necrosed liver cells.

Jaundice is an unusual manifestation.

General health. The patient becomes emaciated.

On examination, the lower border of the *liver* is palpable below the coastal margin and is tender. Liver dullness may extend upwards. The movement of the right side of the chest during respiration is diminished or absent. There may be a marked rigidity of the upper part of the right rectus which will interfere greatly with the palpation of enlarged liver. Occasionally, there may be a bulging of the parieties, indicating the pointing of the abscess. The left lobe of the liver may undergo a compensatory hypertrophy in a very big abscess.

Lung signs. These are due ot the collapse of the right lung base caused by the growing liver abscess. A right-sided pleural effusion may occasionally be present.

Apical impulse. This may be displace upwards and laterally by a large abscess.

Intestinal symptoms, such as diarrhoea or dysentery are absent. On abdominal palpation, areas of thickening of the bowel with tenderness may be elicited.

Course and Termination of Liver Abscess. It may heal up spontaneously leaving an encysted mass, the contents of which may be dried up, fibrosed or even calcified.

With the continued lysis of liver tissue, the abscess may grow in various directions ultimately coming in contact with the neighbouring structures, through which the contents are discharged. Thus a liver abscess may have the following terminations:

(i) A right-sided liver abscess may rupture (Fig. 23A):

    (a) *Externally.* A spontaneous rupture through the parieties is one of the most natural forms of termination of liver abscess. The skin in these cases may be secondarily infected with the trophic forms of *E. histolytica,* forming *granuloma cutis.*

    (b) *Into the Lungs.* The "pus" is expectorated with the sputum giving rise to haemoptysis. Such a sputum will have a viscid consistency and is chocolate brown in colour ("anchovy-sauce pus"). Microscopically, liver cells and trophozoites of *E. histolytica* may be recognised.

    (c) *Into the Right Pleural Cavity*, leading to empyema thoracis.

    (d) *Below the Diaphragm*, producing a variety of subphrenic abscesses.

    (e) *Into the Peritoneal Cavity*, producing a generalised peritonitis.

(ii) A left-sided liver abscess may rupture into (Fig. 23B):

    (a) *Stomach.* The "pus" is vomited out, leading to haematemesis.

    (b) *Pericardial Cavity,* causing purulent pericarditis and ending fatally.

    (c) *Externally,* through the anterior abdominal wall in the epigastric region.

    (d) *Left Pleural Cavity,* causing empyema thoracis.

(iii) A liver abscess situated on the inferior surface may rupture into:

    (a) *Bowel (Transverse Colon* or *Duodenum),* causing diarrhoea and discharge of "pus" in the stool.

    (b) *Peritoneal Cavity*, causing a fatal peritonitis.

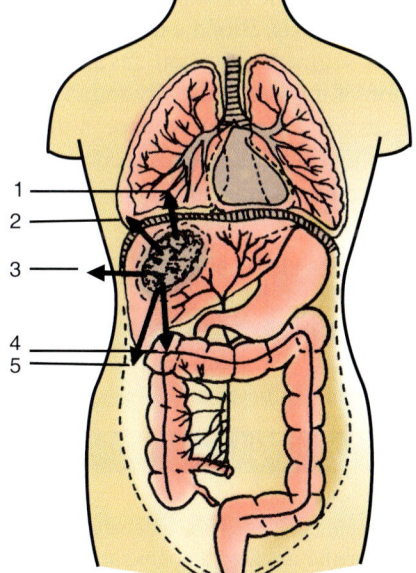
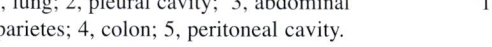

Fig. 23A—Diagram showing the possible sites of rupture of a right-sided liver abscess.
1, lung; 2, pleural cavity; 3, abdominal parietes; 4, colon; 5, peritoneal cavity.

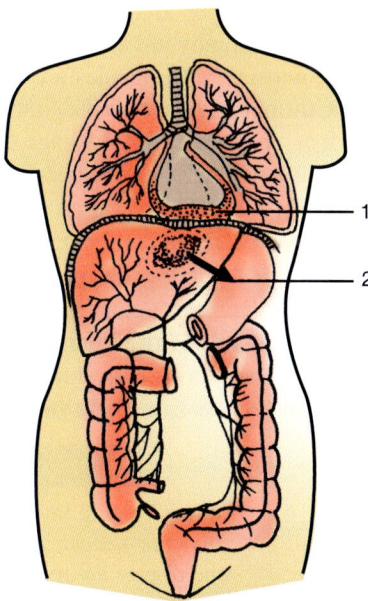

Fig. 23B—Sites of rupture of a left-sided liver abscess.
1, pericardial cavity; 2, stomach.

(iv) A liver abscess situated on the posterior surface may rupture into:
Inferior Vena Cava. Such an occurrence, although rare, is invariably fatal (Fig. 24).

Other *sites* of rupture of a liver abscess which have been recorded by different observers include the common bile duct, the pelvis of the kidney and the perinephric tissues of the lumbar region.

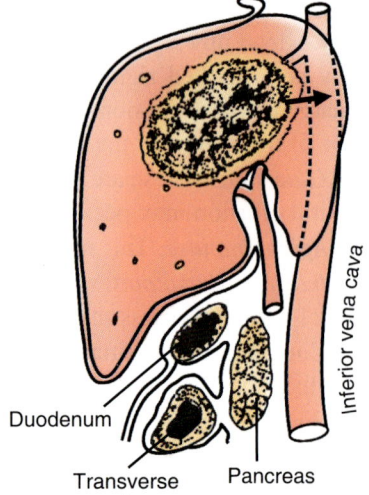

Fig. 24—A liver abscess on the posterior surface may rupture into the inferior vena cava.

METASTATIC LESIONS IN OTHER ORGANS (Fig. 25)

Pulmonary Amoebiasis. Amoebic abscess of lungs may be primary or secondary:

(i) *Primary.* It is a rare condition, occurring independently even without the presence of any hepatic abscess. In these cases, trophozoites of *E. histolytica* gain entrance from the gut-wall *via* the portal circulation into the pulmonary capillaries. Evolution of lung abscess, either single or multiple, occurs in the same way as that of a liver abscess.

(ii) *Secondary.* It arises as a complication of liver abscess by direct extension through the adhesion formed with the diaphragm, the liver and the base of the right lung. In such cases a single abscess, varying in size, may form in the lower lobe of the right lung.

Cerebral Amoebiasis. It is one of the rare varieties of metastatic amoebiasis. In the majority of cases, amoebic brain abscess arises as a complication of either hepatic or pulmonary abscess or both. The abscess is generally single and of small size and is located most commonly in one of the cerebral hemispheres.

Amoebic Pericarditis. Another rare manifestation of amoebiasis is amoebic pericarditis. Recently more cases have been reported in world's medical literature. Pericardial involvement in amoebiasis occurs invariably by direct extension from amoebic abscess of left lobe of the liver. Occasionally, the disease results from an abscess in the right lobe of the liver or lung abscess. High fever, epigastric pain, palpable mass in epigastrium or in left hypochondrium, tenderness over upper abdomen, dyspnoea and pericardial rub are the salient clinical features of the disease. X-ray of chest and upper abdomen show enlarged heart with elevated diaphragm. Ultrasound of upper abdomen and echocardiography are also helpful in making diagnosis. Blood examination reveals anaemia and polymorphonuclear leucocytosis. ECG changes are generalised ST segment elevation, inverted T-waves, or low voltage complexes.

Cutaneous Amoebiasis. Amoebic invasion of the skin is usually found over the region adjoining a visceral lesion, such as, in the areas of drainage of liver abscess or colostomy wound, in the sites of ruptured appendicular and peri-colic abscesses. Extensive necrosis and sloughing of the skin and subcutaneous tissues are caused by the trophozoites of *E. histolytica* in these areas. Besides these granulomatous ulcerations, a granulomatous mass simulating an epithelioma has been seen in the peri-anal region.

Splenic Abscess. It is found in association with hepatic abscess. Transmission of the trophozoites of *E. histolytica* occurs directly through an adherent splenic flexure of the colon.

Amoebiasis of the Penis. Amoebic infections of the penis are extremely rare and clinically mistaken for carcinoma of the penis or ulcerative venereal disease of the penis. A few cases have been reported in world's medical literature. A few cases have been documented from India also.

Enumeration of the Pathological Lesions Caused by *E. histolytica*

I. INTESTINAL LESIONS: Involve the large gut only.
  1. *In Acute Amoebic Dysentery:* Multiple ulcers, deep and extensive. Complications which may arise in the course of the disease are: peri-caecal and peri-colic abscess, amoebic appendicitis, perforation and generalised peritonitis, gangrene of the gut and fistulas.
  2. *In Chronic Intestinal Amoebiasis:*
      (a) Single latent ulcer in the caecum.
      (b) Multiple, small, superficial ulcers scattered throughout the large gut.
      (c) Thickened caecum and colon, with occasional stricture formation.
      (d) Amoeboma in the caecum and other parts of the large gut.
      (e) Pigmented or non-pigmented scars.

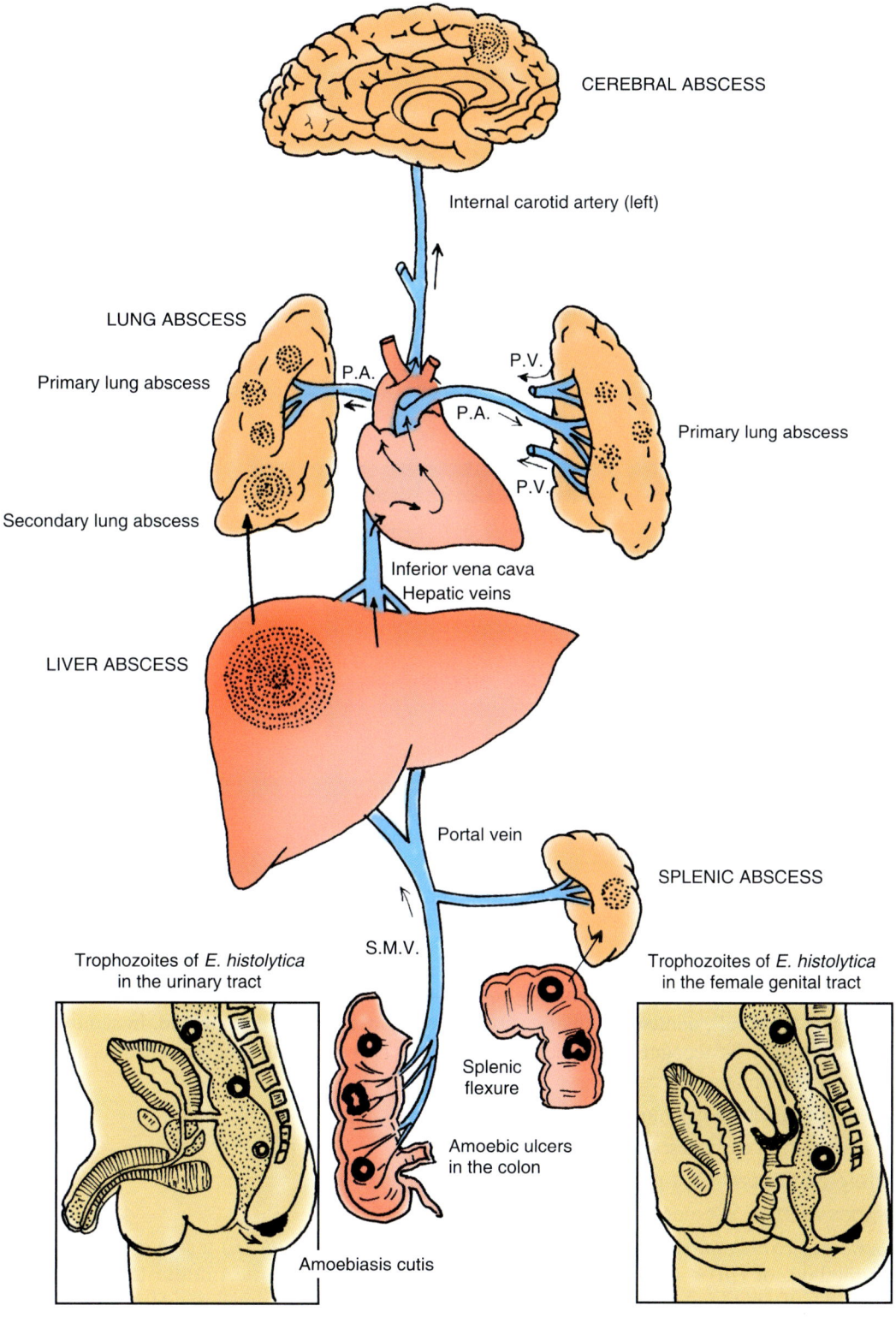

CEREBRAL ABSCESS

Internal carotid artery (left)

LUNG ABSCESS

Primary lung abscess

P.A.

P.V.

P.A.

Primary lung abscess

Secondary lung abscess

P.V.

Inferior vena cava
Hepatic veins

LIVER ABSCESS

Portal vein

SPLENIC ABSCESS

S.M.V.

Trophozoites of *E. histolytica*
in the urinary tract

Splenic
flexure

Trophozoites of *E. histolytica*
in the female genital tract

Amoebic ulcers
in the colon

Amoebiasis cutis

Recto-vesical fistula

Recto-vaginal fistula

Fig. 25—Diagrammatic representation of the evolution of metastatic amoebiasis.

II. EXTRA-INTESTINAL OR METASTATIC LESIONS:

1. *Liver:* In Amoebic Liver Abscess:

    (i) Multiple small abscesses involving the whole organ.

    (ii) A large solitary abscess, usually in the postero-superior surface of the right lobe.

    The term *diffuse amoebic hepatitis* is not widely accepted, because there is no convincing proof that it is due to invasion by *E. histolytica.*

2. *Lungs:*

    (a) Primary: Small, multiple abscesses, may be in one lung or both the lungs.

    (b) Secondary: A single abscess of varying size, situated in the lower lobe of right lung.

3. *Brain:* A small abscess in one of the cerebral hemispheres.

4. *Spleen:* Splenic abscess.

5. *Skin:* Granulomatous ulceration of the skin adjoining a visceral lesion. Granulomatous mass simulating an epithelioma in the peri-anal region.

6. *Uro-genital Tract:* Amoeba gaining entrance either through a recto-vesical fistula or a recto-vaginal fistula. Direct access *via* uro-genital opening may give rise to ameobic vaginitis and amoebic ulcer of the penis but such lesions are extremely rare.

Laboratory Diagnosis of Amoebiasis

The primary aim will be to demonstrate the presence of *E. histolytica* in the material obtained from any particular lesion, such as stool, "pus" of liver abscess and sputum.

Diagnosis of Intestinal Amoebiasis:

(A) SYMPTOMATIC GROUP—Cases of Acute Amoebic Dysentery.

1. EXAMINATION OF STOOL

(a) *Naked Eye or Macroscopic Appearance.* An offensive dark brown semi-fluid stool, acid in reaction, admixed with blood, mucus and much faecal matter is representative of a case of amoebic dysentery.

(b) *General Microscopical Character.* Under this, attention is given to (i) the character of the cellular exudate and (ii) the presence of Charcot-Leyden crystals. The *cellular exudate* is scanty and consists of only the nuclear masses ("pyknotic bodies") of a few pus cells, macrophages and epithelial cells. The red blood cells are clumped and are reddish-yellow or yellowish-green in colour.

Charcot-Leyden Crystals. These are also found in other pathological conditions of the bowel and therefore not pathognomonic of the stool of amoebic dysentery. Their presence only suggests a careful examination of the stool for *E. histolytica.* In saline preparation, they appear as diamond-shaped or whetstone-shaped crystals, clear and refractile. Their sizes vary from 5 to 50 μm.

(c) *Demonstration of E. histolytica* by examining an unstained preparation microscopically. Fresh stool (within 30 minutes after passing the stool), unmixed with any antiseptic or urine, should be examined. In acute cases, the amoebic trophozoites can easily be recognised by their characteristic movement and the presence of ingested red blood cells. A stained preparation is rarely called for.

2. EXAMINATION OF BLOOD shows moderate leucocytosis.

3. SEROLOGICAL TEST. In early cases, it is always negative.

(B) ASYMPTOMATIC GROUP—Cyst-passers or Cyst-carriers.

1. EXAMINATION OF STOOL. Demonstration of *E. histolytica* by:

(a) *Microscopic Examination* of (*i*) a natural stool (formed) for cysts, or (*ii*) a smear (for cysts) prepared by concentration method, or (*iii*) a purged stool obtained after a saline cathartic (motile trophozoites and cysts), or (*iv*) the material collected by the use of sigmoidoscope (trophozoites). Specimen obtained through the sigmoidoscope yields a positive result only when there are visible lesions in the sigmoido-rectal area. At least three consecutive samples of stool should be examined for detection of cyst as excretion of cyst in stool is often intermittent.

(b) *Cultural Examination*. Stools negative microscopically, when cultured, have on various occasions shown the presence of parasites.

(c) *Animal inoculation*. Not used nowadays.

2. BLOOD PICTURE. It is in no way characteristic.

3. SEROLOGICAL TEST. In "asymptomatic carriers" the amoebae, present in the stool, are in the commensal phase with very little or no invasion of the tissues. These cases are sero-negative. But those cases where tissue-invasion without any symptom has existed long enough to stimulate the antibody formation, the serological test may be positive (*vide infra*).

Diagnosis of Hepatic Amoebiasis (Amoebic Liver Abscess):

1. *Diagnostic Aspiration*. Exploratory puncture is one of the most practical methods for confirming the diagnosis of amoebic liver abscess. This may however fail, if it is deep-seated or located in the posterior aspect. The aspirated "pus" may be examined for the demonstration of trophic forms of *E. histolytica (see* p. 26).

2. *Liver Biopsy. E. histolytica* (trophic forms) may be demonstrated in specimens of liver biopsy taken from cases of miliary amoebic hepatic abscess.

3. *Examination of Stool*. Cysts of *E. histolytica* are present in less than 15% cases of amoebic liver abscess and gives information regarding the persistence of intestinal infection.

4. *Examination of Blood* shows leucocytosis, varying from 15,000 to 30,000 per mm^3 of blood. A differential count shows neutrophil granulocytes to be 70 to 75 per cent. Liver function tests show raised alkaline phosphatase level and S.G.O.T. level.

5. *Serological Tests (Immunologic Diagnosis)*. These tests have been in use for the detection of specific antibody and mainly useful in diagnosis of extra-instestinal amoebiasis. Improvement in the production of amoebic antigens, i.e. from axenic cultures as well as in the sero-immunological methods, sero-immunodiagnosis of amoebiasis has become important in the field of laboratory diagnosis. Their value lies in screening for amoebiasis, particularly in the extra-intestinal amoebiasis cases. The tests LAT, IHA, GD, IFA, ELISA, may be usefully employed as additional methods of diagnosis of the disease. Latex fixation test (LAT) is fairly and frequently used. These serological tests are virtually always positive in hepatic abscess, but only about 85% positive in cases of dysentery.

Radioimmunoassay (RIA) and CCIE have also been used in cases of amoebiasis.

AMOEBIC ANTIGEN. It is difficult to get a specific and pure antigen because of microbial associates in cultures of *E. histolytica*. It is however now possible to get such an antigen from the trophozoites of *E. histolytica* grown in an axenic medium. Antigen free from microbial components may be prepared from cysts of *E. invadens* (snake amoeba) which also gives satisfactory results (Yap, Zaman & Aw, 1970).

6. *Intradermal Test* (Leal, 1954). In an infected individual injection of 0.1 ml of an antigen prepared from cultures of *E. histolytica* produces at the site of injection an erythema which manifests after 3 hours, reaching a maximum (9 to 10 cm in diameter) after 20 to 24 hours and disappearing in another 24 to 48 hours.

7. *Radiological Examination*. The right dome of the diaphragm is generally found to be situated at a higher level, because the commonest site of abscess is in the postero-superior surface of the liver. Sometimes there may be a "tenting" of the diaphragm (evidence of basal pleurisy). The actual abscess cavity within the liver cannot usually be visualised radiologically but occasionally it may be detected when it casts a shadow of less opaque area in the substance of the liver.

8. *Radio-isotope tracing of liver*: Recently hepatic photoscan has been introduced to locate the space-occupying lesion in the liver. Tandon *et al* (1966) using I^{131} labelled Rose Bengal as the tracer agent, observed an area of focal filling "defect" in amoebic abscess of liver. They also found that such an investigation was very helpful in detecting concealed and multiple abscesses of the liver and also in studying the progress of healing of this lesion in the liver.

9. Ultrasonography of upper abdomen, CT scan of liver or MRI scan of liver may be found useful for detection of amoebic liver abscess.

Diagnosis of Pulmonary Amoebiasis. Demonstration of the trophozoite of *E. histolytica* in the sputum and by other immunological tests.

When the liver abscess has ruptured through the lung, the material expectorated is typical of the "anchovy-sauce pus" of liver abscess. Microscopically, it will show degenerated liver cells, elements of blood, granular debris and even striated muscle fibres of the diaphragm. The parasites may not be detected in the first expectoration, but will be found in subsequent expectorations. The expectorated "pus" when examined fresh, may demonstrate the motile forms (trophozoites) of *E. histolytica*. The presence of the common, commensal of the mouth *E. gingivalis* in the sputum may cause confusion in the diagnosis.

OTHER METASTATIC LESIONS. In all such cases, the trophozoite of *E. histolytica* should be searched for.

Treatment. Amoebicidal drugs may be grouped as follows:

1. *Tissue Amoebicides.* Drugs acting on the trophozoites of *E. histolytica* in the tissues (invasive amoebae).
   - (a) In the intestinal wall, liver and other metastatic lesions—Emetine and dehydroemetine (DHE). Administered parenterally.
   - (b) In the liver and lungs only—4-aminoquinoline (chloroquine).
2. *Luminal Amoebicides.* Drugs acting on trophozoites and cysts of *E. histolytica* in the lumen only.
   - (a) Direct-acting luminal or Contact amoebicides.
     - (i) Halogenated hydroxyquinolines—Di-iodohydroxyquinoline (diodoquin), iodochlorhydroxyquinoline (clioquinol).
     - (ii) Dichloracetamide group, diloxanide (entamide).
     - (iii) Antibiotics—Paromomycin (humatin).
   - (b) Indirect-acting luminal amoebicides—Antibiotics (tetracycline).
3. *Both Luminal and Tissue Amoebicides.* Drugs acting on the trophozoites and cysts in the lumen and trophozoites of *E. histolytica* in the tissues: Metronidazole (Flagyl) and related compounds like tinidazole and nitroimidazole are administered orally.

Prophylaxis

For Personal Prophylaxis: (i) Use of boiled drinking water, (ii) protection of all food and drink from contamination by flies, cockroaches and rats, (iii) avoidance of use of raw vegetables and fruits, (iv) personal cleanliness and elementary hygienic conditions are to be observed while taking meals.

For Community Prophylaxis: (i) Effective sanitary disposal of faeces, (ii) protection of water supplies from faecal pollution, (iii) avoidance of the use of human excrement as fertiliser, (iv) detection and isolation of carriers.

Species Variation in *E. histolytica*. It is now known that *E. histolytica* shows considerable variation in size, feeding habits and pathogenicity, thereby reflecting that there may be more than one species included under the name *E. histolytica* though genetically different. Some workers are however of the opinion that the differences that exist are due to environmental factors, such as site and associates in the bowel and are not genetically different. The subject-matter thus appears to be complex and the table on next page summarises the various views put forward from time to time.

For reasons not yet understood the non-pathogenic, commensal species of *E. histolytica* may acquire the property of invasiveness and become pathogenic. The tissue invasion is probably influenced by host's diet,* special intestinal flora and enzymatic (proteolytic) activity of the parasite itself.

According to some workers pathogenic (P) and non-pathogenic *E. histolytica* (N.P.) are two different species. *There are lots of controversy regarding these subject matters.* However, several methods like study of migration pattern of 6 isoenzymes, use of monoclonal antibodies against several antigens and use of genetic markers are used to differentiate between pathogenic and non-pathogenic histolytica.

---

* Cholesterol is believed to be a nutritional factor for *E. histolytica* and is also thought to increase its virulence (Biagi *et al.*, 1962).

"Minuta" form of E. histolytica. It is now believed that *E. histolytica* has a commensal phase, living in the lumen of the gut and ingesting bacteria and other contents of the faeces. These amoebae are generally of smaller sizes, trophozoites measuring 12 to 14 μm and cysts measuring below 10 μm. They are derived from the virulent "large race" or the tissue invading forms. These are called "minuta" forms and are often mistaken for *E. hartmanni* (the "small race" of *E. histolytica*).

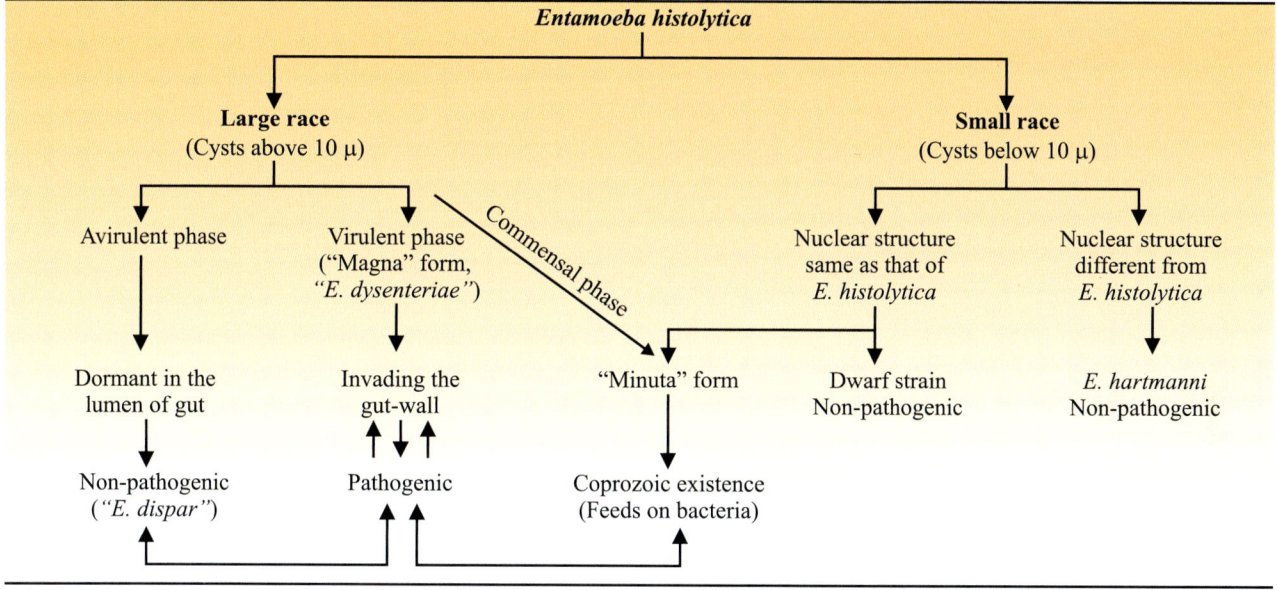

NON-PATHOGENIC SPECIES OF AMOEBIDA

Entamoeba coli (Grassi, 1879) Casagrandi and Barbagallo, 1895

Geographical Distribution. World-wide.

Habitat. Lives in a free state in the lumen of the large bowel.

Morphology. There are mainly two stages in the life cycle: *trophozoite* and *cyst,* with a transitory stage of *pre-cystic form* (Fig. 26).

TROPHOZOITE. It is one of the largest amoeba occurring in the human colon and measures 20 to 40 µm in diameter. It is sluggishly motile. The cytoplasm is not clearly defined. The opaque granular endoplasm is packed with food vacuoles consisting of bacteria and other substances but *never red blood cells.* Because it is richer in chromatin, the nucleus is visible in unstained preparation. In stained preparation the nuclear structure shows a large eccentric karyosome surrounded by a broader halo and coarse chromatin granules lining the thick nuclear membrane.

CYST. It begins with a single nucleus and by repeated nuclear divisions, an octonucleate cyst is formed. It is a rounded body measuring 15 to 20 µm in diameter. In the binucleate stage, there is a large glycogen mass. Chromatoid bodies, if present, are in the form of slender filaments or pointed threads. Neither the glycogen mass nor chromatoid bodies are to be found in a mature cyst.

Life Cycle. Same as that of *E. histolytica.* During excystation, the nuclei of metacystic amoeba do not undergo any multiplication but, on the contrary, the original 8 nuclei may be diminished by as many as 4.

Pathogenicity. Exists as a harmless commensal.

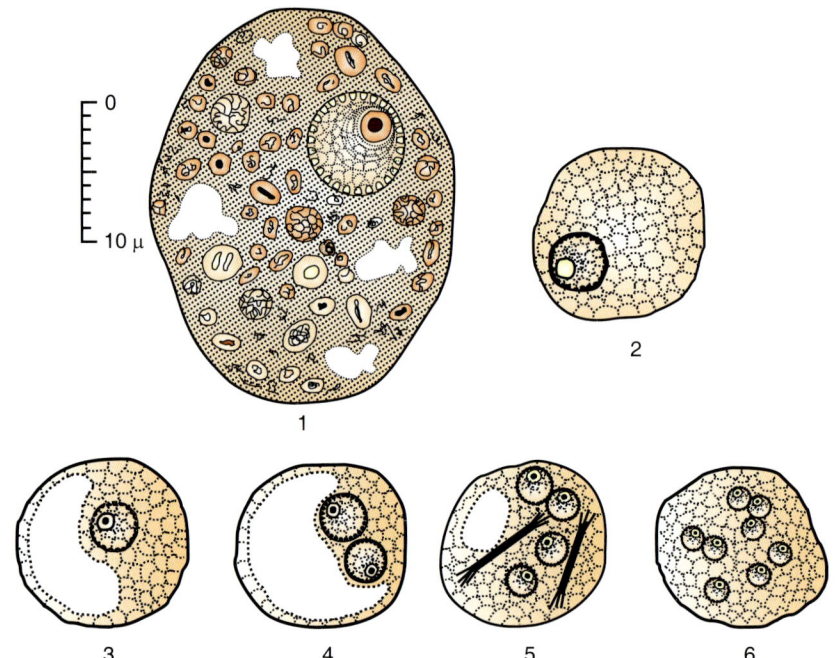

Fig. 26—Three stages of *Entamoeba coli.*
1, trophozoite; 2, pre-cystic form; 3 to 6, cysts with one to eight nuclei. Note the characteristic nucleus with
eccentric karyosome; presence of glycogen vacuoles in 3, 4 and 5; chromatoid bodies in 5.

Diagnosis. As *E. coli* is more commonly found in the dysenteric stool, the morphological difference from the pathogenic species *E. histolytica* is shown in the table below:

Trophozoite and Cyst of *E. histolytica* and *E. coli*

	Entamoeba histolytica	*Entamoeba coli*
TROPHOZOITE:		
Fresh Preparation:		
SIZE:	20 to 30 µm.	20 to 40 µm.
MOTILITY:	Very active	Sluggish.
CYTOPLASM:	Clearly defined into ectoplasm and endoplasm.	Not defined; ectoplasm scarcely seen.

	Entamoeba histolytica	*Entamoeba coli*
CYTOPLASMIC INCLUSIONS:	Red blood cells, leucocytes and tissue debris but *no bacteria*.	Bacteria and other materials but *never red blood cells*.
NUCLEUS:	Not visible in uinstained preparation.	Visible in unstained preparation.
Stained with Iodine:		
NUCLEAR CHARACTER:	Central karyosome; fine chromatin granules line the delicate nuclear membrane.	Eccentric karyosome; coarse chromatin granules line the thick nuclear membrane.
CYST:		
Stained with Iodine:		
SIZE:	6 to 15 µm.	15 to 20 µm.
NUCLEUS:	1 to 4; central karyosome.	1 to 8; eccentric karyosome.
GLYCOGEN MASS:	Visible in uninucleate stage.	Large and visible in the binucleate stage.
Fresh Preparation:		
CHROMATOID BODIES:	Rounded bars.	Filamentous, thread-like with square or pointed ends.

Entamoeba chattoni Swellengrebel, 1914 (*Entamoeba polecki* von Prowazek, 1912). It is commonly found in the large intestine of hog and monkey, rarely in man. The trophozoite resembles that of *E. coli*; the nucleoplasm stains dark and the karyosome is smaller and eccentric. The cyst is uninucleate and shows cytoplasmic condensation and inclusion masses. It is non-pathogenic to man and reservoir hosts.

Entamoeba moshkovskii Tshalaia, 1941. It has been recovered from the sewage but is not known to parasitise man. The trophozoite and cyst resemble those of *E. histolytica* and may cause diagnostic difficulty when treated sewage effluent is examined for the detection of viable *E. histolytica* cysts.

Entamoeba gingivalis (Gross, 1849) Brümpt, 1913. It is a parasite of the human mouth, living as a harmless commensal particularly in the unhealthy tissues around the teeth. It is a small amoeba, measuring 10 to 20 µm in diameter. It is actively motile and when fresh, multiple pseudopodia are seen to protrude. The cytoplasm is divisible into clear hyaline ectoplasm and granular endoplasm. Cytoplasmic inclusions consist of bacteria and other substances but *never red blood cells*. The nucleus is not visible in unstained preparations. When stained, the nucleus shows a well marked karyosome near the centre with delicate achromatic strands extending to nuclear membrane. There is a ring like deposit of chromatin material inside the nuclear membrane (Fig. 27). There is no *cystic phase*.

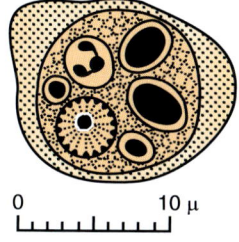

Fig. 27—Trophozoite of
E. gingivalis **showing**
ingested bodies.

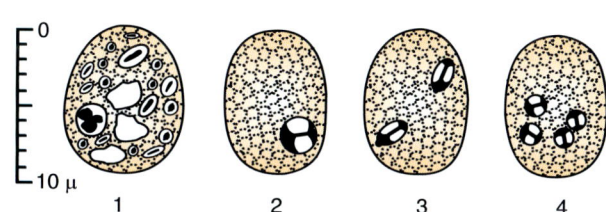

Fig. 28—Morphology of *Endolimax nana*.
1, trophozoite; 2 to 4, cysts with one, two and four nuclei.

Entamoeba hartmanni (von Prowazek, 1912). It is non-pathogenic and closely resembles the "minuta" form of *E. histolytica*. It shows minor morphological differences, having a relatively large nucleus with a large karyosome (may not be central in position) and the peripheral chromatin arranged along a portion of the nuclear membrane either in the form of a single bar or a crescentic granule on one side or discrete granules with wider spaces between them. The glycogen mass in the cyst is smaller and the cytoplasm of the cyst shows small vacuolations. Both trophozoites and cysts are smaller in size. It is neither haematophagus nor histophagus and is restricted to the lumen of the gut. It is difficult to cultivate.

Entamoeba dispar (Brümpt, 1925) According to some workers, *E. dispar* is non-pathogenic species of amoeba and morphologically identical with *E. histolytica*. Cysts of *E. dispar* and *E. histolytica* can not be differentiated under microscope. The trophozoite of *E. dispar* does not contain any ingested red cell.

Endolimax nana (Wenyon and O'Connor, 1917) Brug, 1918. It lives as a harmless commensal in the large intestine of man. It is commonly encountered in diarrhoeic and dysenteric stool. The *trophozoites* are small in size, measuring 8 to 9 µm in diameter and show a sluggish motility. Cytoplasmic inclusions consist of bacteria and other food particles but *never red blood cells*. The nucleus has a large irregular karyosome, lying eccentrically in contact with the nuclear membrane. The *cysts* are oval and are of the same size as the trophozoites. The number of nuclei varies from 1 to 4 but a mature cyst is quadrinucleate. Chromatoid bodies and glycogen vacuole are not seen in any of the stages of cyst formation (Fig. 28).

Iodamoeba bütschlii (Prowazek, 1912) Dobell, 1919. It lives as a harmless commensal in the colon of man. A small (8 to 12 μm) sluggish amoeba, recognised in the *trophozoite* stage by the nuclear character. The size of the nucleus is fairly big (2 to 3.5 μm). The karyosome is a large circular mass, central in position and surrounded by refractile globules. Cytoplasmic inclusions consist of bacteria and other food particles but *never red blood* cells. The trophozoites are rarely seen in the faeces. The *cyst* is a uninucleate body and is either spherical or oval in shape. The cytoplasm contains a large glycogen mass ("iodophilic" body). There are no chromatoid bodies (Fig. 29). The sizes of the cyst and trophozoite are the same.

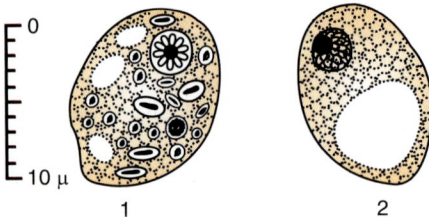

Fig. 29—Morphology of *I. bütschlii.*
1, trophozoite with ingested bacteria and vacuoles;
2, cyst with a large glycogen vacuole and volutin granules.
Note the character of the nucleus.

Blastocystis hominis. As a common inhabitant of human intestine, it was first discovered in 1912. Taxonomy and pathogenicity are still not clear. Now some workers consider it as a protozoon under new suborder of Amoebida. Infection is usually symptomless or may be associated with intestinal symptoms and malabsorption syndrome particularly in patients with AIDS disease.

PATHOGENIC FREE-LIVING AMOEBAE

The free-living amoebae are found in fresh water, mud and moist soil and may infect man. The geographical distributions of pathogenic free-living amoebae are worldwide. They are aerobic unlike other amoebae which are anaerobic. These amoebae are distinct from *E. histolytica*. They belong to the genus Naegleria (with smaller trophozoites and a flagellate phase), genus Acanthamoeba (with large trophozoites and no flagellate stage) and genus Balamuthia (larger trophozoites and no flagellate stage). The species of different genera are as follows:

(a) Genus Naegleria: Species *N. fowleri*

Primary amoebic meningoencephalitis (PAM) is caused by amoebo flagellate *Naegleria. N. fowleri* is thermotolerant and associated with disease, but *N. gruberi* is a free-living non-pathogenic amoeba.

(b) Genus Acanthamoeba: Species *A. castellanii, A. culbertsoni, A. polyphaga, A. rhysodes*

Acanthamoebae are found to cause two diseases: granulomatous amoebic encephalitis (GAE) and chronic amoebic keratitis (CAK).

(c) Genus Balamuthia: Species *B. mandrillaris*

Granulomatous amoebic encephalitis (GAE) is also caused by leptomyxid free-living amoebae, now designated as Balamuthia.

Primary amoebic meningoencephalitis (PAM) and chronic amoebic keratitis (CAK) occur in healthy individuals, whereas granulomatous amoebic encephalitis (GAE) is found in immunodeficient states.

N. fowleri can easily be distinguished from Acanthamoeba by its more rapid movement, temporary free-swimming flagellate stage and rounded cysts. Acanthamoeba has thorn-like process (acanthapoda), moves much more slowly, there is no flagellate stage i.e. free-living form of the parasite and angular double-walled cysts.

Naegleria fowleri

N. fowleri exists in three forms, a trophozoite form or amoeboid form (found on surface of vegetation and mud), a free-swimming flagellate form (rapidly motile bi-flagellate form found in surface layer of the water) and cyst or resting form (found in same location as the trophozoites). There is rapid transformation from one form to the other form. The trophozoites and flagellate forms are infective to man. Only a few organisms are inhaled in contaminated water during swimming and cause infection to man via olfactory epithelium of nose.

Geographical Distribution. Worldwide distribution in warm fresh water and normally feeding on bacteria.

Morphology. The trophozoite form of these free-living amoebae shows brisk progressive movement at 21°C by means of rounded pseudopodia (lobopodia). Their sizes vary from 6 to 15 μm in diameter. They are slug-shaped with one broad and one pointed extremity ("Limex" form). The nucleus is single, large (2 μm) and has a large nucleolus and fine nuclear membrane. There is a perinuclear halo which on close inspection is found to consist of 4 to 6 vacuoles. The trophozoites may be observed in the cerebrospinal fluid and in tissue of the brain.

The flagellate form is a pear-shaped cell with 2 flagella. In water, some trophozoites assume non-replicating flagellate form, which helps in the spread of the parasite to new water bodies. The flagellate form can revert to the trophozoite form for its multiplication. This form is not observed in the cerebrospinal fluid and in brain.

The cysts are uninucleated and possess double cyst wall. Cyst is not found in CSF or in brain.

Life Cycle. *N. fowleri* completes the life cycle in the external environment (Fig. 30A). The life cycle consists of three stages, an amoeboid trophozoite form, a dormant cyst form, and a flagellate form. The soil amoeba gets transformed from trophozoite form to flagellate form in the water. The flagellate form does not multiply. It reverts back to trophozoite form for multiplication. Cyst develops from trophozoite form. Trophozoites multiply by binary fission. They encyst under unfavourable condition, and excyst under favourable condition.

Pathogenicity. Mammalian pathogenicity of these amoebae has been clearly demonstrated. Intranasal inoculation into mice causes meningoencephalitis similar to that of human cases and the animal dies within 5 days.

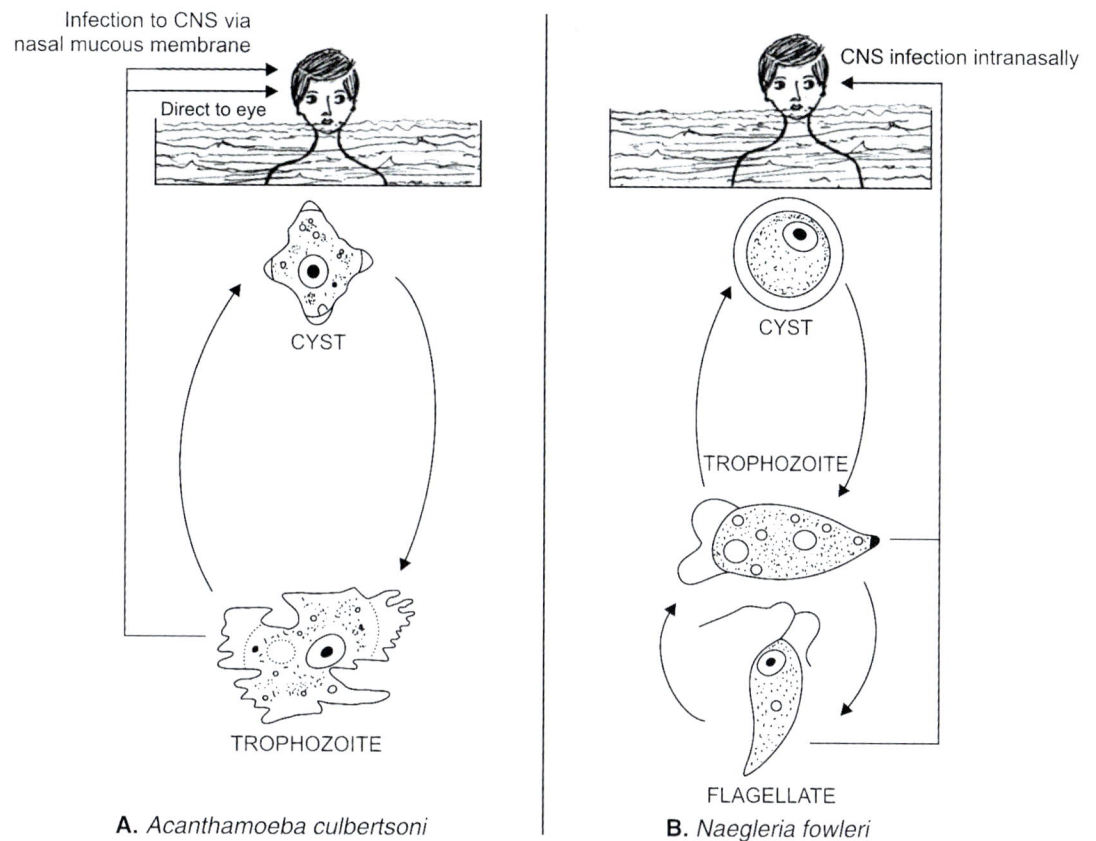

A. *Acanthamoeba culbertsoni*   B. *Naegleria fowleri*

Fig. 30—Life cycle of pathogenic free-living amoebae.

Diagnosis. Examination of wet mount preparation of CSF under microscope demonstrates the motile trophozoites. Staining of CSF smear with Wright or Giemsa stain is also helpful. Fluorescent antibody staining of CSF may demonstrate the amoeba. Proteose peptone glucose medium supports the growth of these free-living amoebae.

Primary Amoebic Meningoencephalitis

This is a new concept in human disease that was first reported by Fowler and Carter in 1965. Cases so far reported were from Australia, Czechoslovakia, USA, Britain and New Zealand. Pan and Ghosh (1971) reported 2 cases from India (Calcutta).

The term 'primary' was used by Butt (1966) to differentiate it from that caused by *E. histolytica*, secondary to lesions elsewhere in the body.

The disease is caused by the free-living amoebae of the genus Naegleria which are found in fresh water, mud, moist soil, polluted warm lake water, streams, ponds, indoor swimming pools. Most of the human infections, though not all, have been caused by *Naegleria fowleri*.

Human infections probably occur either from mesopharyngeal contamination during swimming in water heavily infected with these organisms or other close contact such as from inhalation of particles of decaying animal manure, which supports the growth of these amoebae. The disease shows a preponderance amongst children and young adults and attacks those who enjoy an active life. Incubation period is around 5-7 days. *N. fowleri* does not produce opportunist infection. These amoebae are specifically neurotropic and cerebral invasion takes place through the olfactory nerves; the amoebae have been demonstrated in large numbers in the nerve filaments. The inflammatory exudate was marked in the subarachnoid basal cistern. The cellular component of the exudates comprises of neutrophils and macrophages in equal proportions together with a varying number of amoebae. Sugar and protein levels of cerebrospinal fluid are higher than that found in bacterial pyogenic meningitis. The disease is characterised by acute onset of upper respiratory tract infection followed by symptoms and signs of meningitis.

Fresh unstained preparations are essential to detect motile trophozoites. CSF smear can be stained with Wright or Giemsa stains. Fluorescent antibody staining of CSF can be done. Amoebae may be cultured in non-nutrient agar seeded with *E. coli*. The disease should be considered in the differential diagnosis of every case of acute meningitis, which will then help to establish the diagnosis of *N. fowleri*. The disease follows a rapid and fatal course, if left untreated. The average duration of the illness from the onset of symptoms is 4½ days. The interval between exposures to infection (bathing in an infected pool) and the onset of symptoms is not more than 7 days (Cema *et al.* 1968).

The choice of drug for Naegleria infection at the present moment is large dose of antifungal antibiotic amphotericin-B (1 mg/kg/day I.V. for several days) or ketoconazole (800 mg daily orally for one month).

Acanthamoeba

Several species of *Acanthamoeba* (*A. castellanii, A. culbertsoni, A. polyphaga, A. rhysode*) are pathogenic to man. The important species is *A. culbertsoni*. In immunocompromised people *A. culbertsoni* causes granulomatous amoebic meningoencephalitis (GAE) which terminates to death after weeks or months. *A. polyphaga* can cause corneal ulcer in normal people.

Geographical Distribution. The geographical distribution of *Acanthamoeba* is worldwide. They can multiply on brackish condition. The method of transmission is unknown and not due to contact with warm fresh water.

Morphology. There are two morphological forms: (a) trophozoite, and (b) cyst. Both trophozoite and cyst forms can be the source of infection to man. There is no flagellate stage in parasite.

A trophozoite is 20-50 μm in size (larger than those of naegleria) and it has a rough exterior with several spine-like projections (acanthopoda) which moves slowly. The trophozoite has a single nucleus with large central, dense nucleolus surrounded by halo. Cyst has a winkled outer surface with smooth inner wall with several spores. Cysts are spherical and 15 μm in diameter.

Life Cycle. The cycle is comprised of two stages: trophozoite and cyst stages (Fig. 30B). Man acquires infection by inhalation of dust containing trophozoites, cysts or by direct invasion of traumatised skin or eye. The trophozoites invade the central nervous system through the blood stream producing granulomatous amoebic encephalitis (GAE). The infection of brain is not associated with swimming.

Pathogenicity and Clinical Features. Granulomatous amoebic encephalitis (GAE) occurs in debilitated or chronically ill persons having immunosuppressive therapy or immunocompromised patients such as AIDS patients. Incubation period is more than 7 days. The disease is characterised by focal granulomatous lesion of the brain. The onset of the disease (GAE) is insidious with a prolonged clinical course.

In GAE, cell count in CSF is predominantly lymphocytes and glucose content will not be appreciably lowered. In brain tissues, trophozoites or cysts of acanthamoeba may be found.

Acanthamoeba causes chronic acanthamoeba keratitis which is now a serious problem contact lens user (specially soft ones). It is due to direct inoculation of amoebic trophozoites or cysts into cornea during insertion of contaminated lens.

Diagnosis. Examination of wet mount preparation of CSF or corneal scraping under microscope may show motile trophozoites of *Acanthamoeba*. Trophozoites and cysts forms can be the source of infection to man. The method of transmission is unknown and not due to contact with fresh water. Culture on agar plates seeded with *E. coli* is also helpful. Indirect fluorescent antibody technique (IFAT) may also be used for the diagnosis of disease. Histopathological examination of brain tissue or corneal tissue may demonstrate trophozoites and cysts.

Treatment. There is no effective treatment for granulomatous amoebic encaphalitis caused by Acanthamoeba but ocular lesions caused by acanthamoeba can be treated with enucleation of ulcer and corneal transplant.

Balamuthia

Balamuthia mandillaris (leptomyxid free-living amoeba) produces granulomatous amoebic encephalitis (GAE) in AIDS patients.

Geographical Distribution. Worldwide. Several cases of GAE caused by *B. mandillaris* have been reported from different parts of the world.

Morphology. It has trophozoite and cyst forms. The trophozoites of balamuthia show two forms of pseudopodia either broad lobose or fingerlike. There is no flagellated form of parasite. The trophozoite is 12-60 μm in length and sluggishly motile. The cyst is spherical and 6-30 μm in diameter.

Life Cycle and Mode of Infection. It is similar to that of Acanthamoeba.

Pathogenicity. It causes CNS infection (GAE) in the similar way as produced by Acanthamoeba.

Diagnosis. It can be made by microscopical examination of smear and culture of CSF. The trophozoites can be identified in the CSF whereas both trophozoites and cysts are found in brain tissues. Immunofluorescence may be helpful in the detection of parasite. The trophozoites with pseudopodia can be grown in the tissue culture.

Treatment. Nothing is known about its treatment.

Phylum SARCOMASTIGOPHORA

Subphylum MASTIGOPHORA: Class ZOOMASTIGOPHOREA

The parasites belonging to this group of protozoa possess one or more flagella giving them the power of motility. These are classified, according to their habitat, into two groups:

1. INTESTINAL, ORAL AND GENITAL FLAGELLATES—Infecting the intestinal canal, oral cavity and the genital tract. They are mostly non-pathogenic.

2. BLOOD AND TISSUE FLAGELLATES—Infecting the vascular system and various tissues of the body. Include two genera which are pathogenic to man: (a) *Trypanosoma* and (b) *Leishmania*.

Intestinal, Oral and Genital Flagellates

Order	Genus
Retortamonadida	Chilomastix, Retortamonas
Diplomonadida	Giardia, Enteromonas
Trichomonadida	Trichomonas, Pentatrichomonas, Dientamoeba

Flagellates inhabiting the intestine form the major group. One species (*Trichomonas tenax*) is found in the oral cavity and the other species (*Trichomonas vaginalis*) in the female genital tract. Although none of these flagellates has yet been proved to have any pathogenic role, the clinicians are inclined to implicate *Giardia intestinalis* as a cause of certain diarrhoeic disorder and *Trichomonas vaginalis* as a cause of inflammation of the vaginal mucosa. *T. hominis* possesses five free anterior flagella and is accordingly placed under genus Pentatrichomonas.

Classification. These flagellates contain the following genera:

1. Genus Giardia: *G. intestinalis* (Duodenum).
2. Genus Chilomastix: *G. mesnili* (Caecum).
3. Genus Enteromonas: *E. hominis* (Large intestine—rare species).
4. Genus Retortamonas (Embadomonas): *E. intestinalis* (Large intestine—rare species).
5. Genus Pentatrichomonas: *Pentatrichomonas hominis* (Ileocaecal region).
6. Genus Trichomonas: *T. tenax* (Teeth and gums)
                       T. vaginalis (Vagina).
7. Genus Dientamoeba: *D. fragilis* (Colonic mucosal crypts).

Generic Character. All these flagellates except the Trichomonads, have a trophozoite and a cystic phase. The trophozoites possess multiple flagella which arise from blepharoplasts. An undulating membrane supported at the base by a basal fibre (costa) may or may not be present. The nuclear characters are distinctive in every species. An axostyle (a central supporting rod) and a cytostome representing a rudimentary mouth, are also observed in some species. Reproduction occurs by binary fission of the blepharoplast and the nucleus, followed by longitudinal splitting of the body into two. Encystment is a protective process except for Enteromonas and Giardia. Mature cysts liberated in the faeces are the infective stages of the parasite. The cysts when swallowed with contaminated food, liberate the trophozoites in the small or the large intestine. These flagellates complete their life cycle in a single host, a second host being required only for the continuation of the species. Excepting Giardia these parasites can readily be cultivated in the same medium as used for *E. histolytica*.

Genus Giardia

Giardia lamblia (Lambl, 1859) Alexeieff, 1914

SYNONYM: *Giardia intestinalis, Lamblia intestinalis.*

First seen by Leeuwenhoek (1681) while examining his own stool.

Geographical Distribution. World-wide.

Habitat. Duodenum and the upper part of jejunum of man.

Morphology. Exists in two phases—trophozoite and cyst (Fig. 31).

TROPHOZOITE. When viewed flat, the shape of the trophozoite is like that of a tennis or badminton racket and when viewed side-on it resembles a longitudinally split pear. The dorsal surface is convex and the ventral surface is concave with a sucking disc. The size of the trophozoite is 14 μm long by 7 μm broad. The anterior end is broad and rounded and the posterior end tapers to a sharp point. It is bilaterally symmetrical and all the organs of the body are paired. Thus there are two axostyles, two nuclei and four pairs of flagella.

CYST. The fully formed *cyst* is oval in shape and measures 12 μm long by 7 μm broad. The axostyles lie more or less diagonally, forming a sort of dividing line within the cyst-wall. There are four nuclei which may remain clustered at one end or lie in pairs at opposite poles. The remains of the flagella and the margins of the sucking disc may be seen inside the cytoplasm. An acid environment often causes the parasite to encyst.

Cultivation. Karapetyan (1962) has described a method for the cultivation of *Giardia* together with an yeast, *Candida guillermondi;* it grew well on a medium of chick embryo extract, human serum, Hottinger's digest (tryptic meat digest) and Hank's solution.

Immunology. The disease giardiasis is common in younger age group but uncommon in adult, suggesting that an efficient immunity has developed. Both humoral and cellular mechanisms are important for parasite clearance. The disease usually affects IgA deficient person and anti-IgA

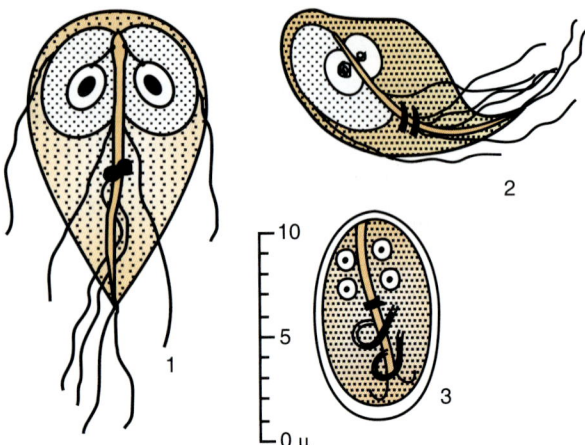

Fig. 31—Trophozoite and cyst of *Giardia intestinalis.*
Surface view (1) and side view or semi-profile view (2) of a trophozoite; (3) cyst.

antibody can be detected on surface of giardia trophozoites, obtained from jejunal fluid and jejunal biopsies. Raised titre of anti-Giardia IgG can be detected in patient with giardiasis for a long time after primary infection. The presence of anti-Giardia sIgA in human breast milk protects breast-fed infants from giardiasis disease.

Life Cycle. In the trophozoite stage, the parasite multiplies in the intestine of man by binary fission. When conditions in the duodenum are unfavourable, encystment occurs, usually in the large intestine. During encystment, a thick resistant wall is secreted by the parasite and the cell then divides into two within the cyst. Infection of man is brought about by ingestion of cysts. Within 30 minutes of ingestion, the cyst hatches out two trophozoites which then multiply in enormous numbers and colonise in the duodenum. To avoid the high acidity of duodenum Giardia often localises in the biliary tract (gall bladder).

Pathogenicity. With the help of the sucking disc the parasite attaches itself on to the convex surfaces of the epithelial cells in the intestine and may cause a disturbance of intestinal function, leading to malabsorption of fat. Consequently, the patient may complain of persistent looseness of bowels, and mild steatorrhoea (passage of yellowish and greasy stools in which there is excess of fat). The parasite is also capable of producing harm by its toxic effect (allergy), traumatic and irritative effect as well as by spoliative action, i.e., by diverting the nutriments. *Clinically* the cases may be divided as follows:

(1) Silent cases without any symptom. (2) Intestinal: Chronic enteritis, acute enterocolitis and malabsorption syndrome. (3) General: Fever, anaemia and allergic manifestations. (4) Chronic cholecystopathy.

The person having hypo- or agammaglobulinaemia and malnourished persons are more susceptible to giardiasis.

Histological studies of mucosal biopsies from the duodenum and proximal jejunum in patients with Giardia infection carried out by Brandborg *et al** (1967) revealed tissue invasion. Trophozoites of *Giardia intestinalis* were found in the mucosal tissues from the epithelium to the submucosa. They caused very little mucosal damage and did not excite any inflammatory reaction.

Laboratory Diagnosis. This includes the following:

(a) A microscopical examination of a freshly passed stool for the demonstration of giardia trophozoites and cysts; the former are found in a diarrhoeic stool or after a purgative. Fluorescent method using monoclonal antibodies and ELISA test, for the detection of giardia antigen in faeces are not in routine use. Sensitivity and specificity of faecal antigen ELISA test are reported to be high.

(b) Giardia trophozoites may be recovered both from aspirates of douodenum and jejunum by *Enterotest*.

(c) Antigiardia antibody detection in serum is not useful in diagnosis of disease.

(d) DNA-based techniques (specific DNA probes for giardia) are available now.

Treatment. Schneider (1961) reported good results with a derivative of imidazole (metronidazole). Metronidazole (250 mg three times daily for 5 days), trimidazole (2 gms once), furazolidone (100 mg 4 times daily for 7–10 days) have been found to be effective for giardiasis.

---

* *Gastroenterology,* 52, p. 143.

Genus CHILOMASTIX MESNILI (Wenyon, 1910) Alexeieff, 1912

A common flagellate living as a harmless commensal in the caecum of man. *Trophozoites* are pear-shaped bodies, measuring 10 to 15 μm in length by 5 to 6 μm in breadth. The round oval nucleus is situated anteriorly and by its side lies the large conspicuous mouth (cytostome). The posterior extremity is drawn out to a fine point. There are three long anterior free flagella and the fourth one is short and lies within the cytostome. There are no undulating membrane and axostyle. The *cysts* are lemon-shaped with a small projection at the anterior end, measuring 7 to 10 μm along its longitudinal axis. The single nucleus lies near the centre. Remnants of the buccal apparatus is also visible (Fig. 32).

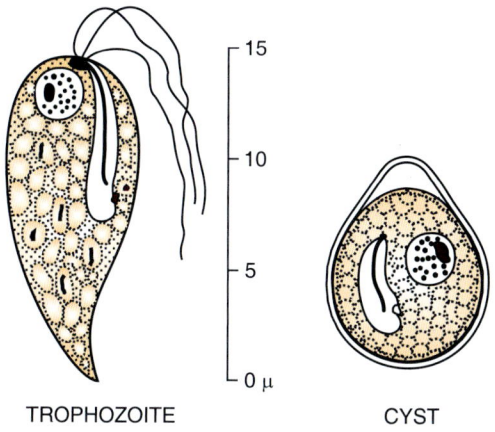

TROPHOZOITE   CYST

Fig. 32—Trophozoite and cyst of *C. mesnili.*

Genus TRICHOMONAS

These are common flagellates of the tropics and are frequently observed in diarrhoeic stools. They exist only in the trophozoite phase and there is *no cystic phase*. The flagellates are pear-shaped bodies and measure 10 to 12 μm in length. The single ovoid nucleus is situated at the round anterior end and a cleft-like depression (cytostome) lies at its side. There are 3 to 5 anterior flagella which are free. A thicker flagellum passes backwards along the side of the body forming the undulating membrane and coming out free at the posterior pointed end. The undulating membrane is supported at the base by a rod-like structure, the costa. The axostyle runs down the middle of the body and ends in the pointed tail-like extremity.

An attempt has been made to classify the genus Trichomonas into the following species according to their habitats (Fig. 33):

1. *Pentatrichomonas hominis* (8 μm)—Inhabiting the ileo-caecal region.
2. *Trichomonas tenax*—Inhabiting the oral cavity, being found around the tartar of the teeth and in pyorrhoeic sockets.

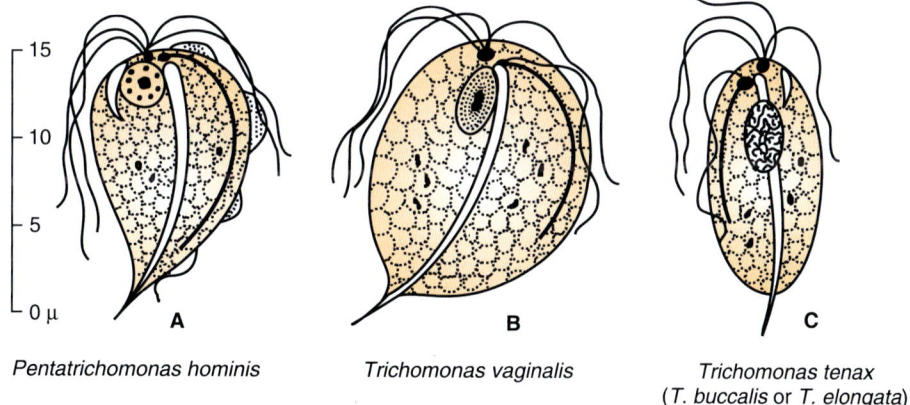

Pentatrichomonas hominis   *Trichomonas vaginalis*   *Trichomonas tenax*
                                                                    (*T. buccalis* or *T. elongata*)

Fig. 33—Intestinal, vaginal and oral Trichomonads. (Exist only in the trophic phase.)

3. *Trichomonas vaginalis* (13 μm)—Geographical distrubution is worldwide. Inhabiting the female genital tract; also found in the urinary tract of both males and females. In this species the cytostome is less conspicuous.

Although certain morphological differences (the length of the parasite, nuclear character and the course of the lateral flagellum) have been pointed out, they are not of sufficient help in the distinguishing of the species. These flagellates are of no pathogenic importance except *T. vaginalis* which is found in large numbers in the leucorrhoeic discharge of females and is regarded by the gynaecologists as the cause of inflammation of the vaginal mucosa. In case of man, *T. vaginalis* infection is a sexually transmitted disease causing urethritis. Infection has also been recorded in newborn female and female children.

Motile tropozoites with jerky movements may be found in microscopical examination of vaginal, urethral discharge and prostatic secretion. Giemsa stain, Papanicolaou stain and culture of specimens on CPLM media are often helpful in the diagnosis of disease. Serological tests like IHA and gel diffusion test are not used routinely.

Molecular methods are other available new tests. Treatment with metronidazole of both sextual partners is often effective and prevents recurrence.

Genus ENTEROMONAS

Enteromonas hominis (da Fonseca, 1915). A rare species, living as a harmless commensal in the small or large intestine of man. *Trophozoites* are small pear-shaped bodies and measure 8 μm long by 4 μm broad. They possess four flagella, three directed anteriorly and lying free, the fourth posteriorly, remaining adherent to the margin of the body and ending in a free terminal lash. The nucleus is situated at the anterior rounded end. The *cysts* are of the same size as the trophozoites and contain 1 to 4 nuclei which may be arranged at opposite poles (Fig. 34).

Genus RETORTAMONAS

Retortamonas (Embadomonas) intestinalis (Wenyon and O'Connor, 1917). It is also known as *Embadomonas intestinalis*. A rare harmless commensal of the intestine (small or large) of man. *Trophozoites* are small oval bodies measuring 5 μm long by 3 μm broad. The nucleus is at the anterior end and by its side lies the cytostome. Flagella are two in number, one directed anteriorly and the other posteriorly passing through the cytostome before becoming free. The *cysts* are small pear-shaped bodies, measuring 4 to 5 μm in length and containing a single nucleus (Fig. 35).

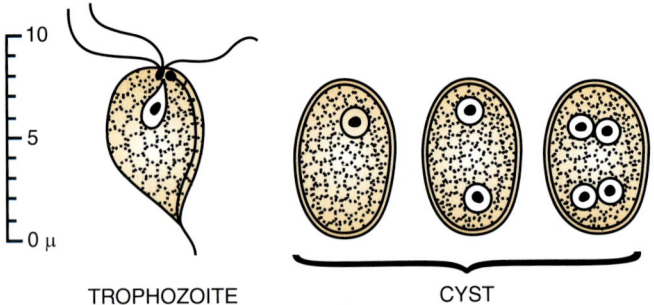

TROPHOZOITE   CYST

Fig. 34—Trophozoite and cyst of *Enteromonas hominis.*

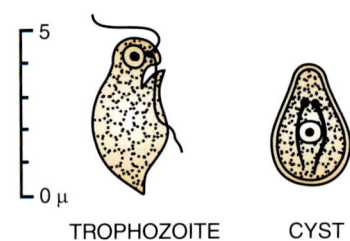

TROPHOZOITE   CYST

Fig. 35—Trophozoite and cyst of
Embadomonas intestinalis.

Genus DIENTAMOEBA

Dientamoeba fragilis (Jeps and Dobell, 1918). This is the smallest (5 to 8 μm) and the rarest of the intestinal amoebae of man. Its name describes its morphology very well, for it is binucleate and its cytoplasm is very fragile. The cytoplasm contains many food vacuoles and bacteria but *never red blood* cells. The nuclear character shows the large chromatin granules, usually 6 in number, forming a star-shaped cluster (Fig. 36). There is no *cystic phase. D. fragilis* was previously believed to be non-pathogenic but now has been associated with intermittent diarrhoea, flatulence, abdominal pain, etc. Life cycle is not fully understood. Based on electronic microscopic feature, *D. fragilis* is reclassified as an aberrant trichomona flagellate (amoeba flagellate).

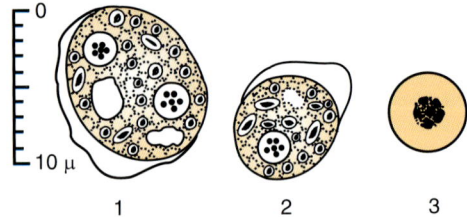

Fig. 36—Morphology of *D. fragilis.*
(Exists only in the trophic phase.)
1, binucleate form; 2, uninucleate form; 3, nuclear character.

Blood and Tissue Flagellates

ORDER KINETOPLASTIDA SUBORDER TRYPANOSOMATINA

These flagellates live in the blood or tissues of man or other animals. They pass through a cycle in the gut of insects which serve as intermediary hosts (vectors). The family includes two genera which are of pathogenic importance to man: *Trypanosoma* and *Leishmania*. These parasites are comparatively complex in structure, having well-developed organelles for locomotion and a nuclear apparatus adapted for special functions. The structural pattern shows the following peculiarities:

1. BODY—The shape varies in the flagellated and non-flagellated stages; in the former the body is elongated, narrow and often curved, while in the latter it is round or ovoid.

2. NUCLEUS—A large rounded or oval structure, usually situated in the centre of the body. As it is concerned with the nutritive functions of the parasite, it is often called trophonucleus.

3. KINETOPLAST—It is a smaller body compared to the nucleus, generally round or rod-shaped and is situated either in front of or behind the nucleus. Hoare pointed out that the kinetoplast is necessary for the development in insect hosts but not for multiplication in the vertebrate hosts.

4. FLAGELLUM—A thin hair-like structure arising from a small granule (basal body) near the kinetoplast and coming out at the anterior end of the body as a free flagellum. The flagellum may be absent in certain types.

5. UNDULATING MEMBRANE—It is a flange or ribbon of protoplasm, formed by the flagellum which while curving around the body, is thrown into a number of folds, the number varying according to the length of the cytoplasmic body.

Developmental Stages of Trypanosomatid Flagellates

In the past, the names of these developmental stages were derived from those genera in which the corresponding stages are the most characteristic forms. Hoare and Wallace* (1966) pointed out that the names, based on genera, are not appropriate, because taxa, being subject to International Code of Zoological Nomenclature, are liable to be changed. They proposed new names which are not in any way connected with the taxa, such as genera, hence a change in the zoological name will not necessarily lead to alteration in descriptive terms. They have utilised the "flagellar characteristics" to serve as a basis for these names. The arrangement of the flagellum in the body, as determined by its starting point (indicated by the position of the kinetoplast), its course and points of emergence, has been considered in describing the various stages. For the terminology, they have used the root "mastigote" (from Greek *mastix*, whip) combined with the appropriate prefixes. The new terms devised (Fig. 37) are as follows:

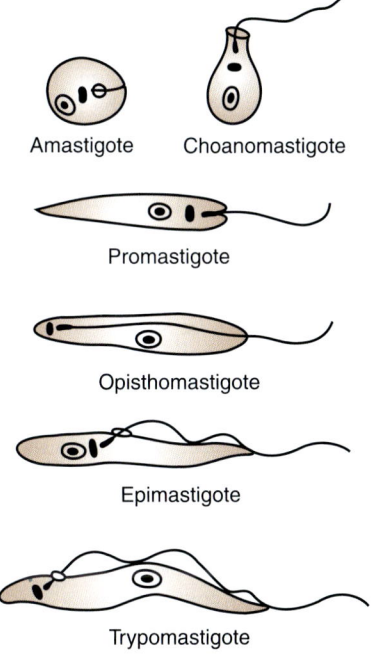

Amastigote   Choanomastigote

Promastigote

Opisthomastigote

Epimastigote

Trypomastigote

Fig. 37—Developmental stages of trypanosomatid flagellates.
(After Hoare and Wallace.)

1. *Amastigote* (for former "leishmanial" stage). Represented by rounded forms without any external flagellum, as in the genus *Leishmania* and others.

2. *Promastigote* (for former "leptomonad" stage). Represented by forms with the kinetoplast lying anterior to the nucleus (antenuclear kinetoplast); the flagellum arising near it emerges from the anterior end of the body, as in the genus *Leptomonas* and others.

3. *Opisthomastigote* (for former "trypanosome" or "trypanomorphic" stage). Represented by forms with the kinetoplast lying posterior to the nucleus (postnuclear kinetoplast); the flagellum arises near it, then passes through the body and emerges from the anterior end (there is no undulating membrane), as in the genus *Herpetomonas* only. This stage is absent in flagellates which infect human being.

4. *Epimastigote* (for former "crithidial" stage). Represented by forms with the kinetoplast lying anterior and close to the nucleus (juxtanuclear kinetoplast); the flagellum arising near it emerges from the side of the body to run along a short undulating membrane, as in the new genus *Blastocrithidia* and in the stages of the genus *Trypanosoma*.

5. *Trypomastigote* for the true "trypanosome" stage; the term is not derived from genus Trypanosoma (Gr. *Trypanon*, to bore; *soma*, body). Represented by forms with postnuclear kinetoplast situated at the posterior end of the body; the flagellum arises near it and emerges from the side of the body to run along a long undulating membrane, as in the genus *Trypanosoma*.

6. *Choanomastigote*, a new term for the peculiar "barley-corn" form, usually with the kinetoplast lying at the anterior end of the body (antenuclear kinetoplast); the flagellum arises near it and emerges at the anterior end of the body through a wide funnel-shaped reservoir, typical of the insect genus *Crithidia*.

Genus TRYPANOSOMA Gruby, 1843

Generic Character. These exist as trypomastigotes in vertebrate hosts (man and animals), some (*T. cruzi*) assuming amastigote forms. They pass their life cycle in two hosts: vertebrate and insect. While developing inside the insect

*Hoare, Cecil A. and Wallace, Franklin G. (1966). Developmental stages of Trypanosomatid flagellates; a new terminology. *Nature,* 212, 1385-86, Dec. 17.

host, they pass through the stages of amastigote, promastigote, epimastigote and metacyclic form of trypomastigote. Multiplication can take place in any of these developmental stages. Transmission is effected from one vertebrate to another by blood-sucking insects. After an infective feed, a certain time must elapse before the insect can infect another individual; any bite before the expiry of this period is non-infective. Infectiveness of an insect depends on the final development of metacyclic form of trypomastigotes.

There are two main types of development:

1. *Anterior Station* (Salivaria)—Ingested trypomastigotes first develop in the mid-gut and then proceed forward to the proventriculus, labial cavity and salivary glands, as in *T. brucei* subgroup. Transmission in these cases is effected by the bite of the insect.

2. *Posterior Station* (Stercoraria)—Ingested trypomastigotes develop in the intestine from where they pass backwards to the hind-gut, as in *T. cruzi* and *T. lewisi*. Transmission occurs by ingestion of faeces of the insect, as in *T. lewisi* or by rubbing the faecal matter into the wound caused by the bite of the insect, as in *T. cruzi*.

Morphology of Trypomastigotes. Accompanying diagram (Fig. 38) shows the general morphological structure of the trypomastigote form of a trypanosome.

Polymorphism of Trypomastigotes. These are forms which differ in the shape and size of the body, presence or absence of a free flagellum and the position of the nucleus. The trypomastigotes of *T. brucei* sub-group are polymorphic.

Method of Reproduction. Reproduction occurs by binary longitudinal fission. It begins with the division of the kinetoplast and the basal body, followed later by

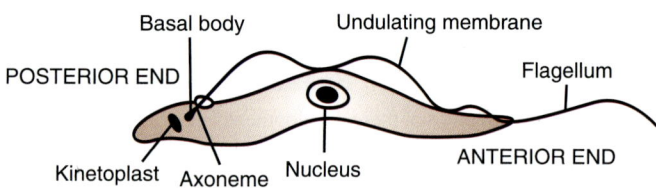

Fig. 38—**Morphology of a trypomastigote form.**

the division of the nucleus. The flagellum with the undulating membrane remains with one of the halves of the basal body, while a new one develops from the other. The cytoplasmic body then splits longitudinally from the anterior end.

Classification. Trypanosomes of Man. The trypanosomes which infect man are the following:

1. *T. brucei* subgroup (human strain)—Causes African trypanosomiasis. *T. brucei gambiense* causes Gambian form of sleeping sickness in West and Central Africa and *T. brucei rhodesiense* causes Rhodesian form of sleeping sickness in East Africa.

2. *T. cruzi*—Causes South American trypanosomiasis (Chagas' disease).

3. *T. rangeli*—A non-pathogenic trypanosome found in the blood of man in Venezuela and also in Colombia.

Trypanosomes of Animals. Besides man, trypanosomes are found in various animals, a few of them are enumerated below:

NON-PATHOGENIC. *T. lewisi* in rat; transmitted by rat fleas.

PATHOGENIC. *T. brucei* (animal strain) found in wild game and domestic animals of tropical Africa; transmitted by *G. morsitans*. Causes "nagana" in some of the domestic animals.

T. evansi, causes "surra" in horses and mules of India; mechanical transmission by blood-sucking fly, tabanid.

T. equiperdum, causes "stallion's disease" (a venereal disease) in horses and asses of Europe, America, North Africa and India; transmitted by coitus.

T. equinum, causes "mal de caderas" amongst horses in South America; transmitted mechanically by tabanid; it has no kinetoplast and no insect cycle.

T. vivax and *T. congolense* cause disease in cattle; transmitted by tsetse flies.

Trypanosoma lewisi Kent, 1880. A natural blood parasite of the common brown and black rats in all parts of the world; hence can be easily obtained for demonstration and study. *Morphology*: It is a long slender parasite, measuring about 25 μm in length. The cytoplasm is free from granules. The nucleus is oval in shape and is placed anteriorly at the junction of the anterior and the middle third of the body. The kinetoplast is rod-shaped, has a transverse position lying at some distance from the posterior extremity. Both ends are sharply pointed and the undulating membrane is not much folded. The species is monomorphic; all the individuals possess a free flagellum. It is non-pathogenic to the rat.

The *life cycle* is passed in two hosts: rat and rat flea. In rat's blood, they live as trypomastigotes and multiply by binary longitudinal fission for a period of 10 days, after which most of the trypomastigotes die. The rat flea becomes infected by sucking rat's blood containing the trypomastigote forms. These penetrate into the cells lining the mid-gut and multiply. The host-cell finally ruptures and the escaping trypomastigotes invade other cells and the process is repeated. Later they migrate into the hind-gut where they change first into epimastigotes and then to metacyclic trypomastigotes, the infective stage of the parasite. These are passed in the flea's excreta and a non-immune rat licking it, becomes infected. The cycle of development in the flea lasts for 5 to 7 days.

Shrivastava *et al* (1974) reported from India (Raipur, Madhya Pradesh) Trypanosoma resembling *T. lewisi* in the peripheral blood of two cases, husband and wife, suffering from short febrile illness (*Trans. Roy. Soc. Trop. Med. & Hyg.*, 68, p. 143).

Trypanosoma rangeli Téjera, 1920. It has been found in the peripheral blood of man in Venezuela. It is a large trypanosome measuring 26 to 34 μm in length and possessing a minute densely staining kinetoplast and is morphologically different from *T. cruzi*. The insect hosts are Panstrongylus dimidiata and *P. geniculatus*. The metacyclic trypomastigotes have been observed in the bug's proboscis and the infection is probably transmitted to the vertebrate hosts (man and dog) by the bite of the insect. The morphology and life cycle of a trypanosome (*T. ariarii*) recovered from the blood of man, in the Ariari Valley, Colombia, resemble those of *T. rangeli*. Both Venezuelan and Colombian forms are non-pathogenic for man.

Note: A rare case of human trypanosomiasis caused by *T. evansi* has been reported in India (Chandrapur district of Maharashtra). [R.M. Power et. al. (2006) Indian Journal of Medical Microbiology (2006) 24(1): 72-4].

Trypanosoma brucei (Plimmer and Bradford, 1899)

The parasite causing African trypanosomiasis in man and nagana in domestic animals.

The parasite was discovered by David Bruce in 1890 and he suggested it to be the cause of "nagana" in cattle in Zululand. It is now known that *T. brucei* in cattle produces a mild or inapparent infection. Hence the correctness of Bruce's observation has been questioned. After a careful study of Bruce's illustration Hoare (1970) is convinced that the strain referred to by Bruce had an admixture of *T. congolense* which was responsible for the disease in the cattle in Zululand.

The trypanosome causing disease in man was first discovered in Gambia by Forde and Dutton in 1902 and in Rhodesia by Stephens and Fantham in 1909.

T. brucei subgroup*

Basing on clinico-epidemiological pattern the African trypanosomiasis (African sleeping sickness) used to be classified as "Gambian" and "Rhodesian" sleeping sickness caused by a sharply characterised species of trypanosomes named as *T. gambiense* and *T. rhodesiense* respectively. Zoologists are of the opinion that there is little justification in giving a species status to each type of the disease.

It is realised that *T. brucei* subgroup comprises a single species containing strains or subspecies of varying host-specificity and virulence. It includes the following:

1. The *animal strain* (previously restricted to the "type species" *T. brucei*). This is widespread throughout the tsetse belt of Africa. This strain does not infect man. It is to be noted that a balanced state of affairs appears to exist between the African trypanosomes and their wild game animals and the adapted organisms do little harm to their hosts.

2. The *human strain* (formerly called *T. gambiense* and *T. rhodesiense*). This is not so widespread. On clinico-epidemiological pattern the following forms are recognised:

(a) "Rhodesian" sleeping sickness, a relatively acute disease.

(b) "Gambian" sleeping sickness, a chronic disease.

(c) "Zambezi" sleeping sickness, although chronic, is more like the acute "rhodesian" form.

Attempts to classify the African sleeping sickness (African trypanosomiasis) strictly in above terms is to be avoided because these African trypanosomes of man are "adapting themselves to their hosts and as such, variations in clinical and epidemiological behaviour are to be expected".

Hoare (1970) suggested that the brucei-rhodesiense-gambiense complex should be regarded as a subspecies of *T. brucei* and may be designated as follows: *T. brucei brucei, T. brucei gambiense; T. rhodesiense* as a virulent nosodeme of *T. gambiense*.

Morphologically, these strains are indistinguishable and can only be differentiated by their behaviour in man (testing infectivity directly in a human volunteer). Rickman and Robson (1970) have introduced a simple sensitivity test (blood incubation infectivity test) by which it is possible to identify whether a strain, isolated from a tsetse fly or a domestic or a game animal, is an animal strain ("*T. brucei*") or a human infectivity strain ("*T. rhodesiense*").

*Blood incubation infectivity test**. The strain of *T. brucei* to be tested is at first inoculated into rats or mice and when the parasitaemia is established a few ml of cardiac blood is withdrawn. About 0.25 ml of this blood is taken in each of the 2 Bijou bottles. To one bottle 2 ml of human blood and an anticoagulant (0.25 mg of 2% pot. oxalate with glucose added to a strength of 3 mg/ml of blood) is taken. This constitutes the *test sample*.

---

* W. E. Ormerod (1967). *Cecil-Loeb Textbook of Medicine*, 12th Ed., W. B. Saunders Co., p. 363.

   L. G. Goodwin (1970). *Trans. Roy. Soc. Trop. Med. & Hyg.*, **64**, p. 797.

** Rickman, L. R. and Robson, J. (1970). The blood incubation infectivity test—A simple test which may serve to distinguish *T. brucei* from *T. rhodesiense*. *Bull. Wld. Hlth. Org.*, **42**, p. 650.

To the other bottle, the human blood is replaced by 2 ml of phosphate-buffered saline (pH 7.4). This represents the *control sample*.

Both the samples after gentle mixing are incubated in a water bath for 5 hours at 37°C. Each of the mixtures is then tested separately by inoculating into a rat. If a later development of persistent parasitaemia occurs in both the rats, the result is said to be positive, i.e., the strain is human infective form and the infectivity to rats having remained unimpaired. If the parasitaemia occurs only in the rat inoculated with the control sample the test is said to be negative, i.e., the strain is of animal origin and inoculation with the human blood having rendered it non-infective to the rat.

Habitat. *T. brucei* is essentially a parasite of connective tissues, where it multiplies readily. It consumes an enormous amount of glucose.

It invades the regional lymph nodes through the lymphatics and also invades the blood stream causing parasitaemia. It finally localises in the brain. It is to be noted that African sleeping sickness is a disease of the central nervous system.

Prevalence of *T. brucei*. As already stated the animal strains of *T. brucei* occur throughout the tsetse belt of Africa but the human strains are not so widespread.

The chronic "gambiense" strain is found mainly in West Africa (from Gambia to the Congo), Central Africa and scattered areas of East Africa, particularly Uganda.

The acute "rhodesiense" strain is distributed only in East Africa, particularly in Tanganyika, Uganda, Zambia, Rhodesia and Malawi.

The chronic "zambezi" strain (pathology similar to "gambiense") is found in Botswana, Rhodesia, Zambia and Portuguese East Africa. The acute "zambezi" strain (resembling "rhodesiense") is found in Tanzania, Uganda and Kenya.

Morphology. *T. brucei* exists in the vertebrate hosts as a trypomastigote form. It is an elongated rather flattened spindle-shaped organism with a blunted posterior end and a finely pointed anterior end. The nucleus is large, oval and central in position. The kinetoplast is small and is situated at the posterior end. The flagellum starts from the posterior extremity near the kinetoplast, curves around the body in the form of an undulating membrane and then continues beyond the anterior end as a free flagellum. The undulating membrane is thrown into folds, the number of which (usually 3 to 4) varies with the length of the parasite. It is an actively motile flagellate.

Polymorphism. The trypomastigotes of *T. brucei* are polymorphic. Individual parasites vary in size and shape in the different stages of their existence. Two main forms are recognised—the one, short, thick, stumpy form (10 µm long by 5 µm. broad) with no free flagellum or having only a very small one; the other, long, slender form (20 µm long by 3 µm broad), having a conspicuously long free flagellum. Between these two forms, intermediate forms are occasionally observed. The first form to appear is a long, slender one and later when the infection is established the short, stumpy form together with the intermediate one appear (Fig. 39).

Antigenic variant. A succession of variants occur in *T. brucei* infection both in animals (rabbits) and man. Each new variant emerges at 3-4 days' intervals, possi-

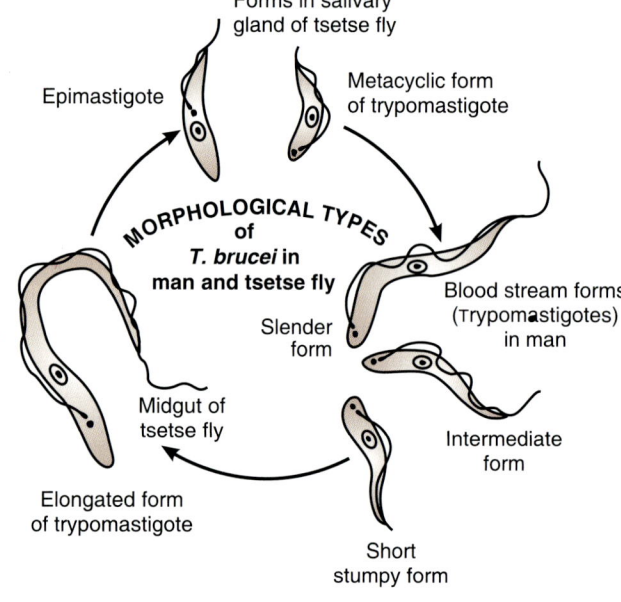

Forms in salivary gland of tsetse fly

Epimastigote

Metacyclic form of trypomastigote

MORPHOLOGICAL TYPES of *T. brucei* in man and tsetse fly

Slender form

Blood stream forms (Trypomastigotes) in man

Midgut of tsetse fly

Intermediate form

Elongated form of trypomastigote

Short stumpy form

[Drawn after Vickerman]

Fig. 39

Trans. Roy. Soc. Trop. Med. and Hyg., **56**, 1962.

bly by selection of mutants. This appears to depend upon the ability of the host's defence mechanism and when the defences fail the final variant multiplies unchecked. Each wave of parasitaemia is accompanied by fever and followed by leucocytosis (monocytosis but not neutrophilia). It may be that the outer proteinaceous coat may protect the organism in escaping from the host's defence mechanism.

Another feature is that the antibodies develop to a series of immunologically distinct type variant in the serum of hosts. Each rise in antibody titre coincides with the disappearance of the homologous variant and when this has been eliminated, a new antigenic type immediately arises.

Occult Visceral Phase. Fantham (1911) observed non-flagellate "latent forms" in the capillaries of internal organs of the vertebrate host. Ormerod and Venkatesan (1971) found amastigotes and sphaeromastigotes (small spherical forms with an undulating membrane and short free flagellum) in the swollen chor-oid plexus of rats inoculated with trypomastigotes of Botswana strain of *T. brucei*. They suggested that these occult visceral forms (the "la-tent forms" of earlier workers) might be the source of relapse strains of trypomastigotes which invade the blood stream. It is also pointed out that the choroid plexus may not be the only site and other site may be in the lungs.

Staining Reaction. When stained with Leishman or some other modifications of Romanowsky stain, the cytoplasm and the undulating membrane appear pale blue; the nucleus reddish purple or red; the kinetoplast and the flagellum dark red (*see* Fig. 40).

Cultivation. N.N.N. medium is not generally suitable for the cultivation of this trypanosome. It has been cultivated in a medium of Ringer's solution with sodium chloride, Tyrode's solution and citrated human blood. Long slender forms of trypomastigote, similar to mid-gut forms of tsetse fly are en-countered in culture.

Animal Inoculation. Laboratory animals, like mice, rats and guinea pigs are generally inoculated for demonstrating the typomastigotes when they are scanty or difficult to find in the pe-ripheral blood of man. In laboratory animals it causes an over-whelming parasitaemia and kills the animal in a few days. When inoculated in rats some of these trypomastigotes (5 to 6 per cent) develop posterior nuclear forms, i.e., the nucleus is situated poste-riorly close to the kinetoplast or behind it (see Fig. 41).

T. brucei in rabbits (syringe transmitted infection) causes a chronic infection lasting a few weeks and most of the animals die after about 4 to 5 weeks.

Immunology. *T. brucei* infection both in animals (rabbits) and man stimulates the output of large quantities of immuno-globulin, most of it is in non-specific IgM (19S) rather than in the IgG (7S) range, having no affinity for the infecting organ-ism. The host is unable to produce specific protective antibody to "large" antigens or the antibody producing cells do not re-ceive any message from macrophages to go into action.

It is also known that infection with this African trypano-some is associated with profound immunosuppressive effects. The humoral immune response is so severely depressed that the patient will not be able to resist any bacterial invasion.

Other serum antibodies found in trypanosomiasis are (1) *ablastin* which prevents multiplication of trypomastigotes and (2) *heterophil antibody*, particularly in *T. br. rhodesiense* infection, which agglutinates sheep erythrocytes and this fact may help in screening types of trypanosomiasis.

Life Cycle. *T. brucei* passes its life cycle in two different hosts (Fig. 42).

The vertebrate hosts (definitive hosts) are man, game and domestic animals.

The insect (intermediate) hosts are several species of the tsetse fly (*Glossina*) and include *G. palpalis, G. tachinoides, G. pallidipes, G. swynnertoni* and *G. morsitans.*

Development in man and other vertebrate hosts. The metacyclic stage (infective form) of trypomastigotes intro-duced by the bite of infected glossina develop into long, slender forms and multiply by binary longitudinal fission at the site of inoculation. These become "stumpy" *via* "intermediate" forms (Fig. 39). Subsequently the parasites invade

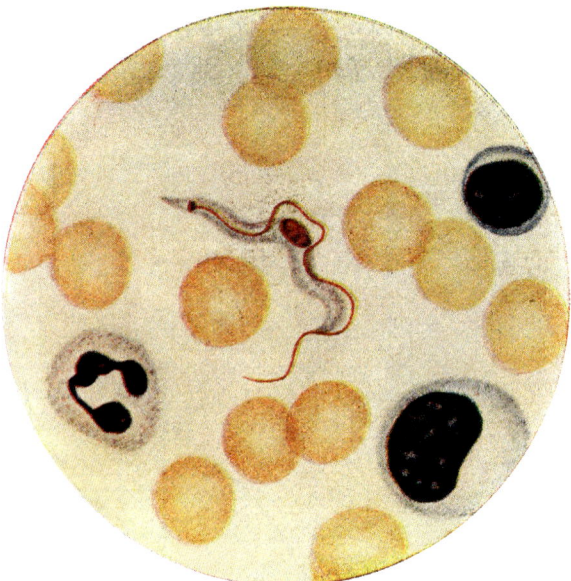

Fig. 40—*Trypanosoma brucei* ("*gambiense*" **strain**) **in the peripheral blood film.**

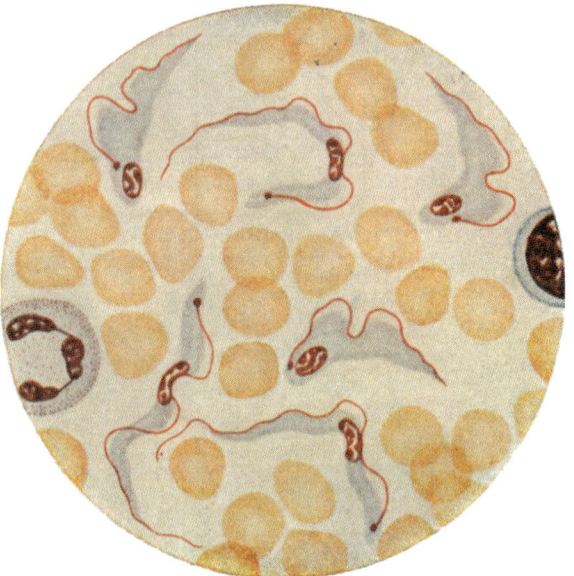

Fig. 41—*Trypanosoma brucei* ("*rhodesiense*" **strain**) **in the peripheral blood of a rodent.**
Note the usual forms and posterior nuclear forms.

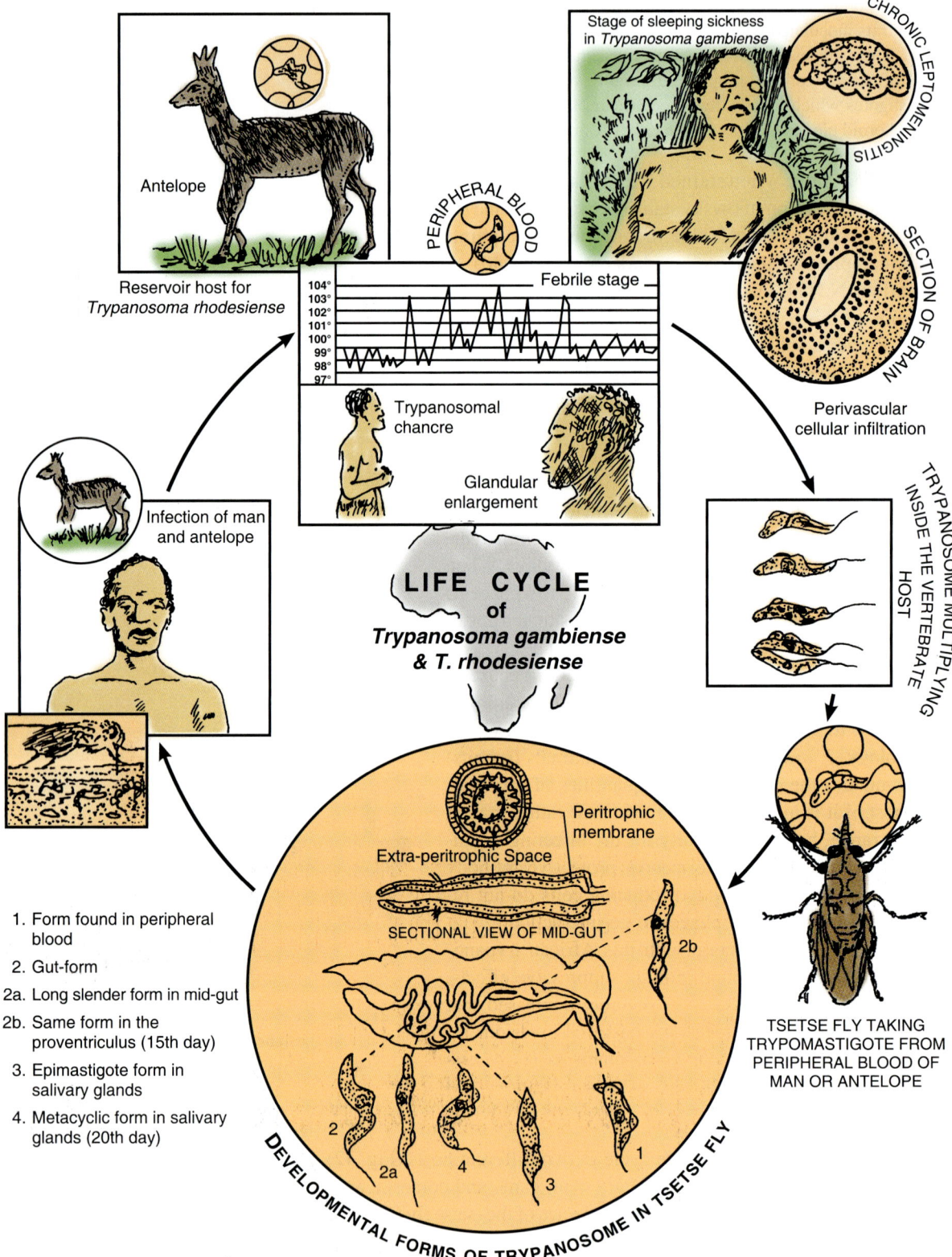

Stage of sleeping sickness in *Trypanosoma gambiense*

CHRONIC LEPTOMENINGITIS

SECTION OF BRAIN

Antelope

Reservoir host for *Trypanosoma rhodesiense*

PERIPHERAL BLOOD

Febrile stage

Trypanosomal chancre

Glandular enlargement

Perivascular cellular infiltration

TRYPANOSOME MULTIPLYING INSIDE THE VERTEBRATE HOST

LIFE CYCLE of *Trypanosoma gambiense* & *T. rhodesiense*

Infection of man and antelope

TSETSE FLY TAKING TRYPOMASTIGOTE FROM PERIPHERAL BLOOD OF MAN OR ANTELOPE

Peritrophic membrane

Extra-peritrophic Space

SECTIONAL VIEW OF MID-GUT

1. Form found in peripheral blood
2. Gut-form
2a. Long slender form in mid-gut
2b. Same form in the proventriculus (15th day)
3. Epimastigote form in salivary glands
4. Metacyclic form in salivary glands (20th day)

DEVELOPMENTAL FORMS OF TRYPANOSOME IN TSETSE FLY

Fig. 42—Life cycle of *Trypanosoma brucei* (*"gambiense"* **and** *"rhodesiense"* **strains**).
Some of the clinico-pathological manifestations are also shown.

the blood stream, resulting in parasitaemia. The trypomastigote forms, particularly the short stumpy forms are taken up by the tsetse fly along with its blood-meal and undergo a series of complex biological development inside the insect host before becoming infective to man.

Development in tsetse fly. The short stumpy forms of trypomastigote ingested by the insect, first change their morphology in the mid-gut. Long slender forms (the kinetoplast lying midway between the nucleus and the posterior end) appear which pass to the posterior end of the extra-peritrophic space (a space between the peritrophic membrane and the epithelial cells), where they continue to multiply for some days. By the 15th day, they escape from the anterior end of this space and enter the lumen of the proventriculus (the proventricular form is the same as that of the mid-gut form). Then they migrate forwards to the buccal cavity, pass on to the hypopharynx and eventually reach the salivary glands through the opening of the salivary ducts. Here they multiply and change their morphology, first into *epimastigote* and then into the *metacyclic* stage (short stumpy forms of *trypomastigote*) which are infective to man.

The time taken for the complete evolution of the infective forms (*metacyclic stage*) inside the tsetse fly is about 20 days. These tsetse flies remain infective for the rest of their lives, a period extending up to 185 days. There is no evidence of a hereditary transmission of trypanosomes in the fly to its offsprings. The tsetse flies produce a single larva and about 6 to 12 larvae during their life span, hence reproduction is very limited.

Transmitting Agents (Vectors) and Reservoirs of Infection (Fig. 43)

The *animal strain* of *T. brucei* is transmitted by *Glossina morsitans* amongst the wild game and domestic animals.

The *"gambiense" strain* of *T. brucei.* The transmitting agents are *Glossina palpalis, G. pallidipes* and *G. tachinoides.* *G. palpalis* (Fig. 44) obtains blood-meal from reptiles, birds and man. *G. tachinoides* feeds on blood of mammals (preferably antelopes) other than man. These are shade- and moisture-loving flies and are found in scrubs and shady trees near water (these are called riverine species). They do not normally travel far from their breeding grounds. Animal reservoirs of infection for this strain are not yet definitely known. Domestic pigs have been known to harbour the strain. So far as the "gambiense" strain is concerned man himself is the reservoir of infection. Interchange of trypanosomes between tsetse fly and man takes place near the water-supply of the village.

The "rhodesiense" strain of *T. brucei.* The transmitting agents are *G. morsitans, G. swynnertoni* and *G. pallidipes.* These flies feed on a wide range of species of game animals but the only important animal reservoir is the bushbuck, *Tragelaphus scriptus.* This antelope lives in close proximity to man and thus forms a link between glossina and man. Zambezi and sporadic rhodesian diseases are spread by this means whereas the epidemic rhodesian strains are spread by direct man-fly-man transmission. Domestic cattle may act as a reservoir of infection. The non-riverine species (*G. morsitans*) are found in more open savannah country than along the shores of rivers and lakes and have a tendency to follow up moving games and other moving objects. When the objects they are following come to rest, they move away and seek the nearest shady place.

Pathogenesis. *Mode of infection.* Inoculative method, by the bite of the infective tsetse fly *Glossina* (both male and female suck blood and can transmit the infection). They bite by daylight, usually in the early morning and evening.

The trypomastigotes (metacyclic stage) are introduced by the fly with the saliva into the subcutaneous pool of blood on which it feeds. Some of the parasites may enter the blood stream direct but the majority becomes entangled in the tissue spaces. The initial growth of the trypomastigotes is in the tissue spaces which form a more favourable nidus or probably here the organisms escape the action of antibodies which might be developed.

It is to be noted that while the trypomastigotes are multiplying in the subcutaneous tissue spaces and causing damage, the organisms are either absent or present in small numbers only in the peripheral blood.

It has been suggested, although unlikely, that the connective tissue damage caused by the trypomastigotes may be due to an exaggerated immune response (autoimmune reaction or massive release of kinin) rather than to any direct effect (mechanical damage due to motility) of this relatively non-toxic organism.

The presence of the trypomastigotes in the subcutaneous connective tissue excites host's response in two ways:

(a) By producing a large amount of non-specific immunoglobulins which are however not capable of sensitising the antigen. Antibodies are produced in response to the secretion of an exo-antigen of the trypomastigote.

(b) By heavily infiltrating the site of infection with macrophages, the cells competent to deal with the invaders. The neutrophils take peculiarly little interest in the defence and are therefore not much in evidence.

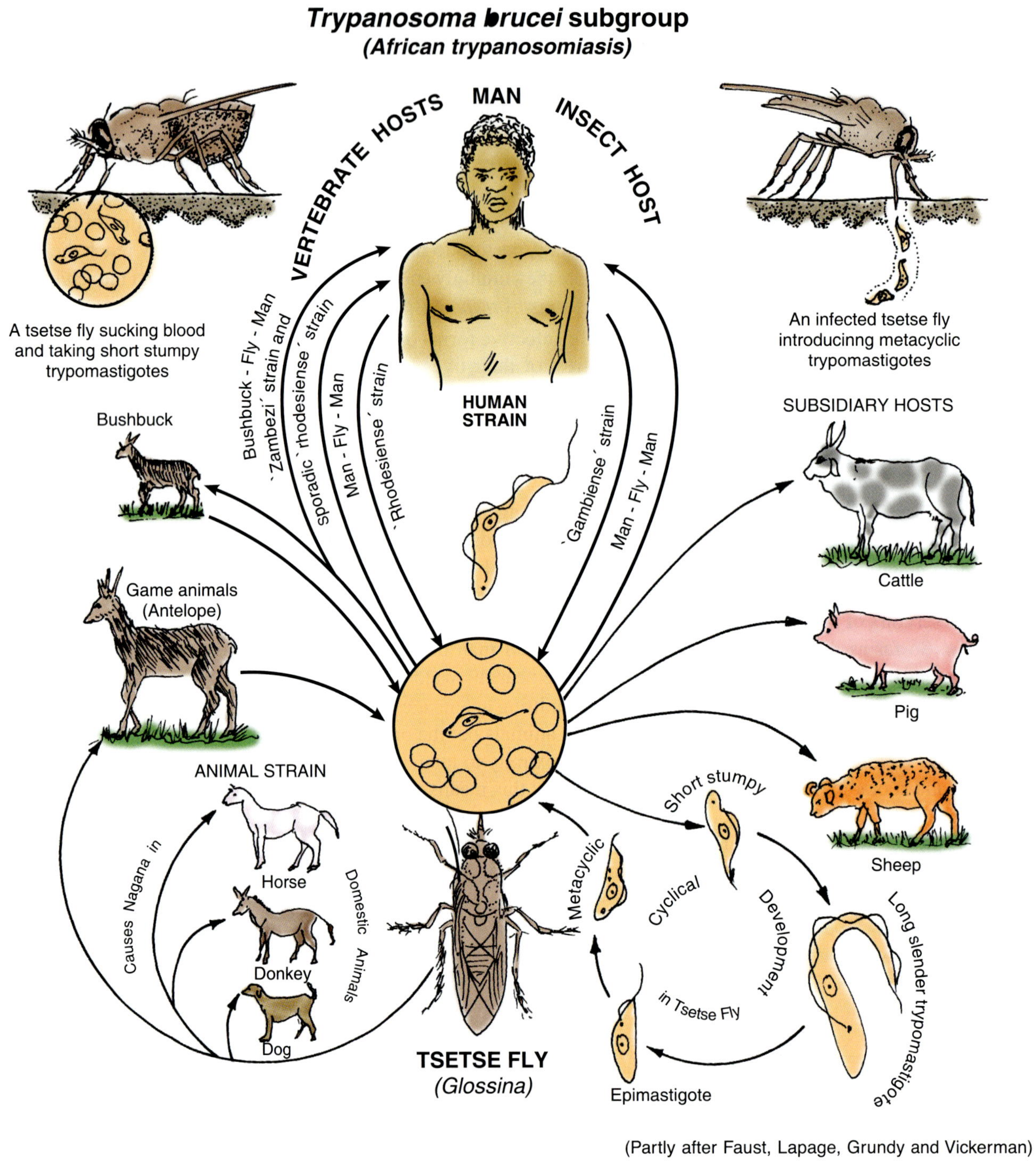

Trypanosoma brucei subgroup
(African trypanosomiasis)

A tsetse fly sucking blood and taking short stumpy trypomastigotes

An infected tsetse fly introducinng metacyclic trypomastigotes

VERTEBRATE HOSTS

MAN

INSECT HOST

HUMAN STRAIN

Bushbuck

Game animals (Antelope)

ANIMAL STRAIN

Causes Nagana in

Horse

Donkey

Dog

Domestic Animals

Bushbuck - Fly - Man 'Zambezi' strain and 'sporadic 'rhodesiense' strain

Man - Fly - Man 'Rhodesiense' strain

'Gambiense' strain

Man - Fly - Man

SUBSIDIARY HOSTS

Cattle

Pig

Sheep

Short stumpy

Metacyclic

Cyclical

Development

in Tsetse Fly

Long slender trypomastigote

Epimastigote

TSETSE FLY (Glossina)

(Partly after Faust, Lapage, Grundy and Vickerman)

Fig. 43

Thus, it will be seen that there is no lack of mobilisation of the host's defensive mechanism but it is the cellular defence which plays the dominant role. The macrophages could be seen to remove the living trypomastigotes in the tissue spaces. The release of kinins may help to attract macrophages; it also increases the capillary permeability of tissues and may explain the oedematous swollen subcutaneous tissue at the site of infection.

Pathogenic lesions. There is severe damage of the perivascular connective tissues. The bundle of collagen fibres are disrupted and the fibroblasts are destroyed.

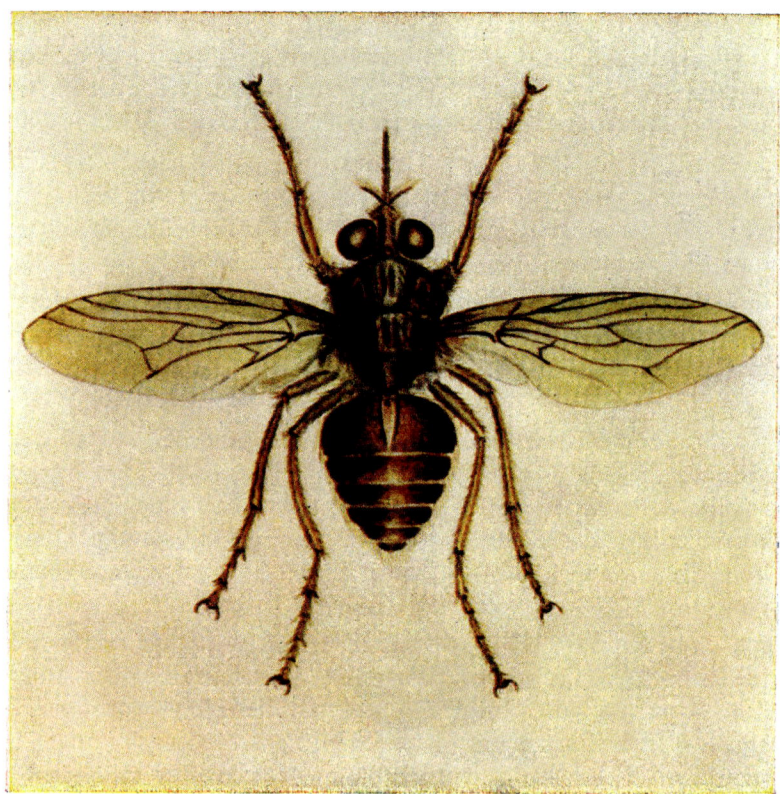

Fig. 44—*Glossina palpalis,* **the insect host for** *"gambiense"* **strain of** *T. brucei.*

The lesions are found mainly in the *lymph nodes* and the *central nervous system.*

The capillary blood vessels of the *central nervous system* are not surrounded by any connective tissue matrix but the nerve cells are embraced by the overlapping fibrous processes of the astrocytes. An increase of glial cells occur throughout the central nervous system and the cerebral perivascular spaces are "cuffed" with mononuclear cells (*perivascular cuffing*). Cerebral softening may result from thrombosis of these "cuffed" vessels. The choroid plexus is severely congested and infiltrated with monocytes, often containing a large number of parasites. There is heavy cellular infiltration in the leptomeninges but slight infiltration in the brain substance.

The *lymph nodes* in early stages show congestion, haemorrhages and marked proliferation of macrophage cells; in the later stages they undergo degenerative changes with extensive fibrosis.

Clinical Pathology

Blood. Leucocytosis (monocytosis) and anaemia.

On account of a high rise of gamma globulin, the erythrocyte sedimentation rate is raised and the serum aldehyde test becomes positive; it also causes an auto-agglutination of red blood cells.

Cerebrospinal fluid. The pressure is raised, the cell count (50 to 100 per mm^3) and protein content (100-150 mg%) are increased. The rise of globulin content gives a "tabetic" type of colloidal gold curve. The parasites may be demonstrated in the CSF. The increased cell count is not sufficient to cause any turbidity of the CSF.

Clinical Features (*see* Fig. 42). A history of exposure to tsetse bite is often available (even a normal tsetse bite causes a severe reaction).

A trypanosomal *chancre* may develop at the site of inoculation of trypomastigotes introduced by the bite of the infected tsetse fly (often passes unobserved or confused with a normal tsetse bite). It is a hard painful nodule and fluid withdrawn from it contains actively dividing trypomastigotes; it subsides in a week or two without suppurating.

In "rhodesian" form the symptoms appear first after 2 weeks of the bite, whereas in "gambian" and "zambezi" forms the symptoms may be delayed for up to a year.

It is characterised by infection of the blood stream, involvement and enlargement of lymph nodes (at first regional, later generalised) and eventually invasion of the central nervous system. The early symptoms are fever (high and fluctuating in "rhodesian" form), severe headache, loss of nocturnal sleep and a feeling of oppression. A fleeting circulate erythematous rash may appear on the chest and shoulders (difficult to detect in coloured skin).

The lymph node enlargement, particularly of the posterior triangle of the neck, is a feature of "gambian" disease whereas the invasion of the central nervous system is rapid in "rhodesian" form. As the central nervous system is involved, the symptoms of meningoencephalitis develop resulting in classical sleeping sickness. In the final stage, the patient becomes thin and wasted, accompanied by various signs of malnutrition.

A patient in whom trypomastigotes have been detected will die sooner or later unless treated. In "rhodesian" disease the patient dies early but with both "zambezi", and "gambian" diseases the patient may survive longer (several years). In "zambezi" disease it may be possible for the patient to overcome the infection naturally and act as "healthy carriers".

Laboratory Diagnosis. This is established by demonstrating the trypanosomes (trypomastigote forms) in any one of the following materials: (a) peripheral blood, (b) bone marrow obtained by sternal puncture, (c) juice aspirated from the swollen lymph nodes (posterior cervical) and (d) the cerebrospinal fluid obtained by lumbar puncture. The methods include (i) a direct microscopical examination of unstained and stained films (Fig. 40), (ii) cultivation and (iii) animal inoculation. If the parasites are scanty and cannot be detected in thin blood film, thick film or concentration method may be employed.

Microscopical examination of a blood film is a useful diagnostic procedure in "rhodesian" form but not so in "zambezi" and "gambian" forms where the organism can easily be isolated by inoculating blood into rats or mice (Fig. 41). Microscopical examination of juice obtained from the swollen lymph nodes may demonstrate the parasite in an early case of "gambian" disease. Examination of the centrifugalised deposit of the CSF may demonstrate the parasite in late cases of "gambian" disease. In wet preparations made from blood (or tissue fluid) the trypomastigotes are seen to be moving actively between the cells. IgM level in the CSF is also increased.

Various concentration methods like microhaematocrit centrifugation method, miniature anion exchange centrifugation technique and buffy coat technique are now used.

Serological tests, such as estimation of IgM levels (reaches a very high level as compared to other protozoal infections) by means of agar gel precipitation, indirect fluorescent antibody test (using *T. brucei rhodesiense* in rats for fluorescence), complement fixation test (with a stable antigen) and ELISA test are now used for the diagnosis and searching cases for further study. Card agglutination test for trypanosomiasis (CATT) and card indirect antigen test for trypanosomiasis (CIATT) are now used for diagnosis of *T. gambiense* infection.

Treatment. Suramin and pentamidine are considered to be the drugs of choice for early acute infection. As they cannot pass the blood-brain barrier, they are not of any value when the central nervous system is involved in which case an arsenical is needed. The arsenical includes, melarsoprol (mel B.). Other effective drug is Eflornithine.

For rhodesian infection IV suramin in a dose of one gm for 1st, 3rd, 7th, 14th and 21st day should be given after a test dose of 100 mg – 200 mg IV.

For gambian infection IM pentamidine in a dose of 4 mg/kg/day for 10 days is recommended.

In case of neurological involvement of both rhodesian and gambian infection melarsoprol in a dose of 2–3.6 mg/kg/day by IV route for 3 days followed by 2nd couse of 3 days at an interval of 7–10 days are prescribed. The dose of the drug in 2nd course is 3–6 mg/kg/day for 3 days. 3rd course can be repeated 15–21 days later.

Eflornithine in a dose of 400 mg/kg/day in four divided doses for 14 days also gives encouraging result in cases of gambian infection with CNS involvement.

Prophylaxis. This consists of the following:

1. Destruction of the habitat of the vector. It is supplemented by the use of insecticides.
2. Game destruction program to eliminate the blood-meal of the fly has no affect on human sleeping sickness.
3. Isolation of the human population from areas known to harbour infective games and treatment of all infected humans. This is much more important in "gambian" disease.
4. *Chemoprophylaxis*. Pentamidine is effective against "gambian" disease. A single intramuscular injection of 4 mg/kg will provide a preventive effect for at least 6 months.

Trypanosoma cruzi Chagas, 1909

SYNONYM: *Schizotrypanum cruzi.*

The parasite causing South American trypanosomiasis or Chagas' disease.

Geographical Distribution. Central and South America.

Habitat. A parasite of muscular and nervous tissues and also of the R.E. system existing in the amastigote form. The trypomastigote forms appear in the peripheral blood from time to time.

Morphology. To main morphological types are found in the human host.

Trypomastigote Forms. In dried and stained film, the parasite appears to be C- or U-shaped. It measures 20 μm in length, has a central nucleus and a large, oval kinetoplast situated at the posterior wedge-shaped end (Fig. 45). Two forms are found in the peripheral blood—one, long and slender and the other, short and broad. Multiplication of the parasite does not occur in the peripheral blood. The trypomastigote forms are either taken up by the insect host or enter tissue cells where they continue to live as amastigote forms.

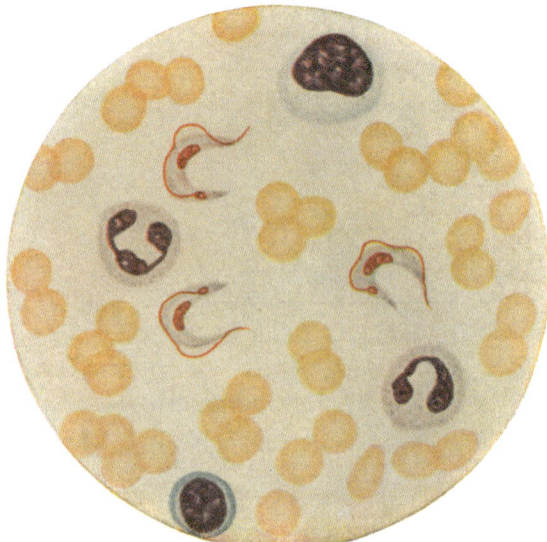

Fig. 45—*Trypanosoma cruzi* **in the peripheral blood film.** Note the C-shaped forms.

Amastigote Forms. These are particularly found inside the cells of striated muscles (heart and skeletal), neuroglial cells of the nervous tissues, as also inside the cells of the reticulo-endothelial system. The amastigote forms are round or oval bodies, measuring 2 to 4 μm in diameter, having a nucleus and a kinetoplast. When fully developed, a large number may be found enclosed in a cystic cavity. Multiplication of the parasite occurs at this stage only.

Staining Reaction. Same as that of other trypanosomes.

Cultivation. Easily cultivated in N.N.N. medium or other modifications thereof.

Immunology. Serum antibodies develop in *T. cruzi* infection but as the parasite continues to grow as amastigote form inside the R.E. cells and parenchyma cells they are not exposed to the action of these antibodies.

Life Cycle. *T. cruzi* passes its life cycle (Fig. 46) in two hosts: one in man or the reservoir host; the other in the transmitting insect, the reduviid bug (*Panstrongylus megistus, Triatoma infestans* and *Rhodnius prolixus).*

Development in Reduviid Bug. The trypomastigote forms are taken up by the bug during the act of biting. In the "stomach" (mid-gut) of the bug they are transformed into amastigote forms and thereafter multiply by binary fission. Later the amastigote forms are transformed into epimastigote forms which migrate backwards to the hind-gut and in turn multiply by longitudinal fission. In 8 to 10 days' time, metacyclic forms of trypomastigote appear and are excreted in the faeces of the bug.

Development in Man. Man is infected either by faecal matter of the bug being rubbed into the wound caused by the bite or by a possible contamination of the conjunctivae and other exposed mucous membranes with the fingers. The

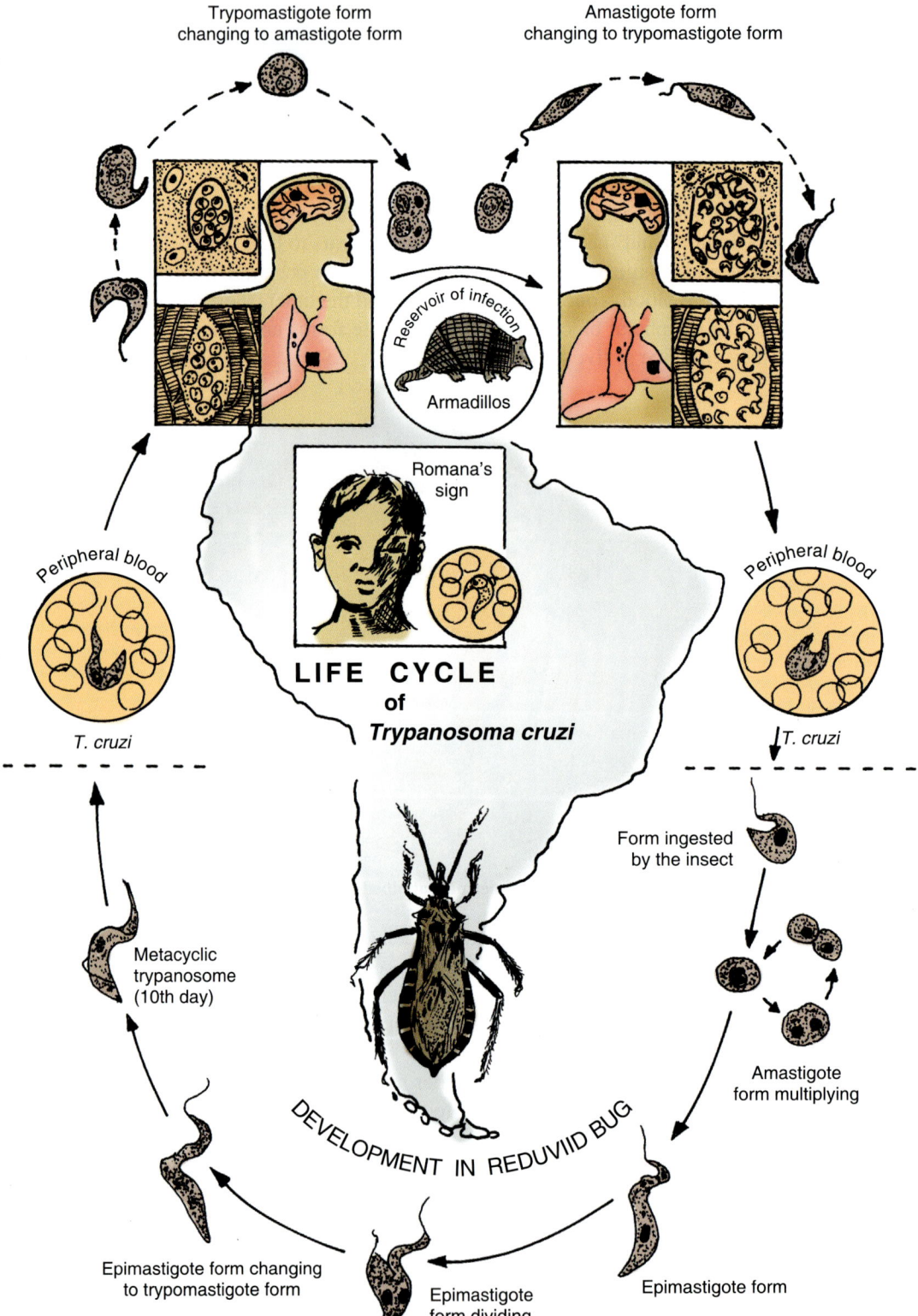

Trypomastigote form changing to amastigote form

Amastigote form changing to trypomastigote form

Reservoir of infection
Armadillos

Romana's sign

**LIFE CYCLE
of
*Trypanosoma cruzi***

Peripheral blood

T. cruzi

Peripheral blood

T. cruzi

Form ingested by the insect

Metacyclic trypanosome (10th day)

Amastigote form multiplying

DEVELOPMENT IN REDUVIID BUG

Epimastigote form changing to trypomastigote form

Epimastigote form dividing

Epimastigote form

Fig. 46—Developmental stages of *Trypanosoma cruzi* in man and reduviid bug.

metacyclic trypomastigotes thus introduced, invade tissue cells and are transformed into amastigote forms. These multiply by binary fission and after passing through promastigote and epimastigote forms are again transformed into trypomastigote forms which are liberated in the blood.

Reservoir Hosts. These are armadillos and opossums. Man is the secondary host. Other animals prone to natural infection are: cats, dogs, bats, wood rats.

Pathogenicity. *Mode of Infection.* Contaminative method, through the agency of a reduviid bug as described above.

Portal of Entry—Skin or conjunctiva.

In the skin a localised swelling "*chagoma*" develops; when the entry is through the conjunctiva an oedematous swelling of eyelids of one eye (*Romana's sign*) develops.

Transmission has also occurred congenitally *via* placenta to newborns, by blood transfusion (donors screened by C. F. test) and accidentally to laboratory workers dealing with *T. cruzi*.

Pathogenic Lesions. The gross lesions are found mainly in the heart (parasitic myocarditis), skeletal muscles and nervous system (thyroid gland in some regions) and are all due to the invasion of the parasites inside the tissue cells. The cells of the reticulo-endothelial system are particularly involved. The parasite multiplies only in the amastigote stage and not in the trypomastigote state. Hence the pathogenic effects are due to the amastigote forms. Parasitic multiplication within the cells leads finally to destruction of the cell. In acute cases, rarely, all cells and tissues may be invaded but in chronic cases major damage affects the cardiac muscle and peripheral ganglion cells.

Clinical Features. *Incubation Period*—7 to 14 days.

Infection with *T. cruzi* causes a disease in South America, known as Chagas' disease. Two clinical types, acute and chronic, are described.

The *acute form* occurs in children and infants. It is characterised by fever, conjunctivitis, unilateral oedema of the face, enlargement of the spleen and lymph nodes, anaemia and lymphocytosis. It lasts for a period of 20 to 30 days, often terminating fatally with symptoms of meningoencephalitis or myocardial failure.

The *chronic form* is seen in adults and adolescents. It is characterised by disturbances of cardiac rhythm (heart block, Adams-Stokes syndrome) and neurological manifestations (spastic paralysis, psychical change). It may last for a period of 12 years.

In endemic areas, a common complication of chronic cases of Chagas' disease is the dilatation of tubular organs (megaoesophagus and megacolon), the basic lesion in such cases being the degeneration of intramural autonomic nerve plexuses by the toxic action of *T. cruzi*—Cardiomyopathy may occur as a complication of Chagas' disease.

A peculiar herniation of the endocardium through loosened myocardial muscle bundles at vortex (apex of left ventricle) has been observed at autopsy in cases of Chagas' disease. The ventricular apical aneurysm is about 2-3 cm in diameter and is often filled with a thrombus; it rarely ruptures. The pulmonary conus is also dilated.

Laboratory Diagnosis

1. By microscopical examination of a stained blood film for the parasite. It is to be noted that the dividing forms of *T. cruzi* are not found in the peripheral blood, a point which helps to differentiate it from *T. rangeli*, a non-pathogenic blood trypanosome found in endemic areas of Chagas' disease. Blood culture is also helpful.

2. By inoculating a guinea pig with patient's blood. This is useful when the trypomastigotes are not found in the peripheral blood.

3. Xenodiagnosis: By allowing a laboratory-bred parasite-free reduviid bug to feed on an individual suspected to be suffering from Chagas' disease and 2 weeks later examining the intestinal contents for the presence of the parasite (xenodiagnosis).

4. By a specific complement fixation test (Machado-Guerreiro test) with antigen obtained from culture of *T. cruzi* and by an indirect fluorescent antibody test (IFAT), by ELISA test and by IHA test. The serological tests will be positive after one month of infection.

5. Detection of parasite DNA by PCR method is now used for detection for positive case with very few parasites in the blood.

6. By an intradermal test. A delayed hypersensitivity reaction is obtained by using an extract "cruzin" prepared from culture of *T. cruzi*.

7. Biopsy of an involved lymph node or muscle (calf or deltoid) may reveal amastigote forms of *T. cruzi*.

Treatment. Nifurtimox (lampit) in a dose of 10 mg/kg/day in three divided doses orally after meal for 92-120 days is used. Alternative drug benznidazole in given orally in a dose of 5-10 mg/kg/day in two divided doses for 30-90 days.

Prophylaxis

(i) Attack on the Parasite. Treating the disease with a specific drug, if available.

(ii) Attack on the Vector. Use of insecticides and use of building materials which are impermeable to the bug.

(iii) Personal Prophylaxis. Avoiding the bites of the insect by using mosquito-nets.

Genus LEISHMANIA Ross, 1903

Generic Character. The genus *Leishmania* was created by Ross, in 1903, to include the parasite of Indian kala-azar, *Leishmania donovani*. Morphologically the flagellates belonging to the genus *Leishmania* are identical to those of the genus *Leptomonas*. Thus both the genera have an amastigote and a promastigote stage and the differences are as follows:

	GENUS LEPTOMONAS	GENUS LEISHMANIA
Life cycle:	Only in insect host. No vertebrate host.	Both in a vertebrate and an insect host.
Transmission:	Ingestion of "cysts".	By intermediate host.

Leishmaniasis is considered to be zoonotic disease, the infection being maintained in endemic areas, in dogs, wild rodents or other mammals. Several leishmanial species (21 species) are responsible for the disease leishmaniasis in man in over 88 countries. The different species are morphologically indistinguishable. They can be differentiated by isoenzyme analysis, DNA sequence analysis, or monoclonal antibodies study. Visceral leishmaniasis is a severe clinical entity in which parasites migrate to vital organs.

Species Parasitic to Man. Under genus Leishmania there are 2 subgenus: (I) Leishmania and (II) Viannia. Under two subgenus, species are as follows.

I. Under subgenus Leishmania:

1. *Leishmania donovani complex*

(a) *Leishmania donovani* causing Kala-azar*. The infection is generalized, and as the parasites are distributed inside the internal organs, the disease kala-azar is also called *visceral leishmaniasis*. The parasite may also cause a variety of skin lesions (dermal leishmanoid) without any visceral manifestations. Kala-azar or anthroponotic visceral leishmaniasis (AVL) is prevalent in Middle East, Africa, India (Bihar, West Bengal, Orissa, Assam, Tamil Nadu, Gujarat, Punjab and Jammu), certain parts of China, South America and Europe. Vectors are *P. argentipes*, and *P. chinesis* in India and China, respectively. Man is the only known reservoir.

(b) *Leishmania infantum* Nicolle, 1908. This is the parasite of infantile kala-azar, occurring in Mediterranean areas, Middle East and China. It causes zoonotic visceral leishmaniasis (ZVL). *P. perniciosus* and *P. ariasi* act as vector in the Mediterranean areas whereas *P. chinensis* and *P. alexandri* are vectors in China. Dogs, foxes and jackals are known reservoirs.

(c) *Leishmania chagasi* da Cunha and Chagas, 1937. It causes zoonotic visceral leishmaniasis (ZVL) in the New world. The vector is *Lutzomyia longipalpis*. Dogs and foxes are animal reservoirs.

(d) *Leishmania archibaldi*. It causes VL in Africa. *P. orientalis* and *P. martini* act as vectors. Rodents and carnivorous animals act as resrvoirs.

Note: According to some workers *L. chagasi* and *L. archibaldi* are not separate species (TVS 793 WHO 1990).

---

* The word *kala-azar* has been derived from two Indian words *kala* and *azar* meaning "black sickness", an illness in which the colour (pigmentation) of the skin turns black. The word *kala* also means "deadly" thereby signifying a fatal illness.

2. *Leishmania tropica complex*

(a) *Leishmania tropica:* It causes a dry type of cutaneous lesion (non-ulcerating type) and has an urban distribution. The incubation period is from 2 months to more than a year. The lesion is usually facial. Man and domestic dog are the reservoirs of infection. It is prevalent in Middle East, Mediterranean areas, N. Africa, N.W. India and Pakistan. It causes VL in exceptional cases.

(b) *Leishmania killicki:* It causes local cutaneous leision.

3. *Leishmania major complex*

Leishmania major: It causes a moist type of local cutaneous lesion (ulcerating type) and has a rural distribution. The reservoir host is the desert gerbil *R. opimus* and other small rodents. Ulcers are found on the extremities with regional lymphadenitis which appear 2-6 weeks after sandfly bite. It is prevalent in Central Asia and Iran. It causes DCL during immunosuppression states.

4. *Leishmania aethiopica complex*

Leishmania aethiopica: It is found in Kenya, Ethiopia, Europe. It causes CL and in exceptional cases it produces DCL.

5. *Leishmania mexicana complex*

(a) *Leishmania mexicana.* It is a benign form affecting the skin without invasion of oro-nasal mucosa. It causes chiclero's ulcer (Bay sore), a chronic lesion occurring at the site of sandfly bite. It is characterised by a single cutaneous lesion on the ear, face or hand which undergoes spontaneous healing and leads to deformities through scarring. It is prevalent in Mexico, Guatemala, Honduras, Belize, Colombia, Costa Rica, Dominion Republic, Ecuador, French Guiana, Panama, Peru, USA and Venezuela. It causes DCL in exceptional cases and VL during immunosuppression states.

(b) *Leishmania amazonensis.* It causes local cutaneous leision and in exceptional cases it produces DCL and VL.

(c) *Leishmania venezuelensis.* It causes local cutaneous leision.

(d) *Leishmania garnhami.* It causes local cutaneous leision.

(e) *Leishmania pifonoi.* It causes a malignant form with extensive lesion in the skin of lepromatous type.

Note: According to some workers *Leishmania garnhami* and *Leishmania pifonoi* are not separate species (TVS 793 WHO 1990).

II. Under subgenus Viannia:

1. *Leishmania braziliensis complex*

(a) *Leishmania braziliensis.* It is a malignant form associated with invasion of skin and oro-nasal mucosa (espundia). It is prevalent in Argentina, Belize, Bolivia, Brazil, Colombia, Costa Rica, Ecuador, French Guiana, Honduras, Mexico, Panama, Paraguay, Peru and Venezuela. The lesion commences as a papulopustular swelling of the skin localised in the region of nostrils, mouth or eyes or widespread on the face, ears, elbows and knees. After a variable time the mucosal surface of the mouth and nose are involved causing destructive and mutilating erosions. Sometimes the whole of nasal septum is destroyed. The lesion generally heals by scarring producing the typical tapir nose or camel nose. It causes DCL and VL during immunosuppressive state.

(b) *Leishmania peruviana.* A benign form without invasion of oro-nasal mucosa and causing dry papule in the skin (a single sore, k.a. uta in Peru). The reservoir host is the domestic dog and the transmitting sandfly is *Lu. noguchi.* It has now been found in Peru and Ecuador.

2. *Leishmania guyanensis complex*

(a) *Leishmania guyanensis.* It is prevalent in Brazil, Colombia, Guyana, Peru, Surinam and French Guiana. It is a benign form affecting cutaneous lesion and in exceptional cases it causes MCL.

(b) *Leishmania panamensis.* It is found in Panama, Colombia and Costa Rica. It usually causes LCL but affects oronasal mucose in exceptional cases. It can cause DCL during immunosuppressive state.

(c) *Leishmania shawi.* It causes CL.

3. *Leishmania lainsoni complex* It causes CL and self-recovery occurs.

4. *Leishmania naiffi complex* It causes CL.

Note: VL means visceral leishmaniasis; CL means localised cutaneous leishmaniasis; DCL means diffuse cutaneous leishmaniasis; MCL means mucocutaneous leishmaniasis.

CLINICAL CLASSIFICATION OF LEISHMANIASIS

1. Visceral leishmaniasis or Kala-azar

(a) Indian Kala-azar caused by *L. donovani* with a human reservoir.

(b) Mediterranean Kala-azar or Infantile Kala-azar also Chinese, Middle East and Russian Kala-azar caused by *L. donovani infantum* with a canine reservoir.

(c) South American Kala-azar caused by *L. chagasi* with a canine reservoir.

(d) African Kala-azar (Sudanese and East Africa) with rodent reservoir.

2. Cutaneous leishmaniasis (CL) and no visceral manifestation: Clinical features of CL vary, between and within regions due to different species of leishmania, type of zoonotic cycle concerned and also due to genetically determined response of the patient. A classical lesion shows as a nodule at the site of inoculation followed by formation of central crust. The crust may fall away exposing a wet type of ulcer. A depressed scar and altered pigment develops on healing of ulcer satellite nodules at the edge of lesion are characteristic features. CL may be presented as a papulonodular lesion covered by superficial scales (dry type of ulcer).

I. Dermal leishmanoid or post Kala-azar dermal leishmaniasis (PKDL) is caused by *L. donovani*. Non-ulcerative skin lesion, is a late sequela to visceral infection. It developes in 10% to 20% of patients suffering from visceral leishmaniasis mainly in India. It is rare in China, Mediterranean areas, central and south America. The lesion develops about 1 to 2 years after recovery from VL. The lesions are of 3 types (macular and hypopigmented lesion, erythematous patch and nodules) and do not heal spontaneously.

II. OLD WORLD (OWCL): This condition is usually caused by *L. major, L. tropica* and *L. aethiopica* infection. The species can be distinguished from each other by the enzyme characterization. Cutaneous lesions due to *L. donovani* are found in Africa and Mediterranean basin.

(a) Anthroponotic or urban cutaneous leishmaniasis (ACL) is caused by *L. tropica*. The infection leads to slow, self-healing, local lesion of skin and as sequela a depressed scar is formed. The ulcer usually starts as small itching papule covered with fine whitish scale which subsequently becomes thick, dark and finally falls off. The lesion may be found on the face, feet, legs and arms. Children are usually affected. It is prevalent in Afghanistan, Greece, North India, Islamic Republic of Iran, Iraq, Israel, Kenya, Kuwait, Lebanon, Morocco, Pakistan, Saudi Arabia, Syrian Arab Republic, Tunisia and Turkey.

Leishmaniasis recidivans (LR). The lupoid or tuberculoid leishmaniasis of the skin is believed to be a sequela of an incomplete immune response to an earlier episode of oriental sore. It caused by *L. tropica*. Slowly progressive type of skin lesion usually on the face is characterized by scar with peripheral activity. Often confused with lupoid vulgaris due to scarcity of amistogote in the lesion. It responds poorly to treatment and may last for many years. The lesion does not heal spontaneously.

(b) Zoonotic or rural cutaneous leishmaniasis (ZCL) caused by *L. major*. It is found in central Asia, Middle East, North Africa, North India and Pakistan. Multiple painless lesions are noticed on the limbs, nose and lips, but do not involve the mucous membrane. Self-healing occurs rapidly. In non-immune person, ulceration and secondary infection occur in the lesion which heals slowly and results in a disfiguring scar.

(c) Cutaneous lesions caused by *L. aethiopica* giving rise to small cutaneous lesion on the face and ulceration is absent. Slow healing occurs within 1-3 years.

Diffuse cutaneous leishmaniasis (DCL) or *leishmaniasis diffusa*. It results from specific deficiency of cell-mediated immunity to leishmania antigen. In new world DCL (South America), the disease is caused by *L. amazonesis*. *Leishmania mexicana* is the parasite most commonly associated with DCL in New World (Dominican Republic) whereas in old world *Leishmania aethiopica* is the causative agent of DCL and has been reported in Ethiopia and Kenya. DCL is characterized by the appearance of nodular infiltrative lesions which are neither destructive nor erosive but most disfiguring. It starts as a single lesion and spreads slowly over the face, ears, extremities and buttocks, until the whole body is affected but there is no ulceration or mucosal involvement. Histologically the nodes consist almost entirely of histocytes with a relative absence of lymphocytes and plasma cells.

Numerous amastigote forms of parasites, free or in macrophages are found in the skin lesions, because of absence of secondary lymphocytic invasion. It is an anergic manifestation characterized by massive dissemination of skin lesions, having a striking resemblance to lepromatous leprosy. The leishmanin skin test is negative. Leishmania (amastigote form) has been recovered both from blood and bone marrow. DCL responds poorly to antimonials and does not heal spontaneously. Pentamidine and amphotericin B have been found to be effective but both have serious side-effects. There is a tendency of relapse after treatment.

III. NEW WORLD (NWCL): The following diseases have been noticed in South and Central America.

(a) CL (*Uta*). Caused by *Leishmania peruviana*. A benign form without invasion of oronasal mucous membrane causes dry papule in the skin (a single sore, k.a. uta in Peru).

(b) CL (*Chiclero's ulcer, or Bay sore*). Caused by *Leishmania mexicana*.

(c) CL (*Pain bios*). Caused by *Leishmania guyanensis*. A benign form affecting oronasal mucous membrane.

(d) CL (*Ulcera da bejulo*). Caused by *Leishmania panamensis*.

(e) CL. Caused by *Leishmania braziliensis*.

(f) CL. Caused by several other species of leishmania such as *L. amazonensis*, *L. venezuelenensis*, *L. lainsoni*. Simple cutaneous lesion is formed and self-recovery takes place.

Note: The term Old World is used for the rest of the world whereas New World refers to the Americas.

3. Muco-Cutaneous Leishmaniasis (MCL) or Espundia caused by *Leishmania braziliensis* and occasionally by *Leishmania panamensis*. It is prevalent in South and Central America. There are two stages, a primary cutaneous lesion, sometimes followed by a secondary mucosal involvement which occurs after a variable time of latency of primary cutaneous lesion. MCL develops in 5% patients suffering from primary cutaneous lesion. No history of primary skin lesion is available in large number of cases. Nasal mucous membrane, pharynx, larynx and upper lip are involved. Sometimes whole of the nasal septum is destroyed. Granulomas develop at mucocutaneous junction followed by gross destruction of soft tissue and cartilage causing disfigurement of nose and mouth. Parasite affects the mucous membrane by lymphatic or haematogenous dissemination. Death may occur from severe respiratory infection due to respiratory acute obstruction.

Leishmania donovani (Laveran and Mesnil, 1903) Ross, 1903

The parasite causing visceral leishmaniasis or kala-azar.

It is named after the discoverers, Leishman and Donovan, both of whom reported on the organism simultaneously; Leishman from London in May 1903 and Donovan from Madras in July 1903.

Geographical Distribution. Endemic in many places in India, China, Africa, Southern Europe, South America and Russia.

In India, it is specially common in Assam and Bengal along the coasts of the Ganges and the Brahmaputra. It is also endemic in Bihar, Orissa, Madras and the eastern parts of Uttar Pradesh as far as Lucknow.

Habitat. Inside the vertebrate host (man) the parasite is always intra-cellular, occurring in the amastigote form. It is essentially a parasite of the R. E. System.

Morphology. The parasite exists in two stages:

1. *Amastigote Stage* (formerly called "leishmanial" form): Occurs in man.
2. *Promastigote Stage* (formerly called "leptomonad" form): Occurs in (a) gut of insect (sandfly) and (b) artificial culture.

AMASTIGOTE STAGE (AFLAGELLAR STAGE). The parasite at this stage resides in the cells of the reticulo-endothelial system of vertebrate hosts (man, dog and hamster).

The characteristics of the amastigote form (Figs. 47 & 48) are as follows:

Shape and *Size*. It is a round or oval body measuring 2 to 4 μm along the longitudinal axis.

Cell membrane is delicate and can be demonstrated in fresh specimens only.

Nucleus measures a little less than 1 μm in diameter. It is oval or round and is usually situated in the middle of the cells or along the side of cell membrane.

Kinetoplast lies tangentially or at right angles to the nucleus. It comprises a DNA-containing body and a mitochondrial structure.

Axoneme (rhizoplast), a delicate filament extending from the kinetoplast to the margin of the body. It represents the root of the flagellum.

Vacuole, a clear unstained space lying alongside the axoneme.

PROMASTIGOTE STAGE (FLAGELLAR STAGE). This stage (Figs. 49 & 50) of the parasite is only encountered in cultures and in insect vectors (sandflies).

Shape and *Size*. The earlier ones are short oval, or pear-shaped bodies, measuring 5 to l0 μm in length by 2 to 3 μm in breadth. The fully developed ones are long slender spindle-shaped bodies, measuring 15 to 20 μm in length by 1 to 2 μm in breadth.

Nucleus is situated centrally. *Kinetoplast* lies transversely near the anterior end.

Eosinophilic vacuole, a light staining area lying in front of the kinetoplast over which the root of the flagellum runs.

Flagellum may be of the same length as the body or even longer, projecting from the front. The flagellum does not curve round the body of the parasite and therefore there is no undulating membrane.

Note: With Leishman's stain the cytoplasm appears blue, the nucleus, pink or violet and the kinetoplast, bright red.

Cultivation. *L. donovani* can be cultured in a medium composed of two parts of salt agar and one part of defibrinated rabbit's blood. The medium was first introduced by Novy and MacNeal, later modified by Nicolle and is

AMASTIGOTE & PROMASTIGOTE FORMS OF *LEISHMANIA DONOVANI*

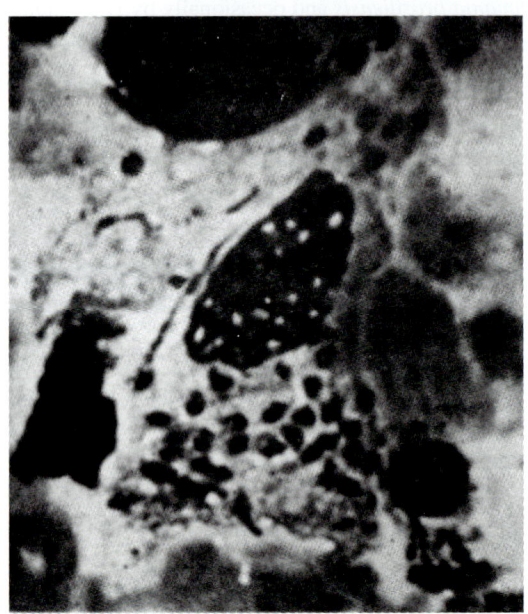

Fig. 47—Amastigote forms of *L. donovani* **inside a macrophage cell.**
Smear from a sternal puncture material.

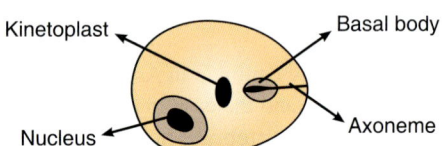

Fig. 48—Diagrammatic representation of the morphology of amastigote form of *L. donovani*.

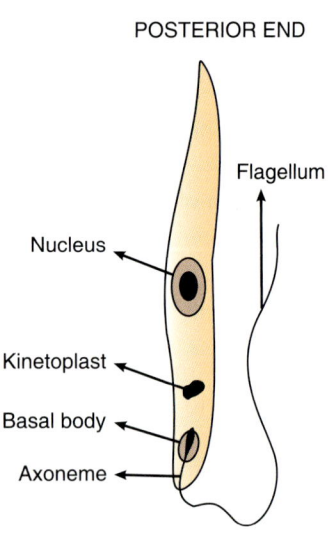

Fig. 49—Diagrammatic representation of the morphology of promastigote form of *L. donovani*.

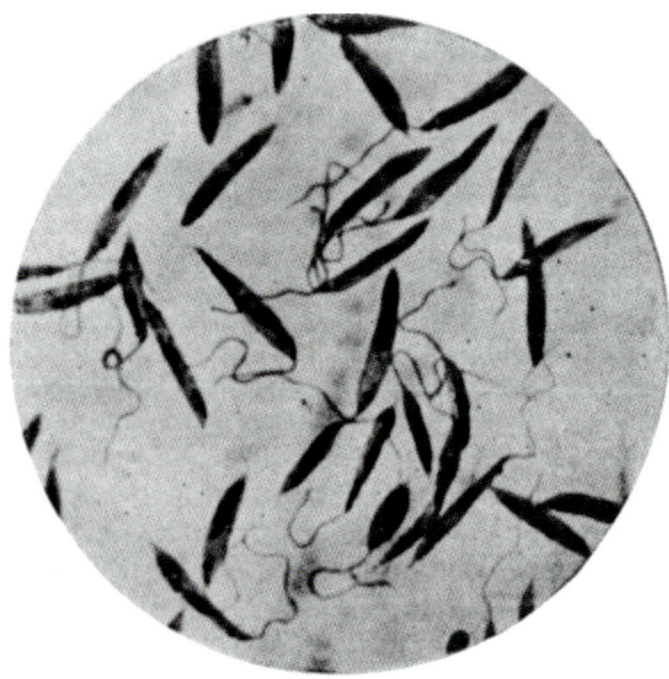

Fig. 50—Promastigote forms of *L. donovani*.
Smear from a culture.

commonly referred to as N.N.N. medium. The material for culture is inoculated into the water of condensation of the medium and incubated at 22° to 24°C. Special care should be taken to avoid contamination with bacteria which would otherwise cause degeneration and death of *L. donovani*. It has been shown that the presence of ascorbic acid and haematin, favours the growth of the parasite. *See Appendix* I

In N.N.N. medium, the amastigote form changes into promastigote form which then multiplies actively by longitudinal fission to produce a large number of flagellates. In the laboratory, a strain may be preserved by making subcultures every 2 or 3 weeks.

The intracellular growth of *L. donovani* can be maintained in tissue culture at 37°C for as long as 32 days.

Susceptible Animals. The dog has been found to be naturally infected with L. donovani in the Mediterranean region and elsewhere, producing a disease resembling in many ways infantile kala-azar.

Common *laboratory animals*, such as mice, rats and guinea pigs are not suitable for transmission of infection. A small rodent of North China, called a *hamster (Cricetulus griseus)* has been found to be very susceptible to *L. donovani* infection. Syrian and European hamsters can also be infected. These animals are used in the laboratory for transferring the infection and working out the details of sandfly transmission. Infected hamsters have also been utilised for testing the efficacy of leishmanicidal drugs.

Immunology. Amastigotes developing from promastigotes excite a cellular reaction comprising histiocytic proliferation followed by invasion of lymphocytes and plasma cells. The former give shelter to *Leishmania* inside which the parasites multiply. The latter help to eliminate the parasites by a process of cell-mediated immunity through sensitised lymphocytes, destroying leishmania-filled macrophages. In *L. donovani* infection, owing to lack of host response due to immuno-suppressive effect, the cell-mediated immunity and delayed hypersensitivity reaction of the skin to leishmanin antigen (a positive intradermal test—Leishmanin or Montenegro reaction) do not develop until the visceral infection has been cured. Hence the cells of the R. E. System of the affected organs proliferate and become heavily parasitised, accompanied by an increase in the IgG fraction of the serum gamma globulin (hyper-gammaglobulinaemia) which however is not protective but is responsible for formol gel reaction. The increase in gamma globulin causes a reversal of albumin-globulin ratio (normally globulin is 2 g and albumin 4.5 g per 100 ml and in kala-azar globulin becomes 4 g and albumin 2.8 g per 100 ml).

Specific antibodies, such as complement-fixing, haemagglutinating and fluorescent antibodies which develop in kala-azar can be used for diagnostic purposes.

Life Cycle. The parasite has two stages (Fig. 51) in its life cycle:
1. The amastigote form, occurring in man (also in dog in some areas).
2. The promastigote form, occurring in sandfly.

The *amastigote form* while residing in the cells of the reticulo-endothelial system, multiplies by binary fission. Multiplication goes on continuously till the cell becomes packed with the parasites. The host-cell is thereby enlarged and eventually ruptures (as many as 50 to 200 or even more may be found embedded in the cytoplasm of the enlarged host-cell). The parasites liberated as a result of the rupture into the circulation are again either taken up by, or invade fresh cells and the cycle is repeated. In this way, the entire reticulo-endothelial system becomes progressively infected. In the blood stream, some of the free amastigotes are phagocytosed by the neutrophilic granulocytes and monocytes (macrophages). A blood-sucking insect draws these free amastigote forms as well as those within the monocytes during its blood-meal.

In certain species of sandfly, these amastigote forms develop into *promastigote forms* which again multiply by binary fission producing an enormous number of flagellates. Multiplication proceeds in the mid-gut of the sandfly and the flagellates tend to spread forwards to the anterior part of the alimentary canal (pharynx and buccal cavity). A heavy pharyngeal infection of the sandfly is usually observed between the 6th and the 9th day of its infective blood-meal. This type of development is known as anterior station development. The transmission is thereby effected through the bite of the infected sandfly (salivary glands are not infected).

Reservoirs of Infection. In Mediterranean areas, China and Brazil, the dog is considered to be the reservoir of infection for man. Canine leishmaniasis does not exist in India where human kala-azar is endemic; hence in India man is the main or only source of infection. In Sudan and East Africa, it is primarily a rodent infection and in Russia (rural areas) the jackals are the reservoirs of infection.

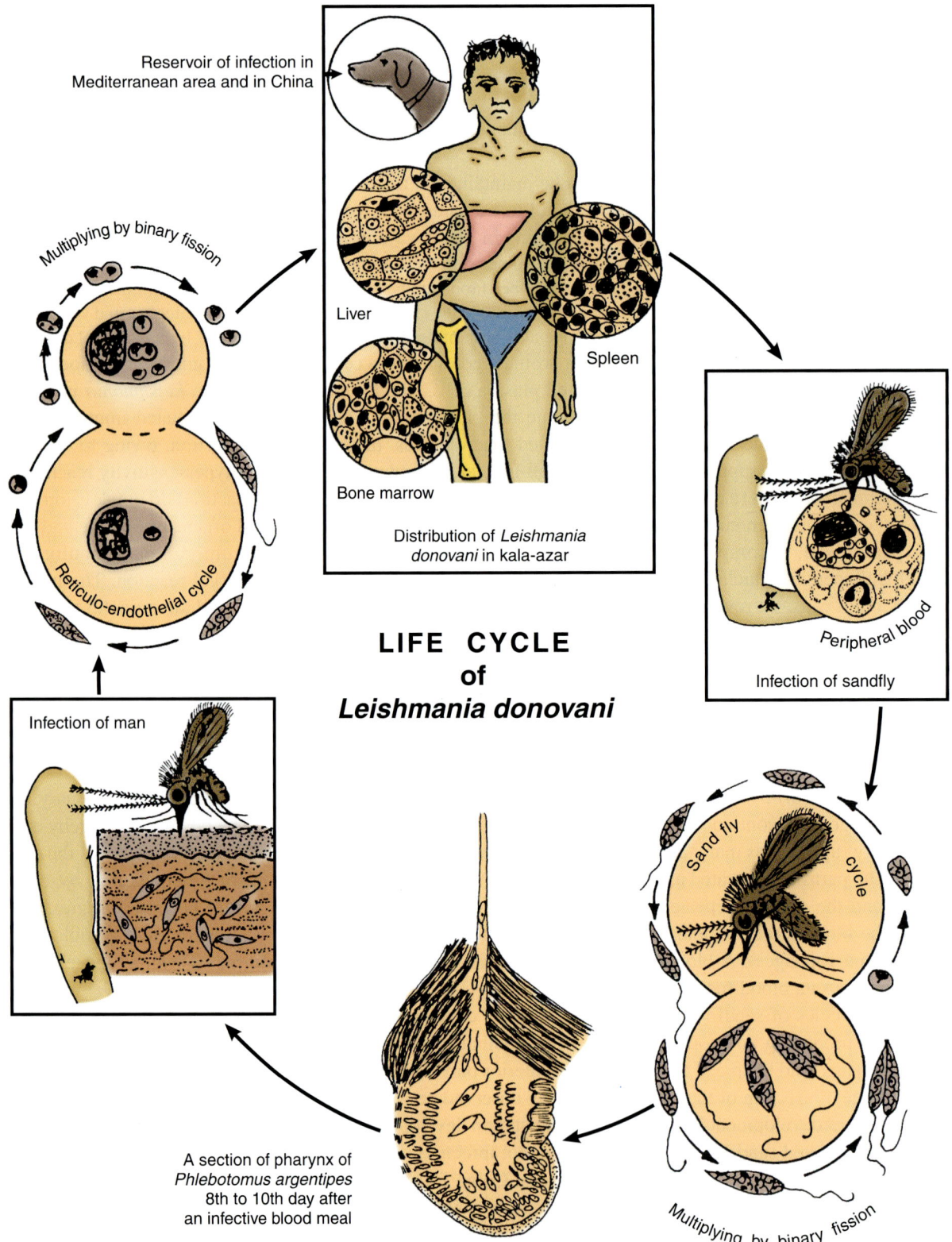

Reservoir of infection in Mediterranean area and in China

Multiplying by binary fission

Reticulo-endothelial cycle

Liver

Spleen

Bone marrow

Distribution of *Leishmania donovani* in kala-azar

LIFE CYCLE of Leishmania donovani

Peripheral blood

Infection of sandfly

Infection of man

Sand fly cycle

Multiplying by binary fission

A section of pharynx of *Phlebotomus argentipes* 8th to 10th day after an infective blood meal

Fig. 51—Development stages of *L. donovani* in man and sandfly.

Method of Transmission. The "natural" transmission of *L. donovani* from man to man is carried out by a certain species of sandfly of the Genera Phlebotomus and Lutzomyia. The species concerned are as follows:

Indian vector—*Phlebotomus argentipes*.

Mediterranean vectors—*Phlebotomus perniciosus* (Italy and Sicily), *Phlebotomus major* (Crete) and *Phlebotomus perniciosus* var. *langeroni* (Sudan).

Chinese vectors—*Phlebotomus chinensis* and *Phlebotomus sergenti* var. *mongolensis*.

Sudanese vector—*Phlebotomus orientalis*.

East African (Kenya) vector—*Phlebotomus martini*.

Brazilian vector—*Lutzomyia longipalpis*.

Russian vector—*Phlebotomus arpaklensis*.

L. donovani undergoes a specific development in various species of sandflies but only where there is a biological relationship, the promastigote forms (flagellates) after multiplying, ascend to the pharynx and enter the proboscis. As already stated, due to the fact that 6 to 9 days elapse before these flagellate forms reach the pharynx and the buccal cavity, it is believed that the sandfly is not infective until that time.

Then again the development of flagellates and their transmission by the female sandflies depend upon whether they have fed on suitable fruit or plant juices before their second blood-meal. The sandfly which subsists on fruit or plant juices after the first blood-meal shows a heavy flagellate infection, its pharyngeal and buccal cavity becoming completely blocked by the flagellates. Bites of such "blocked" sandflies on susceptible persons almost invariably cause infection, as in order to take a blood-meal the sandfly has to liberate the flagellates into the wound caused by its proboscis. Some of the flagellates, thus entering the circulation directly are destroyed while some take refuge inside the cells of the reticulo-endothelial system; here, they change into amastigote forms and undergo slow multiplication. The flagellates remaining in the local depot of the subcutaneous tissues are taken up by the clasmatocytes where the promastigote forms change into amastigote forms and thereafter undergo multiplication. These parasitised cells may also enter the general blood stream as wandering macrophages, leading to a general infection.

Other Methods of Transmission. These include (a) congenital infection* of a child *in utero*, (b) transmission by blood transfusion, (c) transmission by inoculation of cultures of *L. donovani*, and (d) possible transmission during coitus. Regarding the last method, Symmers** (1960) reported a curious case of a woman who had never left England but who developed a leishmanial sore on the vulva, her husband had inadequate treatment of Sudanese kala-azar some years before. Cutaneous leishmaniasis may be transmitted through vaccination*** and through sucking of nipple.****

Pathogenicity of *Leishmania donovani*

Incubation Period. This is the period between the time of the initial infection and the appearance of clinical manifestation. It generally varies from 3 to 6 months, but it may exceed one and sometimes two years.

A primary skin lesion (leishmanioma) preceding visceral disease has been observed in Sudan and Middle Asia but not in India and South America. It has also been observed in Kenya that artificial inoculation into the skin of a culture of promastigotes from either a human, gerbil or ground squirrel strain of *L. donovani* produces a nodule (leishmanioma) about 1 to 1½ inch in diameter in 1 to 3 weeks' time.

Clinical Features. Infection with *L. donovani* produces the disease kala-azar or visceral leishmaniasis, characterised by the following:

Pyrexia is often an early symptom and it may be continuous or remittent in type, becoming intermittent at a later stage. In 20 per cent of cases, pyrexia shows a double rise in 24 hours. Waves of pyrexia may be followed by apyrexial period. Thus, often it becomes very difficult to elicit from the patient the exact duration of fever.

Splenic enlargement is one of the most striking features and the organ progressively enlarges. With the progress of the disease, it extends several inches below the costal margin, often filling up the entire abdomen. However, the rate of spleenic enlargement may not always synchoronise with the duration of illness & moreover the rate of spleenic enlargement may vary from patient to patient.

---

* Banerjee, D. N. (1955). J.I.M.A., **24**, 433.

** Symmers, W.St.C. (1960). Lancet, **1**, 127.

*** Gundors, A.L. (1987). Vaccination: Past and future role in control. *In* Peters, W. and Killick, Kendrick, R. (eds). The Leishmaniasis in Biology and Medicine, Vol. 2, Orlando: Academic Press, 929-941.

**** Marsden, P.D. et. al. (1985). *Leishmania braziliensis braziliensis infection* of the nipple, BMJ; **290**, 433-434.

The liver is also enlarged but not as much as the spleen.

Lymphadenopathy may be observed in African and Chinese form. Recently it has been detected in some cases India also.

General Features. There is no malaise or apathy and the patient may be quite unaware of the high fever. The patient has a good appetite and a clean moist tongue. Epistaxis may be a presenting symptom. In a fully developed case, emaciation and anaemia become noticeable.

The *skin* over the entire body is dry, rough and harsh and is often pigmented (darkened). The hair tends to be brittle and falls out. In African kala-azar warty eruption on the skin and mucocutaneous lesion may appear.

If left untreated, 75 to 95 per cent of the patients die within a period of 2 years. Death in kala-azar is always due to some complications, such as amoebic or bacillary dysentery, pneumonia, pulmonary tuberculosis, cancrum oris (seen in cases of severe neutropenia) and other septic infections.

It is to be noted that a profound immuno-suppressive effect has been observed in kala-azar and this may lead to secondary bacterial invasion, which the patient will not be able to resist.

Globally leishmaniasis has become a common oppertunistic infection in HIV infected persons (mainly among injectable drug users). Atypical features of the disease like involvement of CNS, lung, intestine, etc. are found in those patients and the disease is also refractory to treatment. Dermal leishmaniasis is less found during immunosuppressive state.

Distribution of Parasites. The parasite (*L. donovani*), after entering the host, invades the cells of the reticulo-endothelial system where it resides and multiplies. Thus, the parasites are distributed all over the body and are particularly found in tissues rich in reticulo-endothelial cells. Localisation of parasite inside these macrophage cells constitutes an actual pathological "block-ade" as produced experimentally by intra-vitam methods of staining with certain non-toxic dyes, such as Indian ink, carmine and trvpan blue. The essential lesion in *L. donovani* infection therefore, consists of proliferation of reticulo-endothelial tissue of the spleen, liver, bone marrow and lymph nodes, which become heavily parasitised.

Pathogenic Lesions

CHANGES IN THE SPLEEN

Macroscopic Appearance (Fig. 52):

(i) The organ is enormously enlarged.

(ii) The capsule of the enlarged spleen is often thickened due to perisplenitis.

(iii) The organ is soft in consistency and cuts easily without any resistance, as if the knife were passing through a muscle or liver.

(iv) The cut surface shows marked congestion and has a dull red or chocolate colour. In fresh specimens, it shows small alternate areas of elevation and depression.

(v) The substance of the splenic tissue is friable and can easily be broken down by the pressure of the thumb, signifying the absence of any fibrosis.

Microscopic Appearance (Fig. 53):

(i) The vascular spaces are widely dilated and engorged with blood.

(ii) The reticular cells of Billroth cords are markedly increased and are packed with amastigote forms of *L. donovani*; the sinus lining cells (littoral cells) do not contain any parasite.

(iii) There is no evidence of fibrosis in the parenchyma but there may be a slight increase of reticulin fibrils to give support to the proliferating cells.

(iv) The trabeculae are thin and atrophic.

(v) The Malpighian corpuscles disappear almost completely due to the pressure of the hyperplastic pulp tissue.

(vi) There is often an increase of plasma cells.

CHANGES IN THE LIVER. The organ is enlarged and congested. The cut surface may show a nutmeg appearance. Microscopically (Fig. 54), it shows the following changes:

(i) The Kupffer's cells are greatly increased in size and number and their cytoplasms are packed with amastigote forms of *L. donovani*.

(ii) The sinusoidal capillaries are dilated and engorged with blood.

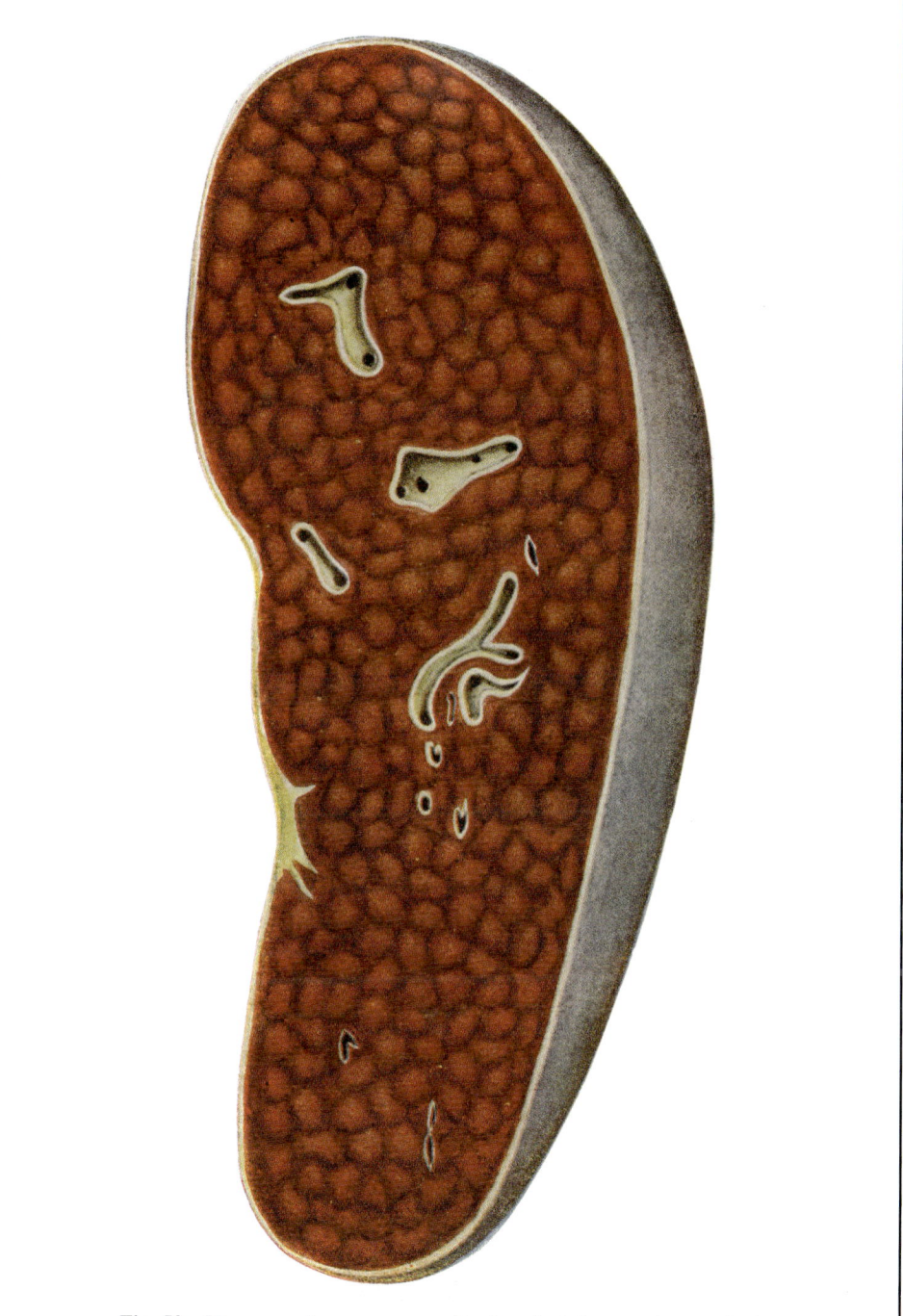

Fig. 52—Macroscopic appearance of spleen in kala-azar (*cut section*).
Showing a greatly enlarged and intensely congested organ with alternate
areas of elevation and depression.

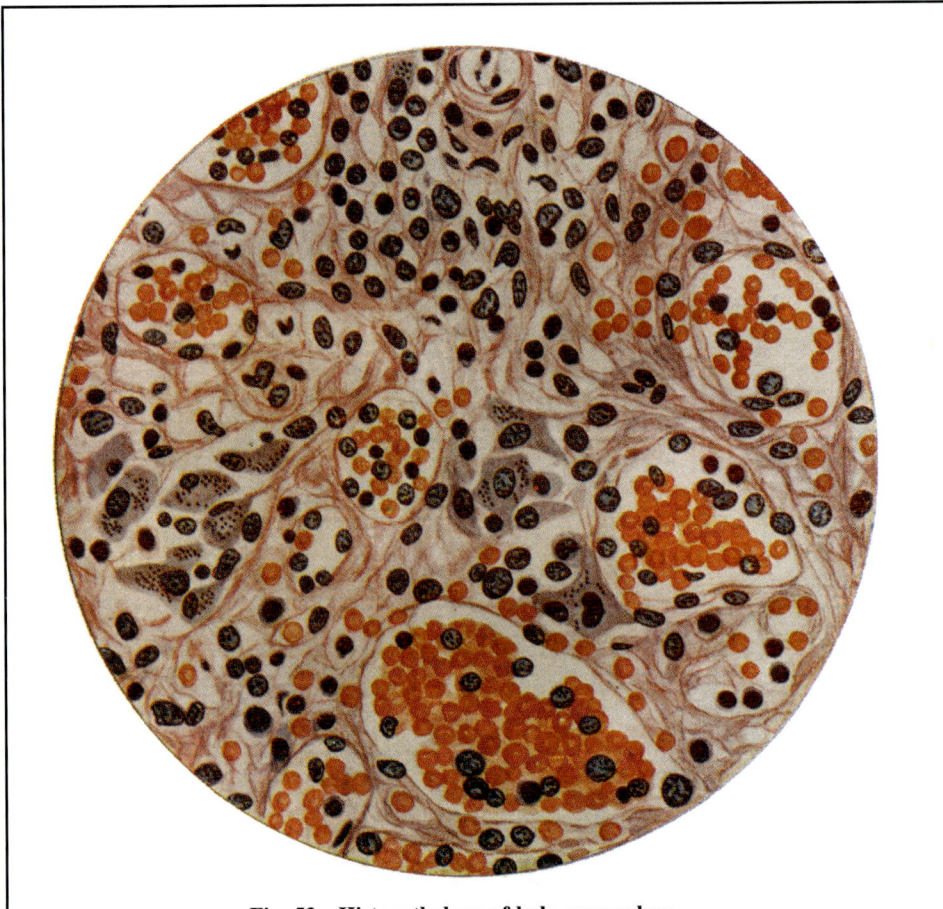

Fig. 53—Histopathology of kala-azar spleen.
An area of pulp tissue showing proliferated reticulo-endothelial cells,
some of which contain *L. donovani*. Sinusoids are dilated and congested.
(Stained with iron-haematoxylin and eosin; seen with oil-immersion lens.)

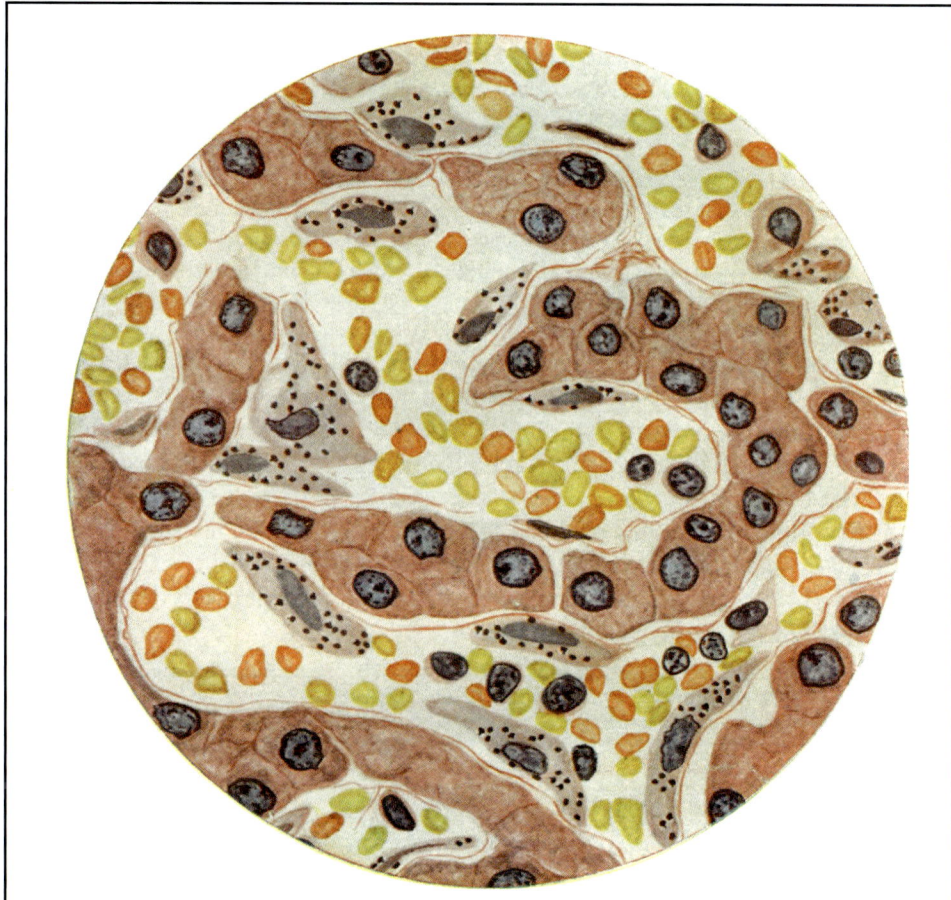

Fig. 54—Histopathology of kala-azar liver.
Showing dilatation and congestion of sinusoidal capillaries, healthy liver cells and parasitisation
of Küpffer's cells (stained with iron-haematoxylin and eosin; seen with oil-immersion lens).

(iii) The liver cells are free from parasitisation. They may undergo thinning and atrophy due to the pressure of dilated sinusoidal capillaries. A certain amount of fatty change may be present.

(iv) Fibrous tissues in the liver are not increased to any great extent, but there is a slight increase of reticulin fibrils developing as a result to reticulo-endothelial proliferation.

JAUNDICE IN KALA-AZAR. Unless the liver is greatly damaged, jaundice does not appear as a manifestation of kala-azar.

CHANGES IN THE BONE MARROW. The reticulo-endothelial tissue undergoes extensive hyperplasia under the stimulus of leishmania infection. This produces a profound disturbance of the haemopoietic activities in the bone marrow, particularly of the leuco-blastic elements resulting in leucopenia (neutropenia) which progressively increases with the advance of the disease. *Microscopically* the marrow reveals a considerable replacement of the haemopoietic tissues, by the proliferated and parasitised macrophage cells (Fig. 55); an increase of plasma cells is also noticeable (see Fig. 57). Demonstration of amastigote forms of the parasite in a smear preparation of the marrow obtained by sternal or iliac crest puncture is utilised for the diagnosis of kala-azar.

Anaemia in kala-azar. A profound anaemia with haemoglobin level 5-10 g/100 ml may occur in kala-azar. The cause of this anaemia in the past was thought to be due to marrow hypoplasia resulting from "crowding out" of erythropoietic tissue by proliferation of parasitised reticulo-endothelial cells. More careful studies of bone marrow however revealed that the erythropoiesis is hyperplastic. Ferrokinetic studies carried out by radioactive isotopic technique demonstrated that in kala-azar the newly formed erythrocytes incorporated the radioactive iron ions in almost normal amounts. Hence, it is unlikely that the marrow hypoplasia is the main cause of anaemia. Haemolysis as a possible mechanism (red cells sequestered and destroyed in the spleen) is now thought to play an important part in the production of anaemia in kala-azar. The presence of a short erythrocyte life span (the survival time of red cells reduced by 50%), anti-red cell antibody, positive Coombs' test (coating of red cells with a complement-containing complex) and antibodies against white cells and platelets suggests an autoimmune basis for the pancytopenia observed in kala-azar (Woodruff, A. W. *et al. Br. J. Haemal.,* **22**, 319, 1972).

CHANGES IN THE LYMPH NODES. These being part of the reticulo-endothelial system are also expected to be involved, but the changes are not constant. Parasites have been observed in the lymph nodes from cases occurring in China and Mediterranean areas* but usually not in those from India. Only two cases of lymphadenopathy in Indian kala-azar with numerous parasites in the aspirated smear have so far been reported (Sen Gupta, 1961; Sen Gupta and Mukherjee, 1968).

CHANGES IN THE INTESTINES. Intestinal lesions are not a feature of kala-azar. The intestinal ulcers found in cases of kala-azar are due to secondary infection, and not to *L. donovani.*

Laboratory Diagnosis. The various laboratory procedures adopted for the diagnosis of kala-azar are shown in the table below:

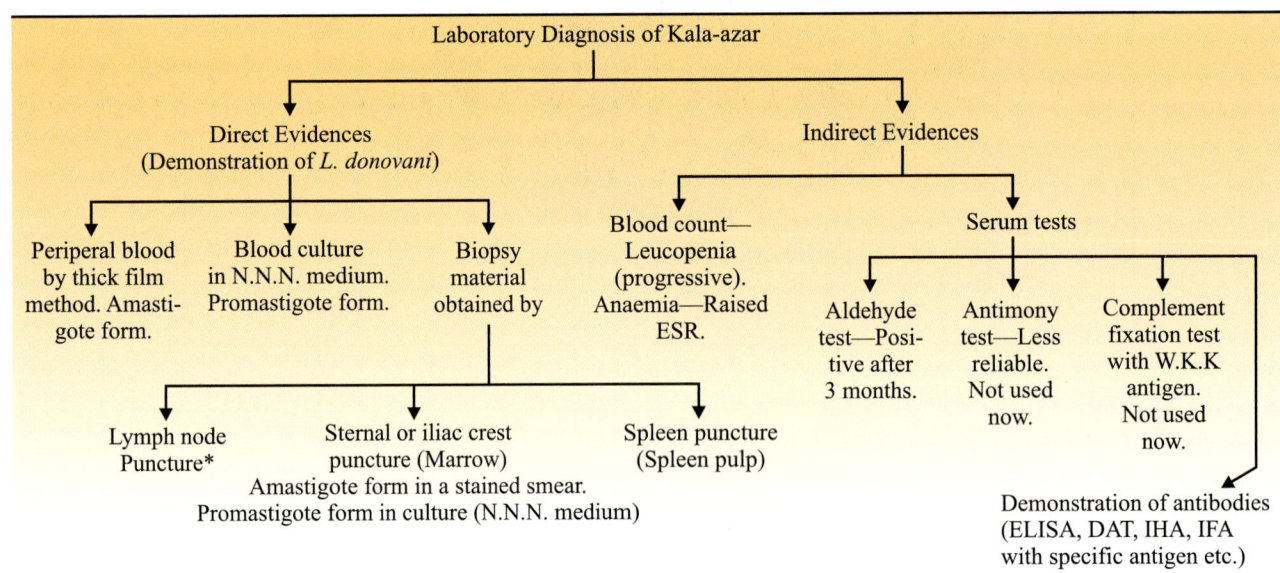

*In cases of Chinese and Mediterranean kala-azar, but rarely in cases of Indian kala-azar.

Leishmanin Test. A killed culture (0.1 to 0.2 ml of a suspension containing 6 to 10 millions of the promastigotes per ml) is injected intradermally. A positive reaction (an area of induration after 72 hours) is produced in cured kala-azar cases 6 to 8 weeks after recovery and represents a delayed hypersensitivity reaction accompanied by cell-mediated immunity. The test is positive in African kala-azar, but not in Indian and Mediterranean kala-azar. The test is negative in untreated kala-azar and post-kala-azar dermal leishmaniasis (P.E.C. Manson-Bhar, 1961).

Adler's Test. The development of the promastigote forms of *Leishmania* in Locke's serum agar can be inhibited by a specific immune serum, but can take place in a heterologous serum. Thus, the three species of Leishmania, *L. donovani, L. tropica* and *L. brasiliensis* can be differentiated serologically to a certain extent, although morphologically, culturally or by animal inoculation they are indistinguishable.

1. Direct Evidences. One of the most conclusive evidences in the diagnosis of kala-azar is the demonstration of the parasite. A parasitological diagnosis may be achieved in one of the following ways: (*a*) Microscopical examination of a stained film, and (*b*) cultural examination.

Materials to be Examined:

   (i) Splenic pulp tissue: Biopsy material obtained by splenic puncture.

  (ii) Marrow: Biopsy material obtained by sternal or iliac crest puncture.

 (iii) Blood: Blood film and blood culture.

 (iv) Lymph node: Lymph node aspirates or biopsy. (See Appendix I)

SPLEEN PUNCTURE. When the organ is considerably enlarged, *it is one of the most valuable methods for establishing the diagnosis*. The amastigote forms (Fig. 56) are found in stained films and promastigote forms in culture. The only risk of spleen puncture is that bleeding might continue from the puncture wound in the soft and enlarged spleen, resulting in death. The risk of such a haemorrhage can be avoided, if the blood is previously examined to exclude haemorrhagic diathesis and leukaemias.

BONE MARROW BIOPSY (from the sternum or iliac crest). It offers a certain method for diagnosis of kala-azar, particularly in early cases, where the spleen is not sufficiently enlarged as to be punctured. Compared to the spleen puncture, it is a safer procedure, as the risk of haemorrhage is greatly minimised, but it is more painful. Its disadvantage over spleen puncture is that when the parasites are scanty, the examination of aspirated marrow may give a negative result. The amastigote forms (Fig. 57) of parasite can readily be demonstrated in a stained film. The promastigote forms (Fig. 58) are demonstrated when the material obtained is cultured in N.N.N. medium.

Blood. A microscopical examination of a *stained blood film* has often been successful in demonstrating the presence of amastigote forms of the parasite in the peripheral blood. Owing to the small number of leishmania parasites present in the peripheral blood, a casual examination of a thin blood film is often attended with a negative result. The chances of finding *L. donovani* are greatly increased by adopting any one of the following procedures:

   (i) *By making a thick blood film* as recommended for malarial parasites.

  (ii) *By producing a straight leucocytic edge*. While a thin blood film is being drawn and before the blood is almost exhausted, the spreading slide is abruptly lifted off. This will not produce any tailing of the film but a straight edge which will contain a large number of white blood cells. It is only necessary to examine this area for the amastigote forms of *L. donovani*.

 (iii) *By centrifuging citrated blood*. The sediment at the bottom of the tube is withdrawn by means of a capillary pipette, then smeared, dried and stained.

BLOOD CULTURE. It is least sensitive method for diagnosis. A positive result may be obtained in a large number of cases. The only disadvantage of this method is that it is slow and takes a long time (about a month). About 1 to 2 ml of blood is taken aseptically from a vein and diluted with 10 ml of citrated saline solution (0.85 per cent normal saline containing 2 per cent sodium citrate). The cells are then either allowed to settle in a cool incubator (22°C) overnight or centrifuged. The cellular deposit is then inoculated into the water of condensation of N.N.N. medium, and incubated at 22°C for 1 to 4 weeks. At the end of each week, a drop of condensation fluid is examined for promastigote forms.

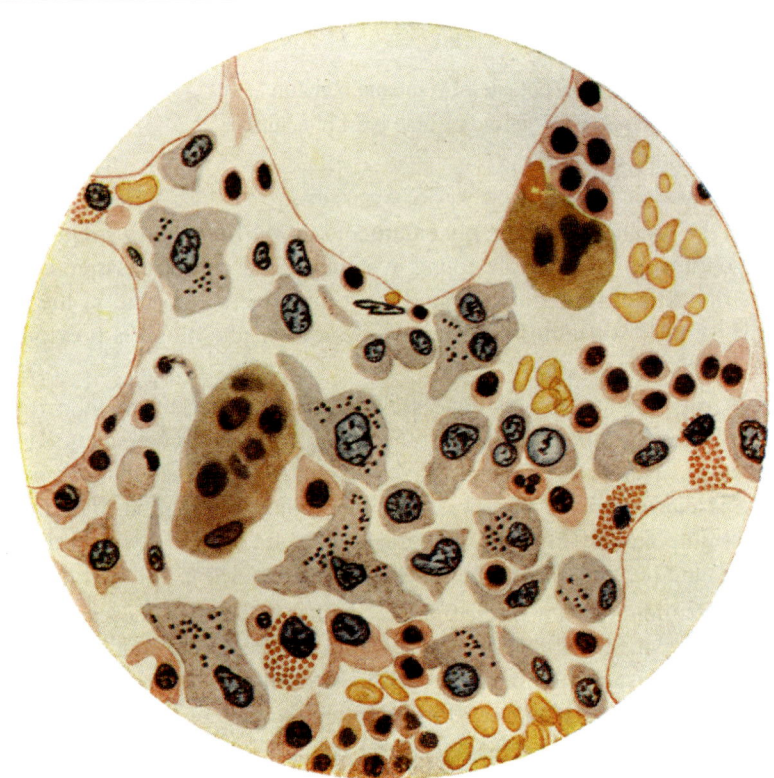

Fig. 55—Histopathology of kala-azar bone marrow.
Showing the diminution of granulocytic elements with increase of erythroblastic tissue
and increase of macrophages which are parasitised. Two megakaryocytes and fat cells
can also be seen. Stained with iron-haematoxylin and eosin; seen with oil-immersion lens.

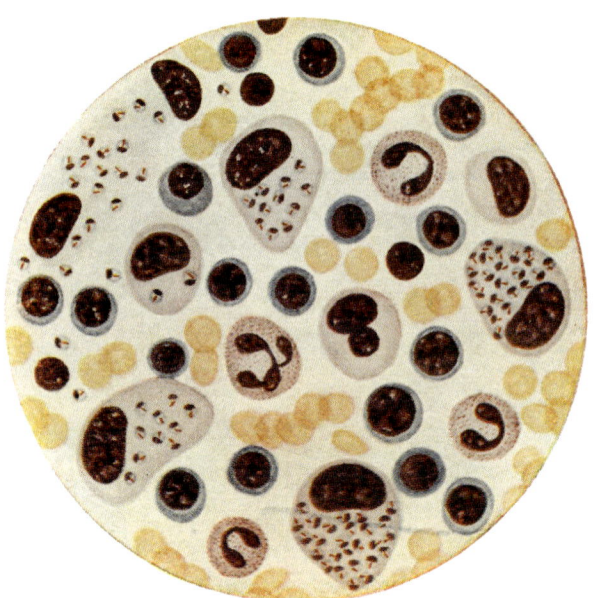

Fig. 56—Smear from material obtained by spleen puncture.
The cytoplasm of macrophage cells is filled with amastigote forms of *L. donovani*.
A few extra-cellular parasites can also be seen. (Leishman's stain)

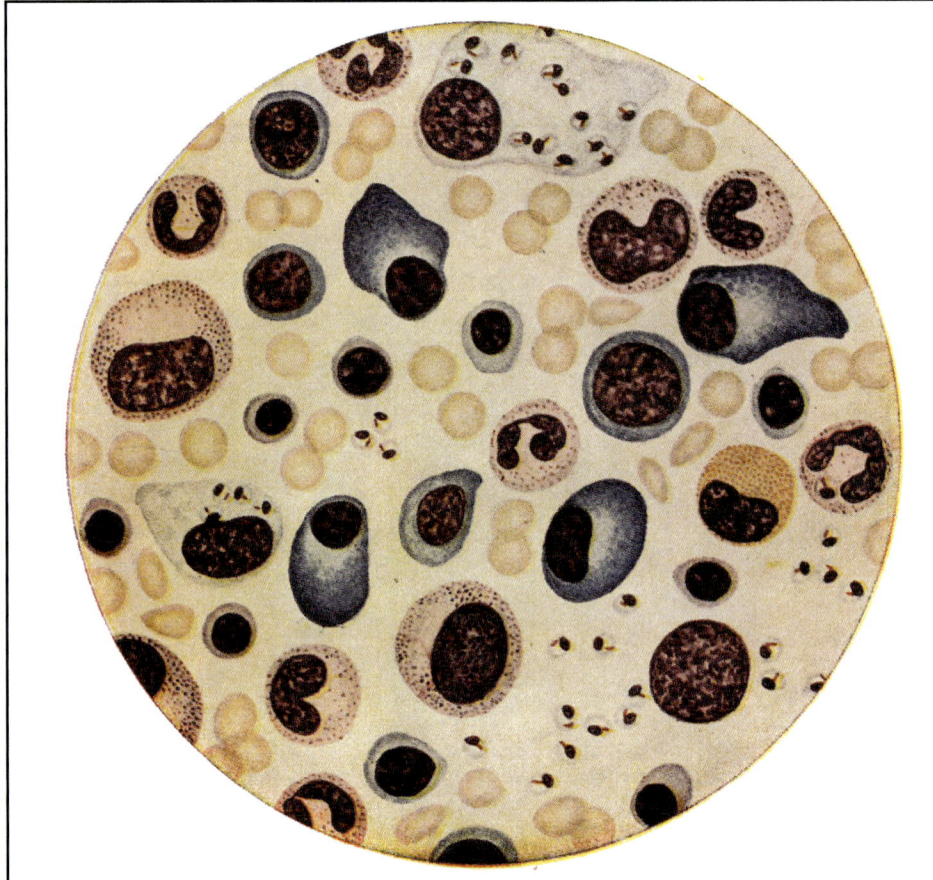

Fig. 57—Smear of marrow fluid obtained by sternal puncture.
Free and phagocytosed *L. donovani* can be seen. Note the different types of
marrow cells and also a few plasma cells. Leishman's stain.

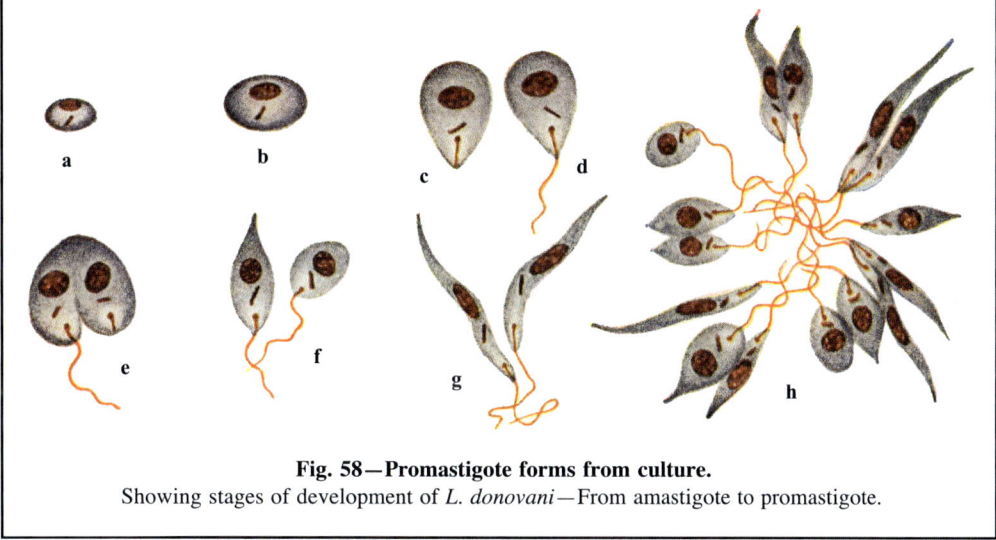

Fig. 58—Promastigote forms from culture.
Showing stages of development of *L. donovani*—From amastigote to promastigote.

2. Indirect Evidences. Infection with *L. donovani* induces certain changes which may be taken as an indication of its presence. They include the following:

 (i) Changes in the blood picture, as revealed by blood count,
 (ii) Changes in the serum resulting from—
   (a) Rise of gamma globulin, detected by aldehyde and antimony tests.
   (b) Development of certain immune bodies, detected by complement fixation test and other tests.

(i) BLOOD COUNT. Examination of leucocyte count reveals *leucopenia* (neutropenia) with a marked diminution of neutrophil granulocytes accompanied by a relative increase of lymphocytes and monocytes. Eosinophil granulocytes are practically absent. The average total count is 3,000 per mm^3 of blood and there is a progressive diminution during the course of the disease, the count falling to 1,000 per mm^3 of blood or even below that. *Agranulocytosis*, an extreme reduction in the granulocytes, although not common, has been reported in a small number of cases.

Erythrocytes are also decreased in number but less so as compared with the neutrophil granulocytes. The proportion of leucocytes to erythrocytes is greatly altered and may be about 1 : 2,000 or 1 : 1,000, the normal being 1 : 750.

(ii) SEROLOGICAL TESTS. (a) *Aldehyde (formol gel) Test* (Napier). Test for rise of gamma globulin: The test depends upon an increase of serum gamma globulin*. About 1 to 2 ml of a serum from a case of kala-azar is taken in a small glass test tube and to it is added a drop or two of 40% formalin. A positive result is indicated by *jellification of milk-white opacity* like the white of a hard-boiled egg. If it occurs in the course of 2 to 20 minutes, the reaction is said to be strongly positive. The aldehyde test is not positive till the disease is of at least three months' duration. The test has also been found to be positive in infections with *S. japonicum* and *T. brucei* (African trypanosomiasis); it is positive in multiple myeloma and cirrhosis liver. The test is negative in cases of cutaneous leishmaniasis.

(b) *Antimony Test* (Chopra *et al.*). This also depends upon a rise of serum gamma globulin. A positive test is indicated by the formation of a *profuse flocculent* precipitate when a 4 per cent urea stibamine solution in distilled water comes in contact with whole serum or a serum diluted 1 in 10 from a kala-azar patient. A negative result is indicated when the two fluids mix without precipitation. As a diagnostic aid antimony test is less reliable than the aldehyde test. Not used nowadays.

(c) *Complement Fixation Test with W.K.K. Antigen.* This test depends upon the presence of certain immune bodies in blood sera of kala-azar patients. The reaction should be considered non-specific in character, as the antigen used is prepared from human tubercle bacillus by Witebsky, Klingenstein and Kuhn, hence called W.K.K. antigen (*Leishmania* and *Mycobacteria* share a common antigen). The test is of distinct advantage in the early diagnosis of the disease, becoming positive within 3 weeks of the infection. The test is positive also in cases of leprosy (particularly lepromatous type), pulmonary tuberculosis and tropical pulmonary eosinophilia. The test is now carried out with an antigen prepared from Kedrowsky's acid-fast bacillus. Not used nowadays.

The tests based on raised globulin level have limited value in diagnosis of VL.

OTHER SEROLOGICAL TESTS. Various serological tests to detect circulating specific antibodies for diagnosis of VL have been developed. Immunoenzymatic technique, immunoblot, countercurrent immunoelectrophoresis, IHA, IFA (most commonly used) are costly and sophisticated. tests for detection of anti-leishmanial antibodies. Other easy tests for detection of anti-leishmanial antibodies include ELISA (dot-ELISA and fast-ELISA), direct agglutination test and Latex particle agglutination test.

Molecular diagnosis (PCA and DNA method of detection) from various types of sample including bone marrow, spleen and blood is a non-invasive method for diagnosis of the disease (VL and CL).

Diagnosis of Acute Kala-azar. For the diagnosis of a case of *acute kala-azar* (an early case of kala-azar of 2 to 6 weeks' duration) one has to depend on the following:

 (i) *Blood count.* The total leucocyte count is diminished (leucopenia) and if the count is made every week, it will show a progressive diminution (progressive leucopenia).
 (ii) *Test for rise of gamma globulin. The aldehyde test* however is negative and it becomes positive only when the disease is of at least 3 months' duration.
 (iii) *Demonstration of parasites*
   (a) In the peripheral blood by a thick film method and by blood culture.
   (b) In the material obtained by a bone marrow biopsy from the sternum or the iliac crest.

---

*Changes in plasma proteins in kala-azar are hypoalbuminaemia and hypergammaglobulinaemia (a gamma globulin which on electrophoresis moves more slowly than the normal gamma globulin).

Note: At this stage, the spleen is not always sufficiently enlarged as to be punctured. Needle aspirated material from spleen is more sensitive method demonstration of the parasite.

A composite diagram showing the clinical, haematological, serological and parasitological findings in a *case of chronic kala-azar* is depicted in Fig. 59.

Treatment. The specific chemotherapeutic drugs include the following:

1. Antimony compounds: Pentavalent antimony compound is now the drug of choice and includes sodium-antimony-gluconate (SAG 600 mg daily for 6-10 days is usually given by IV route. Larger doses 20 mg/kg/day IV for 3-4 weeks may be required in severe cases).

2. Synthetic non-metallic compound: Pentamidine isethionate (4 mg/kg/day IM for 10 days).

Prophylaxis. The preventive measures include the following:

1. *Attack on the Parasite*. In India, control measures should be treatment campaign, whereas in China and Mediterranean areas the campaign should be directed against dogs serving as reservoirs of infection.

2. *Attack on the Vector*. This consists of measures directed against the sandfly, the transmitting agent.

3. *Personal Prophylaxis*. Use of mosquito-net or screen (of 22 meshes to the square inch), voiding the ground floor for sleeping purposes and periodic fumigation of sleeping quarters.

It has been observed in Kenya that intradermal or subcutaneous inoculation of a living promastigote culture of an animal strain isolated from a gerbil or ground squirrel produces an immunity to human strain of *L. donovani*, thereby suggesting the possibility of an active immunisation of a population for the prevention of kala-azar (P. E. C. Manson-Bhar, 1961).

DERMAL LEISHMANOID
(Post-kala-azar Dermal Leishmaniasis)

This is a type of non-ulcerative cutaneous lesion prevalent in endemic areas of kala-azar in India, chiefly in Bengal, less so in Madras and Assam. It develops in about 10 per cent of kala-azar patients generally, one or two years after completion of antimonial treatment for the original disease, when the visceral infection disappears but the skin infection persists. Recently, its incidence appears to have greatly increased. It has also been found in cases of spontaneously cured kala-azar. It is also found in Africa (about 2 %) but rare in China. No cases have been reported from Mediterranean areas and Central and South America.

The clinical manifestations of these dermal lesions may be of three types:

1. DEPIGMENTED MACULES. These are the earliest lesions. The usual sites of distribution of these macules are the trunk and extremities; the face is less commonly affected. The loss of pigmentation is not as complete as is found in the depigmented patches of tuberculoid (neural) leprosy.

2. ERYTHEMATOUS PATCHES. These are also early lesions which appear on the nose, cheeks and chin, often having a butterfly distribution ("butterfly erythema"). They are very photosensitive, becoming prominent towards the middle of the day.

3. YELLOWISH PINK NODULES. These replace the earlier lesions and occasionally appear from the very beginning. The nodules are generally found on the skin and rarely on the mucous membrane of the tongue and eyes. They appear mostly on the face, but may appear on any part of the body. The nodules are soft, painless granulomatous growths of varying sizes (Fig. 60A). The absence of ulceration of the nodules is a characteristic feature as distinct from Oriental sore and espundia.

Sen Gupta and Mukherjee (1968) reported the recurrence of kala-azar in cases associated with dermal leishmanoid and the incidence was found to be 1 in 700 (5 out of 3430 cases). These cases were found to be resistant to antimony treatment.

Diagnosis is established by a microscopical examination of leishman-stained smear prepared from the biopsy material obtained from nodular lesions and demonstrating the amastigote forms of leishmania parasites. Direct smear examination from the depigmented macules does not generally reveal any parasite.

Treatment. Administration of pentavalent antimony compound given in double the doses used for visceral lesions, cures the condition. If a second course is necessary, it should not be repeated within 2 months of the first course. It is to be noted that cases of dermal leishmanoid which developed after being treated for kala-azar, appear to be more

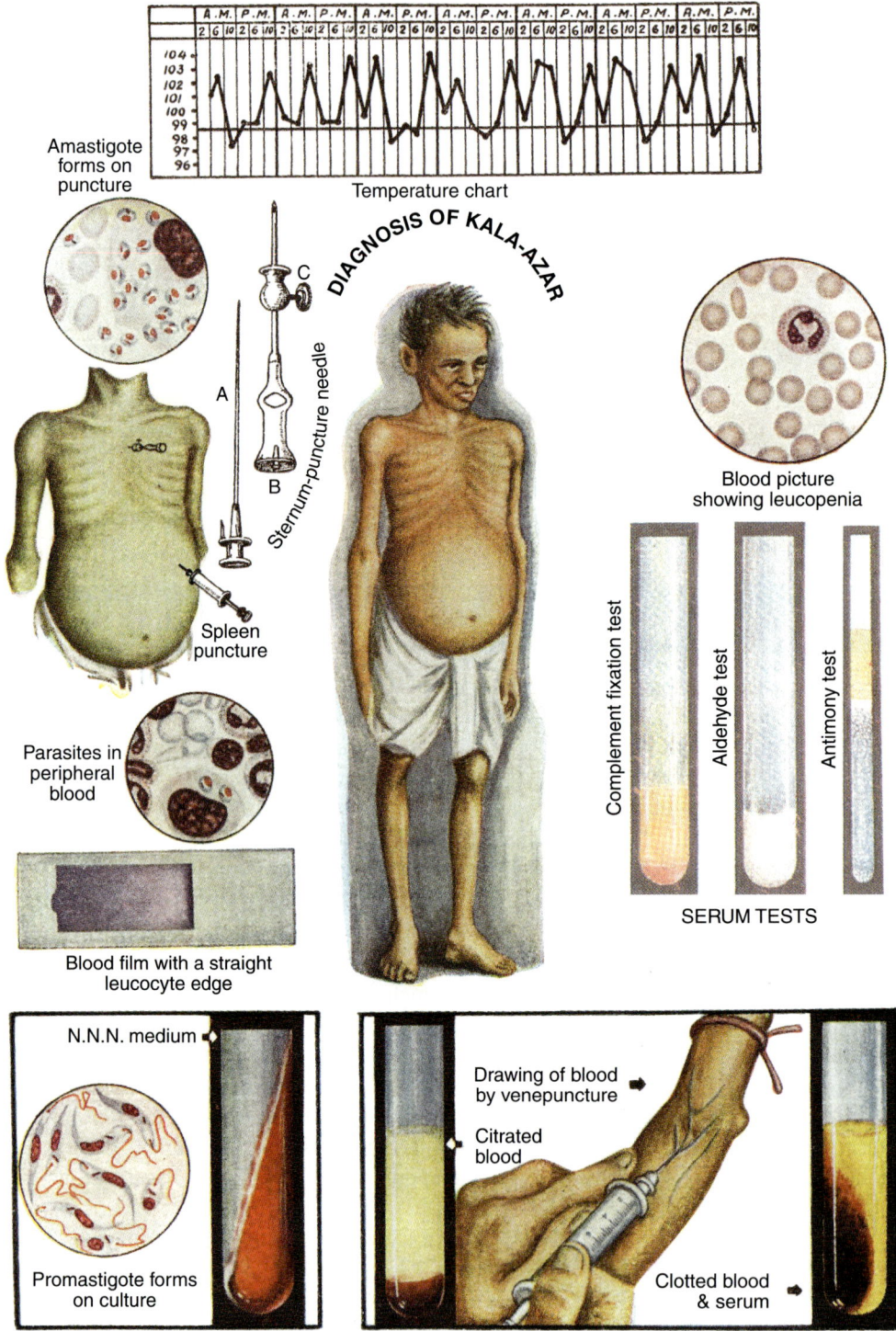

Temperature chart

Amastigote forms on puncture

DIAGNOSIS OF KALA-AZAR

Sternum-puncture needle

A

B

C

Spleen puncture

Parasites in peripheral blood

Blood film with a straight leucocyte edge

Blood picture showing leucopenia

Complement fixation test

Aldehyde test

Antimony test

SERUM TESTS

N.N.N. medium

Promastigote forms on culture

Drawing of blood by venepuncture

Citrated blood

Clotted blood & serum

Fig. 59—A composite diagram showing the methods of diagnosis of a case of chronic kala-azar.

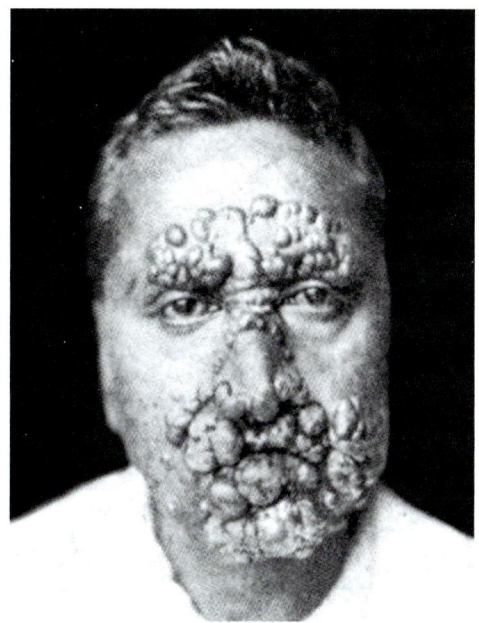

Fig. 60A — A case of dermal leishmanoid.
Showing extensive nodular lesions, resembling a case of lepromatous leprosy.
A very resistant case. Cured after a long continued treatment.

resistant and require higher doses, but cases where no such history is available, the dermal lesions clear up rapidly with a smaller number of injections. In case of failure to treatment with SAG several courses of amphotricin-B infusions are required.

Leishmania tropica (Wright, 1903) Lühe, 1906

The parasite causing cutaneous leishmaniasis or Oriental sore.

Cunningham (1885) first observed the parasite in the tissues of a Delhi boil in Calcutta, but misinterpreted it. Borovsky (1898) and Wright (1903) both gave an accurate description of its morphology and it was Lühe (1906) who gave the name *Leishmania tropica*.

Geographical Distribution. The parasite is found along the shores of Mediterranean, through Syria, Arabia, Mesopotamia; Persia to Central Asia, the drier parts of Central and Western India and also in many places of Central Africa.

Relationship to kala-azar. It is to be noted that although *L. tropica* exists in many countries where *L. donovani* is prevalent, the two parasites are not found in the same locality, and kala-azar is very rare from places (Iraq and Iran) where Oriental sore is endemic. It may be pointed out that in India, kala-azar is confined to moist eastern parts of the country, whereas Oriental sore is limited to dry western parts. In Central Asia and Eastern Mediterranean, they may be found side by side in a single family.

Habitat. Inside the clasmatocytes (cells of R.E. System) of the skin.

Morphology. The amastigote form occurs in man, while the promastigote form is found in cultures and in sandflies. Morphologically, *L. tropica* (Fig. 61) is indistinguishable from *L. donovani*.

Cultivation. The parasite can be easily cultivated in N.N.N. medium (technique same as for *L. donovani*). Cultures can be kept indefinitely by sub-inoculation.

Susceptible Animals. Laboratory animals can be easily infected with *L. tropica*. In Syrian hamsters and occasionally in mice, intraperitoneal inoculation produces a visceral infection.

Human Oriental sore can be reproduced in the spermophile, *Citillus citillus*.

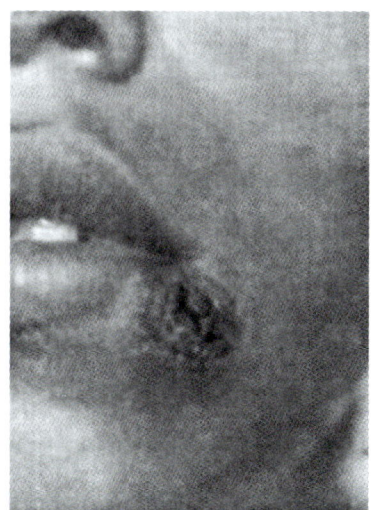

Fig. 60B — Oriental sore on the face of an Indian boy.
Note the granulomatous ulcer near the angle of the mouth.

Immunology. In *L. tropica* infection, a well marked cell-mediated immunity appears early without any serum antibodies but accompanied by the development of a delayed hypersensitivity reaction and elimination of parasites. A single attack of Oriental sore gives life-long immunity. Two conditions in which cell-mediated immune response is ineffective in clearing cutaneous parasites are *leishmaniasis recidiva* and *leishmaniasis tegumentaria diffusa*.

Life Cycle and Method of Reproduction. It is exactly the same as that of *L. donovani* except that the amastigote form resides in the large mononuclear cells of the skin (Fig. 62) and not in the viscera. The amastigote form in man and the promastigote form in sandflies, both divide by binary fission.

Reservoirs of Infection. In endemic areas dogs serve as reservoirs of infection. In desert areas of Central Asia gerbils (*Rhombomys opimus,* a rodent) are the main source of infection.

Mode of Transmission. Sandflies play the role of transmitting agent. They become readily infected by feeding upon cases of Oriental sores. The promastigote forms appear in the buccal cavity of the sandfly in about 3 weeks' time. Infection is transmitted to man either by direct inoculation through the bite of the sandfly or by crushing of the infected sandflies into the punctured wound caused by the bite.

Contamination of the abraded skin with the infected material by direct contact does produce the infection, but this is not the usual mode of transmission.

Species of sandfly responsible for the transmission of the disease in their respective zones:

Phlebotomus papatasii in North Africa and Eastern Mediterranean areas.

Phlebotomus sergenti in Iraq, India and Persia.

Phlebotomus caucadcus and *P. papatasii* in Central Asia.

Pathology. The nature of lesion caused by *L. tropica* is characterised by a chronic infective granuloma with fibrosis. In the early stage, proliferation of the cells of R.E. system (monocytes or macrophages) forms the primary reaction, inside which the parasites are found in large numbers. Later, round cell infiltration (lymphocytes and plasma cells) associated with a marked reduction in the number of parasites and development of a delayed hypersensitive skin reaction (leishmanin reaction) occur.

Clinical Features. Infection with *L. tropica* produces a cutaneous lesion called Oriental sore (tropical sore) or Delhi boil (Fig. 60B). The incubation period varies from a few weeks to 6 months and in some cases, it may be one to two years. The *lesion* begins as a raised nodule about one inch in diameter. In majority of cases, it ulcerates, having a clean-cut margin with a raised indurated edge, surrounded by red areola. The parasite at this stage is not to be found on the floor of the ulcer but along the red margin. The sore has a tendency to heal spontaneously but slowly, taking about 6 months or more. The ulcer is filled up by granulation tissues and a depressed white scar is often left.

The sores are *distributed* on the exposed parts of the body, particularly on the face and extremities. The sores are usually limited to 2 or 3 in number, but sometimes there may be single sore.

Note: Solitary and multiple small, round, painless subcutaneous nodules containing parasites are sometimes found in the draining area of cutaneous lesion. It is due to lymphatic dissemination and is mainly reported with *L. major, L. brasiliensis, L. guyanensis* and *L. panamensis.*

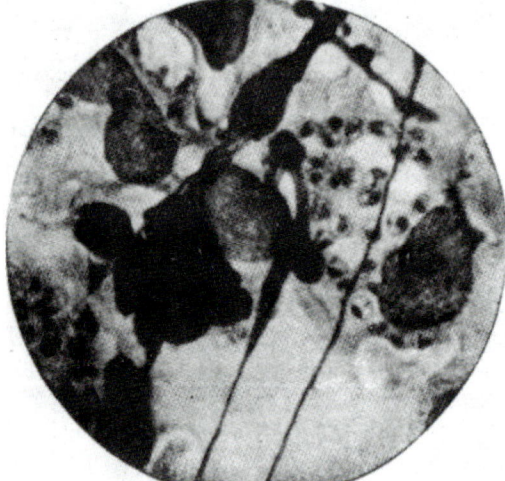

Fig. 61—Morphology of *Leishmania tropica.* Amastigote forms of parasite can be seen inside macrophage cells.

Blood picture shows a normal leucocyte count. Serum aldehyde test is negative and serum gamma globulin normal.

Leishmaniasis recidivan. This is a relapsing form of skin lesion appearing after healing of Oriental sore with a characteristic cellular infiltration resembling cutaneous tuberculides (lupus vulgaris). It is seen in Asia Minor. It is an allergic manifestation without complete immunity in which leishmanin reaction is positive. Histologically, the cutaneous lesion (nodules and papules) consists of epitheloid cells surrounded by lymphocytes, forming typical delayed hypersensitivity granulomas. The parasites are numerous within the epitheloid cells and are thus inaccessible in such granulomatous lesions. This chronic form of leishmaniasis is occasionally due to *L. brasiliensis* in the New World.

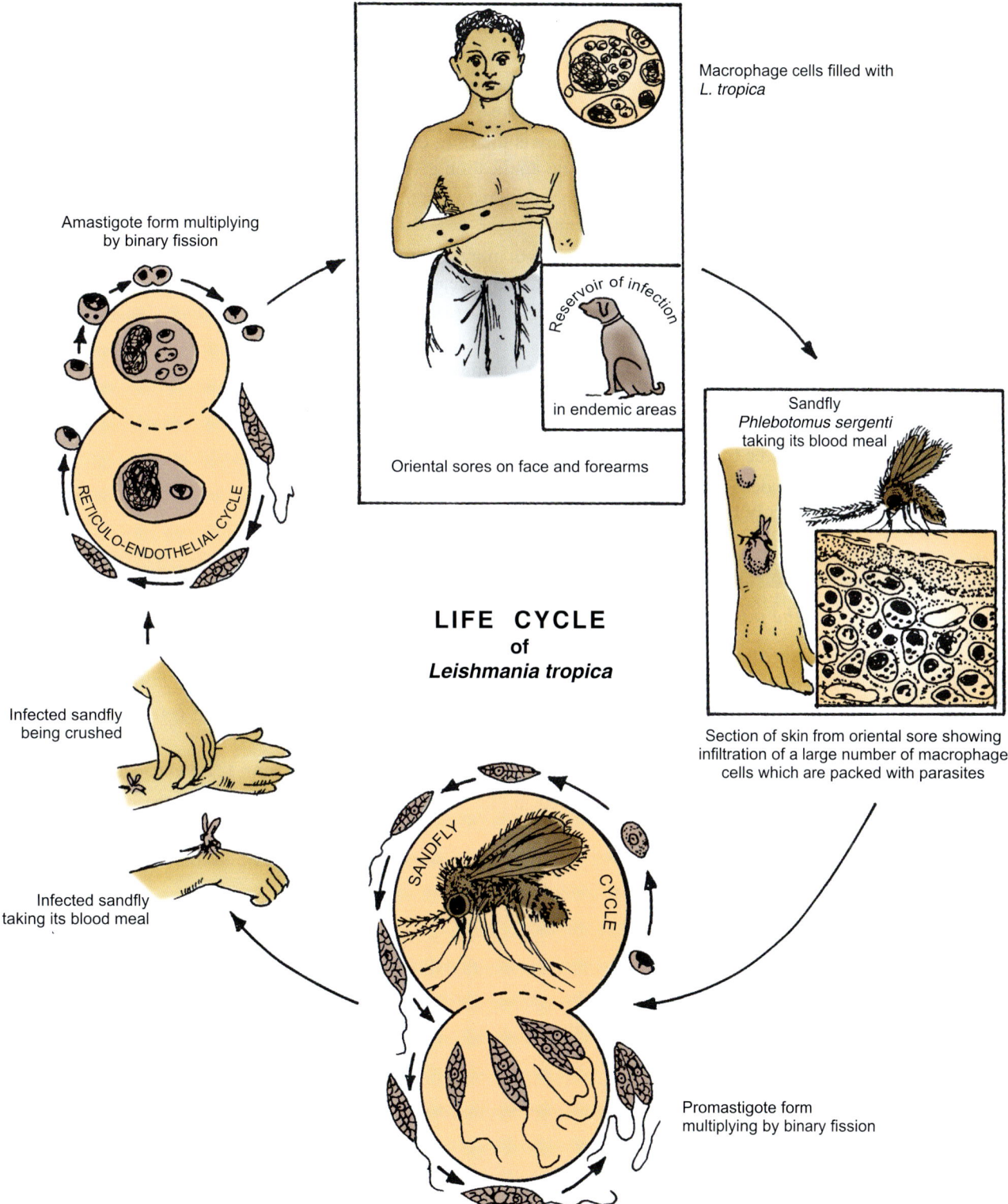

Macrophage cells filled with *L. tropica*

Amastigote form multiplying by binary fission

Reservoir of infection in endemic areas

Oriental sores on face and forearms

RETICULO-ENDOTHELIAL CYCLE

LIFE CYCLE
of
Leishmania tropica

Infected sandfly being crushed

Infected sandfly taking its blood meal

Sandfly
Phlebotomus sergenti
taking its blood meal

Section of skin from oriental sore showing infiltration of a large number of macrophage cells which are packed with parasites

SANDFLY CYCLE

Promastigote form multiplying by binary fission

Fig. 62—Developmental stages of *L. tropica* in man and sandfly.

Laboratory Diagnosis. This consists of a microscopical examination of a smear made from the material obtained by a puncture of the indurated edge of the sore and stained by Leishman's method. Amastigote form of the parasite will be found in large numbers inside the macrophage cells. If the smear is negative, cultures should be made on N.N.N. medium.

Skin Test (*Leishmanin Reaction*). Intracutaneous injection of leishmanin (a suspension of promastigotes) of *L. tropica* gives a positive skin test in cases of Oriental sore.

Treatment. A pentavalent preparation of antimony is the drug of choice. Amphotericin-B and ketoconozole are alternative drugs. Aminosidine ointment and dry heat application give satisfactory result.

Most of the cases with small single lesion heal spontaneously in a few months. Multiple disfiguring lesions require energetic treatment to avoid permanent disfigurment.

Paranteral SAG in a dose of 20 mg/kg/day for 20 days or more is used for treatment of cutaneous lesion. Chest X-ray should be done before starting of paranteral SAG as the drug may lead to flaring up tuberculous lesions, if present.

Local infiltration with SAG in a dose of 1 ml per lesion has been used with encouraging result. It can be repeated for three occasions at the interval of 3-5 days.

Ketonazole (600 mg daily for 4 weeks), fluconazole (200 mg daily for 6 weeks) and itraconazole (200 mg daily for 6 weeks) are also alternative effective drugs and produce good result in cutaneous lesion.

Refractory cutaneous lesion and mucotaneous lesion should be treated with amphotericin-B or liposomal amphotericin-B. Small lesion may be treated by surgical execision and curettage or freezing with liquid nitrogen.

Prophylaxis. This includes (i) elimination of the reservoir hosts (if possible), (ii) control of sandflies, (iii) individual protection from sandfly bites, and (iv) prophylactic immunisation with a culture of *L. tropica*.

*Leishmania braziliensis**

The parasite causing espundia or muco-cutaneous leishmaniasis.

* Carini (1911) first observed the organism **Leishmania brasiliensis** and Vianna (1911) described it as a new species.

Geographical Distribution. Confined to Central and South America.

Habitat. It occurs as an intracellular parasite (amastigote form) inside the macrophage cells of the skin and mucous membrane of the nose and buccal cavity.

Morphology. *L. braziliensis* is morphologically and culturally indistinguishable from *L. donovani* and *L. tropica*.

Cultivation. The parasite can be easily cultivated in N.N.N. medium. It can be grown on the chorio-allantoic membrane of the chick embryo.

Susceptible Animals. Inoculation of cultures into Syrian hamsters causes a local skin lesion only and even intraperitoneal inoculation does not produce any visceral infection.

Life Cycle. It is now known that the insect host of this parasite is a wild species of sandfly (Genus *Lutzomyia*) commonly found in the regions where this parasitic infection prevails. Hence, as in other leishmanias, the sandfly plays the role of the transmitting agent. The life cycle and method of reproduction appear to be identical with those of other types of leishmania.

Reservoir Hosts. These are small forest rodents.

Transmission. South American leishmaniasis is a zoonosis, affecting the skin of small forest rodents and is maintained by a variety of sandflies feeding on them. Man is infected by the bite of anthropophilic sandflies. The disease is auto-inoculable and can also be inoculated from man to man; hence, direct contact plays an important part in the transmission of the infection.

Immunology. In *L. braziliensis* infection associated with metastasis in the skin and mucous membrane, the cell-mediated immunity does not develop until metastasis has taken place.

Pathology. There is no essential difference between the pathology of the skin lesions caused by *L. tropica* and *L. braziliensis*. The initial lesion in American cutaneous leishmaniasis, unlike Oriental sore, has a tendency to enlarge radially forming an ulcer with a clean-cut margin and a weeping surface. *Histological* examination of the skin and the mucous lesion shows infiltration of lymphocytes, plasma cells and large mononuclear cells and necrosis of tissues. The parasites (amastigote forms) are found in large numbers inside the clasmatocytes and monocytes at the periphery of the lesion.

Clinical Features. *The incubation period* is unknown, probably a few days to a few weeks. The clinical manifestation comprises a specific ulcerative granuloma of the skin followed by involvement of the mucocutaneous area in some cases.

Diagnosis. This is confirmed by demonstrating the amastigote forms of *L. braziliensis* in skin and mucocutaneous lesions (smear or biopsy specimen) and an intradermal skin test (a delayed hypersensitivity reaction) using cultures of *L. brasiliensis*.

Leishmaniae are scanty in skin smears in cases of chicle ulcer (Bay sore) and uta, hence biopsy of skin lesion is required. In espundia and DCL amastigotes of *L. braziliensis* can readily be demonstrated in a skin smear or a biopsy specimen.

Treatment. A pentavalent preparation of antimony is the first drug of choice. In resistant cases, amphotericin B may be tried.

Prophylaxis. As it is a zoonotic disease, it is difficult to control the source of infection. Forest workers should therefore take measures to protect themselves against sandfly bites.

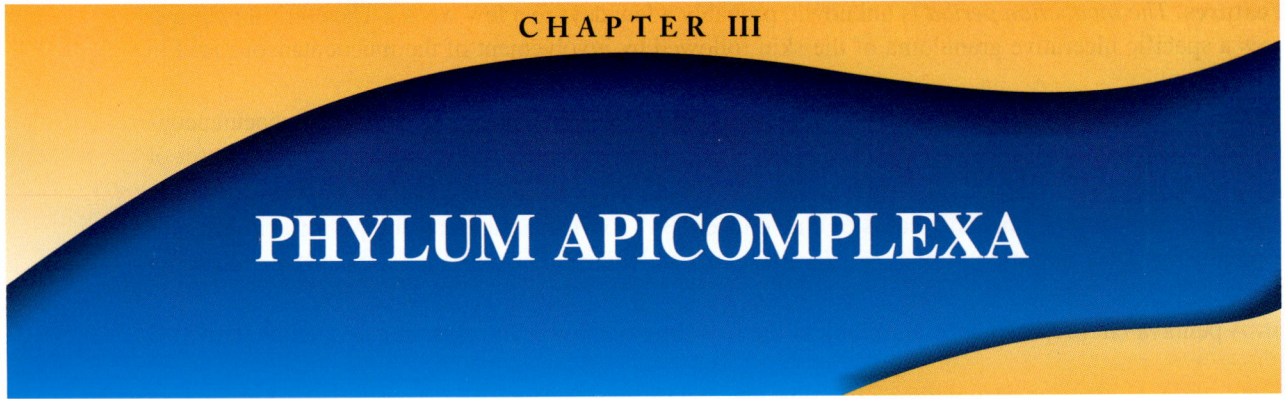

CHAPTER III

PHYLUM APICOMPLEXA

Generic Character. The parasites belonging to this group of protozoa do not possess any special organs of locomotion, such as flagella or cilia. They show only slight amoeboid change of form. They reproduce asexually by schizogony followed by sexual union or syngamy; this is known as alternation of generation. In case of Plasmodia, these two stages of life cycle take place in alternate hosts, so there is not only an alternation of generation but also an alternation of host. The sporozoa infecting man are divided into two main groups:

1. *Intestinal Parasite.* Here, after the sexual union, the development of oöcyst occurs in the passed faeces on the soil and infection is transmitted by contamination.

2. *Blood-inhabiting Parasite.* Here, the sexual union takes place inside the insect host and the infection is transmitted by inoculation.

Systematic Classification of Apicomplexa. Phylum Apicomplexa is classified as follows: class Sporozoea, subclass Coccidia, order Eucocciida. Order Eucocciida has suborders of medical importance: (i) Eimeriina and Haemosporina. Suborder Eimeriina has genera: (a) Eimeria, (b) Isospora, (c) Toxoplasma, (d) Sarcocystis. Suborder Haemosporina has genus Plasmodium.

The genera Cyclospora and Cryptosporidium are recognised, under subclass Coccidia, as new parasites of medical importance and cause parasitic infection in human beings particularly in AIDS patients, like other genera (Isospora, Toxoplasma and Sarcocystis).

Suborder HAEMOSPORINA

Genus PLASMODIUM Marchiafava and Celli, 1885

Generic Character. The parasites belonging to this Genus possess a life cycle which shows an alternation of generation accompanied by an alternation of host. Asexual cycle (cycle of schizogony) occurs inside the red blood cells of the vertebrate host and sexual cycle (cycle of sporogony) occurs in an invertebrate host. The product of schizogony is called a *merozoite* and the product of sporogony is called a *sporozoite*. The gametogony (formation of gametocytes) really starts inside the red blood cells of the vertebrate host and is completed in various species of blood-sucking mosquitoes with the production of sporozoites, the forms infective to the vertebrate host. The malarial parasites of man and other animals belong to this Genus.

Species Parasite of Man. Four recognised and distinct species are: (1) *Plasmodium malariae* (Laveran, 1881), Grassi and Feletti, 1890, (2) *Plasmodium vivax* (Grassi and Feletti, 1890), (3) *Plasmodium falciparum* (Welch, 1897), and (4) *Plasmodium ovale* (Stephens, 1922).

Malarial parasites of primates capable of infecting man. These are:

(i) BENIGN TERTIAN TYPE: (a) *P. cynomolgi* Mayer, 1907, (b) *P. cynomolgi bostianellii* Garnham, 1959, (ii) OVALE TERTIAN TYPE: *P. simium* Fonseca, 1951, (iii) QUARTAN TYPE: (a) *P. inui* (Halberstädter & von Prowazek, 1907), (b) *P. brasilianum* (Gonder & von Berenberg-Gossler, 1908), (c) *P. shortii* Bray, 1963, (*iv*) QUOTIDIAN TYPE: *P. knowlesi* Sinton & Mulligan, 1932.

Species Parasitic to Animals. There are a large number of species which parasitise higher apes, monkeys, birds (sparrows, canaries, domestic fowls, ducks), rodents, bats and cold-blooded animals like lizards. Transmission of malarial parasites of man and monkey is effected by anopheline mosquitoes, while transmission of malarial parasites of bird is effected by culicine mosquitoes. A large amount of experimental work has been carried out with bird malaria, rodent malaria and monkey (simian) malaria.

Landmarks in the Evolution of the Knowledge of Malaria. The name of the disease malaria was given as far back as 1753. It is interesting to note that the treatment of the disease became first established (in the middle of the seventeenth century) before anything was known about its etiology and how the disease was transmitted. Another curious fact is that before the discovery of the plasmodia, the presence of pigment (black material) in organs with malarial infections had been observed by Meckel (1847) and Virchow (1849). The pigmented appearance of spleen and brain in malaria post mortem was however noted also by Lancisi in 1716 and Bright in 1831.

1880   Laveran discovered the malarial parasite in an unstained preparation of fresh blood.

1883   Marchiafava used methylene blue for the staining of malarial parasite.

1885   Golgi demonstrated the erythrocytic schizogony (also known as Golgi cycle) of quartan malarial parasite.

1886   Golgi demonstrated the erythrocytic schizogony of benign tertian malarial parasite; also differentiated the benign and quartan species.

1891   Romanowsky introduced the staining method of malarial parasite.

1897   Ross in Secunderabad found oöcysts on the stomach wall of an anopheline mosquito which had previously fed on a malaria patient.

1898   Ross in Calcutta worked out the mosquito cycle with the parasite of bird malaria, whereas Bignami *et al* demonstrated the same with the parasite of human malaria.

1900   Patrick Manson proved the theory of mosquito transmission.

1934   Tissue phase of malarial parasite was demonstrated in avian malaria.

1948   Shortt and others worked out the pre-erythrocytic schizogony of malarial parasite in the parenchyma cells of liver, first with cynomolgi malaria then with vivax malaria. They also demonstrated the exo-erythrocytic schizogony of malarial parasite in cynomolgi malaria.

1949   Shortt and others demonstrated the pre-erythrocytic schizogony of *P. falciparum*.

1952   Jeffery *et al* demonstrated a three days' old pre-erythrocytic schizont of *P. falciparum* in the human liver.

1954   Garnham *et al* discovered the pre-erythrocytic schizogony of *P. ovale*.

MALARIAL PARASITES OF MAN

(*Plasmodium vivax, Plasmodium falciparum, Plasmodium malariae, Plasmodium ovale*)

Geographical Distribution. Malarial parasites are found in all countries, extending from 40°S to 60°N. The tropical zone is the endemic home of all malarial parasites. While *P. malariae* is a parasite of subtropical zone, *P. vivax* is the prevailing species of the temperate zone. The distribution of *P. ovale* has mainly been reported from East Africa, West Africa especially Nigeria, and Philippines.

Habitat. The malarial parasites infecting man, after passing through a develop mental phase in the parenchyma cells of the liver, reside inside the red blood corpuscles and are carried by the circulating blood to all the organs.

Life Cycle. The malarial parasite passes its life cycle (Fig. 63) in two different hosts.

1. IN MAN: The parasite residing inside the liver cell and the red blood corpuscle reproduces by asexual method (schizogony). Hence man represents the *intermediate host* of the malarial parasite.

2. IN FEMALE ANOPHELINE MOSQUITO: For the initiation of the mosquito cycle, sexual forms (male and female gametocytes) are first developed inside the human host. These are then transferred to their insect host, where they develop further and are transformed into sporozoites. These sporozoites are infective to man. On account of this sexual method of reproduction, mosquito represents the *definitive host* of the malarial parasite.

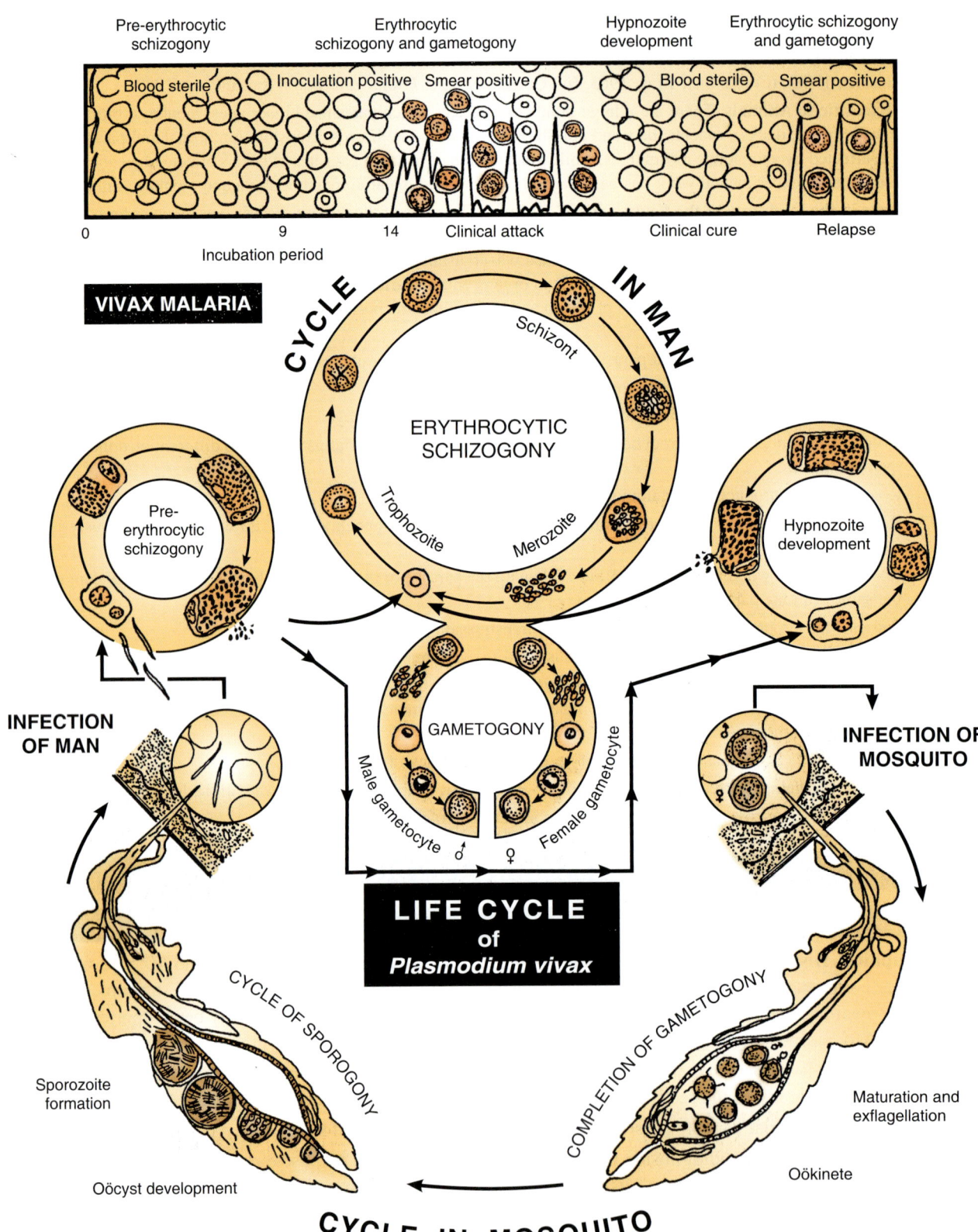

Pre-erythrocytic schizogony

Erythrocytic schizogony and gametogony

Hypnozoite development

Erythrocytic schizogony and gametogony

Blood sterile   Inoculation positive   Smear positive   Blood sterile   Smear positive

0   9   14   Clinical attack   Clinical cure   Relapse

Incubation period

VIVAX MALARIA

CYCLE IN MAN

ERYTHROCYTIC SCHIZOGONY

Schizont

Trophozoite

Merozoite

Pre-erythrocytic schizogony

Hypnozoite development

INFECTION OF MAN

GAMETOGONY

Male gametocyte ♂   Female gametocyte ♀

INFECTION OF MOSQUITO

LIFE CYCLE of Plasmodium vivax

CYCLE OF SPOROGONY

COMPLETION OF GAMETOGONY

Sporozoite formation

Maturation and exflagellation

Oökinete

Oöcyst development

CYCLE IN MOSQUITO

Fig. 63

HUMAN CYCLE

Human cycle starts with the introduction of sprozoites by the bite of an infected anopheline mosquito. It comprises the following stages:

(i) PRE-ERYTHROCYTIC or PRIMARY EXO-ERYTHROCYTIC SCHIZOGONY. Sporozoite* does not directly enter into a red blood corpuscle to start its erythrocytic schizogony, but undergoes a developmental phase inside the tissues of man. This phase of development has been referred to as pre-erythrocytic schizogony and consists of only one generation of pre-erythrocytic schizont, the cycle lasting approximately 8 days in *P. vivax*, 6 days in *P. falciparum* and 9 days in *P. ovale*. The pre-erythrocytic schizogony occurs inside the parenchyma cells of the liver. The liberated merozoites are called *cryptozoites*. The smaller ones (*micromerozoites*) enter the circulation and the larger ones (*macromerozoites*) re-enter the liver cells.

Neither any clinical manifestation nor any pathological damage is produced by the parasite while developing inside the liver. During the pre-erythrocytic schizogony, the parasites are not found in the peripheral blood and inoculation of such blood does not produce any infection, i.e., the blood is sterile.

(ii) ERYTHROCYTIC SCHIZOGONY. During this phase, the parasite resides inside the red blood corpuscle and passes through the stages of *trophozoite, schizont* and *merozoite*. These asexual forms of parasites can be demonstrated in the thick smears of the peripheral blood 3 to 4 days after the completion of pre-erythrocytic schizogony, i.e., in *P. vivax* infection about 12 days and in *P. falciparum* infection about 9 days after exposure. Each cycle of erythrocytic schizogony lasts 48 to 72 hours; in *P. vivax, P. ovale* and *P. falciparum* it is 48 hours, whereas in *P. malariae* it is 72 hours. The parasitic multiplication during the erythrocytic phase is responsible for bringing on a clinical attack of malaria (overt malaria). The schizogony cycle may be continued for a considerable period, but in course of time the infection tends to die out either due to exhaustion of asexual reproductive capacity or to the spontaneous destruction of the parasites.

(iii) GAMETOGONY. After the parasites have undergone erythrocytic schizogony for a certain period (which varies with the different species), some of the merozoites, instead of developing into trophozoites and schizonts, give rise to forms which are capable of sexual function after leaving the human host. These are called *gametocytes* and develop in the red blood cells of the capillaries of internal organs (spleen and bone marrow). Only the mature *gametocytes* are found in the peripheral blood. The maturation is completed in about 96 hours (4 days), i.e., twice the time taken by an erythrocytic schizont to attain full maturity. Gametocytes do not cause any febrile reaction in the human host and are produced for the propagation and ultimate continuance of the species. The individual who harbours the gametocytes is known as a "carrier".

(iv) LATENT STAGE (HEPATIC). After the establishment of blood infection, the initial tissue phase (pre-erythrocytic phase) disappears completely in *P. falciparum*, whereas in *P. vivax* and *P. ovale*, it persists in the liver cell as dormant form (resting phase). This resting phase of parasite (latent stage) is known as *hypnozoite*, which is capable of developing into *merozoits*. This form never arises from asexual parasites of erythrocytic schizogony and are now held to be responsible for relapses of vivax, ovale. In the absence of fresh infection this form is the source of asexual parasites.

Note: There are mainly two phases of development in the human host:
  1. Inside the Liver (Tissue Phase):
     (i) Pre-erythrocytic (or Primary Exo-erythrocytic) Schizogony—No clinical symptom and no pathological damage.
     (ii) Hypnozoite stage— Cause of relapse.
  2. Inside the Red Blood Cell (Erythrocytic Phase):
     (i) Erythrocytic Schizogony—Cause of malarial paroxysm.
     (ii) Gametogony—Infects mosquito.
  The essential difference between the tissue phase and erythrocytic phase of development is that the pigment granules are absent in the former but present in the latter.

---

* *Sporozoite*. It is a minute thread-like curved organism, tapering at both ends. It measures 9-12 ftm in length, has a central elongated nucleus and does not contain any pigment (as seen under light microscope).

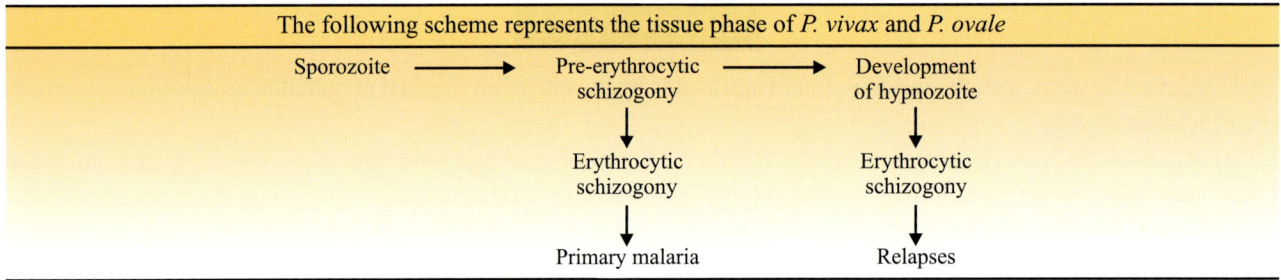

The following scheme represents the tissue phase of *P. vivax* and *P. ovale*

Sporozoite → Pre-erythrocytic schizogony → Development of hypnozoite

Erythrocytic schizogony → Erythrocytic schizogony

Primary malaria → Relapses

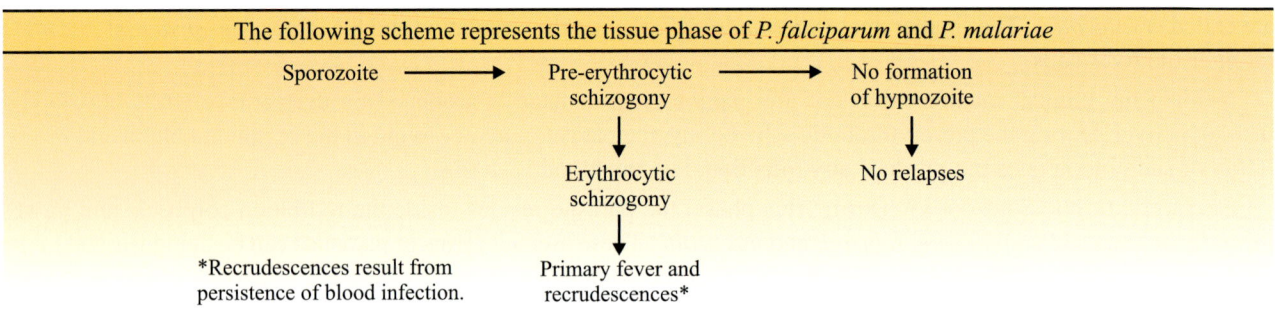

The following scheme represents the tissue phase of *P. falciparum* and *P. malariae*

Sporozoite → Pre-erythrocytic schizogony → No formation of hypnozoite

Erythrocytic schizogony → No relapses

*Recrudescences result from persistence of blood infection.

Primary fever and recrudescences*

MOSQUITO CYCLE

(SEXUAL CYCLE OF MALARIAL PARASITE)

The sexual cycle of malarial parasite first starts in the human host by the formation of gametocytes which are then transferred to the insect host where further development proceeds. A female *Anopheles* during its blood-meal from an infected person, ingests both the sexual and asexual forms of parasite but it is only the mature sexual forms which are capable of development; the rest die off immediately. It has been estimated that in order to infect a mosquito, the blood of a human *carrier* must contain at least 12 gametocytes per mm^3 of blood and the number of female gametocytes must be in excess of the number of males.

The first phase of development occurs inside the mid-gut ("stomach") of the mosquito. From one microgametocyte, 4 to 8 thread-like filamentous structures, *microgametes* are developed. As this process of development can be observed outside in a moist preparation of blood, it is called *ex-flagellation*. The macrogametocyte does not show any flagellation and from one *macrogametocyte* only *one macrogamete* is formed, the maturation occurring by a process of nuclear reduction and extrusion of polar bodies. The crescents of *P. falciparum* at first become rounded in shape and the rest of the maturation process is the same as with the gametocytes of other species. The gametes are ready for fertilisation and by a process of chemotaxis microgametes are attracted towards the macrogametes. One of the male gametes attaches to the periphery of the female gamete at the site of a small protrusion and penetrates inside the body. Fusion takes place between the male and female pronuclei and the resulting body is called a *zygote*. This form is developed in 20 minutes to 2 hours after the mosquito's blood-meal.

In the next 24 hours, the zygote lengthens and matures into an *oökinete* (formerly called a *vermicule*). In the past, it has been a difficult problem to explain the passage of oökinete through the gut-wall of the mosquito. Howard (1906), however suggested that the mucosal cell actually engulfs the oökinete. A study by electron microscope by Garnham *et al* (1962) has given a clue to the mechanism involved (Figs. 64 & 65).

The oökinete first comes to lie in contact with the peritrophic membrane. It passes this barrier and pushes aside the brush border of a mucosal cell and its anterior end comes close to the host cell membrane. The entry of the oökinete into the cell is made possible by the secretion of some proteolytic substance through a slit at the anterior end of the oökinete, which causes lysis of the cell membrane. Later, it is found in the middle of the cell and finally rests against the external border of the cell and basement membrane, where it develops into an *oöcyst*.

The *oöcyst* is a spherical mass surrounded by a structureless capsule; it measures 6 to 12 μm in diameter, containing a single vesicular nucleus and pigment granules of the macrogamete. As the oöcyst matures, it increases in diameter from 6 to 60 μm and meiotic and mitotic divisions follow to form a large number of haploid *sporozoites* (varying from a few hundreds to thousands). The number of oöcysts in the stomach wall varies from a few to more than a hundred. When fully mature, i.e., on or about the 10th day of infection, the oöcyst ruptures, releasing sporozoites in the body cavity (haemocele) of the mosquito. The sporozoites are distributed through the circulating fluid into various organs and tissues of the mosquito (except the ovaries). They have a special predilection towards the salivary glands and ultimately reach a maximum concentration in the ducts. The mosquito at this stage is capable of transmitting infection to man. A single bite of the mosquito is sufficient for this purpose. For determining the species of *anopheles* concerned in the spread of malaria, the presence of sporozoites in the salivary glands is to be taken as a positive proof of the development of the human malarial parasite in the species of *Anopheles* mosquito, provided it is anthopophilus.

Different species of malarial parasites can develop in the same mosquito and such an infected mosquito can transmit the infection to man giving rise to cases of "mixed infection", the commonest being *P. falciparum* with *P. vivax*.

Electron Microscope Studies of Oökinete and Sporozoite

Structure of Oökinete. The electron microscope studies of Garnham *et al** (1962) revealed the following:

1. It is enclosed in a 2-layered envelope, consisting of an outer corrugated and inner smooth layer.
2. Anteriorly the inner layer appears more dense and to split, producing what looks like a mouth.
3. Just internal to the envelope lie the hollow peripheral fibrils, 55 to 65 in number.
4. There is a granular nucleus with nucleolus.
5. There is no micropyle.
6. Among cytoplasmic inclusions are crystalloid structures, mitochondria, lysosomes and irregular masses of black pigment granules lying in vacuoles of the cytoplasm.

Structure of Sporozoite. The electron microscope studies of the sporozoite of Haemamoeba (= Plasmodium) gallinacea by Garnham *et al*** (1960) revealed the following (Fig. 66):

1. There is a thick double membrane, the outer corrugated and the inner stout.
2. At the anterior end, there is a cup-like structure lying in an apical depression.
3. Twelve hollow peripheral fibrils are attached to the cup. These fibrils are found to be contractile or tensile in function. These have a locomotory function.
4. A long bulbous paired organelle, presumed to secrete a proteolytic enzyme to facilitate sporozoite's penetration of cells in both hosts.
5. The nucleus lies in a well-marked pit, *micropyle*.
6. Inside the cytoplasm are numerous mitochondria, which provide a source of energy.

Garnham *et al**** (1961, 1963) later studies the sporozoites of human and simian parasites and observed that they resemble those of avian parasite, showing only some minor variations as follows (Fig. 67):

(i) The pellicle consists of 3 layers and an intermediate zone can be distinguished, which was not prominent in avian parasite. The pellicle is continuous over the whole organism except at the anterior end and at the base of the micropyle.

(ii) The anterior cup is more elaborate with concentric rings (probably 3) in human form.

(iii) The peripheral fibrils in *P. falciparum* are 15 in number (14 + 1), in *P. vivax* 11 (10 + 1), in *P. ovale* 13 (12 + 1) and in *P. cynomolgi bastianellii* 11 (10 + 1).

---

* Garnham, P. C. C., Bird, R. G. and Baker, J. R. (1962). III. The ookinetes of Haemamoeba and *Plasmodium. Trans. Roy. Soc. Trap. Med. & Hyg.,* **56**, 116-120.

** Garnham, P. C. C, Bird, R. G. and Baker, J. R. (1960). Electron microscope studies of motile stages of malarial parasites. I. The fine structure of the sporozoites of *Haemamoeba (=Plasmodium) gallinacea. Trans. Roy. Soc. Trop. Med. & Hyg.,* **54**, 274-278.

*** Garnham, P. C. C, Bird, R. G., Baker, J. R. and Bray, R. S. (1961). II. The fine structure of the sporozoites of *Laverania (=Plasmodium) falcipara. Trans. Roy. Soc. Trop. Med. & Hyg.,* **55**, 98-102.

Garnham, P. C. C., Bird, R. G. and Baker, J. R. (1963). IV. The fine structure of the sporozoites of four species of *Plasmodium. Trans. Roy. Soc. Trop. Med. & Hyg.,* **57**, 27-31.

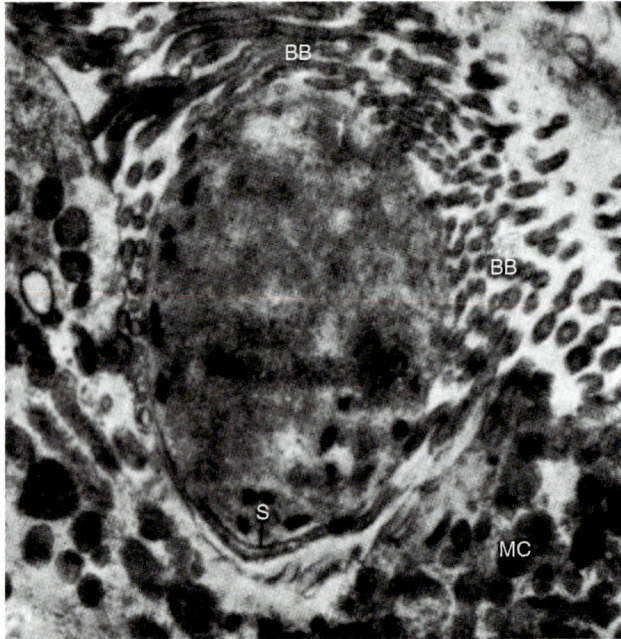

Fig. 64—Penetration of mosquito gut cell by oökinete of *Plasmodium cynomolgi bastianellii*; **pushes aside the brush border of the mucosal cell.**
BB, brush border; MC, mosquito gut cell; S, anterior slit.

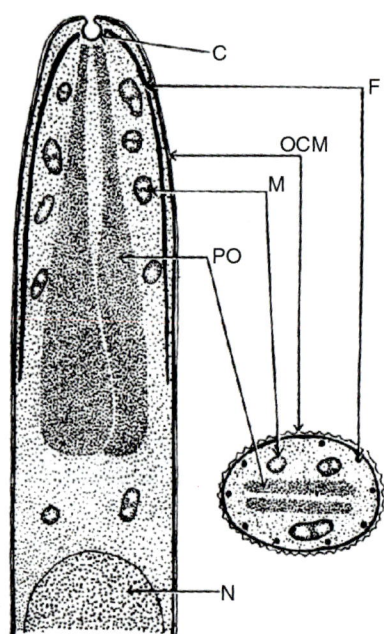

(Longitudinal and transverse sections)

Fig. 66—Sporozoite of *P. gallinaceum* (*Haemamoeba gallinacea*).
C, apical cup; F, peripheral fibril; OCM, outer surface membrane; M, mitochondria; PO, paired organelle; N, nucleus.

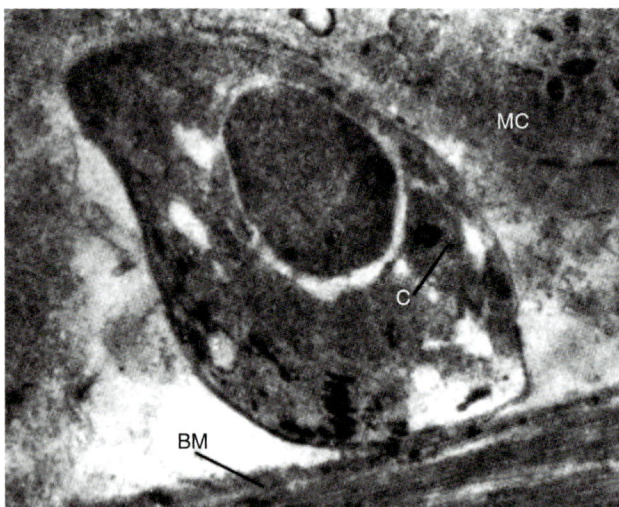

Fig. 65—The oökinete of *Plasmodium cynomolgi bastianellii* **is lying against the external border of the cell and the basement membrane.**
BM, basement membrane; MC, mosquito gut cell; C, crystalloids.

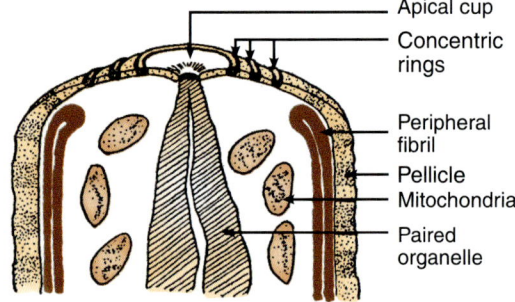

(Longitudinal section)

Fig. 67—Anterior end of the sporozoite of *P. falciparum* (*Laverania falcipara*).

[Garnham *et al*, *Trans. Roy. Soc. Trop. Med. & Hyg.*, 1960, 1961, 1962]

(iv) The paired organelle is long, narrow and sinuous in *P. falciparum*, whereas it is narrow in others.

The structural peculiarity of the sporozoite shows that it possesses some means of locomotion and penetration, has a source of energy and is provided with a sense of direction. Through the micropyle comes out the "sporoplasm" to initiate the pre-erythrocytic schizogony in the liver cell. Before starting its growth, the "sporoplasm" assumes a spherical form.

The oökinete has to undertake a much easier journey and hence, there is no need of an elaborate apparatus.

MORPHOLOGY OF MALARIAL PARASITES

Plasmodium vivax (Grassi and Feletti, 1890)

The parasite of benign tertian or vivax malaria.

The specific name "vivax" is derived from *L. vivere*, to live, and indicates the activity of movement.

Pre-erythrocytic Schizogony (Fig. 68). This phase of development occurs inside the parenchyma cells of the liver and the parasite multiplies by the asexual method (schizogony). It comprises a single cycle and lasts approximately 8 days. The fully developed pre-erythrocytic schizont measures 42 μm in diameter and contains a large number of merozoites (about 12,000). The merozoites consist of a fragment of chromatin with very little of cytoplasmic mass. These merozoites may either enter into a red blood cell* to start their erythrocytic schizogony or re-enter into the parenchyma cell of the liver to continue the exo-erythrocytic schizogony.

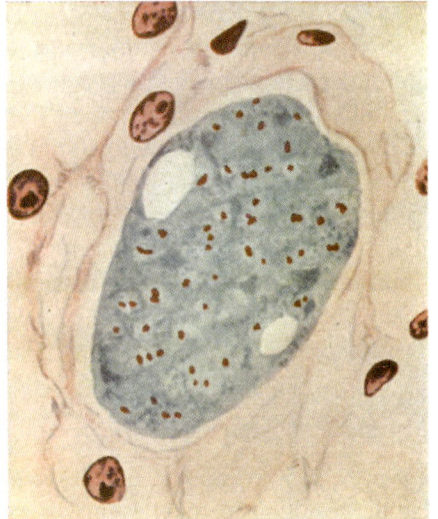 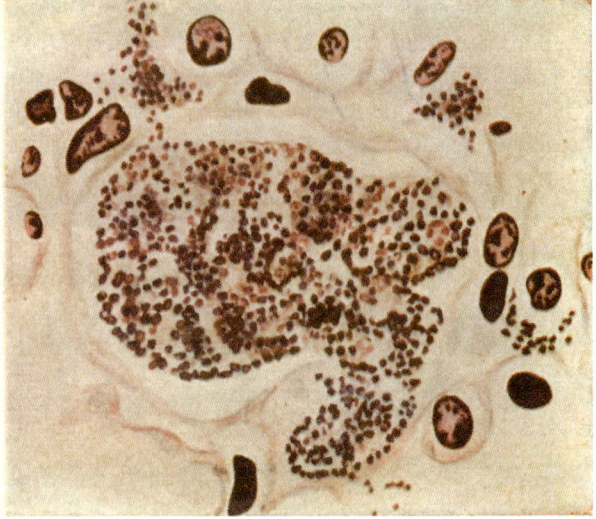

20 μ

A—7th day schizont.
B—7th day schizont, more advanced stage showing release of merozoites.

Fig. 68—Pre-erythrocytic schizogony of *P. vivax* **inside the parenchyma cell of human liver.**
[*After Shortt & Garnham*, 1948; *Trans. Roy. Soc. Trop. Med. & Hyg.*]

Erythrocytic Schizogony. The parasite performs various nutritive functions for its growth and development inside a red blood cell. It reproduces by asexual method of multiplication. It is now known that *P. vivax* shows a greater tendency to invade younger red blood cells (which are usually of greater diameter) and reticulocytes than mature erythrocytes. During erythrocytic schizogony, the parasite passes through the following stages: *trophozoite, schizont* and *merozoite*. The cycle of erythrocytic schizogony lasts approximately 48 hours (2 days) and is completed mainly in the peripheral circulation. Each red blood cell is generally invaded by a single parasite and no more thin 1 or 2 per cent red cells are involved.

TROPHOZOITE. Early trophozoite with Leishman's stain appears to consist of a blue cytoplasmic ring, a red nuclear mass and an unstained area called nutrient *vacuole*.** The diameter of the ring is 2.5 to 3 μm, i.e., about one-third the

---

* The method of entry of merozoites into the red cells is not clear, because the envelopes remain intact after the merozoites have entered.

** Under electron microscope, it is seen to be lined by a double membrane, presumably derived from the plasma membrane of the parasite. The erythrocytic material is incorporated inside these vacuoles and the pigment granules (haematin) are also found within the double membrane of the vacuole. The trophozoite feeds on the host cell by the process of *phagolrophy* or may ingest the erythrocytic material *via* a cytostome, a structure resembling the micropyle of the sporozoite.

size of a red blood cell which is 7.2 μm. One side of the cytoplasmic ring is thicker than the other and the nucleus is situated on the thinner part of the ring. The trophozoite possesses a very active amoeboid movement and constantly thrusts out pseudopodia inside the red blood cell, giving rise to diverse forms. After a period of growth of about 10 hours, yellowish brown pigment granules appear in the cytoplasm of the parasite. While developing, the parasite induces the following changes in the *infected red blood cell*:

(i) It enlarges and becomes double its original size.

(ii) It becomes greatly distorted in shape becoming rhomboidal or irregular in outline.

(iii) It has a washed-out appearance and becomes pale and almost colourless.

(iv) The portion of the cytoplasm unoccupied by the parasite shows a dotted or stippled appearance, called Schüffner's dots, after the name of its discoverer. With Leishman's stain they appear as pinkish granules.

According to the stage of growth, the trophozoites have been described as early trophozoites and late or growing trophozoites.

SCHIZONT. This form appears after a period of growth of about 36 to 40 hours and represents the full-grown trophozoite, ready to divide. At this stage, the parasite has become rounded in shape and has lost all amoeboid activities. The vacuole has disappeared and the pigment granules are still scattered throughout the cytoplasm. The nucleus is large and lies at the periphery. In size, it is larger than a red blood cell, measuring 9 to 10 μm in diameter. In the next 6 to 8 hours, the nuclear division is completed and about 12 to 24 (on an average 16) daughter-individuals are produced. These are called merozoites which arrange themselves in the form of a "rosette" (usually in 2 rows) with the pigment granules at the centre, giving the parasite a mulberry-like appearance. When the maturation is completed, the red blood cell, unable to hold the parasite any longer, bursts. This gives rise to the malarial paroxysm synchronising with the completion of schizogony. According to the stage of maturity, the schizonts have been described as immature schizont (nucleus not divided) and mature schizont (nucleus divided).

MEROZOITE. This consists of an oval mass of cytoplasm with a central nucleus and measures about 1.5 to 1.75 μm in length and 0.5 μm in breadth. It has no pigment. The free merozoites attack new red blood cells and continue their erythrocytic schizogony repeating the cycle every 48 hours.

Gametogony. Certain schizonts become modified biologically and the resulting merozoites, instead of undergoing schizogony, are differentiated into sexual forms. Merozoites of a single schizont become either all males (microgametocytes) or all females (macrogametocytes). Changes in the infected red blood cells (increase in size, pallor and Schüffner's dots) are also seen during the gametocyte development.

The differences between a microgametocyte and a macrogametocyte are as follows:

	Microgametocyte	Macrogametocyte
Size:	9 to 10 μm.	10 to 12 μm.
Cytoplasm:	Stains light blue.	Stains deep blue.
Nucleus:	Diffuse, large; lies laterally.	Small, compact; lies peripherally.

Gametocytes of *P. vivax* appear in the peripheral blood from the first day of fever (16 days after inoculation of sporozoites), i.e. 4 to 5 days after the initial appearance of the asexual parasites in thick smears. Gametocytes, not taken up by the insect host, do not live for more than a week in the human blood.

Latent stage (hepatic). Morphologically hypnozoite (latent parasite in liver) cannot be distingused from the schizonts leading to first clinical attack. The latent hepatic stage is maintained throughout the course of *P. vivax* infection independent of erythrocytic schizogony and lasts for several years. Thus, a single infection with *P. vivax* exists in the human body up to several years and is characterised by short-term and long-term relapses, after which the infection generally dies out. As long as the hypnozoite (latent stage) persists, it can help to maintain erythrocytic schizogony.

Plasmodium falciparum (Welch, 1897)

The parasite of malignant tertian or falciparum malaria.

The specific name "falciparum" (Latin *falx*, a sickle) is derived from its sickle-shaped gametocytes.

Pre-erythrocytic Schizogony (Fig. 69). This comprises a single cycle and lasts 6 days. The youngest pre-erythrocytic form of *P. falciparum* observed inside the parenchyma cells of the liver probably represented three days' growth, measuring about 15 µm in diameter. The mature pre-erythrocytic schizont measures 60 µm in length and 30 µm in breadth and contains numerous small merozoites (about 40,000), measuring 0.7 µm across. The merozoites are liberated on the seventh day of infection and enter into red blood cells to start their erythrocytic schizogony. It is now known that they do not re-enter into the liver cells and the pre-erythrocytic schizonts disappear completely without giving rise to late tissue phase (exo-erythrocytic forms).

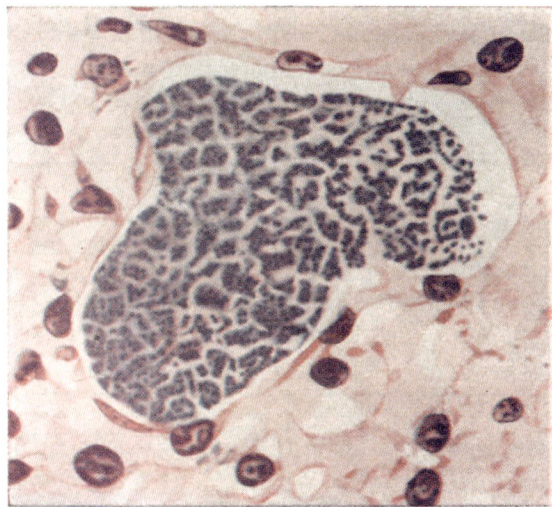 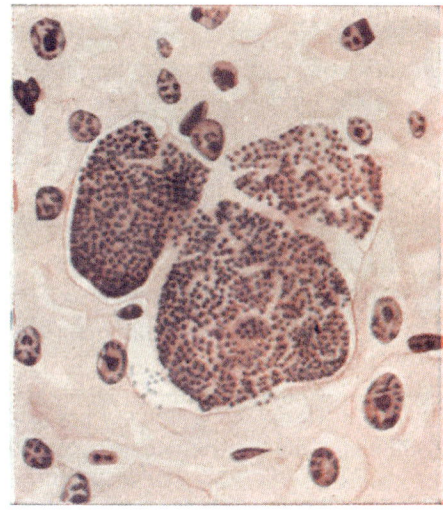

A—6th day form.   B—Mature schizont, ready to burst.

Fig. 69—**Pre-erythrocytic schizogony of** *P. falciparum* **inside the parenchyma cell of human liver.**
[*After Shortt et al*, 1951; *Trans. Roy. Soc. Trop. Med. & Hyg.*]

Erythrocytic Schizogony. *P. falciparum* does not show special affinity for any particular type of red blood cell but invades both the reticulocytes and erythrocytes (young and old). Schizogony occurs inside the capillaries of the internal organs (spleen, liver and bone marrow), hence only the ring-forms (not the growing trophozoites and schizonts) are found in the peripheral blood. The cycle of schizogony is completed in about 36 to 48 hours. Multiple infection of the red blood cell, i.e., more than one parasite (from 2 to 6) invading a single red blood cell is very common with this species.

TROPHOZOITE. The early ring-form measures 1.25 to 1.5 µm in diameter. It consists of a fine and uniform cytoplasmic ring with a nucleus often projecting beyond the ring or lying outside the ring. The parasite often attaches itself to the margin or the edge of the host-cell, the nucleus and a small part of the cytoplasm remaining almost outside. This is known as *form appliqué or accolé.* The nucleus is often divided into two parts which may either remain close together or be situated at opposite poles.

The *pigment granules* formed by the parasite are dark brown or black in colour and collect into a single mass at an early stage.

The *infected red blood cells* remain unaltered, but the cells containing the large-sized rings occasionally show a crenated appearance at the periphery. The colour of the cell is reddish violet. Schüffner's dots are not seen, but in their place 6-12 Maurer's dots or clefts (staining brick-red with Leishman's stain) are seen.

As soon as the pigment appears in the cytoplasm of the parasite and the size of the ring increases to about 4 μm in diameter, it is filtered out by the capillaries of the internal organs. Here, the vacuole disappears and the parasite assumes a compact solid form, containing a single nucleus with the pigment granules collected into a single dark brown or black mass.

SCHIZONT. As the growth continues, the nucleus divides into several masses, varying from 8 to 32 in number. The cytoplasm also divides into the same number as the nuclear masses, forming as many segments arranged around the central pigment mass. The mature schizont measures 4.5 to 5 μm in diameter and occupies about two-thirds of the invaded red blood cell.

MEROZOITE. It measures 0.5 to 0.7 μm in diameter and is small in size. The average number is between 18 and 24.

Gametogony. The gametocytes of this species are sickle-shaped and are called "crescents". Gametogony occurs inside the capillaries of bone marrow and spleen. With the growth of gametocyte, the red blood cell is gradually used up and only its skin remains in the form of a sheath enclosing the parasite. The size of the mature gametocyte is about one and a half times larger than the red blood cell harbouring it, hence the latter is stretched beyond recognition and its remains can only be recognised on the concave side of the parasite projecting outward in the form of an arched rim. The differences between a microgametocyte and a macrogametocyte are as follows:

	Microgametocyte	Macrogametocyte
Shape:	Broader, shorter; ends blunt.	Longer, narrower; ends pointed.
Size:	8 to 10 μm by 2 to 3 μm.	10 to 12 μm by 2 to 3 μm.
Cytoplasm:	Stains light blue.	Stains deep blue.
Nucleus:	Scattered in fine granules over a wide area.	Condensed into a small compact mass at the centre.
Pigments:	Scattered throughout the cytoplasm.	Aggregate like a wreath round the nucleus.

In primary infection, the gametocytes appear in the peripheral blood about 10 days after the appearance of asexual parasites in thick smears, i.e., about 21 days after inoculation of sporozoites. When "crescents" are not taken up by the insect host, they persist in the peripheral blood for a long period (30 to 60 days or even longer).

Latent stage (hepatic): This is completely absent, hence relapses are not a feature of this infection. Recrudescence may occur.

Note: The parasitaemia caused by *P. vivax and P. ovale* is suppressed by concurrent *P. falciparum* infection.

Plasmodium malariae (Laveran, 1881) Grassi and Feletti, 1890

The parasite of quartan malaria.

Laveran (1880) first studied this species and gave the specific name malariae which is still retained.

Pre-erythrocytic Schizogony. Although the tissue phase has not yet been observed in man, it may be inferred that a pre-erythrocytic schizogony also exists in this species. The probable duration of the cycle may be assessed as 15 days.

Garnham (1951) observed the pre-erythrocytic schizogony of *P. inui* (a quartan parasite of the monkeys), the length of the cycle being 11 days. Bray (1960) demonstrated the pre-erythrocytic schizont of *P. malariae* in the liver of a chimpanzee by intravenous inoculation of sporozoites obtained from the salivary glands of 110 mosquitoes (*A. gambiense*) infected with the gametocytes of *P. malariae* in the blood of a Liberian child. The pre-erythrocytic schizont was observed in the liver from the 7th to 12th day. The earliest stage is 5.5 μm in diameter with 5 nuclei; the mature schizont is about 22 μm with over 2,000 merozoites.

Erythrocytic Schizogony. *P. malariae* shows a special tendency to invade mature and older erythrocytes (less than 1 per cent of red cells are infected). The cycle of schizogony is completed in approximately 72 hours (3 days) and occurs mostly in the peripheral circulation.

TROPHOZOITE. The young ring-form has the same signet-ring appearance as that of *P. vivax*. A characteristic feature of *P. malariae* is that the parasite often stretches right across the red blood cell, assuming a band-like appearance*. When the parasite is 6 to 8 hours' old, coarse pigment granules, dark brown or black in colour, appear in its cytoplasm. The invaded red blood cell is not enlarged, does not show any alteration of colour and is undotted (after prolonged staining Ziemann's dots are seen).

SCHIZONT. It is circular in outline and measures 6.5 to 7 µm in diameter. After 48 to 54 hours' growth the nuclear division starts. When the segmentation is complete, the merozoites numbering 6 to 12 arrange themselves around the central pigment mass giving the parasite a "daisy-head" appearance.

MEROZOITE. It measures 2 to 2.5 µm in diameter.

Gametogony. The evolution of gametocytes proceeds in the same way as that in *P. vivax*. The gametocytes are round and measures 7 to 7.5 µm in diameter; females are comparatively large. The maturation of gametocytes is completed in 6 days. The mature gametocytes appear in the peripheral blood a few days after the first attack of fever. The morphological differences between the male and the female gametocytes are the same as described under *P. vivax*. The host-cell is not enlarged.

Latent stage (hepatic). Nothing is known about the hypnozoite, but recrudescence can occur after the disappearance of the erythrocytic stage of the parasite and may occur up to 55 years. It is also known that in *P. malariae* infection parasitaemia can perhaps persists for life.

Plasmodium ovale (Stephens, 1922)

The parasite of ovale tertian malaria.

The specific name of the parasite is derived from its oval shape and also the shape of the infected red blood cell which is rendered oval.

Pre-erythrocytic Schizogony (Fig. 70). The length of the cycle is 9 days. Fifth-day and ninth-day schizonts have been discovered in sections of human liver (obtained by open operation). A mature schizont measures about 70 to 80 µm in length by 40 to 50 µm in breadth and contains about 15,000 merozoites which are large (about 1.8 µm) spherical bodies with the nucleus on one side.

Erythrocytic Schizogony. The schizogony cycle is completed in about 48 hours and occurs mostly in the peripheral blood. It combines the features of *P. malariae* and *P. vivax*; morphologically it resembles the former, whereas its effect on the host-cell and duration of schizogony cycle are similar to that of the latter.

TROPHOZOITE. The ring-form measures 2 to 2.5 µm in diameter and resembles more closely that of *P. malariae* but the band-form is not seen. The pigment granules are coarse and dark brown in colour. Even at the early ring-stage of the parasite, the infected red blood cell shows granules like Schüffner's dots and take a violet tinge; these are named James's dots. Practically, every infected cell shows this eosinophilic stippling. The infected red blood cell is slightly enlarged, often oval (about 24 per cent) with fimbriated edges in thin films (distorted by spreading).

SCHIZONT. It is round or oval in shape, measuring 6.2 µm in diameter. The nuclear material is divided into 6 to 12 masses (usually 8); in relapses the number may be doubled.

MEROZOITE. It measures 2 to 2.5 µm in diameter. The nucleus is crescentic.

Gametogony. Development of gametocytes occurs from the merozoites in the same manner as in other species. The gametocytes are distinguished from those of *P. malariae* by the oval shape of the infected cells and the presence of James's dots, and from those of *P. vivax* by the smaller size of the infected cells and irregular outline.

Latent stage (hepatic): The hypnozoite forms have been discovered in the liver, and relapses occur in ovale tertian malaria.

---

* This is considered to be an artefact, because it is not seen in thick drops.

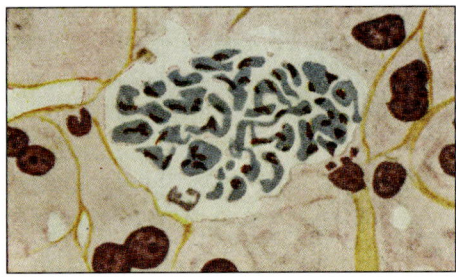

a, 5th day form.

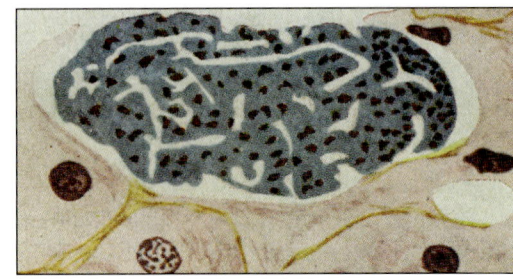

b, Immature form with clefts.

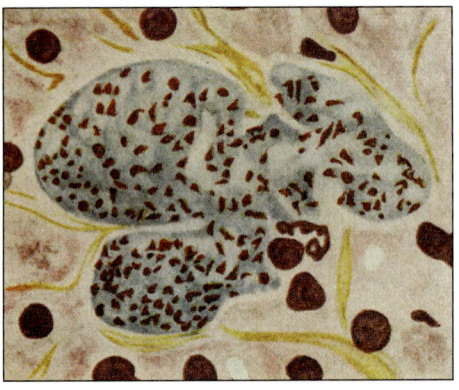

c, Lobular form with large nuclei.

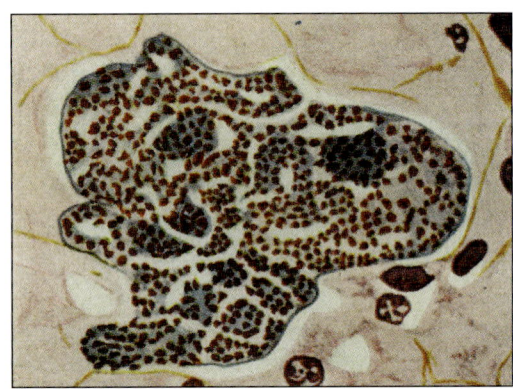

d, Immature form showing whorls and "pallisade" nuclei.

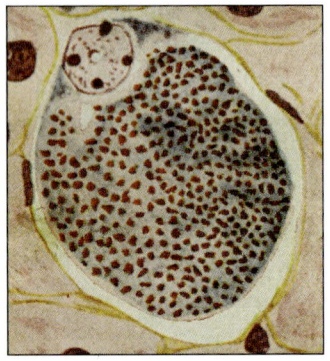

e, Immature form of regular outline.

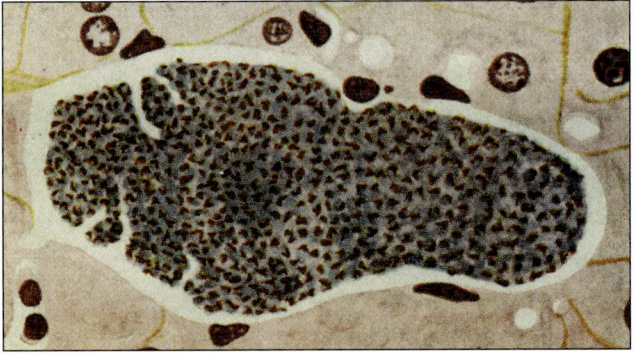

f, Mature form (9th day form) packed with merozoites.

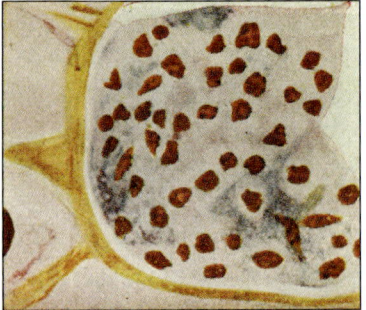

g, Portion of fig. c showing
structure of nuclei.

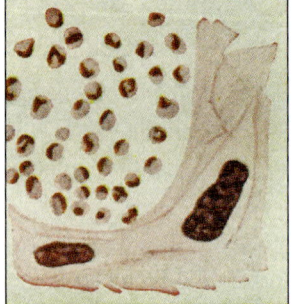

h, Portion of fig. f showing
arrangement of merozoites.

Fig. 70—Pre-erythrocytic schizogony of *P. ovale* **in the parenchyma cell of human liver.**
[*After Garnham et al*, 1955; *Trans. Roy. Soc. Trop. Med. & Hyg.*]

MALARIAL PARASITES OF MAN
Differential Characters of Erythrocytic Phases (Fig. 71)

	P. vivax	P. falciparum	P. malariae	P. ovale
SCHIZOGONY:	48 hours.	48 hours or under.	72 hours.	48 hours.
FORMS IN PERIPHERAL BLOOD:	Trophozoites, schizonts and gametocytes.	Rings and crescents only. Growing trophozoites and schizonts rarely.	Trophozoites, schizonts and gametocytes.	Trophozoites, schizonts and gametocytes.
TROPHOZOITES: RING-FORM:	Size, 2.5 μm. Cytoplasm opposite the nucleus is thicker.	Size, 1.25 to 1.5 μm. Cytoplasm fine and regular in outline. Often with 2 nuclei. Form *accolé*. Multiple infection.	Same as *P. vivax*.	Same as *P. malariae*.
GROWING FORM:	Irregular with a vacuole. Actively amoeboid.	Assumes a compact form. Pigments collect into a single mass early.	Band-like. Slightly amoeboid. Vacuole disappears early.	No ribbon shape. Slightly amoeboid.
SCHIZONT (MATURE)	Size, 9 to 10 μm. Regular, almost completely fills an enlarged red blood cell.	Size, 4.5 to 5 μm. Fills two-thirds of a red blood cell which is not enlarged.	Size, 6.5 to 7 μm. Regular, almost fills a normal-sized red blood cell.	Size, 6.2 μm. Fills about three-quarters of a red blood cell which is slightly enlarged.
MEROZOITES:	12 to 24. Arranged in an irregular grape-like cluster.	18 to 24 or more. Arranged in a grape-like cluster.	6 to 12, usually 8. Arranged around a central mass of pigment like a "daisy" or a "rosette".	6 to 12, usually 8. Irregularly arranged.
MALARIAL PIGMENTS:	Yellowish-brown; fine granules.	Dark brown or blackish; one or two solid blocks.	Dark brown coarse granules.	Dark yellowish brown; coarser than *P. vivax*.
INFECTED R.B.C. (HOST-CELL):	Enlarged, pale. Schüffner's dots present.	Usually unaltered. Crenation, reddish violet colour and Maurer's dots.	Not enlarged, not pale and no dots. Ziemann's dots on prolonged staining.	Slightly enlarged, oval shape, fimbriated. James's dots appear early.
GAMETOCYTE:	Spherical or globular. Much larger than a red blood cell. Host-cell enlarged with Schüffner's dots.	Crescentic. Larger than a red blood cell. Host-cell hardly recognisable.	Round or oval. Size of a red blood cell. Host-cell not enlarged.	Oval. Size of a red blood cell. Host-cell slightly enlarged with James's dots.

Female: Cytoplasm stains blue; nucleus, small and compact.

Male: Cytoplasm stains pale blue or reddish; nucleus, large and diffuse.

Tissue Phases of Mammalian Malaria Parasites
(Pre-erythrocytic Schizogony: Figs. 72 & 73)

Disease	Species of Parasites	Length of Pre-erythrocytic Schizogony	Size of Mature Schizont	Number of Merozoites	Year of Discovery
MONKEY MALARIA					
Tertian Periodicity	P. cynomolgi	8 days	38 μm	Under 10,000	Shortt & Garnham, 1948
Quartan Periodicity	P. inui	11 days	24 μm	2,000	Garnham, 1951
HUMAN MALARIA					
Benign Tertian	P. vivax	8 days	42 μm	12,000	Shortt & Garnham, 1948
Malignant Tertian	P. falciparum	6 days	60 by 30 μm	40,000	Shortt et al, 1949
Ovale Tertian	P. ovale	9 days	80 by 50 μm	15,000	Garnham et al., 1954
Quartan	P. malariae	7 to 12 days (in the liver of chimpanzee)	22 μm	2,000	Bray, 1960

Exo-erythrocytic Schizogony: First discovered in cynomolgi malaria of monkey in 1948 by Shortt and Garnham. Ex-erythrocytic schizonts of *P. vivax* (Rodhain, 1956) and *P. ovale* (Bray, 1957) have been observed in chimpanzee's liver after inoculation of sporozoites of respective parasites.

MALARIAL PARASITES OF MAN
Differential Characters of Erythrocytic Phases

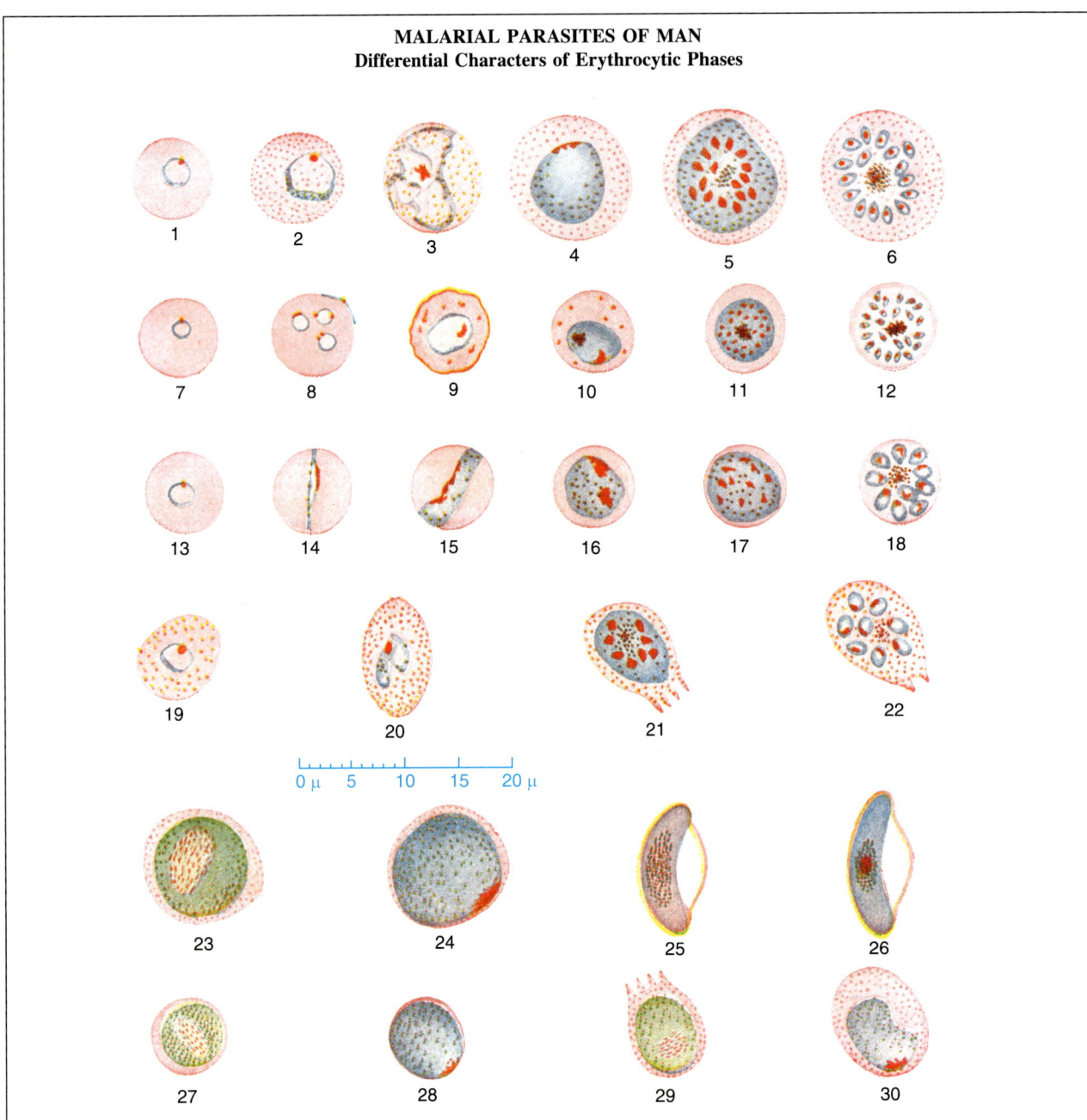

Fig. 71

1 to 6, *P. vivax*. 1, 2, 3, trophozoites (1, early ring-form, 2 & 3, large ring-forms with Schüffner's dots, 3, amoeboid form); 4, 5, 6, schizonts—early to mature (rosette) stage.

7 to 12, *P. falciparum*. 7, 8, 9, trophozoites; 10, 11, 12, growth of a schizont (inside the capillary of internal organ); 8, showing multiple infections with form "accolé"; 9 & 10, showing Maurer's dots in the host-cell. Note the normal size of the infected cell.

13 to 18, *P. malariae*. 13, ring-form; 14, 15, band-form; 16, 17, 18, growth of a schizont. Note the normal size of the host-cell and undotted erythrocytes.

19 to 22, *P. ovale*. 19, 20, trophozoites; 21, 22, developing schizonts. Note James's dots in all the stages as also the irregular and oval shape of the enlarged host-cell.

23 to 30, mature gametocytes of *P. vivax* (23 male, 24 female), *P. falciparum* (25 male, 26 female), *P. malariae* (27 male, 28 female) and *P. ovale* (29 male, 30 female).

TISSUE PHASE OF MALARIAL PARASITE

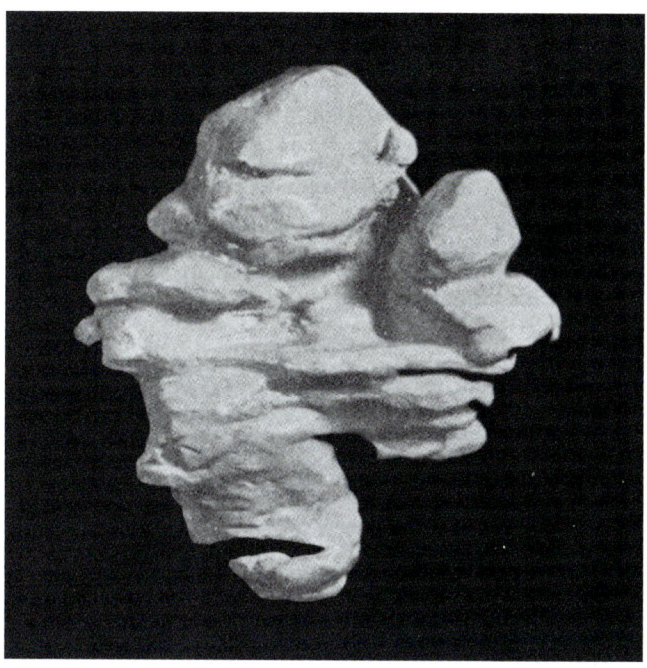

Fig. 72—The outline of a complete single pre-erythrocytic schizont of *Plasmodium falciparum.*
The photograph is taken from a plasticine model reconstructed from the camera lucida drawings of 17 serial sections.
[*After Shortt et al, 1951; Trans. Roy. Soc. Trop. Med. & Hyg.*]

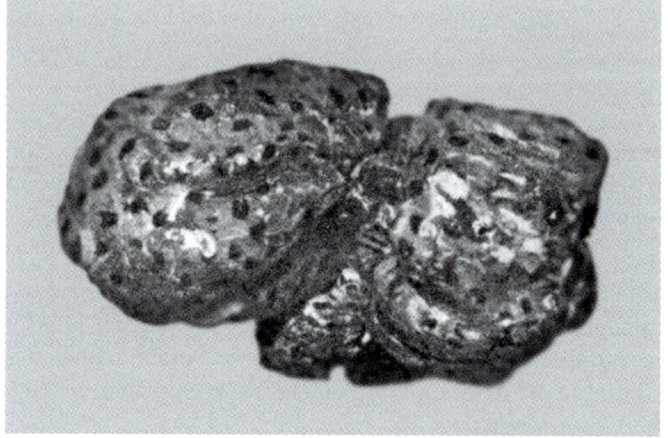

Fig. 73—The outline of a complete single pre-erythrocytic schizont of *Plasmodium ovale.*
The photograph is taken from a plasticine model recons tructed from the camera lucida drawings of 13 serial sections.
[*After Garnharn et al, 1955; Trans. Roy. Soc. Trop. Med. & Hyg.*]

Comparison of the Course of Natural Infection of *P. vivax* and *P. falciparum* in Man		
	P. vivax	*P. falciparum*
PRE-ERYTHROCYTIC SCHIZOGONY:	Consists of one cycle; lasts 8 days. Number of merozoites produced by each schizont: about 12,000.	Consists of one cycle; lasts 6 days. Number of merozoites produced by each schizont: about 40,000.
ERYTHROCYTIC ERYTHROCYTIC:	Each cycle lasts 48 hours. Appearance* of parasites in thick smears on 12th day of infection. First rise** of temperature on 16th day of infection. Primary attack lasts 3 to 4 weeks.	Each cycle lasts 36 to 48 hours. Appearance* of parasites in thick smears on 10th day of infection. First rise** of temperature on 12th day of infection. Primary attack lasts 10 to 14 days.
GAMETOGONY:	Gametocytes in peripheral blood on 16th day of infection (1st day of fever: 4 days after the appearance of asexual parasites in peripheral blood).	Gametocytes in peripheral blood on 21st day of infection (after 9 days of fever: about 10 days after the appearance of asexual parasites in peripheral blood).
LATENT HEPATIC STAGE:	Present; continuing for a period not exceeding 3 years. Relapses often occur.	Absent. Relapses do not occur.
A SINGLE INFECTION:	Lasts up to 3 years.	Generally lasts a month but may last up to a maximum of one year. (Recrudescence occurring as a result of incomplete sterilisation.
HYPNOZOITE REACTIVATION:	Present Absent	Absent. Present, occurs due to renewed multiplication of low level persistent asexual parasite in blood.

* *Appearance of Parasites.* This depends upon the density of the parasites in the peripheral blood. The *microscopic density* is in the neighbourhood of 10 parasites per mm^3 of blood.

** *First Rise of Temperature.* This depends upon the density of the parasites. The *pyrogenic density* (fever threshold) is in the neighbourhood of 50 parasites per mm^3 of blood.

Staining Method. The structural details of malarial parasites are best studied by using any of the modifications of the *Romanowsky's stains* such as Leishman's and Gemsa's stains. The former is prepared by dissolving the dry powders in acetone-free pure methyl alcohol and is used in strength of 0.15 per cent; whereas the latter is obtained as a readymade watery solution. Hence, fixation of the film with alcohol is only necessary when Giemsa's stain is used.

Principle of Romanowsky's Stains. These stains are not single stains but compound stains formed by the interaction of medicinal (not pure) methylene blue and eosin. With ageing or exposure to acids, alkalis or ultraviolet light, a number of oxidation products (methylene azures) are formed from methylene blue. By this process a series of loosely combined chemical bodies (methylene blue eosinate, methylene azure eosinate etc.) are formed which give contrast colour staining. The eosin stains the red blood cells pink, methylene blue stains the cytoplasm of malarial parasite blue and azure with eosin stains nuclear chromatin red.

Field's Stain. This is used for thick films without fixation and the staining process is done quickly within a few seconds (4 seconds). *See Appendix I.*

Cultivation. Culture methods have been evolved to observe the erythrocytic schizogony of malarial parasite as it occurs in man. Only the development of one generation can be studied. Hence, it is not a "culture method" in the truest sense but in reality a "concentration method". Bass and John's technique with a slight modification was used for the cultivation of malaria parasite in artificial culture media. Trager and Jensen (1976) successfully cultivated human malaria parasite in in *Vitro. See Appendix I.*

Animal Inoculation. Human species of malarial parasites can now be transferred to several species of primates. Similarly, certain species of malarial parasites of monkeys, when inoculated into man, are able to establish themselves in the human host. Two questions now arise, whether an animal reservoir of human malaria exists and whether a natural monkey-to-man transmission can take place.

Accidental laboratory infections of man with the simian parasite, *P. cynomolgi bastianellii* (Bastinelli strain of *P. cynomolgi*) have been reported (Eyles *et al*, 1960) although the naturally acquired infections of simian malaria in man appears to be rare.

Immunology. Development of immunity in malaria is manifested by tolerance to infection (cessation of clinical phenomenon despite parasitaemia) which is the result of active immunity (both cellular and humoral) consequent upon the concomitant presence of the parasites. The phagocytic activity of the cells of the reticulo-endothelial system (particularly those in the spleen and liver) helps in the development of immunity to malarial infection and the parasites are destroyed and kept at subclinical levels (Figs. 74, 75 and 76). Hence, it has been suggested that the immunity in malaria depends upon a persistent latent infection, known as *infection immunity or premunition*. Shortt and Garnham showed that the immunity in malaria may be complete and may occasionally persist for some time, even after disappearance of the parasites or termination of the infection.

It is now known that plasmodial antigens derived from asexual erythrocytic phases of the parasite stimulate the appropriate cells of the body to produce specific antibodies, both protective and precipitating, which are present in the IgG and IgM fractions of the serum gamma globulin. The malarial antibodies promote phagocytosis of antibody-bound parasites by making them acceptable to macrophages. They do not act on sporozoites and therefore do not prevent superinfection.

The cellulo-humoral anti-parasitic defence mechanisms of the host is only effective against the asexual erythrocytic parasites (mature schizonts and free merozoites), but not against the gametocytes and the hypnozoit forms. The merozoites released from the latent hepatic stage source serve to infect the red blood cells and may bring about a clinical attack of malaria in the absence of re-infection. As long as the immunity mechanism is effective, the merozoites released by the liver-schizonts into the circulation are at once destroyed and so, cannot invade the erythrocytes (those which re-enter the liver cells are however unaffected). It is only when this immunity mechanism fails that the merozoites escaping from the liver-schizonts succeed in invading the erythrocytes and so produce a parasitic relapse (Shortt, 1950).

Plasmodial Antigens. These are soluble antigens and are present in the sera of infected persons which can be detected by Ouchterlony double diffusion precipitation techniques. They can also be extracted from infected erythrocytes. Wilson *et al*[*] (1969) classified *P. falciparum* antigen on the basis of heat susceptibility test as (i) a labile (L) antigen destroyed by heating at 56°C for 30 minutes, (ii) a resistant (R) antigen stable at 56°C for 30 minutes, and (iii) a stable (S) antigen not destroyed at 100°C for 5 minutes. The L antigens have been further subdivied into 2 subclasses—La (4 antigens) and Lb (3 antigens).

Malarial Antibodies and Immunoglobulins. Protective malarial antibodies exist in IgG (7S) fraction of immune sera whereas precipitating antibodies have been shown to exist in both IgG and IgM components (McGregor and Wilson,[**] 1971). Antibodies to La antigen are all in IgG fraction of serum gamma globulin. They can cross the placenta and appear in the sera of infants born from an immune mother (almost all newborn infants in Gambia, a hyperendemic *P. falciparum* area showed specific IgG antibodies in their sera). These protective antibodies persist for months or years and tend to die away if there is no re-infection. Persistence of the immunity thus depends on the frequency of antigenic stimulation.

Antibodies to S antigen are mostly present in IgM (19S) fraction of serum gamma globulin and are mostly precipitating antibodies. They do not cross the placenta, persist for brief periods and are present in the sera of adults but not in young children.

Immunological Consequences of Malarial Infection.[***] These may be considered under the following:

1. *Protective immunity*. Newborn infants derive a passive immunity (congenital immunity) for a short period (for the first 6 months of life) from the immune mother by the passage of specific IgG antibodies *via* milk and across the placenta. The older age group derive an "antitoxic" immunity (no antiplasmodial effect but the "toxic" products of parasite metabolism are neutralised).

2. *Initiation of pathological states*. These are (i) malarial nephrosis, particularly in *P. malariae* infection in children, (ii) idiopathic tropical splenomegaly syndrome (big spleen disease) in adults, (iii) an autoimmune haemolytic anaemia (auto-antibody against erythrocytic antigen) seen in pregnant women with *P. falciparum* infection (the anaemia is disproportionate to parasitaemia and the anaemia cannot be explained merely by the destruction of parasitised red cells), and (iv) abnormal immune responses.

3. *Immunosuppressive effect towards other antigenic stimuli*. This explains the less frequent occurrence of autoimmune diseases in malarial infections. McGregor and Burr[****] (1962) demonstrated that tetanus toxoid failed to produce an antitoxin response in Gambian children with malarial parasitaemia.

There is now increasing epidemiological evidence that Burkitt's lymphoma in man is the result of a synergic action between Plasmodial and Oncogenic viral infections. Malarial infection by its immunosuppressive effect allows virus proliferation or interferes with immune reactions to neoplastic cells.

A definite antagonism exists between visceral leishmaniasis and malaria in man and may be the result of an increase in immunologically competent cells (Adler[*****], 1963).

---

* Wilson, R. J. M. *et al* (1969). *Lancet,* **2**, 201.

** McGregor, I. A. and Wilson, R. J. M. (1971). *Trans. Roy. Soc. Trop. Med. & Hyg.,* **65**, 136.

*** McGregor, I. A. (1972). *Br. Med. Bull.,* **28**, 22.

**** McGregor, I. A. and Burr, M. (1962). *Trans. Roy. Soc. Trop. Med. & Hyg.,* 56, 364.

***** Adler, S. (1963). *In Immunity to Protozoa*, pp. 235-245, Oxford: Blackwell.

IMMUNITY IN MALARIA : CELLULAR DEFENCE

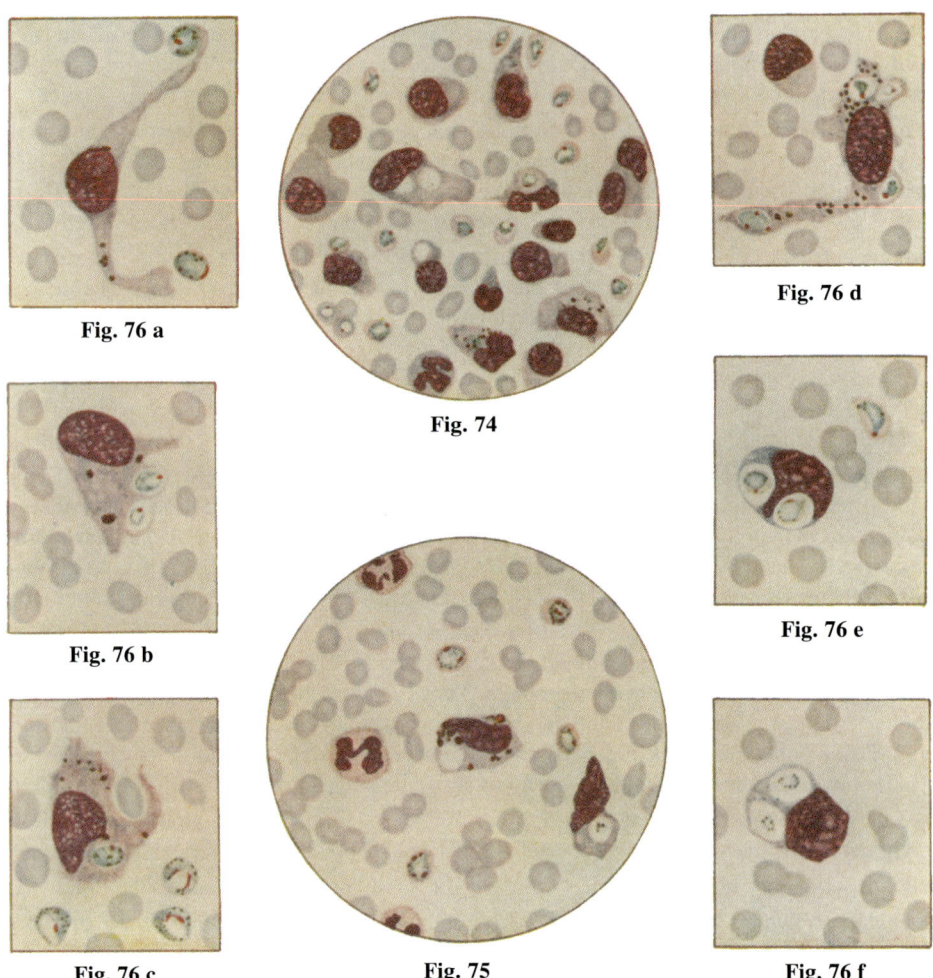

Fig. 76 a

Fig. 74

Fig. 76 d

Fig. 76 b

Fig. 76 e

Fig. 76 c

Fig. 75

Fig. 76 f

Fig. 74—*Plasmodium knowlesi* infection in a *rhesus* monkey, showing phagocytosis of malarial parasites in the peripheral blood. Note the shower of large phagocytic cells (monocytes).

Fig. 75—Blood film from the same animal about four hours after the previous film. Note the decreasing number of parasitised erythrocytes.

Figs. 76 a, b, c, d, e & f—Various stages of phagocytosis of malarial parasites by the monocytes and their ultimate digestion. Ingested malarial pigments can also be seen inside these monocytes (drawings made from different areas of the blood film depicted in the figure 74).

Reservoirs of Infection. Human species of malarial parasites are not harboured by any of the lower animals. Hence man, particularly the children in an endemic area, acts as the only reservoir of infection. In some parts of Africa, chimpanzees may act as reservoir for *P. malariae.*

Method of Transmission (Mode of Infection). The female anopheline mosquitoes act as intermediaries in transmitting infection to man. The malarial parasites undergo developmental changes in the mosquito and some time (about 8 to 10 days) elapses before the mosquito becomes infective; this is the period required for the sporozoites to develop and reach the salivary glands. The infection is transmitted by the *inoculative method.* During the act of biting, the mosquito's proboscis pierces the skin and the salivary secretion is injected into the puncture wound. This droplet carries a large number of sporozoites which are directly introduced into the blood stream but cannot be found in it after about half an hour.

Transmitting Agent—Female anopheles. Ten species of Anopheles are considered to be of importance in malaria transmission in India: *A. culcifacies, A. stephensi, A. philippinensis, A. fluviatilis, A. varuna, A. minimus, A. annularis, A. leucosphyrus (A. balabacensis), A. sundaicus, A. jeyporiensis canctidiensis.*

Infective Forms—Sporozoites.

Portal of Entry—Skin.

Site of Localisation—First in liver cells, then in erythrocytes.

OTHER METHODS OF TRANSMISSION

Injection of an emulsion of salivary glands containing the sporozoites will also induce infection. This is called *sporozoite-induced malaria.*

Injection of blood from a malarial patient containing the asexual forms of erythrocytic schizogony will also induce malaria in man. This is called *trophozoite-induced malaria* and the following are examples:

(i) TRANSFUSION MALARIA. Occurring during the course of blood transfusion* when infected persons (having latent malarial infection) are used as donors (screened by indirect immunofluorescent test).

(ii) CONGENITAL MALARIA. Transmission of infection to foetus in utero through some placental defect (a physiologically healthy placenta offers a barrier to the passage of malarial parasites to the foetus).

(iii) MALARIA IN DRUG ADDICTS. Through the use of the same syringe*, when one of them is infected.

Therapeutic Malaria. Malarial infection has been artificially induced for the treatment of neuro-syphilis (general paralysis of the insane). The methods employed are:

(i) By inoculating blood of an infected donor.

(ii) By allowing laboratory-bred infected mosquitoes to bite the recipient.

(iii) By injecting emulsion of salivary glands containing sporozoites.

The species of malarial parasite used is *P. vivax.*

There exist some differences between malaria induced by trophozoites and malaria induced by sporozoites and they are as follows:

	Sporozoite-induced Malaria	*Trophozoite-induced Malaria*
PRE-ERYTHROCYTIC SCHIZOGONY:	Present.	Absent.
INCUBATION PERIOD:	Long.	Short.
LATENT STAGE (HEPATIC):	May be present.	Absent.
RELAPSES:	May occur.	Do not occur.
SCHIZONTICIDAL DRUGS:	No radical cure; because of the presence of latent stage (hepatic)	Can be radically cured; no latent stage (hepatic)

Spread of Malaria. The factors responsible for the spread of malaria include the following: (1) The presence of a gametocyte carrier (source of malarial parasite), (2) existence of a suitable Anopheles vector, and (3) a susceptible person.

If this cycle or chain (Fig. 77) can be broken at any point, the occurrence of malaria can be prevented.

Pathogenicity. Infection with the *Plasmodia* causes intermittent fevers which are known as malaria**. Each of the four species causes a characteristic fever and the diseases are designated as follows:

---

* Other common hazard of these practices is viral hepatitis due to type B virus; also called hepatitis associated antigen (HbsAg) or Australia antigen, because it was first detected in the serum of an Australian aborigine.

** The word *"malaria"* was derived from two Italian words *mala* and *aria,* meaning "bad air". It was the belief at the time (as far back as 1753) that the air transmitted the disease and inhalation of poisonous gases emanating from a marshy place was supposed to be the chief factor.

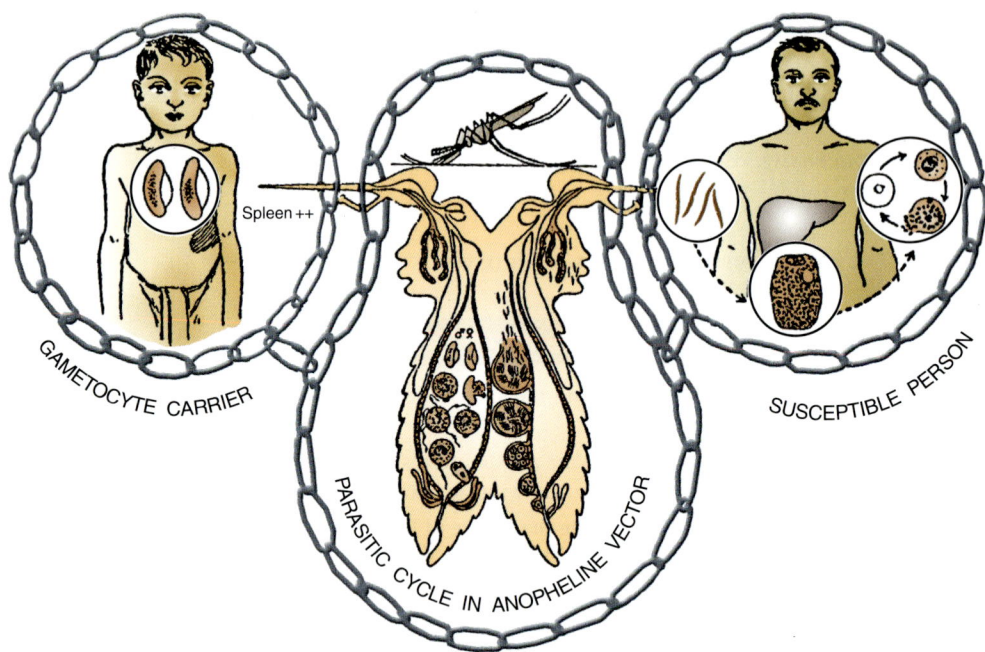

Fig. 77—**Spread of malaria, showing the life cycle of** *P. falciparum.*

P. vivax—Vivax malaria (Benign tertian malaria).

P. malariae—Quartan malaria (Malariae malaria).

P. falciparum—Falciparum malaria (Malignant tertian malaria); it is also responsible for pernicious malaria. Blackwater fever is also a special manifestation of falciparum malaria and is discussed separately.

P. ovale—Ovale malaria.

Incubation Period. The sporozoite after gaining entrance into the human body undergoes a developmental cycle first in liver and then in the red blood cell. With the commencement of the erythrocytic schizogony the parasite multiplies in geometrical progression and on reaching a sufficient concentration in the blood, brings about the onset of fever. This period of development is called the *incubation period* which varies with different species as follows:

In *P. vivax, P. ovale* and *P. falciparum* it is 10-14 days and in *P. malariae* it is 18 days to 6 weeks.

A long incubation or latent period of about 38 weeks has been observed particularly with *P. falciparum,* European strains of *P. vivax.* It is suggested that the number of sporozoites injected may have some relation to this long incubation period. It is also seen in persons who have taken antimalarial suppressant.

Clinical Features of Malaria. The main clinical manifestations in a typical case, are a series of febrile paroxysms, followed by anaemia and splenic enlargement.

1. FEBRILE PAROXYSM. The malarial paroxysm starts generally in the early afternoon but actually it may start at any time. Each paroxysm shows a succession of 3 stages: (i) the cold stage (lasting 20 minutes to an hour), (ii) the hot stage (lasting 1 to 4 hours), and (iii) the sweating stage (lasting 2 to 3 hours). Thus the *total duration* of the febrile cycle is from 6 to 10 hours, varying however with the species of *Plasmodia.*

Types of Fever. The febrile paroxysm synchronises with the erythrocytic schizogony of the malarial parasite:

(a) With a 48-hour cycle the fever recurs every third day, *tertian fever* (Figs. 78 & 79) and

(b) with a 72-hour cycle the fever recurs every fourth day, *quartan fever* (Fig. 80).

(c) Fever recurring at intervals of 24 hours, quotidian periodicity (Figs. 81 & 82) has also been observed in infections with *P. vivax* or with *P. malariae.* This is due to the maturation of two generations of tertian parasites on two successive days (*tertiana duplex*) or three generations of quartan parasites maturing on three successive days (*quartana triplex*). When two generations of quartan parasites mature on successive days, the fever occurs on two successive days followed a day of apyrexia (*quartana duplex*).

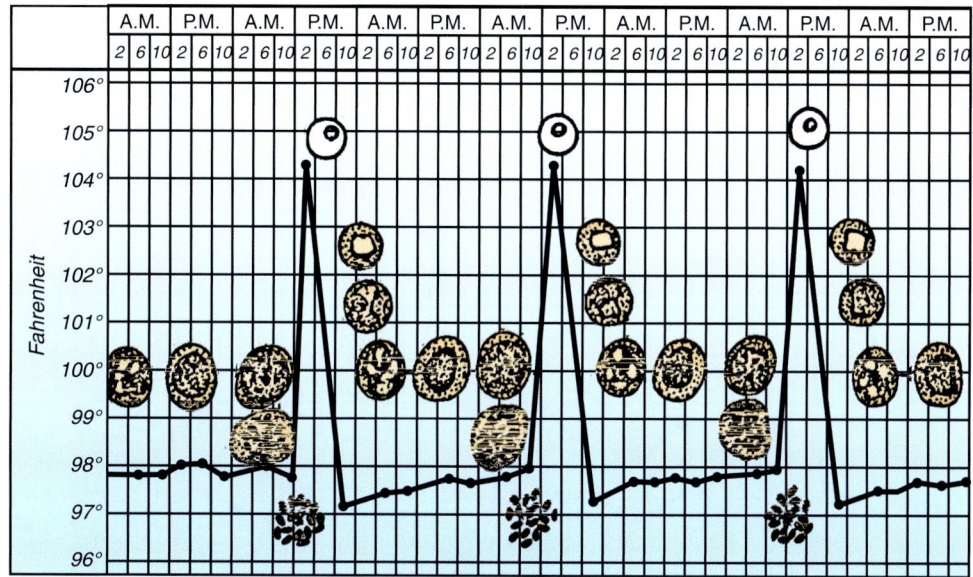

Fig. 78—Fever with tertian periodicity, in vivax malaria.
Developmental phases of the parasite with a 48-hour cycle are also shown.

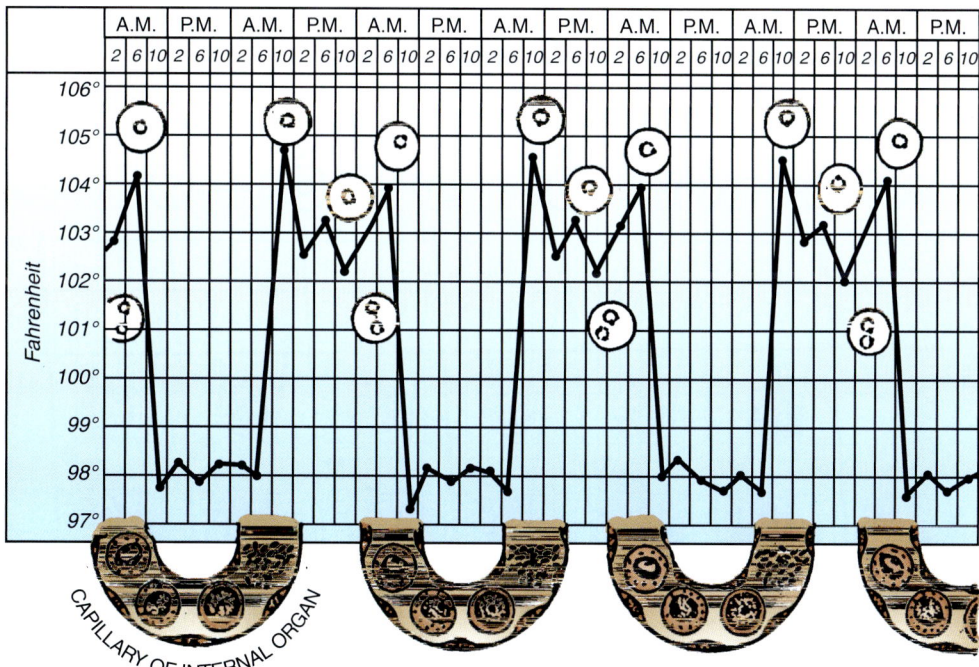

Fig. 79—Fever with tertian periodicity, in falciparum malaria.
Note the prolonged paroxysm. Developmental phases of the parasite with a 48-hour cycle are also shown.

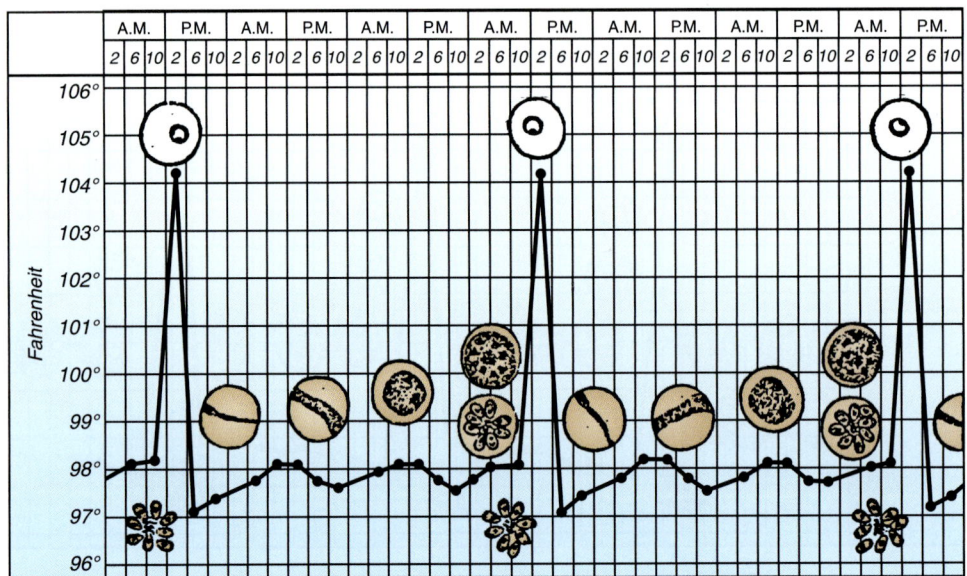

Fig. 80—Fever with quartan periodicity, in quartan malaria.
Developmental phases of the parasite with a 72-hour cycle are also shown.

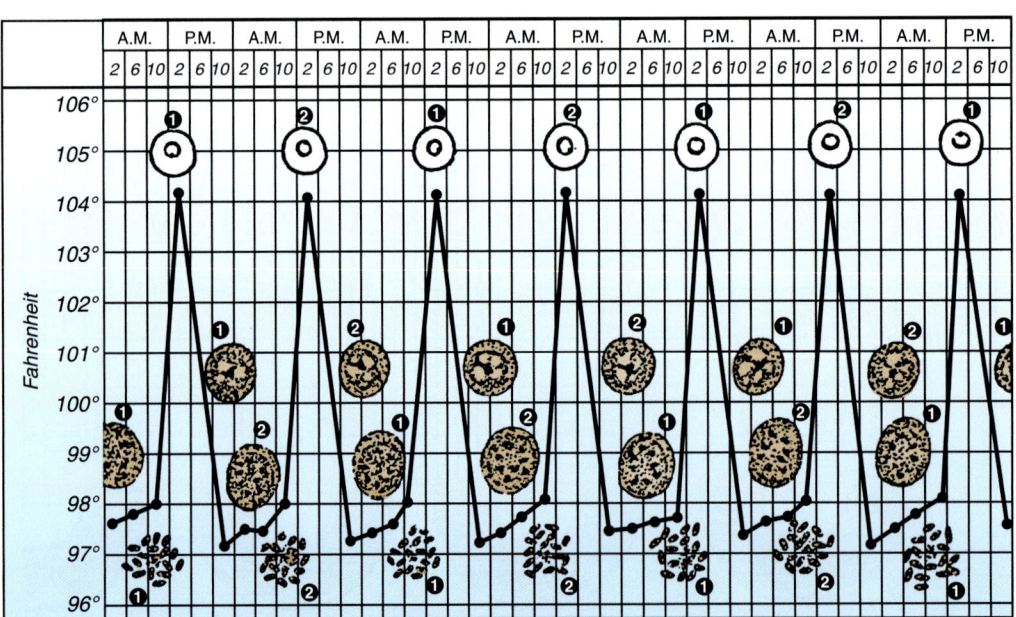

Fig. 81—Fever with quotidian periodicity, in *Plasmodium vivax* infection.
Showing developmental phases of two generations of parasites.

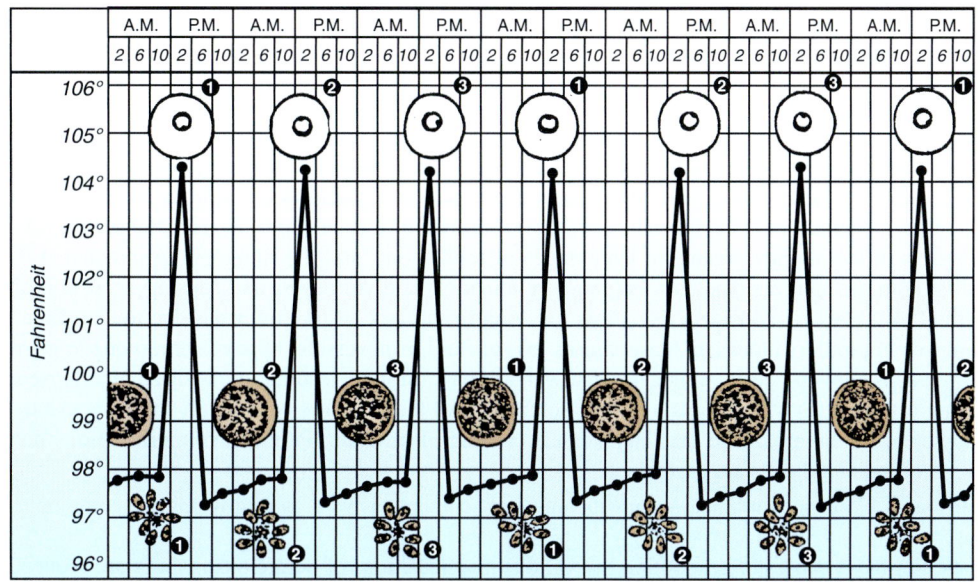

Fig. 82—Fever with quotidian periodicity, in *Plasmodium malariae* **infection.**
Showing developmental phases of three generations of parasites.

In *vivax malaria* (benign tertian malaria) the characteristic intermittent periodic fever becomes established only in the later stages, the initial pyrexia generally being continuous, quotidian or remittent. In early stages, two broods of parasites undergo schizogony on alternate days, thereby releasing two generations of merozoites with a febrile reaction each day. Later, one brood drops out and the febrile curve becomes certian.

In *quartan malaria* the intermittent periodic fever starts from the very beginning.

In *falciparum malaria* the febrile paroxysm may not show the three successive cold, hot and sweating stages. The fever in such cases, instead of being intermittent, may be continuous or remittent. This has been explained by the fact that several generations of the parasite are multiplying at different intervals. After the first paroxysm, there is no remission of fever and the temperature may remain at the same level (continuous) or may show a drop (remittent) towards the latter part and then merge on to the next paroxysm, which comes on before the period of 48 hours has elapsed. *Pyrogenic density* is the number of parasites in blood at which fever develops. It is higher in *P. falciparum* than that of other species.

2. ANAEMIA. After a few paroxysms, anaemia[*] of a microcytic or a normocytic hypochromic type develops as a result of breaking down of red blood cells during segmentation of parasites.

3. SPLENOMEGALY. Enlargement of the spleen is one of the important physical signs in malaria. In primary cases, the enlargement is so slight as to escape detection by palpation. After some paroxysms, and usually by the second week, it is definitely enlarged and palpable.

Relapses in Malaria. It is the renewed clinical manifestation or parasitaemia and may result from the following:

(i) *Persistence of blood infection* in which the surviving population of erythrocytic forms are increased. This is k.a. *recrudescence* and is a feature of *P. falciparum* infection. It may occur mostly up to 1 year.

(ii) *Persistence of hypnozoite forms* in the liver in which erythrocytic schizogony commences again. This is k.a. recurrence or true relapse and is a feature of *P. vivax* and *P. ovale* infections. In these cases, there is no erythrocytic schizogony in the latent period.

Note: Malaria infection following blood transfusion is due to the presence of erythrocytic form of the parasites in the donor's blood. The true relapse does not occur as sporozoites are not involved in it.

---

[*] In malarial infections in animals anaemia has also resulted from autoimmune haemolytic reaction.

Definition. The term "pernicious malaria" is referred to a series of phenomena occurring during the course of an infection of *P. falciparum* which, if not effectively treated, threatens the life of the patient within 1 to 3 days.

Pathogenesis. The serious complications that may develop in "pernicious malaria" (acute falciparum malaria) are the result of capillary blockage consequent upon decreased effective circulating blood volume. It has long been thought that *the blockade of the capillary blood vessels* of the internal organs arises from agglutination of parasitised erythrocytes. This has been attributed to certain peculiar biological features of *P. falciparum*, such as (i) recession of asexual parasites from the peripheral circulation to the capillary blood vessels of the internal organs for later stages of schizogony, and (ii) stickiness of infected erythrocytes (coated with fibrin) in relation to vascular endothelium, helping agglutination of erythrocytes and causing occlusion of capillary blood vessels. Maegraith (1967) however considers that stasis resulting from vasoconstriction, itself due to sympathetic hyperactivity, plays an important role in capillary blockage. Stasis means loss of fluid from vessels (hypovolaemia) due to increased permeability of the endothelial cells allowing heavy molecules and water to pass through, leading to increased blood viscosity and concentration of circulating erythrocytes which contain mature schizonts. All these factors collectively are responsible for the accumulation of erythrocytes in the lumen of the capillary vessels causing obstruction. Pernicious manifestations may be anticipated when more than 5% of red blood cells are parasitised.

Note: The peripheral blood shown a heavy parasitaemia and schizonts as well as ring-forms are commonly present in large numbers.

Clinical Types. For the purposes of description the various manifestations of pernicious malaria are grouped as follows:

1. CEREBRAL MALARIA—Manifested by hyperpyrexia, coma, paralysis.

2. ALGID MALARIA—Characterised by cold and clammy skin with vascular collapse leading to peripheral circulatory failure. Along with this there may be either vomiting (gastric type) or watery diarrhoea (choleraic type) or passage of blood in faeces (dysenteric type).

3. SEPTICAEMIC MALARIA—Characterised by high continued temperature (resembling typhoid fever), bilious remittent fever, pneumonia, cardiac syncope. Severe malaria should be considered in any non-immune patient with a parasite count greater than 2%.

PATHOLOGY OF MALARIA

General Considerations. The malarial parasite resides inside the red blood cell of the human host. The schizogony cycle is completed within the host-cell in which it is parasitic, ultimately resulting in the destruction of the cell. During the process of growth, it produces a pigment (haematin) from the haemoglobin and also multiplies asexually to form daughter-individuals (merozoites). Thus on completion of schizogony, the following substances are liberated into the blood stream: merozoites, pigment granules, unused portion of the cytoplasm of the infected red blood cells and "malaria toxins".

Although it has not yet been possible to identify any "malarial toxin", Maegraith (1967) obtained evidence of a soluble factor (inorganic phosphate and lactic acid) which depresses respiration and halts cellular metabolism by interfering with mitochondrial activity (*cytotoxic anoxia*).

In malarial infection, oxygen-carrying function of blood is not disturbed and general *anoxic anoxia* does not occur.

It is to be noted that shock in plasmodium infection may be related to liberation of kinins.

MALARIAL PIGMENT (haematin). The term "hazmozoin" is not recommended (W.H.O., 1963).

The pigment granules, liberated in the plasma at the time of rupture of segmenting parasites, are filtered out from the circulating blood by the activity of the cells of the reticulo-endothelial system and inside these cells they may be found in any amount. Hence the organs rich in reticulo-endothelial cells become densely pigmented and assume a colour varying from slate-grey to black, giving the *characteristic pigmentation* of organs in malarial infection. The malarial pigment, although it contains iron, does not give the Prussian blue reaction when stained with the potassium ferrocyanide but takes a black stain instead.

Besides the malarial pigment, other pigments are found as a result of extensive blood destruction and are therefore not specific products of malarial parasites. These are mainly two: one containing iron, the *haemosiderin* and the other iron-free, the *haematoidin* which later is converted into bile pigment (*haemobilirubin and cholebilirubin*).

Red Blood Cell Physiology in Malaria. The red blood cell physiology in malaria is disturbed, because of the growth and development of the parasite inside the red blood cell. Its direct effect is reflected on the blood and erythropoietic function of the

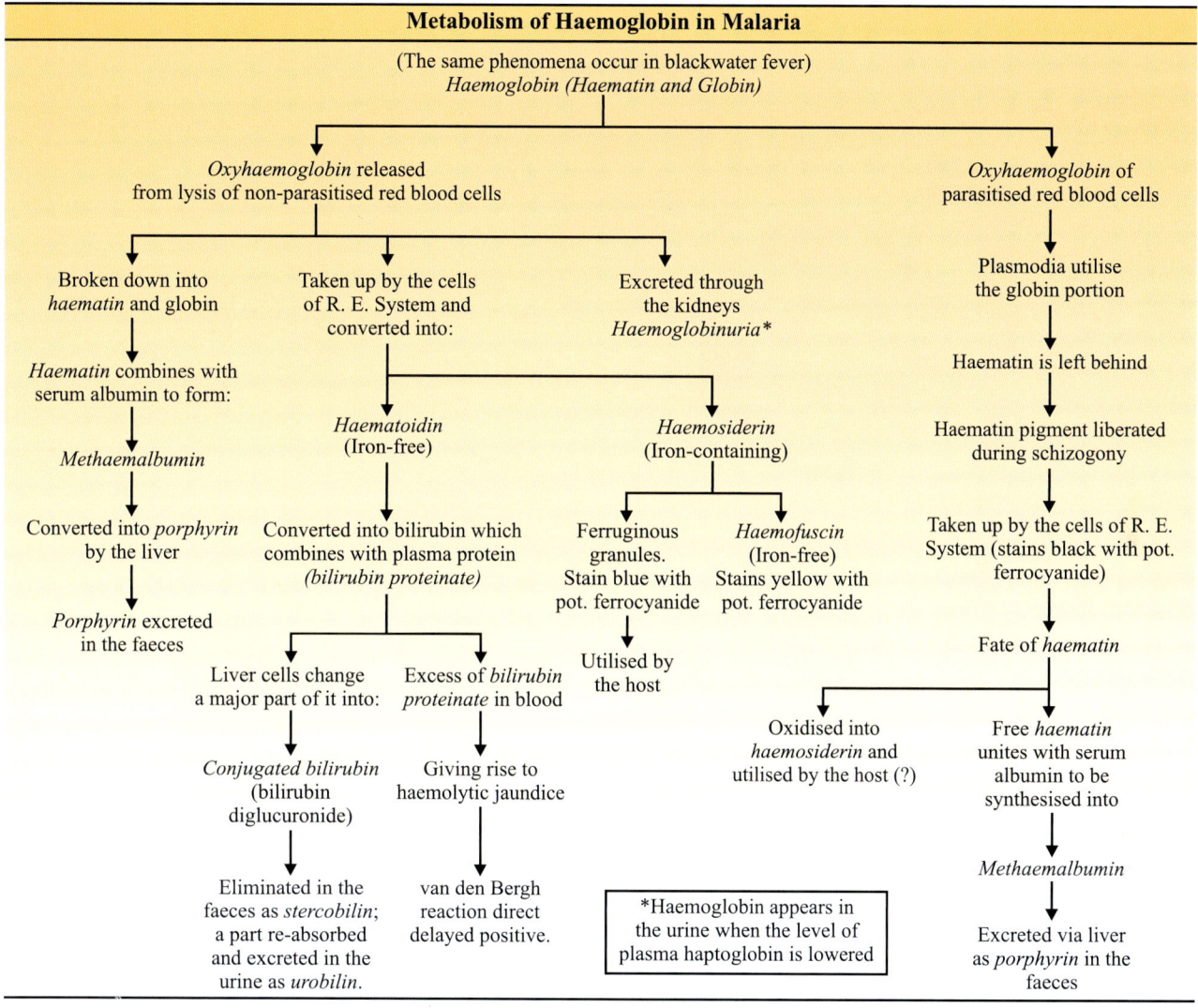

Metabolism of Haemoglobin in Malaria

(The same phenomena occur in blackwater fever)
Haemoglobin (Haematin and Globin)

Oxyhaemoglobin released from lysis of non-parasitised red blood cells

Oxyhaemoglobin of parasitised red blood cells

Broken down into *haematin* and globin

Taken up by the cells of R. E. System and converted into:

Excreted through the kidneys *Haemoglobinuria**

Plasmodia utilise the globin portion

Haematin combines with serum albumin to form:

Haematin is left behind

Methaemalbumin

Haematoidin (Iron-free)

Haemosiderin (Iron-containing)

Haematin pigment liberated during schizogony

Converted into *porphyrin* by the liver

Converted into bilirubin which combines with plasma protein (*bilirubin proteinate*)

Ferruginous granules. Stain blue with pot. ferrocyanide

Haemofuscin (Iron-free) Stains yellow with pot. ferrocyanide

Taken up by the cells of R. E. System (stains black with pot. ferrocyanide)

Porphyrin excreted in the faeces

Liver cells change a major part of it into:

Excess of *bilirubin proteinate* in blood

Utilised by the host

Fate of *haematin*

Conjugated bilirubin (bilirubin diglucuronide)

Giving rise to haemolytic jaundice

Oxidised into *haemosiderin* and utilised by the host (?)

Free *haematin* unites with serum albumin to be synthesised into

Eliminated in the faeces as *stercobilin*; a part re-absorbed and excreted in the urine as *urobilin*.

van den Bergh reaction direct delayed positive.

*Haemoglobin appears in the urine when the level of plasma haptoglobin is lowered

Methaemalbumin

Excreted via liver as *porphyrin* in the faeces

---

bone marrow. During erythrocytic schizogony and gametogony, the parasite performs various nutritive functions. It derives nutrition from the oxyhaemoglobin of the red blood cells inside which it grows. It takes oxygen readily from the oxyhaemoglobin of the infected red blood cells and the amount of oxygen consumed increases with the growth of the parasite. The protein material (globin*) of the erythrocytes is broken down and resynthesised into parasitic protein, the waste product being iron porphyrin (haematin or ferrihaemic acid) and its disposal is associated with the pigmentation of various organs which deal with it. The protein metabolism of the parasite is closely linked to the oxidation of glucose which provides energy requirements of the growing plasmodia. The glucose is converted first into pyruvic acid and then into carbon dioxide and water; with incomplete oxidation lactic acid is produced. Glucose-6-phosphate dehydrogenase (G-6-PD), an enzyme present in erythrocytes is an important requirement for plasmodium, hence those with G-6-PD deficiency may have some protection against plasmodium infections.

Note: Para-aminobenzoic acid (PABA) is necessary for the full metabolism of malaria parasites, particularly of the *erythrocytic* phase and its deficiency inhibits their growth. Mother's milk is deficient in PABA (it may also contain malarial antibodies from the immune mother) and may thus protect the infant from malaria infection.

During schizogony not only the unused haemoglobin of parasitised red blood cells, but also haemoglobin from the lysis of non-parasitised red blood cells is liberated. The metabolism of these liberated haemoglobins is shown in the table on page 92. The figure 83 represents a composite diagram to show the various changes associated with the disorder of red blood cell physiology in malaria.

---

* In sickle cell anaemia, the protein fraction of the haemoglobin molecule (Hb S) differs from the normal haemoglobin (Hb A) whereas in thalassaemia, there is interference with the synthesis of normal haemoglobin and the foetal haemoglobin (Hb F) persists. Individuals possessing Hb S and Hb F gene are protected against *P. falciparum* malaria.

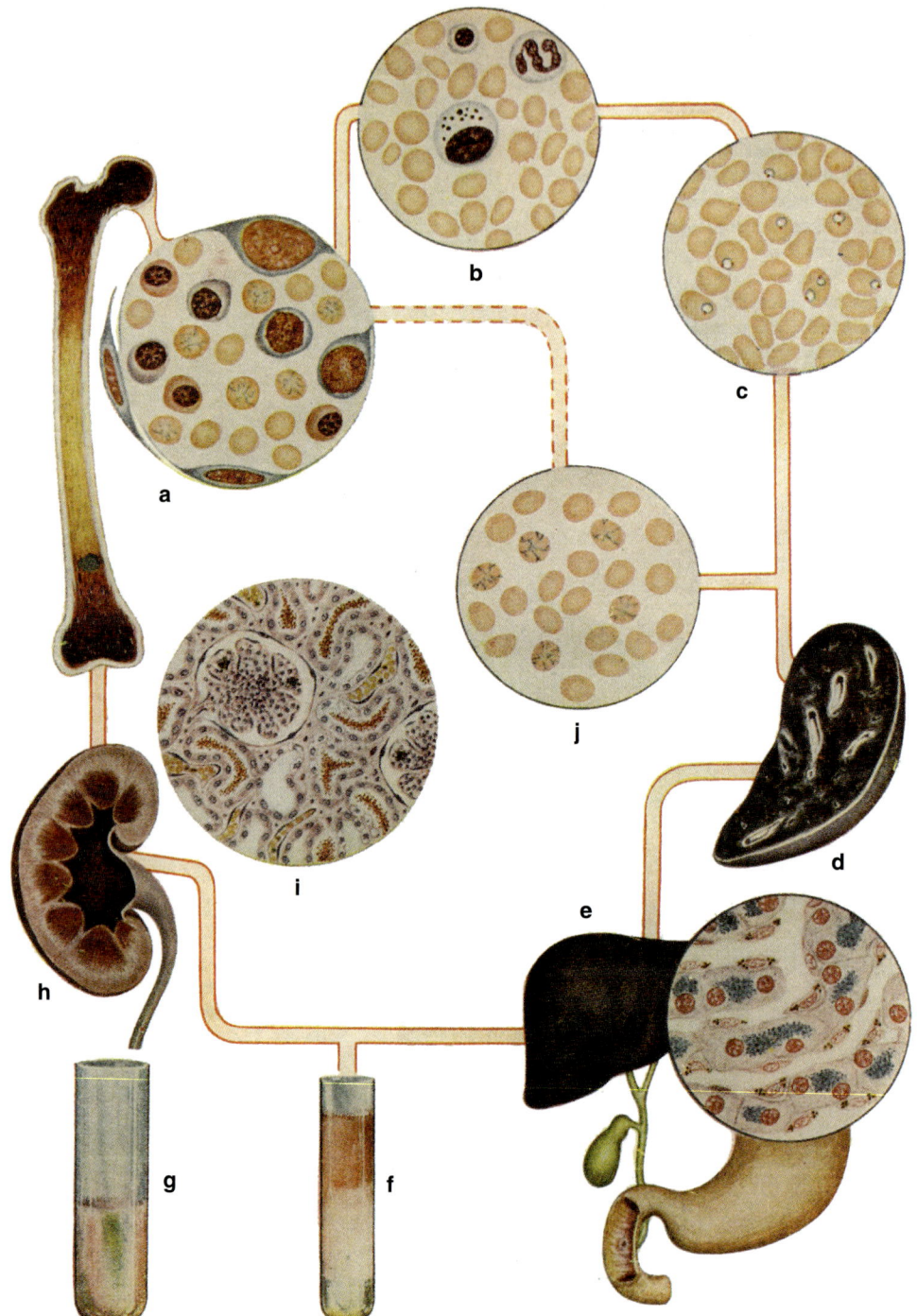

Fig. 83—Red blood cell physiology in malaria.

(The same phenomena occur in blackwater fever.)

a, bone marrow showing a normal erythropoiesis (reticulocytes are not readily released); b, haemogram depicting a normocytic hypochromic blood picture (malarial pigment inside a monocyte); c, parasitised erythrocytes containing ring-form of *Plasmodium falciparum*; d, pigmented spleen; e, pigmented liver, a section of liver treated with potassium ferrocyanide showing Prussian blue reaction of haemosiderin pigment while the malarial pigment is stained black and the biliary tract through which excess of the bile flows into the duodenum; f, direct delayed or immediate positive van den Bergh reaction (note the purple colour); g, urobilin test in urine positive (note the green fluorescence); h, kidney in malaria and blackwater fever; i, section of the kidney showing haemoglobinuric nephrosis; j, blood picture showing a reticulocytosis and disappearance of malarial parasites (occurring within 6 to 8 days after specific chemotherapy).

Main Features of Malarial Pathology

1. Pigmentation of various organs, giving the characteristic slate-grey or black colour. The malarial pigment is always found within the cells of the reticulo-endothelial system. The pigment granules are physiologically inert and take no part in the pathogenesis of malaria.

2. Hyperplasia of the reticulo-endothelial system (proliferation of cells and reticulin fibrils) resulting from increased activity in order to deal with the *Plasmodia* and their effete products (haematin, toxins etc.).

3. Parasitised erythrocytes filling the lumina of the capillaries of the internal organs. This is particularly seen in *P.falciparum* infection as the later stages of schizogony is mainly completed in the internal organs.

4. Vascular changes consisting of congestion and dilatation of sinusoidal vessels. Perivascular haemorrhages resulting from the damage to the capillary endothelium are seen in falciparum malaria.

5. Degenerative changes of parenchyma cells due to hypoxic state resulting from capillary blockage (seen in acute falciparum infection).

6. Mesenchymal reaction does not take any active part in the pathology of malarial infection and any fibrosis observed is the result of reparation of the local damage but the fibrosis is never so extensive as to cause, fibrosis of the organ.

7. Immunosuppression has been noticed in malarial infection and this may lead to secondary bacterial invasion.

Pathological Changes in Various Organs

(Common to all Species)

Spleen. The spleen functions, in malaria, as a filter for removing the parasites as well as the product of their schizogony from the blood stream. The parasites are found in abundance in all stages of development (erythrocytic schizogony and gametogony) in the spleen in all forms of malaria, particularly *falciparum* malaria. Malarial parasites and haematin pigments are actively phagocytosed in the spleen by macrophages mainly by the cells of Billroth cords (red pulp). The littoral cells of the venous " sinuses (sinus lining cells) do not take any active part, except in overwhelming infections.

A normal histological picture of the red pulp of the spleen is shown in Fig. 84.

MACROSCOPIC APPEARANCE (Fig. 85)

(i) The organ is moderately *enlarged*; even in chronic cases it never assumes such unusually big* proportions as may be seen in cases of kala-azar and other splenomegalic conditions prevalent in the tropics.

(ii) The *colour* is slate-grey or black, depending on the amount of pigmentation.

(iii) The *capsule* is thin and stretched in acute falciparum malaria but in chronic cases, it may be thickened due to associated perisplenitis.

(iv) The *consistency* of the organ (pulp substance), in acute cases is soft whereas in chronic cases it is fairly firm, for which reason chronic malarial spleen is termed "ague cake".

(v) The *cut surface* appears as a homogeneous black area with scattered white fibrous bands (trabeculae) and greyish white spots (Malpighian corpuscles).

Occasionally, haemorrhages under the capsule and in the substance of the spleen have been observed in acute falciparum malaria and cases are on record where spontaneous rupture of the organ has occurred.

HISTOPATHOLOGY. Microscopical examination (Fig. 86) reveals the following:

(i) Congestion of splenic sinusoids.

(ii) Enormous amount of pigments, both haematin and haemosiderin, are found to be scattered all over. Under the low power of the microscope these appear as so many precipitates; under higher magnification, the malarial pigment (haematin) is found inside the macrophage cells of the red pulp.

(iii) The number of macrophage cells are greatly increased.

(iv) Malpighian corpuscles (white pulp) are free from pigments and parasites.

---

* "Big spleen disease" (idiopathic tropical splenomegaly syndrome) found in adults in certain hyper-endemic malarial areas has been shown to be related to an abnormal immune response to plasmodial antigen (although the malarial parasites are absent from the blood). It is associated with hepatomegaly (liver biopsies reveal sinusoidal lymphocytosis), anaemia, leucopenia, increased serum IgM concentrations and high malaria antibody titres (Pitney, 1968). Continuous malaria chemoprophylaxis over many months caused a gradual reduction in the spleen size together with clinical improvement, but cessation of prophylaxis resulted in reappearance of the syndrome (Williams-Watson & Allan, 1971).

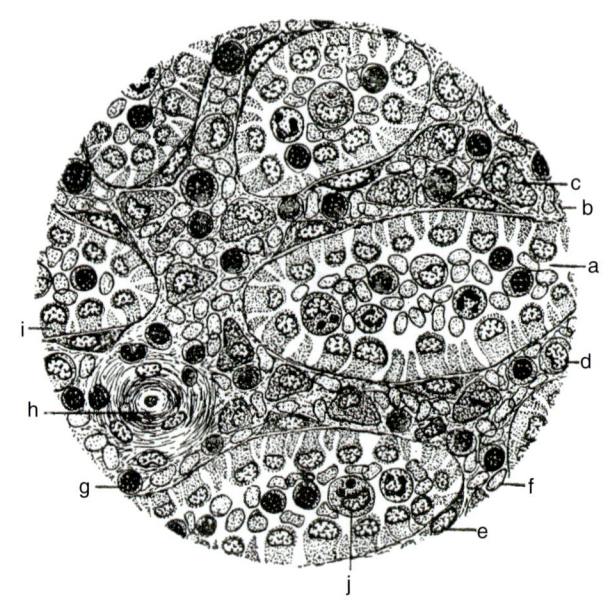

Fig. 84—Normal histological picture of the red pulp of the spleen.

a, venous sinus; *b*, cells in the Billroth cord; *c*, fixed macrophage; *d*, monocyte; *e*, reticular cell; *f*, erythrocyte in the Billroth cord; *g*, lymphocyte; *h*, sheathed artery; *i*, sinus-lining cell (littoral cell); *j*, free macrophage with erythrocytes (phagocytic) inside the venous sinus.

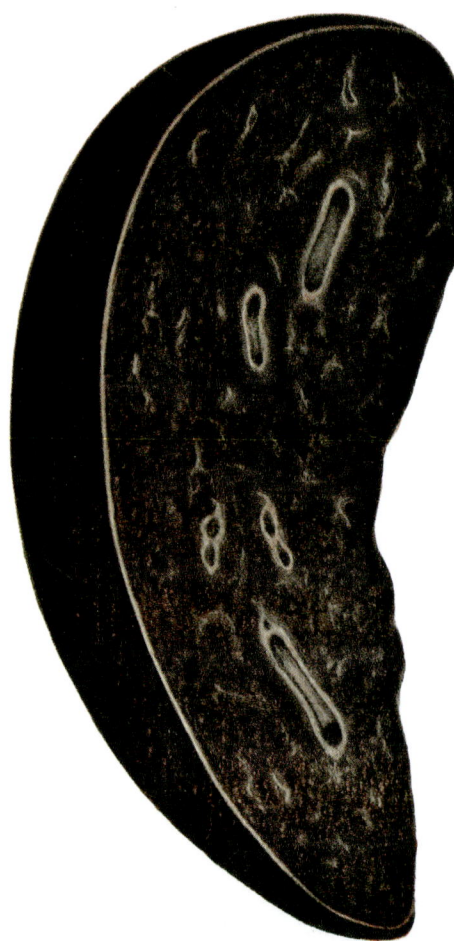

Fig. 85—Macroscopic appearance of a malarial spleen (*cut section*).
Showing the characteristic pigmentation (bronze black colour) of the organ.

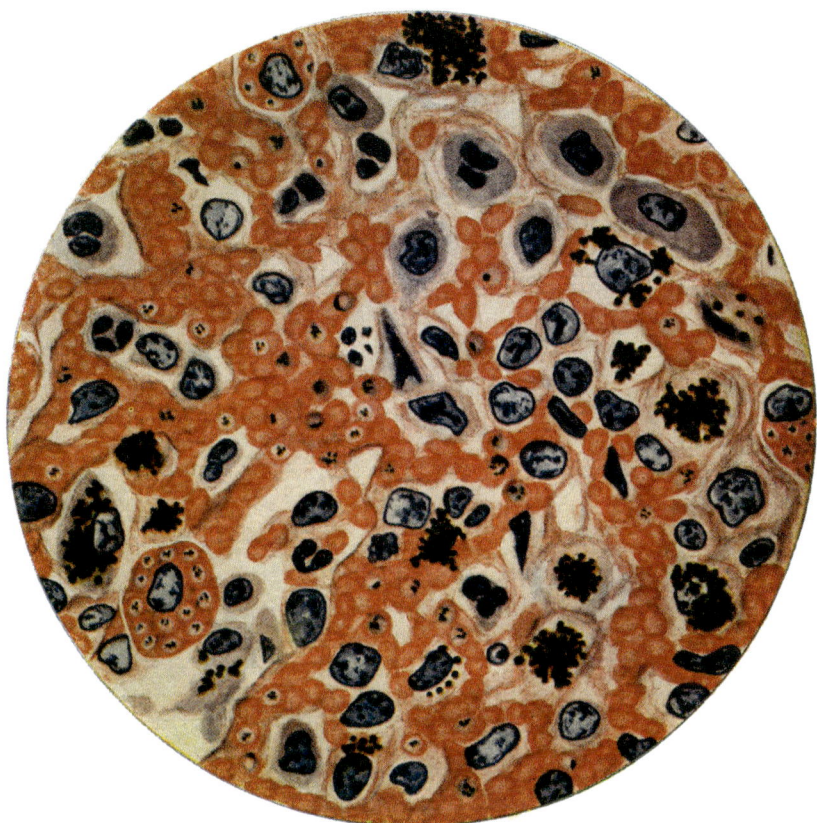

Fig. 86—Microscopic appearance of a malarial spleen, showing various pathological changes (*see text*) Haematoxylin and eosin stain.

(v) The parasites can be differentiated as black dots in the red blood cells when the sections are stained with haematoxylin and eosin.

(vi) The reticulin fibrils may be increased in chronic cases.

Liver. Macroscopic Appearance. The organ is uniformly *enlarged* due to the vascular congestion and proliferation of reticulo-endothelial cells. The colour varies from dark chocolate-red to slate-grey or even black, and depends upon the stage of congestion and the amount of haematin pigment. The *cut surface* shows dilated lobular veins; where the fatty change is limited to the central zone of the lobule, it stands out as a yellowish area against a brownish red background.

HISTOPATHOLOGY. Microscopical examination reveals the following:

(i) The central veins of the lobules and sinusoidal capillaries are dilated and filled with red blood cells, many of which are parasitised.

(ii) The Küpffer's cells are increased in number and their cytoplasms are filled with malarial pigment (haematin) and parasitised erythrocytes.

(iii) The parenchyma cells of the liver lying in the central zone show fatty degeneration, atrophy and necrosis (centrilobular necrosis). This has been attributed to hypoxia resulting from interference with the escape of hepatic venous blood (hepatic "sluice" reflex of Maegraith).

(iv) The parasites are found in various stages of development and may lie within the red blood cells, free in the lumen of the sinusoids or phagocytosed by the Küpffer's, cells (Fig. 87).

(v) Fibrous tissue is not increased to any great extent. Any fibrous tissue that may be observed in the portal zone or in the central zone is to be regarded as secondary to the process of degeneration.

Bone Marrow. In *acute cases* the marrow of the long bones undergoes very little change. In chronic cases the upper and lower thirds of the long bones are reddish-brown in colour and may even be slate-grey or black. The yellow fatty marrow becomes gradually replaced by the vascular cellular tissue (red formative marrow).

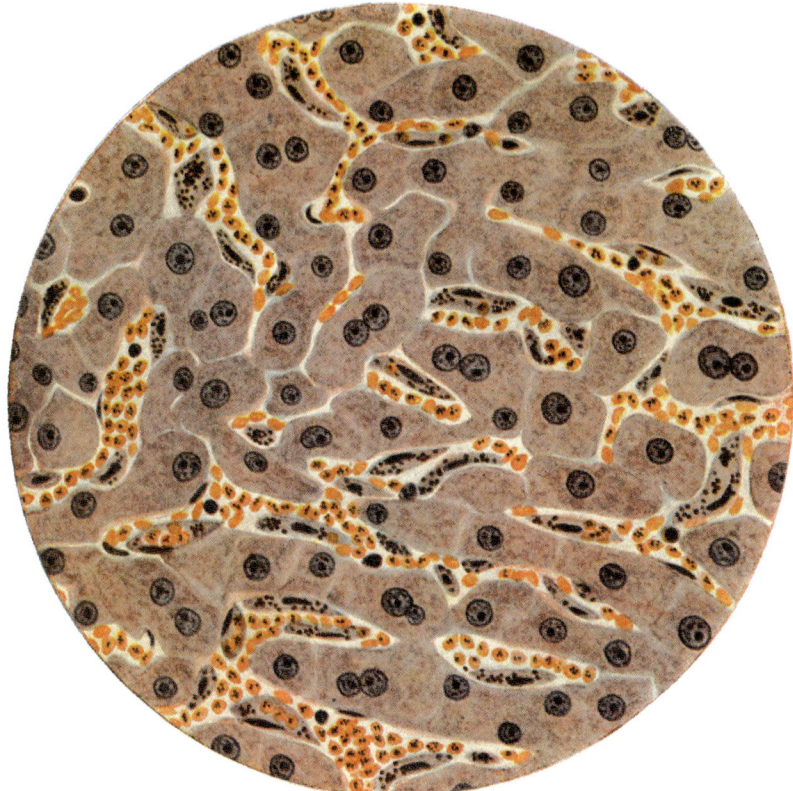

Fig. 87—Microscopic appearance of a malarial liver (Haematoxylin and eosin stain).
Note the sinusoidal capillaries filled with parasitised erythrocytes and the Küpffer's cells
containing malarial pigment, parasitised and non-parasitised erythrocytes.

MICROSCOPICAL EXAMINATION shows parasitised red blood cells, hyperplasia of reticulo-endothelial cells which are laden with the malarial pigment (haematin) and an erythroblastic reaction of the normoblastic type (increase in the number of nucleated red blood cells and reticulocytes) with some depression of myeloblastic activity (as evidenced by decrease in the granulocytes of the blood).

Kidneys. The renal manifestations in malaria may be divided into two groups:

(i) Those found during an attack of acute falciparum malaria and also in blackwater fever is the renal anoxia syndrome characterised by oliguria or anuria and acute uraemia; it is also k.a. renal tubular vascular syndrome or "lower nephron nephrosis".

(ii) Those found in relapsing quartan malaria, resembling nephrotic syndrome. The nephropathy associated with quartan malaria is the result of immunological reaction arising from antigen (*P. malariae*) and antibody complexes deposited on the glomerular capillary basement membrane. The glomerular injury is caused by complement (β_1, G globulin) activation and release of enzymes from the granules of leucocytes (Giglioli, 1962; Cameron, 1972).

Pathological Changes in Pernicious Malaria

(Changes in Organs in Pernicious Types of Falciparum Malaria)

Pathology of Cerebral Malaria

Brain. The entire capillary network of the brain tissue is distended and often occluded or "plugged" by the parasitised erythrocytes (Fig. 88); these are more prominent in the grey matter than in the white matter and the distribution is even and uniform in all locations. Occasionally, the distribution of parasitised erythrocytes associated with the blocking of the blood vessels may be regional which may account for certain focal symptoms. All stages of the erythrocytic cycle may occur in the brain capillaries and although the trophozoites and schizonts are the forms most commonly seen in cerebral cases gametocyte formation has also been observed.

MACROSCOPIC APPEARANCE. Pial and cerebral blood vessels are markedly congested. The *cut surface* of the brain shows slate-grey colour of the cortex associated with multiple punctiform haemorrhages in the subcortical white matter (Fig. 89). Areas of small infarcts may be seen in the brain substance.

HISTOPATHOLOGY. Microscopical examination may reveal the following:

(i) Dilatation and congestion of cerebral capillaries filled with parasitised erythrocytes.

(ii) Perivascular haemorrhages, having the appearance of "ring haemorrhages". These occur around the plugged vessel. The red blood cells of haemorrhages are not parasitised.

(iii) Scattered areas of softening due to degeneration of the nerve tissue.

Later the softened areas are invaded by glial cells forming the so-called "malarial granulomas" of Dürck, result of a reparative reaction to local damage. A full developed "granuloma" consists of a collection of proliferated glial cells radially arranged around the occluded blood vessel. When the lesion has advanced to the stage of "granuloma", some permanent damage in the form of multiple sclerotic areas may remain in the brain as a sequel to malarial infection. The psychotic syndrome which sometimes follows the illness after an apparent recovery may be correlated to such pathological lesions. The evolution of a "malarial granuloma" is depicted in Figs. 90-93.

Pathology of Algid Malaria

Gastro-Intestinal Tract. The mucous membrane shows pigmentation of a slate-grey colour. Occasionally, there may be punctiform haemorrhages but ulcerations are not present. The intestinal contents may be watery or dark-brown with very little mucus. Microscopically, the mucosal and submucosal capillaries are congested and packed with parasitised erythrocytes, but the capillaries of muscular and serous layers contain very few parasites.

Peripheral Blood Vessels. Generalised vascular collapse (peripheral circulatory failure) resulting from adrenal damage or arising independently, accounts for death in these cases. The heart in such cases does not show any significant damage (Fig. 94).

Adrenal Glands. The essential histopathological changes in the adrenal glands are necrosis of *Zona fasciculata* and haemorrhages with congestion of *Zona reticulata*. Parasitised erythrocytes and pigmented phagocytes are found in the sinusoidal capillaries of the adrenal glands (Fig. 95).

Pathology of Septicaemic Malaria

Heart. Macroscopic appearance of the heart does not show any abnormality. Microscopical examination reveals intensely congested coronary blood vessels filled with parasitised erythrocytes. Fatty degeneration and necrosis of heart muscle are also observed (Fig. 96).

Lungs. Cases having pneumonic symptoms show small areas of haemorrhages with patches of oedema and collapse. Microscopically, alveolar capillaries are found to be congested and filled with parasitised erythrocytes. Lung alveoli contain extravasated red blood cells and pigmented monocytes (Fig. 97).

Blood. A high degree of parasitaemia is a feature of this type of malaria and both schizogony and gametogony occur in the peripheral circulation (Fig. 98) and also inside the capillaries of the internal organs. On account of heavy infection of red blood cells, a severe type of anaemia quickly develops.

CLINICAL PATHOLOGY

Changes in Blood. An individual suffering from an attack of malaria, after a few paroxysms, becomes temporarily anaemic. The *anaemia* is not due to any depression of the erythropoietic function of the bone marrow, but is the result of destruction of the infected red blood cells during each cycle of schizogony. It is therefore an example of haemolytic anaemia. The reduction in red blood cells is greater in *P. falciparum* infection than in infections with *P. vivax* and *P. malariae*, because this species invades young and mature erythrocytes and the infection rate of red blood cells (parasitaemia) is also greater. The red blood cell count in acute falciparum malaria may be as low as 1 million per mm^3 of blood; whereas in relapsing vivax and quartan malaria, it may be 2 to 3 millions per mm^3 of blood. Anaemia, in malaria, is of the normocytic and hypochromic type. An autoimmune haemolytic mechanism has also been postulated to explain anaemia in malaria.

Leucocyte count is increased (may even be 10 to 20 thousand per mm^3) during the period of rising temperature of the malarial paroxysm but it quickly comes down to normal after the paroxysm is over (the fall is actually noticed as soon as the temperature reaches its acme). With recurring paroxysms, leucopenia becomes established, the total count ranging from 3,000 to 5,000 per mm^3 of blood. The neutrophil granulocytes are diminished, ranging from 50 to 70 per cent; monocytes show an actual increase ranging from 10 to 20 per cent. Both the monocytes and neutrophils are often found to contain ingested haematin pigment.

In pernicious malaria, the characteristic blood picture is a mild leucopenia, the average count being 5,200 per mm^3 of blood.

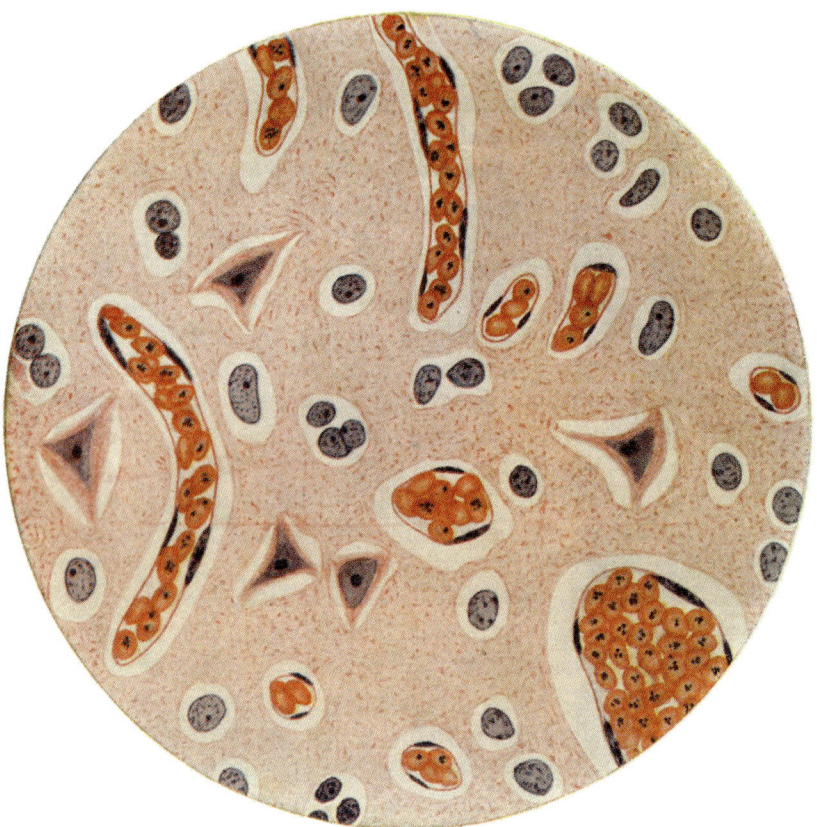

Fig. 88—Microscopic appearance of brain in acute falciparum malaria.
Showing the entire capillary network filled with parasitised erythrocytes.

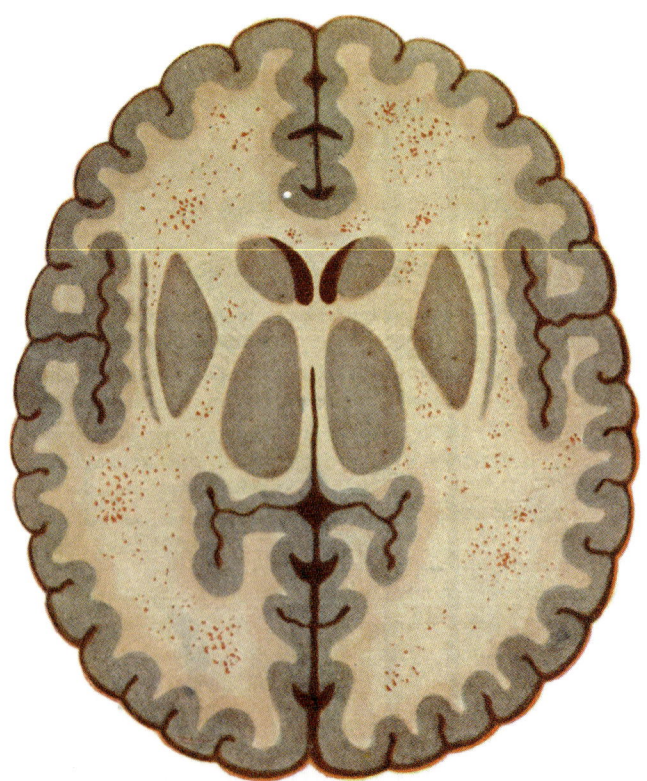

Fig. 89—Brain in acute falciparum malaria.
Showing petechial haemorrhages in the sub-cortical white matter and slate-grey colour of the cerebral cortex and the basal ganglia.

EVOLUTION OF SO-CALLED "MALARIAL GRANULOMA"

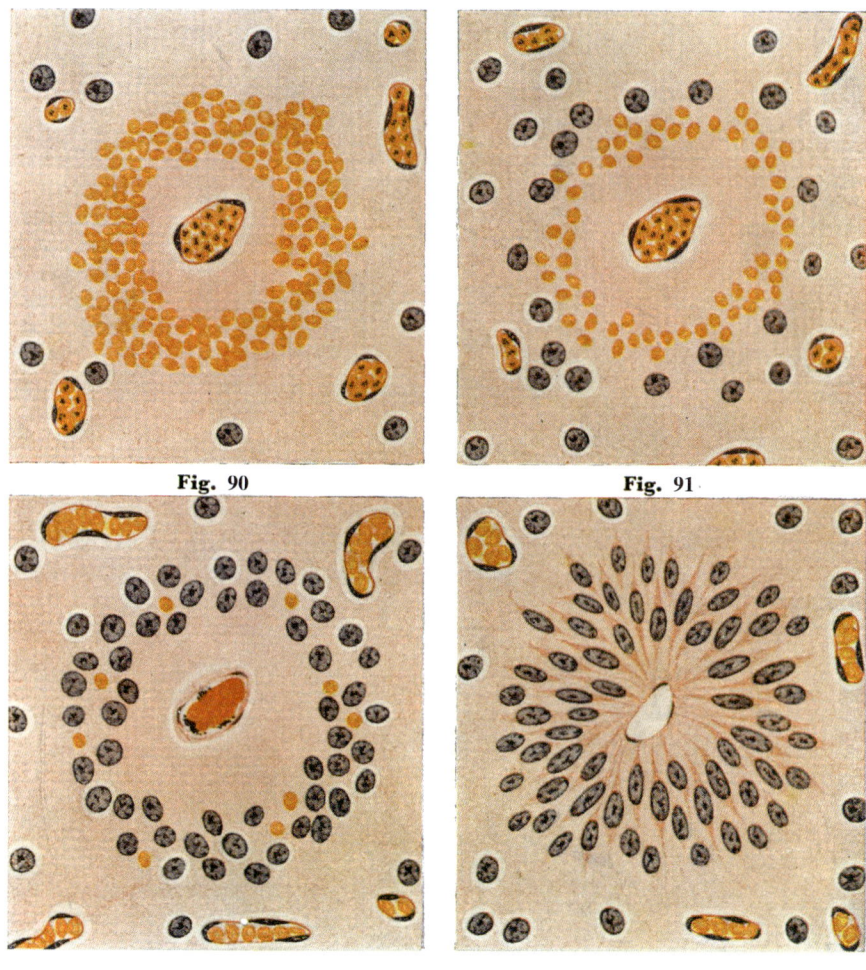

Fig. 90   Fig. 91

Fig. 92   Fig. 93

Fig. 90—Ring haemorrhage with central "plugged" capillary vessel. Erythrocytes of the haemorrhage are non-parasitised.

Fig. 91—Demyelinisation of the central necrotic area surrounding the "plugged" capillary vessel; a few red blood cells persisting in the peripheral zone.

Fig. 92—Central thrombosed capillary vessel with parasite pigment at the periphery, necrotic intermediate zone and neurological cells mixed with non-parasitised erythrocytes in the peripheral zone.

Fig. 93—Proliferated glial cells arranged radially around the central capillary vessel —a reparative reaction.

Chemical Changes in the Blood in Malaria

1. Plasma albumin is reduced; may be related to liver dysfunction. Increase of serum gamma globulin accounts for various specific and non-specific serologic tests. Albumin/globulin ratio is reversed.

2. Cholesterol level rises during rigor and falls during apyrexial period.

3. Rise of blood sugar is probably correlated to adrenal function. Low blood sugar in falciparum malaria.

4. Rise of plasma potassium resulting from destruction of red blood cells.

5. ESR is raised. It is related to plasma protein and change in the surface of the red blood cells.

6. A fall of pH and a loss of alkali reserve, due to increase of pyruvates and lactates.

7. Indirect reacting bilirubin is increased.

8. Pathological haemoglobinaemia is unusual.

9. Biological changes in erythrocytes comprise increase in cellular sodium with equivalent decrease in cellular potassium.

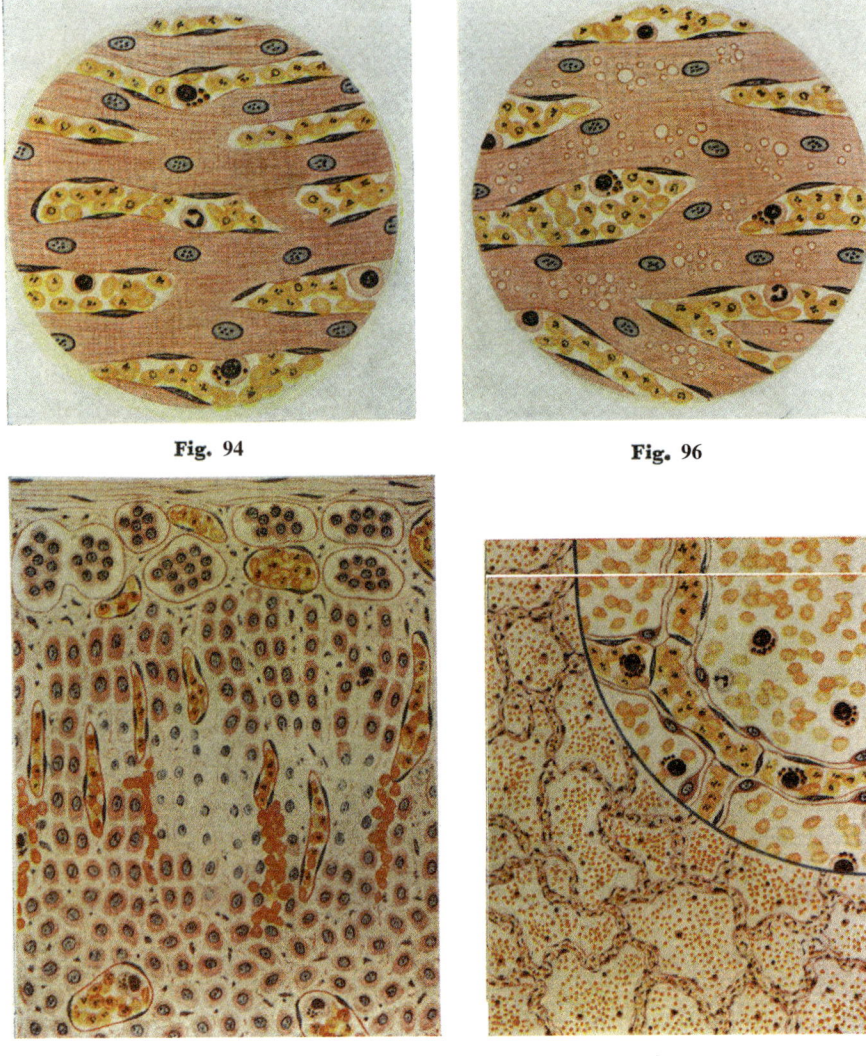

Fig. 94

Fig. 96

Fig. 95

Fig. 97

Fig. 94—Heart in *falciparum* malaria (algid type). Capillaries are filled with parasitised erythrocytes. No significant pathological change in the myocardium can be observed.

Fig. 95—Adrenal gland in *falciparum* malaria. Capillaries are filled with parasitised erythrocytes. Haemorrhages and necrosis can be seen in the zona fasciculata.

Fig. 96—Heart in *falciparum* malaria (septicaemic type). Capillaries are filled with parasitised erythrocytes. Fatty degeneration of the myocardium can be seen.

Fig. 97—Lungs in *falciparum* malaria. Alveoli contain non-parasitised erythrocytes and a few pigmented monocytes. Alveolar capillaries are filled with parasitised erythrocytes (a magnified view is given in the inset).

Laboratory Diagnosis of Malaria

A microscopical examination of a blood film forms one of the most important diagnostic procedures in malaria. In the majority of cases of symptomatic malaria, a careful examination of thin film will invariably show the plasmodia provided no antimalarial drugs have been administered prior to the taking of blood films; thick films are rarely called for. It is a good practice to take both thin and thick films, at the same time, either on the same slide or on two different slides so that the parasite may be quickly detected in the thick film and then the thin film examined for identifying the species. Sometimes, it may be necessary to administer antimalarial drugs as soon as the clinical diagnosis has been

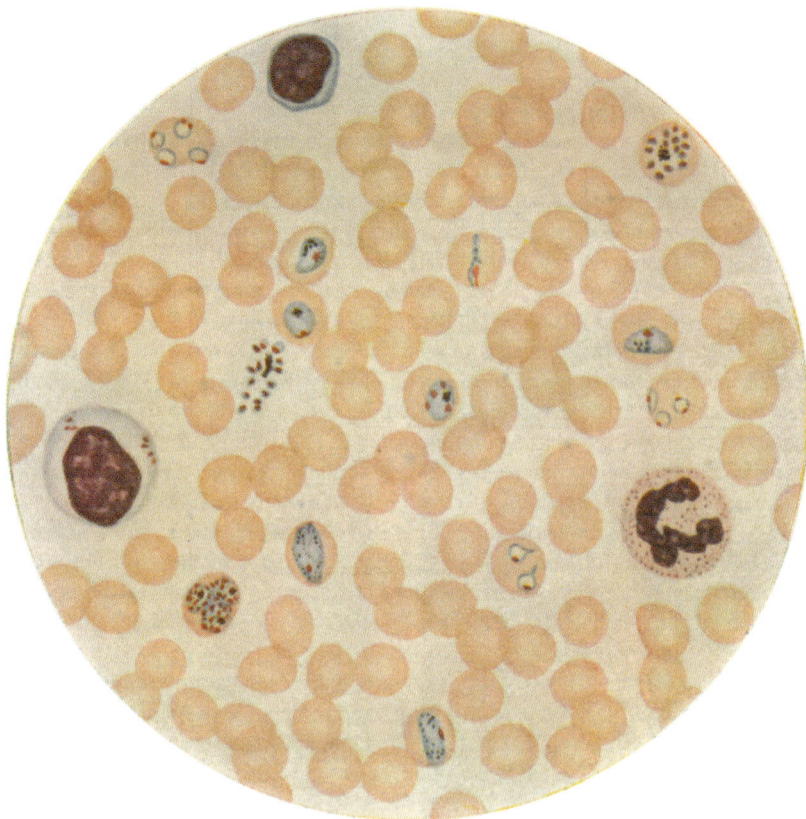

Fig. 98—Blood-film from a case of "septicaemic type" of pernicious malaria, showing schizogony and gametogony of *P. falciparum* **in the peripheral blood.** (The patient developed haemoglobinuria. Cured with antimalarial treatment.)

made and in these cases, blood slides should immediately be taken, if necessary, by the clinician himself and sent to the laboratory for examination. For the technique of preparation and staining of blood films, *see Appendix I.*

In a well-stained film, if parasites are numerous, the species can be easily identified but the possibility of mixed infections should always be remembered. Difficulty in identifying the species may be experienced when only a few ring-forms are encountered. In such cases, however the blood should be examined a few hours later to arrive at a correct diagnosis. Use of fluorescent staining method and examination of stained slide under fluorescent microscope and QBC test (quantitative buffy coat test) are new methods for identification of parasite.

Difficulties in Detecting the Malarial Parasite:

  (i) Blood films taken after an antimalarial drug.

 (ii) Blood films taken during the apyrexial interval of *falciparum* malaria.

(iii) In all cases of primary infection, during the first 2 to 3 days.

OTHER METHODS IN DIAGNOSIS:

Cultural Examination. This is not required for diagnosis except only in special circumstances, when there is a difficulty in differentiating the trophozoite (ring-form) of *P. vivax* from that of *P. falciparum.*

Blood Count. This has very little importance in the diagnosis of malaria. The significant change in chronic malaria is moderate leucopenia (neutropenia) with monocytosis (15 to 20%). The presence of pigmented monocytes is a good evidence of past or present malarial infection. In acute falciparum malaria the blood picture is either normal or shows a leucopenic trend.

Serological Tests. These are not necessary for the diagnosis of acute infection, but are used for studying immunological aspects of populations living in highly endemic areas and detecting latent infection in subjects who are used as blood donors.

IMMUNOFLUORESCENCE TEST (direct and indirect). The fluorescent dye used in the test conjugates with the gamma globulin of the serum to be tested. If such conjugated gamma globulin contains malarial antibody, it will adhere to the relevant malarial parasite and will be recognised as glistening particles under the fluorescent microscope.

GEL PRECIPITATION TEST. The antigen from *P. falciparum* is used. The incidence of positive result is very high in hyperendemic areas.

Other serological tests are IHA, ELISA and agar gel deffusion test. No serological tests can be compared with the sensitivity and specificity of microscopical detection of malaria parasite.

Other methods include DNA probes and Dot blot assay for diagnosis of malaria.

RAPID DIAGNOSTIC TESTS (dip stick test or test strip test). These tests are based on detection of antibody of two antigens in blood sample (histidine rich protein 2 (P*f*HRP2) and parasite lactate dehydrogenase (P*F*LDH). These test provide good diagnosic sensitvity and helpful diagnostic method where microscope examination for malaria parasite is not possible. P*F*LDH is cleared rapidly from the blood within days of onset of treatment. P*f*HRP2 clears very slowly form the blood and takes almost one month for complete disapreance after acute infection. Histidine-rich protein (P*f*HRP2) is specific of *P. falciparum*. Parasite lactate dehydrogenase (pLDH) of all plasmodium species, infecting man can be detected by the use of rapid tests also. These tests are rapid test and take about 15-20 minutes. Several commercial kits (Parasight F, Paracheck F) are available.

Sternal Puncture. This is not popular in the diagnosis of malaria, because in cases where bone marrow biopsy demonstrates the presence of malaria parasites, an examination of the peripheral blood will also show the presence of the parasites.

Treatment. The various antimalarial drugs are grouped as follows:

1. *Essentially therapeutic* (Clinical cure): 4-aminoquinolines such as chloroquine artemisinin compounds, quinine (for drug-resistant *P. falciparum*) and mefloquine. These are potent drugs having action on early erythrocytic phases of the parasite.

For radical cure an 8-aminoquinoline, primaquine is used after the clinical cure. It acts on the latent stage of parasites in the liver, hence prevents relapses. It also acts on gametocytes, but has little action on asexual blood parasites.

2. *Protective or prophylactic*: Proguanil (chlorguanide), pyrimethamine and trimethoprim. These are dihydrofolate reductase inhibitors and are mostly used to "suppress" clinical manifestations. These drugs can destroy pre-erythrocytic phase of the parasite in the liver (causal prophylaxis) and inactivate gametocytes, thereby preventing further development in the mosquitoes. They act on the dividing schizonts.

Chloroquine may be used where local strains are resistant to proguanil and pyrimethamine; quinine, if other drugs are not available. Cycloguanil, a metabolite of proguanil, may be used as a long-acting injectible prophylactic.

3. *Synergists* (potentiate the action of schizonticidal drugs): Sulphonamides and sulphones (dapsone) are often used in combination with dihydrofolate reductase inhibitors. *See Appendix II.*

Note: Emergence of drug-resistant parasites (*P. falciparum*) necessitates the use of multiple drug regimen.

Prophylaxis. FOR PERSONAL PROPHYLAXIS: (i) Protection against mosquito bites, and (ii) systematic use of antimalarial drugs as a prophylactic measure (chemoprophylaxis).

FOR COMMUNITY PROPHYLAXIS: (i) *Prevention of carrier* by antimalarial drugs having a destructive effect on the gametocytes; the only drug possessing such action is 8-aminoquinoline. This being a toxic drug cannot be used for mass prophylaxis however, (ii) *Anti-mosquito measures.* These may be directed towards adult mosquitoes and their larvae, (a) Destruction of adult mosquitoes can be carried out by spraying with insecticides, such as D.D.T. or gammexane. (b) Anti-larval measures consist of elimination of breeding places of the mosquitoes and use of larvicides (oil, parish green, D.D.T. dissolved in oil). (iii) Use of pyrethroid treated bednets and mosquito repellants are fruitful personal prophylactic measures.

Note: Emergence of insecticide-resistant mosquitoes (vectors) and drug-resistant Plasmodia (parasites) have caused a serious setback in several successful eradication programmes of malaria. The aim is effective control instead of malaria eradication. The objectives are: (i) to prevent death from malaria which is possible, because of availability of new powerful drugs; (ii) to see that the industrial and agricultural progress do not suffer; (iii) to see that there is no fresh outbreak in such areas.

Malaria Vaccine: Research on malaria vaccine is going on. It is hoped that vaccines may prevent death, and infection may be attenuated only, but the disease cannot be prevented.

BLACKWATER FEVER

Definition. It is a manifestation of falciparum malaria occurring in previously infected subjects and is characterised by sudden intravascular haemolysis followed by fever and haemoglobinuria. The disease is now rare as new synthetic antimalerial drugs have replaced quinine.

Etiology. It is associated with infection by *Plasmodium falciparum*, most commonly observed amongst the non-immune (non-indigenous) individuals who have resided in malarious countries for 6 months to 1 year and have had inadequate doses of quinine for both suppressive prophylaxis and treatment of repeated clinical attacks. In these cases, quinine often acts as a precipitating factor. Other factors which have been known to precipitate an attack of blackwater fever are: cold, exposure to the sun, fatigue, trauma, pregnancy, parturition and X-ray treatment of the spleen. Patient with G6PD deficiency may develop this condition, after taking oxidant drugs.

Pathogenesis. Intravascular haemolysis.

MECHANISM OF HAEMOLYSIS. The exact mechanism of haemolysis in blackwater fever is not yet clearly known. There appears to be some haemolytic agent involved whereby the red blood cells undergo lysis and liberate a large quantity of oxyhaemoglobin into the blood stream. In falciparum malaria, intravascular haemolysis occurs periodically at the time of schizogony. This probably stimulates the R.E. system to form antibodies of the nature of haemolysin and lecitholysin. Thus, in repeated malarial attacks a hypersensitised state (pre-blackwater fever state) is produced which when stimulated by any factor, such as heavy *P. falciparum* infection of homologous or heterologous strain, administration of quinine and other precipitating factors leads to an explosive output of haemolysin resulting in the haemoclasic crisis of blackwater fever. Recent studies indicate that individuals having glucose-6-phosphate dehydrogenase deficient red blood cells are particularly susceptible to such haemolysis.

EFFECT OF INTRAVASCULAR HAEMOLYSIS. The excess of haemoglobin liberated in the circulating blood as a result of intravascular haemolysis is either catabolised into methaemalbumin, or converted by P. E. System into bilirubin and haemosiderin, or excreted through the kidneys. The following effects are observed:

(i) *Methaemalbuminaemia.* Oxyhaemoglobin in blood is broken down into globin and haematin (ferrous); the latter, after oxidation (ferric state), combines with serum albumin forming methaemalbumin which is not excreted in the urine (unable to pass through the renal glomeruli), but retained in the plasma causing methaemalbuminaemia.

(ii) *Hyperbilirubinaemia.* The bilirubin formed by R.E. System is far in excess of what the liver can excrete and is thereby retained in the plasma, causing hyperbilirubinaemia.

(iii) *Haemoglobinuria.* An excess of haemoglobin remains in the circulating blood and when the haptoglobin, a protein of the plasma, is unable to bind the free haemoglobin, it is excreted through the kidneys causing haemoglobinuria. Oxyhaemoglobin may be converted into methaemoglobin in the renal tubules or deposited in the tubules as acid haematin.

PIGMENTS IN BLOOD AND URINE: *Blood.* Oxyhaemoglobin, methaemalbumin and bilirubin. Van den Bergh reaction gives an indirect positive. *Methaemoglobin is not present in the blood.*

Urine. Oxyhaemoglobin (gives red colour), methaemoglobin (gives dark-brown or black colour), haematin, urobilin. *Methaemalbumin is not present in the urine.*

Parasites in Blood. In the majority of cases, the *parasites* (*P. falciparum*) are not detected in the peripheral blood either during or after the attack, as they are destroyed by the haemolytic crisis. Though the parasites disappear during the attack, they usually re-appear within a week or a fortnight after the haemolytic crisis.

Pathology. The morbid anatomy and histopathology of blackwater fever is practically the same as that of a severe type of falciparum malaria. The changes are specially noticeable in the kidneys and liver. The *kidneys* are large and dark in colour (due to congestion and pigmentation) and microscopically, degenerative changes are noticeable in the distal convoluted tubules which are blocked with eosinophilic granular debris (haemoglobin casts). Parasitised erythrocytes may or may not be detected inside the renal capillaries. The liver is enlarged and soft and is stained intensely yellow (due to haemosiderin); necrotic changes in the parenchyma cells are most marked in the central zone of the liver lobule. The *gall bladder* is filled with dark green viscid bile. The *spleen* is enlarged and coloured black due to the malarial pigment.

In blackwater fever there is excessive deposit of haemosiderin pigment in the liver, spleen and kidneys.

Clinical Features. The attack begins with fever and rigor, followed by aching pains in the loins, haemoglobinuria, icterus, bilious vomiting, circulatory collapse and acute renal failure. The haemolytic episode is generally only one or two.

Clinical Pathology

BLOOD CHANGES

Cytology (Blood Picture). R.B.G. count is 1 to 2 millions per mm^3 (normocytic anaemia) and haemoglobin percentage drops down to 10. There may be normoblast, polychromasia and basophilic stippling of red blood cells. During recovery, reticulocytosis is marked. W.B.C. count shows neutrophilic leucocytosis of a moderate degree.

Biochemical Alteration. Blood urea is increased and blood cholesterol is diminished. Plasma haptoglobin is very much lowered.

Parasites and Pigments. Vide supra.

URINARY CHANGES. The colour of the urine varies from red to dark brown (portwine) and is acid in reaction. When allowed to settle, there is a heavy brown amorphous deposit at the bottom. Albumin is excreted in large amounts; urobilin test shows a marked reaction. Microscopical examination shows haemoglobin casts and haematin crystals but *no red blood cells*. Haemoglobin pigments excreted in the urine (*vide supra*) are recognised by their characteristic absorption bands in the spectrum.

Complications. Renal failure (uraemia), acute liver failure and circulatory collapse.

Sequelae. Anaemia, pigment calculi.

Treatment. If parasites are detected in the peripheral blood, antimalarial chemotherapy should immediately be instituted and the drug of choice is chloroquine (for chloroquine resistant *P. falciparum* strain, as in South-East Asia, other drugs should be used). A fatal outcome in blackwater fever is often due to renal failure which is of the reversible renal anoxic type, hence it is treated with the help of artificial kidney or by peritoneal dialysis. Blood transfusion may be called for and care should be taken in cross-matching donor and recipient bloods. Both red blood cells and plasma are to be cross-matched for each specimen of blood transfused. Intravenous glucose saline was formerly used to replace lost fluid but it is risky in patients who have oliguria and anuria. Administration of large doses of alkalies was also given up because it was found to be harmful to kidney function.

Prophylaxis. With the advent of modern drugs for treatment and prophylaxis of malaria in place of quinine the indigenous inhabitants are protected from blackwater fever. If possible the subject of BWF should leave the endemic area and must not come back to it or reside in any malarial locality.

Class SPOROZOEA: Subclass COCCIDIA
Order EUCOCCIDIIDA: Suborder EIMERIINA

The family Eimeriidae comprises of two genera of medical importance *Isospora* and *Eimeria*. These are intracellular parasites, living inside the epithelial cells of intestinal mucosa. These two genera are differentiated by the character of mature oöcyst.

(a) In Isospora, the oöcyst contains 2 sporocysts each with 4 sporozoites.

(b) In Eimeria, the oöcyst contains 4 sporocysts each with 2 sporozoites.

The members of family Sarcocystidae differ from those of the family Eimeriidae mainly in having heteroxenous life cycle. The oöcysts contain two sporocysts each with 4 sporozoites. The genera *Toxoplasma* and *Sarcocystis* belong to this family.

The genera *Isospora*, *Toxoplasma* and *Sarcocystis* are causing parasitic infection amongst human beings particularly in AIDS patients.

Life Cycles of Eimeriidae. This shows an alternation of generation, one asexual and the other sexual, both of which are passed in the same host (Fig. 99).

INSIDE THE HUMAN OR ANIMAL HOST. The parasite while undergoing asexual schizogony inside the epithelial cells of intestine passes through the stages of trophozoite, schizont and merozoite. At the end of each cycle, a number of merozoites (motile, fusiform bodies) are liberated in the lumen of the gut. Each merozoite invades an epithelial cell and continues its asexual cycle of development as before, which is repeated for several generations.

With the onset of the sexual cycle, some of the merozoites become sexually differentiated into male and female forms, known as microgametocytes and macrogametocytes respectively. After maturation of gametocytes, one male gamete penetrates a female gamete and fertilises it. The resulting body is called a zygote.

OUTSIDE THE HUMAN OR ANIMAL HOST (in the soil). The zygote, formed after the sexual union, is discharged in the faeces in an encysted stage, known as oöcyst. These oöcysts are colourless oval bodies, consisting of a distinct cyst-wall with a protoplasmic mass inside. They measure 32 µm by 16 µm. In *Isospora* out side the human host, the nucleus of oöcyst divides into two, forming two ovoid uninucleate *sporoblasts*. Within each sporoblast, four uninucleate sausage-shaped sporozoites are developed; this is now known as sporocyst. Each sporozoite measures 14 µm by 7 µm.

The infection of a new host usually occurs by the oral route through ingestion of food or drink contaminated with faeces containing the mature sporocysts. On entering the intestine, the sporocyst ruptures in the lumen of the gut, liberating sporozoites; the latter invade the epithelial cells to start their asexual cycle of schizogony.

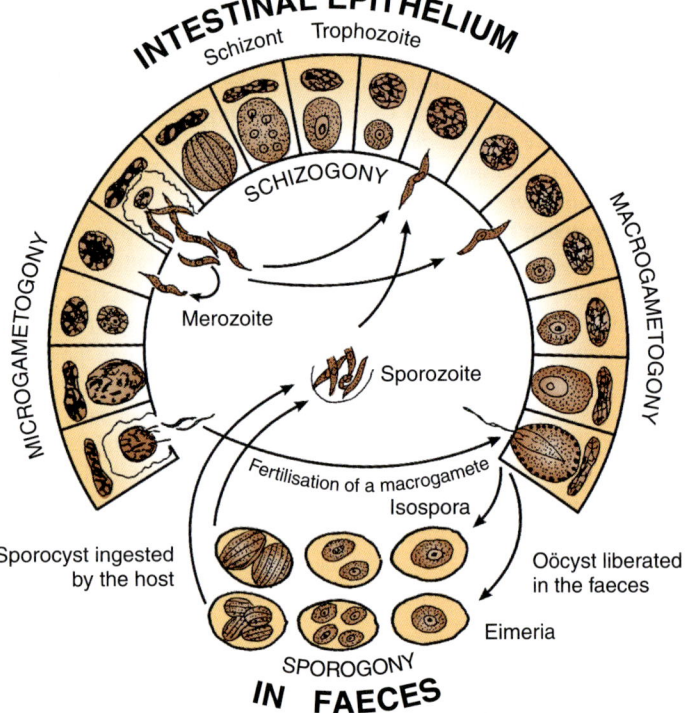

Fig. 99—Life cycle of intestinal sporozoa.
(Modified after Dobell and O'Connor, 1921)

Genus ISOSPORA

Isospora belli Wenyon 1923

Isospora belli, a parasite causing Isosporiasis is reported from man particularly patient with AIDS disease.

Geographical distribution: It is distributed throughout the world, but most prevalent in Africa and South America.

Morphology: Each oöcyst is elongated and measures 22 µm by 15 µm. The oöcyst is surrounded by a cyst-wall having two layers. Immature oöcyst, passed in human faeces, contains two sporoblasts which mature into sporocysts. Each sporocyst contains four sporozoites which are crescent-shaped.

Habitat: It inhabits in the small intestine of man (lower part of the ileum) and may cause intestinal symptoms.

Life cycle: Life cycle completes in one host. Isospora belli has two cycles, sexual sporogony and asexual schizogony in the epithelial mucosa of the only host, man. Infection is by faecal-oral route following ingestion of oöcysts. Immature oöcysts in fresh faeces is elongated (tapered extremity) with a thin clear, colourless double layered hyaline-wall containing an unsegmented zygote. On further development after 48 hours, two ovoid sporoblast are formed each of which develops into two sporocysts. Each sporocyst contains four crescent-shaped sporozoites which is infective.

Sporozoites excyst and invade the epithelial cells of jejunum and duodenum and undergo asexual multiplication to form trophozoites. These trophozoites mature into schizonts which spilt up into merozoites. With the rupture of host cells, merozoites invade fresh cells to repeat the cycle. The merozoites develop into (multicellular) male gametocytes or (unicellular) female gametocytes. The male gametocyte ruptures and liberates many male microgametes which fertilize the female macrogametes to form immature oöcyst containing unsegmented zygote. This oöcyst passed out in the faeces and sporulates after 48 hours to become infective.

Clinical features: Incubation period is 7 to 11 days. Most infections are asymptomatic. In symptomatic infection, the features of malabsorption follow a benign self-limited course lasting for a few weeks to many months. Several deaths have been reported in case of Isosporiasis in AIDS patient.

Diagnosis: Diagnosis is made by finding the immature oöcyst in faeces and in duodenal aspirates or by duodenal biopsy. 50% patients with isosporiasis have eosinophilia.

Treatment: Combined therapy with Sulfadiazine 4 gm, Pyrimethamine 75 mg, in four divided doses daily for 3-7 weeks is curative. Trimethoprim (160 mg) and Sulphamethoxazole (800 mg) – twice daily for 2–3 weeks are also effective.

Genus TOXOPLASMA
Toxoplasma gondii Nicolle and Manceaux, 1908

The parasite was discovered by Nicolle and Manceaux in 1908 in a small rodent, gondii (*Ctenodactylus gundi*) of Africa. Human importance of the organism was realised 30 years after, i.e., from the year 1939 (although 2 cases were reported in the interval, one in 1914 by Castellani from Sri Lanka and the other in 1923 by Janku from Prague). It is a small protozoon being widely distributed in man and animals all over the world.

Life Cycle. *Toxoplasma gondii* is now believed to be a coccidian parasite but an unusual one, having an intestinal phase in its homologous host, such as cat of the Family Felidae, particularly *Felis catus* (domestic cat) and an extra-intestinal phase in its heterologous host, such as mouse, man and other animals (Fig. 100).

ENTERIC CYCLE. Hutchison *et.al.* (1970, 71) observed schizogonic and gametogonic stages (microgametocytes and macrogametocytes) of *T. gondii*, resembling the endogenous cycle of a coccidia, inside the epithelial cells of the small intestine (ileum) of domestic cats fed on mouse brain containing "cysts" (tissue cysts) of *T. gondii*. Large numbers of oöcysts, resembling those of the *Isospora* were found in the infected cat's faeces. Schizogony and gametogony occurred in the epithelium of the tips of intestinal villi. They usually develop in the ileum (the commonest site of infection), but the whole of the small intestine can be affected. All stages of schizogony and gametogony may be found together and multiple infections of the host cells are common. The parasite develops in a vacuole lying between the brush border and the nucleus of the intestinal epithelial cells. About 4-29 merozoites are found inside a schizont and they form a cluster around a residual body and may appear to radiate fan-wise from it. The merozoites (4.9 × 1.5 µm) liberated from the rupture of schizont may continue their cycle of schizogony, while others develop into micro- and macrogametocytes. Each microgametocyte contains 12-32 microgametes (*B.M.J.*, **1**, 142, 1970; *Trans. Roy. Soc. Trop. Med. & Hyg.*, **65**, 380, 1971).

EXOENTERIC CYCLE. The oöcysts containing 2 sporocysts are excreted in cat's faeces for about 1 to 2 weeks. On maturation (after about 1-5 days), the sporocysts develop into 4 sporozoites resembling trophozoites and become infective to man and other animals (mammals and birds). The oöcysts after ingestion liberate sporozoites which in heterologous hosts penetrate mucosal cells of the intestine (ileum) and are carried by the blood and lymph stream first to the mesenteric lymph nodes (lymphoid-macrophage system) and then to distant organs, such as brain, eyes, liver, spleen, lymph nodes, heart, skeletal muscles and placenta of pregnant uterus. In all these places, they form *pseudocysts* and the parasite inside the cyst is known as *endozoite* (the nucleus is central in position). Cells parasitised subsequently rupture and the endozoites escape to continue their intracellular multiplication. It multiplies by internal budding (endogeny), hence termed endozoite (Vivier, 1970). A pseudocyst may contain 50 to 100 organisms. The pseudocyst represents the proliferative stage of the parasite and is responsible for causing extensive damage to the tissues in which it develops.

Some of the sporozoites and also the endozoites tend to localise in the central nervous system and the musculature where they are transformed into tissue cysts inside which the parasite also multiplies. The parasite inside the tissue cyst is known as the *cystozoite** (the nucleus is situated at the rounded end). Its method of endogeny is also different. A tissue cyst may reach 100 µm in size and contain hundreds of cystozoites. It does not cause any damage to the tissues and is not associated with any symptoms and signs.

Both the pseudocyst and the tissue cyst are infective and animals can acquire infection by cannibalising other infected animals (mammals and birds). This is also true of man.

---

* Hoare, C. A. (1972). The developmental stages of Toxoplasma. *J. Trop. Med. & Hyg.*, **75**, 56-8.

ENTERIC CYCLE
IN HOMOLOGOUS HOST (CAT)

EXOENTERIC CYCLE
IN HETEROLOGOUS HOST (MAN)

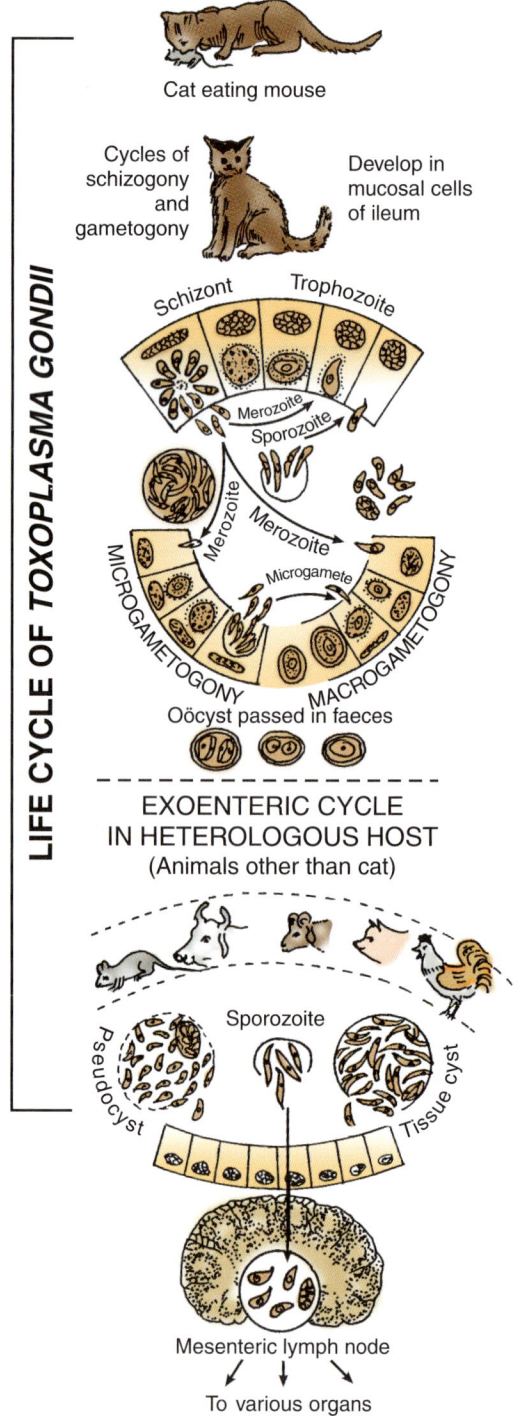

LIFE CYCLE OF *TOXOPLASMA GONDII*

Cat eating mouse

Cycles of schizogony and gametogony

Develop in mucosal cells of ileum

Schizont   Trophozoite

Merozoite
Sporozoite
Merozoite
Merozoite
Microgamete
MICROGAMETOGONY   MACROGAMETOGONY

Oöcyst passed in faeces

EXOENTERIC CYCLE
IN HETEROLOGOUS HOST
(Animals other than cat)

Sporozoite
Pseudocyst
Tissue cyst

Mesenteric lymph node

To various organs

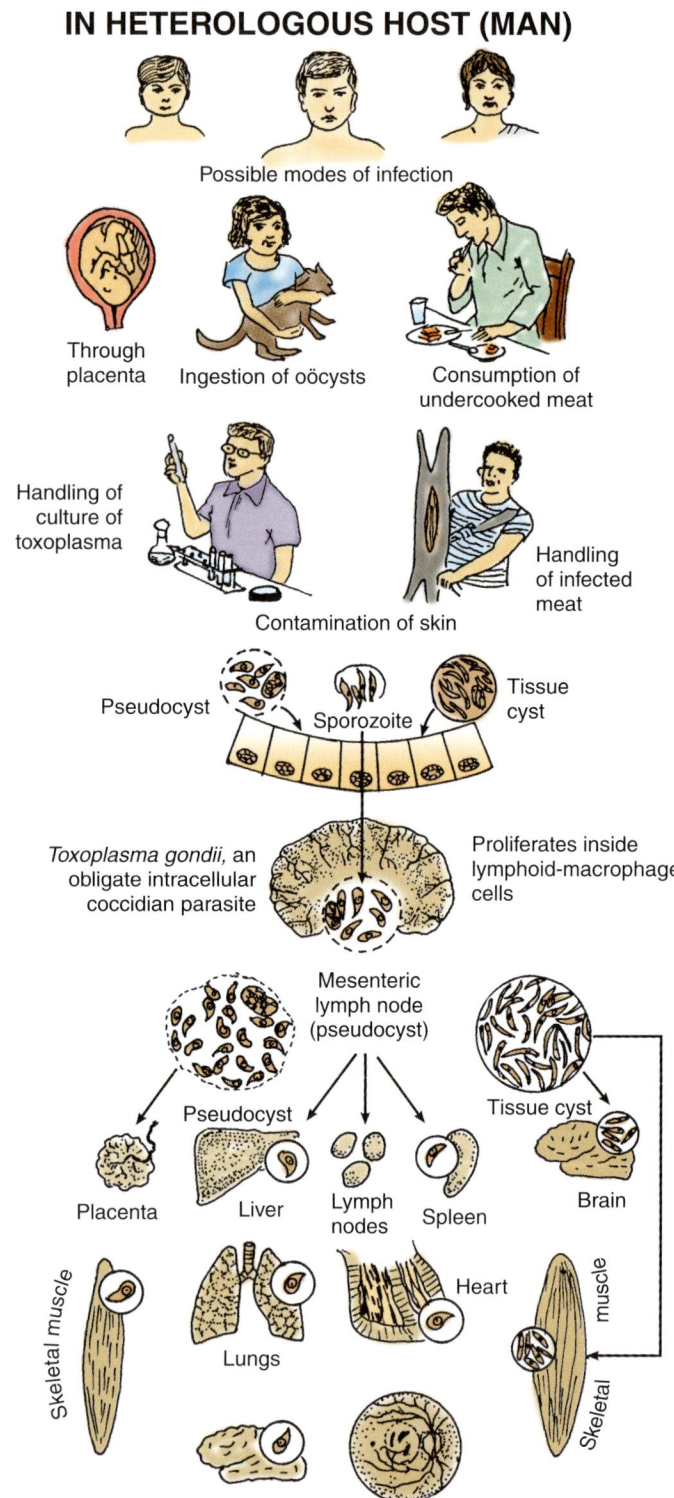

Possible modes of infection

Through placenta   Ingestion of oöcysts   Consumption of undercooked meat

Handling of culture of toxoplasma

Handling of infected meat

Contamination of skin

Pseudocyst   Sporozoite   Tissue cyst

Toxoplasma gondii, an obligate intracellular coccidian parasite

Proliferates inside lymphoid-macrophage cells

Mesenteric lymph node (pseudocyst)

Pseudocyst

Placenta   Liver   Lymph nodes   Spleen   Brain

Skeletal muscle

Lungs   Heart   Skeletal muscle

Brain   Chorioretinitis

Fig. 100

Morphology. Two forms of Toxoplasma are found in man (also in mammals and birds)—Pseudocyst (proliferative stage) and tissue cyst.

Tissue Cyst or Extra-cellular Form. It may be found free in the tissue fluids. It is often found to be embedded in the central nervous system and the musculature, where it is surrounded by a resilient membrane, forming the wall of the tissue cyst. The cystozoite is a slender crescent-shaped organism, one end rounded and the other pointed. The single nucleus is situated at the rounded end.

Pseudocyst or Intra-cellular Form. It is found in the cells of the R.E. System and many nucleated cells. The endozoite is often crescent-shaped but may be oval and the nucleus is central in position. It measures 4 to 6 μm in length by 2 μm in breadth.

Staining Reaction. It stains readily with alkaline methylene blue. When stained with Giemsa's stain the cytoplasm appears blue, the nucleus reddish-purple and paranuclear body red.

Cultivation. It can be cultivated in association with living tissues (in chorioallantoic membrane of the developing chick embryo). The parasite multiplies only in the presence of living cells.

Pathogenicity. In the majority of cases, the infection may pass unnoticed but dissemination of the parasites occurs through the blood stream ultimately localising in various organs such as brain, spinal cord, eyes, lungs, liver, spleen, bone marrow, lymph nodes, heart muscle and skeletal muscles.

The pathological lesion is characterised by an area of focal necrosis, surrounded by inflammatory cells (monocytes, plasma cells and lymphocytes). A large number of parasites may be found inside the cell which is enlarged, forming what is known as pseudocyst.

The *Toxoplasma* parasite penetrates* the cell membrane of macrophages or host cells by the anterior tip and remains within a vacuole. It may be degraded and digested after the uptake or may remain alive and multiply. The parasites which survive within the vacuole do so by blocking the fusion of lysosomes of the host cells. It is suggested that some parasitic factors (a membrane active substance) may be responsible for inhibition of lysosomal fusion with vacuole which helps the survival of the parasites within the host cells. In the absence of this parasitic factor, the parasites are killed and digested (Kean, 1972).

Incidence. Human infections of toxoplasma have been reported from European countries, Middle East, Sri Lanka, United States of America, Australia, Hawaii and many other places. The infection appears to be cosmopolitan.

Clinical Features. The disease toxoplasmosis has been recognised both as a neonatal infection and as an acquired infection in children and adults. Congenital toxoplasmosis is generally fatal and lesions are widespread, having a special predilection for the developing nervous system of the foetus.

The various lesions found in acquired toxoplasmosis may be grouped as follows:

(1) *Cerebrospinal*. Characterised by encephalomyelitis, hydrocephalus, calcification of cerebral lesions; chiefly found in infants and children.

Eyes. Focal chorioretinitis (pigment-ringed scar) near macula; anterior uveitis occasionally.

(2) *Lymphatic*. Fever with generalised lymphadenitis (Slim's disease); found between the ages of 5 and 15 years. The parasite shows a peculiar affinity for the posterior cervical lymph nodes.

(3) *Skin* (Exanthematous). Maculopapular rash, resembling rashes of typhus fever; chiefly found in adults.

(4) *Lungs*. Interstitial pneumonia, resembling an atypical virus pneumonia.

(5) *Heart*. Myocarditis (pseudocyst in muscle fibres).

(6) *Liver* and *Spleen*. Enlarged.

(7) *Uterus*. Abortion.

Note. Congenital infections are always symptomatic. Acquired infections on the other hand are usually asymptomatic, occurring in adults as latent infections and detected by laboratory tests.

Immunology. Both cellular and humoral immunity develop after infection. Humoral antibodies which develop in Toxoplasma infection are demonstrated by various serological tests (*vide infra*). Of the immunoglobulins both IgG and IgM are present. IgM antibody can be demonstrated by immunofluorescence test and its presence in newborn indicates congenital infection. Serological tests are most helpful when they are negative or when a rising titre can be demonstrated, hence two samples of blood at 3-4 weeks' interval are to be examined.

---

* Zaman, V. and Colley, Fredrick, C. (1972). Ultrastructural study of penetration of macrophages by *Toxoplasma gondii*. *Trans. Roy. Soc. Trop. Med. & Hyg.*, **66**, 781-82.

Changes in Blood and Cerebrospinal Fluid

Blood. Leucocytosis (about 12,000 per mm^3 of blood). Relative increase of lymphocytes and monocytes. In many cases, an increase of eosinophils (about 20 per cent) has been observed.

C. S. F. In meningo-encephalitis cases, the colour is yellow, protein is increased and leucocytes are present in large numbers.

Mode of Infection (Transmission). Human toxoplasmosis may occur in two ways:

(1) *Congenital.* Foetus is infected *in utero* through the transplacental route. The organism is transmitted from the infected mother who may not show any symptoms of the disease. Infection occurring in early months of pregnancy results either in abortion or stillbirth of the foetus. If infection occurs in later months of pregnancy, the foetus is free from any sign of the disease which however develops 2 to 3 months after birth. If the mother is infected during the puerperium, a breast-fed infant may acquire the infection through mother's milk.

(2) *Acquired.* The infection may occur in children and also in adults. The organism may enter by the following routes:

(a) By ingestion of underdone meat (containing pseudocyst), cow's milk and eggs (pseudocyst has been found in the ovaries of hen). It is possible that many patients are infected by swallowing oöcysts discharged in the faeces of infected reservoir animal (cat).

(b) By inhalation (droplet infection)—The organisms are found in the bronchial secretions and sputum. Pneumonitis is a common feature of toxoplasmosis in animals.

(c) By inoculation (through skin)—Contact with infected tissues of animals. Toxoplasma can penetrate through cracks and small abrasions in the skin.

Note: Sheep and swine may be a likely source of infection for man. The infection in these animals is generalised in the skeletal muscles, hence handling and testing meat prior to cooking or eating it uncooked facilitates the spread of infection to man (Work, 1971). It appears that the dog does not play any part in the epidemiology of the disease in man.

Laboratory Diagnosis: Direct Evidences. Demonstration of *Toxoplasma gondii*, although not always possible, may be carried out as follows:

(a) *Microscopical* examination of stained smears of the material obtained from bone marrow puncture and splenic puncture or centrifuged deposit of C.S.F. and smears made from any tissues removed by biopsy (preferably lymph node or muscle) or at autopsy.

(b) *Inoculation* of the suspected material in laboratory-bred mice, guinea pigs and hamsters.

Indirect Evidences. Serodiagnosis is important in pregnant women and AIDS patients. These include the following:

(a) *Indirect haemagglutination* and (b) Fulton's agglutination tests are useful diagnostic methods. The use of the live organisms is not required.

(c) *Indirect fluorescent antibody* test (IFA), is now well accepted.

(d) *Fluorescent stain for Toxoplasma* (Goldman's test). The organism appears brightly fluorescent when treated with fluorescin-tagged globulin fraction of homologous antiserum. It can be used to find parasites in tissue smears and sections.

(e) *Methylene blue dye test of Sabin and Feldman.* The method consists in finding out a cytoplasm-modifying antibody in the patient's serum. If the patient's serum contains the specific antibody, less than 50 per cent of free toxoplasma do not accept the stain and the cytoplasm remains colourless (those in intact cells however accept the stain). In a negative serum 90 to 100 per cent of the free toxoplasma accept the stain. The technique is as follows: Equal amounts (0.1 ml) of diluted patient's serum (1 : 16, 1 : 64, 1 : 128 and 1 : 256 dilutions), toxoplasma suspension obtained from the peritoneal exudate of infected mice and normal human serum (for "accessory factor") are incubated for 1 hour at 37°C in a water bath. To each of the tubes is then added one drop of saturated alcoholic solution of methylene blue at pH 11. A drop of the mixture is then put on a slide, covered with a coverslip and examined under the high power lens of the microscope. The number of extra-cellular (free) toxoplasma with stained and unstained cytoplasm is counted. The highest dilution of the serum in which 50 per cent or more of the organism have unstained cytoplasm is taken as the titre. The dye test (due to persistent antibody) is positive early, persists longer and does not disappear completely.

It is now known that the dye test gives positive reactions with sarcocystis, *Trichomonas vaginalis*, *Trypanosoma lewisi* and probably other parasites. Hence, a dye test positive with a titre of 1 : 128 should be taken as diagnostic of active toxoplasmosis.

(f) *Neutralising antibody test of Sabin and Ruchman.* The method consists of intracutaneous injection of patient's serum with living toxoplasma into a rabbit. Failure to develop any skin reaction (erythema with oedema) after 3 to 5 days indicates a positive test.

(g) *Complement fixation test of Sabin and Warren*. This develops 3 to 4 weeks after infection. Antigen is obtained from chick-embryo cultures. A titre less than 1 : 8 is not indicative of active toxoplasmosis. The C.F. test (due to shorter lived antibody) is positive late in the course of infection and becomes negative sooner.

(i) *Toxoplasmin skin test of Frenkel*. Suitable dilutions of toxoplasmin are injected intradermally. Appearance of an area of erythema with an induration of over 10 mm after 48 hours indicates positive reaction (a delayed type). Not so reliable as the serological test.

(j) ELISA test is very informative as it provides the titre of IgM and IgG separately and is now used routinely.

(k) PCR of the amnoitic fluid used to detect toxoplasma specific DNA and helpful in diagnosis of the disease.

Treatment.Pyrimethamine (daraprim) combined with sulphadiazine have been found to be an effective remedy. The useful regimen for an adult is as follows:

(i) Pyrimethamine 50 mg orally, 6-8 hours later 25 mg on first day, followed by 25 mg daily for 2-4 weeks. In severe cases, the treatment may be prolonged up to 6 months with occasional interruption of chemotherapy for a week at a time and checked by a blood count at frequent intervals. Should be avoided in pregnant women during the first trimester.

(ii) Sulphadiazine 2 g orally, Stat; followed by 1 g 6-hourly for the same period.

Folic acid and vitamin B complex should be administered concurrently. Prednisolone is given in ocular toxoplasmosis.

The alternate drug includes the antibiotic spiramycin (3-4 gm/day for 3-4 weeks) either alone or in combination with other drugs.

Prophylaxis. Measures should be directed against the possible methods of transmission.

No female workers of child-bearing age, with a negative Sabin-Feldman dye test, should be employed in a laboratory on work involving live cultures of Toxoplasma.

Toxoplasmosis in immuno-deficient states. Toxoplasma infection occurring in patients receiving large doses of immunosuppressive agents causes high and prolonged fever (not responsive to usual antibiotics) associated with diffuse encephalitis. The symptoms readily subside with anti-toxoplasmic therapy. The manifestations of toxoplasmosis may result from an exacerbation of pre-existing infection or most probably a newly acquired infection (opportunist infection) developing as a consequence of diminished immune responses of the patient (Kean, 1972)*.

Genus SARCOCYSTIS

As the name suggests, *Sarcocystis* is a parasite which forms cyst in the muscle.

Sarcocystis infection has worldwide distribution but has comparatively low incidence in man. Three species namely *S. hominis*, *S. suihominis*, and *S. lindemanni* can produce two distinct clinical entities: (a) Intestinal sarcocystosis, (b) Muscular sarcocystosis.

Intestinal sarcocystosis: Intestinal sarcocystosis is caused by *S. hominis* (or *S. bovihominis* or *Isospora hominis*) and *S. suihominis*, in which man is the definitive host. As the specific names indicate, cattle (oxen) and pig act as an intermediate host of *S. hominis* and *S. suihominis*, respectively.

Morphology: There are three morphological forms of intestinal sarcocystis namely (a) oöcyst, (b) sporocyst and (c) sarcocyst. Each oöcyst contains two sporocysts and four sporozoites are present in each sporocyst. Oöcyst is thin-walled and colourless. It is 13–19 μm in diameter in *S. hominis*, whereas it measures 10–13 μm in *S. suihominis*. Sporocyst is oval and measures 8–10 μm in diameter. It contains four banana-shaped sporozoites. It is passed in human faeces and is the infective form of parasite. Sarcocysts of *S. hominis* and *S. suihominis* are spindle-shaped structures with thick striated wall and found along the length of the muscle fibres (diaphragm, oesophagus and cardiac muscle) of cattle and pig, respectively. This sarcocyst is also known as muscular cyst and divided into many compartments containing bradyzoites.

Life cycle: Life cycles of *S. hominis* and *S. suihominis* are passed in two hosts, one definitive host and other intermediate host. Man is the definitive host and cattle and pigs are intermediate hosts of *S. hominis* and *S. suihominis* respectively. Man becomes infected by eating undercooked or raw beef or pork containing sarcocysts of *S. bovihominis* or *S. suihominis*, respectively. After ingestion by man sarcocyst bursts in small intestine and liberates numerous bradyzoites which penetrate the intestinal epithelium to sub-epithelial space where they undergo development forming microgametes and macrogametes. The microgamete escapes in the gut lumen where it fertilizes macrogametes to form zygote and an oöcyst develops from the zygote. Oöcyst containing two sporocysts is known as sporulated oöcyst. Each sporocyst contains four sporozoites. The sporulated oöcysts are shed into the lumen of the small intestine and rupture to release sporocysts in the faeces of man (definitive host). Sporocysts passed in human

---

* B. H. Kean (1972). Clinical toxoplasmosis—50 years. *Trans. Roy. Soc. Trop. Med. & Hyg.*, **66**, 549-567.

faeces are infective to intermediate host. Contaminated food or water containing sporocysts are ingested by cattle or pig and they become infected. Sporozoites are released from sporocyst in the small intestine and enter the blood stream and produce two generations of schizonts. Merozoites are released from schizonts and these merozoites migrate to skeletal and cardiac muscles and develop into sarcocyst containing numerous bradyzoites. The raw or undercooked beef and pork containing this sarcocyst is ingested by man and the life cycle is repeated.

Diagnosis: This can be made from demonstration of mature sporocysts or occasionally oöcyst in human faeces. Two species of sarcocyst are difficult to be differentiated on the basis of sporocyst examination. Serological tests such as IHA, IFA and ELISA are helpful in the diagnosis of the disease.

Muscular Sarcocystosis: It is caused by *S. lindemanni* and man is rarely infected. Besides other countries, a few cases of human sarcocystis have been reported from India also.

Life cycle: Man is an intermediate host and cats and dogs or other carnivorous animals are definitive hosts of *S. lindemanni*. The possible mode of entrance of infection in man is by ingestion of food or drink contaminated by sporocysts of *S. lindemanni*, excreted in faeces of definitive host (cat, dog or other carnivorous animals). Sporocyst liberates sporozoites which invade intestinal wall and then disseminated to skeletal muscle to cause subcutaneous and muscular inflammation. Life cycle of *S. lindemanni* is similar to that of *S. hominis* and *S. suihominis*, but it differs only from the pattern of the hosts.

Clinical features: Muscular sarcocystosis is often asymptomatic and sarcocyst in muscle of man presents as a localized painful muscular swelling (1–3 cm in diameter) accompanied by slight fever, muscle pain, muscular weakness, bronchospasm, and eosinophilia (40%). The subcutaneous and muscular inflammation lasts for several days.

Diagnosis: This can be made by muscle biopsy which shows sarcocysts and by radiology which shows faint shadows in the leg and arm muscles.

Treatment: No specific treatment is available for the treatment of both intestinal and muscular sarcocystosis in man. Intestinal and muscular sarcocystosis can be prevented by avoidance of ingestion of raw or undercooked beef or pork and avoidance of contamination of food and drink with faeces of cat, dog and other carnivorous animals.

Genus : CYCLOSPORA

Cyclospora cayetanensis: It is a newly recognized protozoan parasite and causes disease named as cyclosporiasis in man, particularly in patients with AIDS. First human case was reported in Peru in 1985, although the organism was known since 1929.

Geographical distribution: It has worldwide distribution particularly reported from Nepal, India and South America.

Life cycle: Life cycle is not completely established but it is thought to be similar to that of *Cryptosporidium* species. The parasite requires a single host and possibly has both sexual and asexual stage. Man is infected by ingestion of food and water contaminated with faeces. The unsporulated oöcyst in faeces sporulates outside the host. Excystation of the sporocyst releases two sporozoites which infect the small intestine causing diarrhoea.

Habitat: The parasite dwells in its life cycle intra-cellularly (within the epithelial cells of gastrointestinal tract of the host).

Morphology: Oöcyst is spherical in shape and 8–10 μm in diameter. It contains two sporocysts. Each sporocyst contains two sporozoites. Sporozoites are semilunar in shape and 9 μm by 1.2 μm in size.

Clinical features: The incubation period is around a week. The disease starts with acute watery diarrhoea with nausea, loss of appetite, abdominal pain, fever, fatigue, weight loss, and illness is found in immuno-compromised patients specially in AIDS patients. In more severe form of the disease, the diarrhoea may be prolonged and associated with muscle pain, vomiting, dehydration and substantial weight loss. The illness may last six weeks before self-limiting. If the disease is left untreated, the illness may relapse.

Diagnosis: This is done by detection of oöcyst in stool under microscope. To detect oöcysts in faeces, concentration of faeces by floatation technique is required. By modified Ziehl-Neelsen staining, the oöcysts are stained red in colour as they are acid fast. The parasite can be demonstrated in small bowel biopsy material by electron microscope.

Treatment: Co-trimazole (trimethoprim, 160 mg and sulfamethoxazole 600 mg twice daily for seven days) is the drug of choice.

Genus : CRYPTOSPORIDIUM

Cryptosporidium parvum causes cryptosporidiosis, a parasitic disease of birds, reptiles and fishes. It was first described in a laboratory mouse by Tyzzer in 1907. Cryptosporidiosis is now reported from reptiles, birds and many mammals including man. Human case of cryptosporidiosis was first reported in 1976. The disease has been found in immunologically deficient or compromised individuals. Recent occurrence of cryptosporidial diarrhoea in AIDS patients has attracted attention to this protozoal infection. A number of human cases of cryptosporidial diarrhoea have now been reported in those with the history of contacts with domestic bovids (calves), clearly indicating that cryptosporodiosis as zoonosis. Amongst several species of cryptosporidium only *C. parvum* infects man.

Geographical Distribution: Worldwide.

Habitat: The parasite is intra-cellular and found in distal parts of jejunum, ileum and also the colon.

Morphology: Oöcyst is the infective form of the parasite. The oöcyst exists in two forms, namely one thick-walled (80%) and other thin-walled (20%). Oöcysts are spherical or oval, colourless, measuring 1.5-5 μm in diameter, highly refractile and are shed in the stools. Four elongated sporozoites are present in both thick-walled and thin-walled oöcysts. The thick-walled oöcyst is excreted in the faeces and thin-walled oöcyst causes auto-infection.

Life cycle: Parasite *C. parvum* undergoes both sexual and asexual cycle in a single host (monoxenous). Infection is caused by the faecal oral route by ingestion of oöcyst in contaminated food or drink. After ingestion, thick-walled oöcyst becomes excysted and four sporozoites come out from each oöcyst in the lumen of the small intestine. Sporozoites invade the brush border of epithelial cells and convert into trophozoites, which remain within the brush border of intestine. The trophozoite undergoes asexual multiplication and produce first generation schizogony with formation of 8 merozoites. These merozoites in turn enter neighbouring epithelial cells and produce second generation schizogony with formation of 4 merozoites. The released merozoites differentiate into microgametocytes and macrogametocytes. The microgametocyte undergoes several divisions producing numerous microgametes (one microgametocyte produces 12–16 microgametes), whereas macrogametocytes transform to macrogametes (one macrogametocyte produces only one macrogamete). After fertilization of a macrogamete by a microgamete a zygote develops which differentiates into a unsporulated oöcyst. It undergoes sporogony to form sporulated oöcyst containing four sporozoites. Sporulated oöcyst passes in the faeces and transfers the infection from one person to another. Some thin-walled oöcysts infect the same host by autoinfection and maintain the life cycle of the parasite, without repeated exposure to thick-walled oöcysts that are present in the environment.

Clinical features: Besides gastrointestinal infection (acute watery diarrhoea, anorexia, nausea, vomiting and abdominal pain) extra-intestinal infection of respiratory tract (respiratory cryptosporidiosis), cholecystitis and hepatitis have been reported in severely immunocompromised patient. It can also cause infection in immunocompetent person.

Diagnosis: This can be made by demonstration of oöcyst of the parasite in faeces, also in sputum of respiratory cryptosporidiosis and in duodenal aspiration. Sometimes, oöcyst cannot be demonstrated even after examination of three consecutive wet mount preparations of faeces. In that case, Sheather's sugar concentration technique is used successfully for demonstration of oöcyst in faeces. Three staining methods such as auramine staining, modified Ziehl-Neelsen staining and immunofluorescence staining are commonly used. Ziehl-Neelsen technique reveals the internal structure of the oöcysts as acid fast. IFAT and ELISA test have been developed for detection of serum antibody to oöcyst antigen but are not used routinely. ELISA test for detection of parasite *C. parvum* antigen in faeces by using monoclonal antibody is highly sensitive and specific. PCR method for detection of DNA in faeces and biopsy material is helpful. Intestinal biopsy material demonstrates various stages of *C. parvum*.

Treatment: Disease is self-limiting but sometimes, particularly in AIDS patient, effective treatment with nitazoxanide, in a dose of 500 mg twice daily for 3–5 days is required.

Genus PNEUMOCYSTIS

Taxonomic status of *P. carinii* is uncertain. According to some workers, it has close relationship with fungi as molecular biological techniques show that it is a fungus. Based on its morphology and lack of response to antifungal drugs, *P. carinii* has been regarded as protozoan by some workers. *P. carinii* was first identified by Chagas in the lungs of guinea pig in 1909. The *P. carinii* infection in lung in man was reported in 1911.

Geographical distribution: Worldwide.

Habitat: *P. carinii* is an extracellular parasite found in interstitial tissues of the lungs and their alveoli of wild animals, dogs and man. The disease caused by *P. carinii* is known as *pneumocystosis*.

Morphology: *P. carinii* has three morphological forms : (a) trophozoite, (b) precyst, and (c) cyst. Trophozoites measure 1–5 μm and are amoeboid in shape and covered by a pellicle 10 to 40 μm thick. They have small tubular expansion known as filopodia. Precysts are 3–5 μm long, oval in shape with a cluster of mitochondria in their centre but with a few filopodia. The nucleus in the precystic stage undergoes three divisions. Precystic stage is a transitional stage between trophozoite and cystic stages. A mature cyst is thick-walled, 10 μm in diameter and spherical in shape. There are eight infective young trophozoites in each cyst and has a pellicle 70 to 140 μm thick.

Clinical features: Two distinct types of pneumocystosis, (a) epidemic, in premature, malnourished and debilitated infants during the early months (i.e. 2–6 months) of life, and (b) sporadic pneumocystosis in hypoimmune children and adults, i.e., immune-compromised hosts, have been described.

Latent pulmonary infections (interstitial pneumonia) in apparently healthy man and many species of laboratory, domestic and wild animals have been reported. The idea of transmission of infection from dog or other domestic animals to man is considered much less important than inter-human spread. Generally, *P. carinii* infection is rare in immunocompetent individual and usually asymptomatic. It is common in patients with impaired immune mechanisms (patients with corticosteroid therapy, in AIDS patients etc.) and causes death of the patients.

The common presenting symptoms of *P. carinii* pneumonia (PCP) are fever, non-productive cough, shortness of breath, cyanosis and if left untreated the disease causes death of the patient. Extrapulmonary pneumocystosis is rare. Various factors such as AIDS, malnutrition oropharyngeal candidiasis, anti-malignant therapy, prolonged steroid therapy, premature birth, predispose to *P. carinii* infection.

Life cycle: Complete life cycle is not known but presumably it is similar to that of other members of the genus. The inhaled cyst in the alveoli becomes excysted and releases sporozoites which are converted into trophozoites. They become encysted and produce eight daughter trophozoites, which are known as intracystic body, arranged in a rosette pattern within the cyst. The intracystic body is 1 to 1.5 μm in size, spherical, crescent-shaped or amoeboid. On rupture of the cyst, each intracystic body releases the trophozoites which initiate another cycle of multiplication either in the same host or in the different host. Both trophozoite and cyst are found in the alveoli of the infected lung tissue.

Diagnosis: This is done by demonstration of parasite in sputum, tracheobronchial lavage and tracheobronchial biopsy or lung biopsy specimen. The cyst is stained by Giemsa or methamine silver technique. Immunofluorescence is also used to detect the cyst. ELISA test demonstrates parasitic antigen. Diagnosis can be confirmed by chest X-ray showing characteristic widespread pulmonary infiltration of lung. Pulmonary function tests indicate reduction in vital capacity and total lung capacity. Lung scanning is a sensitive screening method. Histopathological examination of lung biopsy material shows thickened alveolar septa and alveoli are infiltrated with mononuclear cells and plasma cells. The *Pneumocystis carinii* organisms are found in the alveoli.

Treatment: For specific chemotherapy several drugs are usually chosen. The antifolate compound (trimethoprim and sulfamethoxazole) is drug of choice. Other medicines such as pentamidine, dapsone, atovaquone-primaquine, clindamycin are used either alone or in combination with other drugs. Severe pneumocystis carinii pneumonia (PCP) may be treated with pentamidine isotheonate in the dose of 4 mg/kg body weight daily by intramuscular route for 12–14 days.

Subclass : PIROPLASMIA Levine 1961
Order : PIROPLASMIDA Wenyon 1926

Members of order Piroplasmida are small parasites of ticks and mammals which do not produce spore, flagella, cilia, and true pseudopodia. Their locomotion is helped by both flexion or gliding. The intracellular pigments are not produced in any stage. Asexual reproduction occurs by binary fission or schizogony in erythrocytes or other blood cells of mammals. Sexual reproduction occurs in some species.

Genus BABESIA Victor Babes, 1888

Victor Babes, Romanian biologist, first identified the parasite in the blood of sheep and cattle in 1888. The name Piroplasma was given to Babesia due to its pear-shaped structure and disease caused by parasite is known as piroplasmosis. Babesiosis is another name of the disease.

Geographical distribution: Since 1957 human infections have been reported from various parts of the world (Yugoslavia, North Ireland, Scotland, France, USSR, USA etc.). Human cases of babesiosis have also been reported from Mexico, Europe, Southern and Western USA.

Habitat: The parasite is found inside erythrocytes and resembles the ring-form of *Plasmodium falciparum*, causing diagnostic problem.

Morphology: The species of *Babesia* are intraerythrocytic, non-pigment-producing parasites of various vertebrates— amphibians, reptiles and many mammals including man. Ticks of various types are the vectors as well as the reservoirs of *Babesia*. *Babesia* causes important infection in cattle, causing lethal haemoglobinuric fever, red-water fever, or Texas fever of cattle. They are usually described from their stages in the red blood cells of vertebrates. They are pyriform, round or oval-shaped parasites.

Generally, three species *B. divergens* and *B. bovis* from cattle and *B. microti* from rodents have been reported to infect man. *B. divergens* and *B. bovis* so far have been reported in splenectomized persons, whereas human cases of *B. microti* have so far been reported from the north-east coast of the USA, and in persons with intact spleen. *B. bovis* is 2.4 μm by 1.5 μm, *B. divergens* is 0.4 μm by 1.5 μm and *B. microti* is 2 μm by 1.5 μm in size. Sporozoites are infective for man and other vertebrates. They enter the erythrocytes and get converted into trophozoites. Trophozoites appear in ring-forms and 2–4 μm in diameter with scanty cytoplasm and small chromatin dot. They multiply asexually by budding to form merozoites which infect fresh erythrocytes and repeat the life cycle.

Clinical features: *Babesia* infection in man may lead to a rapid onset of high fever, nausea, vomiting, haemolytic anaemia and red-coloured urine, leading within a few days to jaundice, haemoglobinaemia, haemoglobinuria, then renal insufficiency or failure, culminating into death. The human infection with *Babesia* may mimic mild malaria-like fever. However, disease takes severe form in splenectomized person and HIV positive person, self-limiting febrile illness is caused by *B. microti* whereas *B. bovis* and *B. divergens* produce severe and fatal illness in splenectomized person.

Diagnosis: This may be attempted in any patient with a fever and possible history of tick bite. Examination of thin blood films stained with any Romanowsky stains may reveal the parasite simulating *P. falciparum* rings without any pigmentation. Diagnosis is made by IFA test, animal (hamster) inoculation and PCR method. PCR detects the *babesia* antigen within 24 hours.

Life cycle: Two hosts are required to complete the life cycle (principal host is the tick and secondary host is human being). After the bite of Ixodid tick, the sporozoites present in the salivary gland of tick are inoculated into the vertebrate and enter the blood stream to invade erythrocytes. They transform into trophozoites which appear as ring-form, resembling the ring form of *P. falciparum*. The trophozoites multiply asexually by budding to form merozoites. The released merozoites infect new erythrocytes and cycle is repeated. The ticks are infected by ingestion of merozoites containing erythrocytes through feeding on vertebrates. Some of the intraerythrocytic merozoites become isogametes (ray bodies) in tick's intestine and by fusion of two isogametes produce zygote and later it becomes kinete. Further development occurs outside the intestine in a variety of tissues. Through schizogony, sporozoites are developed which after few days, migrate to salivary gland of ticks. The sporozoites are injected to new host by bite, through saliva of infected ticks. The salivary gland and ovary are most important for transmission.

Treatment: Clindamycin with oral quinine and atovaquone with azithromycin have been found effective against Babesiosis. Human *B. microti* infection appears to be self-limiting, deserves only symptomatic treatment.

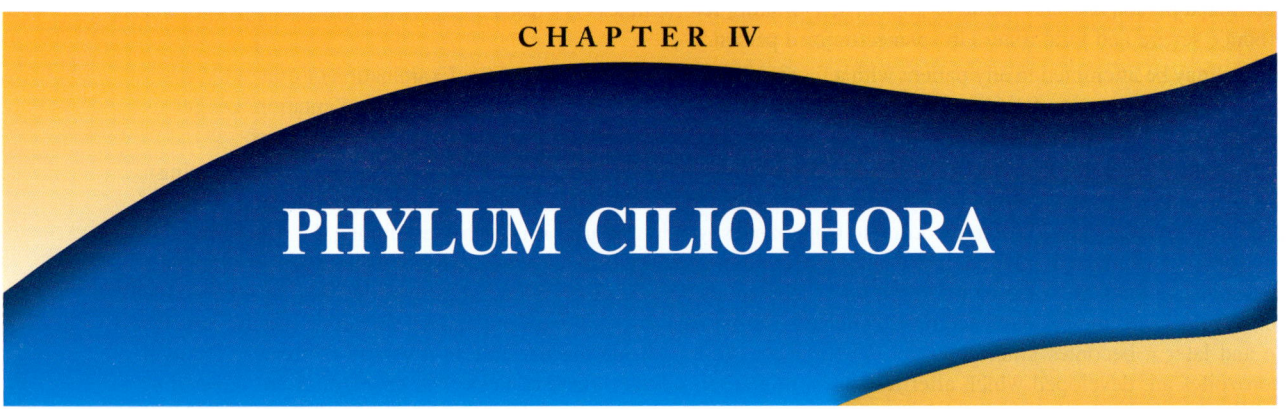

CHAPTER IV

PHYLUM CILIOPHORA

Class KINETOFRAGMINOPHOREA; Subclass : VESTIBULIFERIA

Order : TRICHOSTOMATIDA; Suborder : TRICHOSTOMATINA

The body of the parasite is covered with cilia (hair-like processes). There are two morphologically distinct nuclei. The shape of the body is defined by a cell membrane.

Genus BALANTIDIUM

The species pathogenic to man is *Balantidium coli.*

Balantidium coli (Malmsten, 1857) Stein, 1862

The parasite causing dysentery in man (ciliate dysentery or balantidiasis).

Geographical Distribution. World-wide.

Habitat. It is the largest protozoal parasite inhabiting the large intestine of man. It is also found in pigs and monkeys. The pig is the common reservoir of infection but the parasite is harmless to this host.

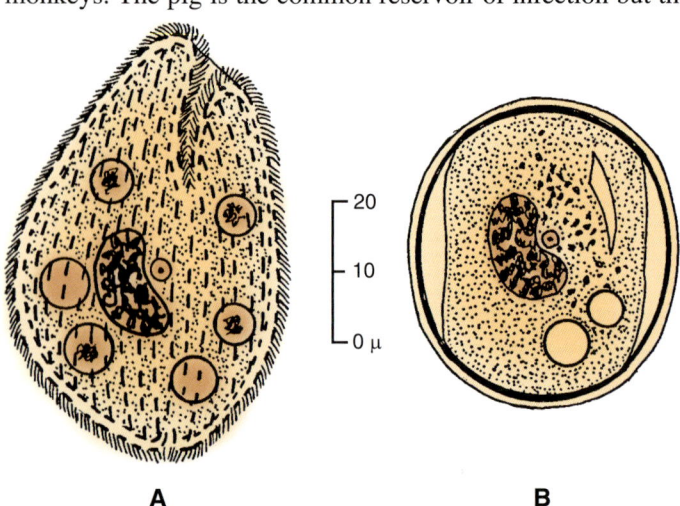

Fig. 101—Morphology of *Balantidium coli.*
A, trophozoite stage; B, cystic stage.

Morphology. The parasite exists in two stages (Fig. 101).

1. Trophozoite Stage: Found in dysenteric stools.

2. Encysted Stage: Found in chronic cases and carriers.

TROPHOZOITE. In *shape*, it is an oval body. The size is variable, the average measurement being 60 to 70 μm in length and 40 to 50 μm in breadth. The *body* is covered with a delicate pellicle showing longitudinal striations. The *cilia* are short and delicate and are of uniform length but those that line the mouth part appear to be longer and are called "adoral cilia". Underneath the pellicle is a thin layer of clear ectoplasm. The body is mainly composed of granular endoplasm. At the anterior end is situated a groove (*peristome*) leading to a mouth (*cytostome*) terminating in a short funnel-shaped gullet (cytopharynx) extending up to one-third of the body. There is no intestine. At the posterior end is a permanent anus called the *cytopyge*. The internal structure consists of the following:

(a) Two nuclei: a large kidney-shaped macronucleus situated in the middle of the body and a small round micro-nucleus lying in the concavity of the macronucleus.

(b) Two contractile vacuoles: one near the middle of the body and the other at the posterior end.

(c) Many food vacuoles consisting of debris from host's gut-content and occasionally tissue debris, R.B.C. and W.B.C.

CYST. It is slightly smaller than the trophic form, measuring 50 to 60 µm in diameter. The cytoplasm is granular and contains the macronucleus, the micronucleus and a refractile body. The contractile vacuoles may remain active for some time during encystment. The cyst is surrounded by a thick transparent double-layered wall.

Cultivation. *B. coli* can be grown in the same medium as *E. histolytica*.

Life Cycle and Method of Reproduction

Note the following:

B. coli passes its life cycle in two stages, but in one host only (Fig. 102).

Pig—The natural host. *Man*—Rare and incidental host.

Cyst—The infective stage of the parasite.

Portal of Entry—Mouth, by ingestion.

Transmission occurs from pig to pig, pig to man, man to man and man to pig.

The cyst when ingested, liberates trophozoites in the large intestine and from each cyst a single individual is formed. The trophozoite may remain in the lumen or enter into the submucous coat of the large intestine, where it

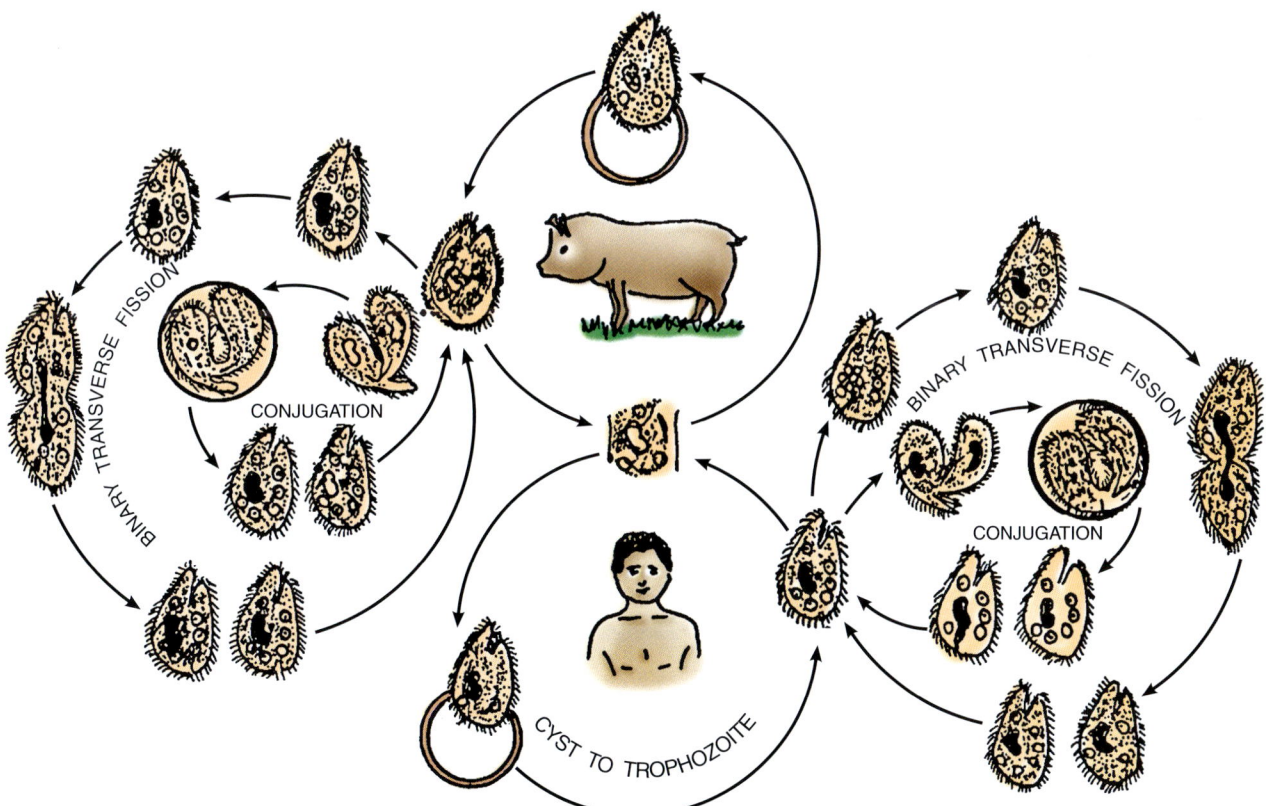

Fig. 102—Life cycle of *Balantidium coli* **in pig and man.**
(Modified after Brümpt)

grows and multiplies by binary transverse fission. With each division two daughter-ciliates are produced and by successive divisions, large numbers of trophozoites are formed. First the micronucleus divides into two, then the macronucleus and finally the body splits into two by a transverse partition. The daughter-individual formed from the anterior half retains the cytostome of the original parasite but reconstructs the posterior end of the body, whereas the one formed from the posterior end develops its own cytostome and other structures. After a period of growth and multiplication, the trophozoite undergoes encystment particularly when it finds conditions unsuitable for vegetative existence.

Conjugation. During this process, the two trophozoites are enclosed in a cyst. An exchange of nuclear materials occurs, after which the individuals separate.

Pathogenicity. MODE OF INFECTION. The pig serves as the usual source of infection to man. Persons having an occupational contact with these animals are thus liable to contract the infection. Transmission is effected through the. ingestion of food contaminated by cysts obtained either from the faeces of a pig or man.

PATHOGENESIS. The parasite thrives mainly on starchy food found in abundance in pig's intestine. Hoare stated that in the presence of abundant starchy food, the parasite does not invade the epithelial cells of the intestine. This probably explains its harrrlessness in the pig. The scarcity of starchy food in the human bowel also explains the rarity of balantidial infection in man.

LESION. This consists of ulceration of the colon, indistinguishable from amoebic ulcers. The diagnosis cannot be established until the specific parasite has been detected in the tissues. The necrotic process generally extends through the mucous and sub-mucous coat and at times may even extend to the muscular coat. *The parasite is not known to invade the liver.*

The clinical manifestation associated with this parasitic infection is characterised by the passage of blood and mucus in the stool. The condition is afebrile.

Diagnosis. Clinically balantidial dysentery cannot be differentiated from other forms of dysentery. It can only be diagnosed by a microscopical examination of the stool showing the presence of the trophozoites of *B. coli*. The technique for stool examination is the same as for the other intestinal protozoa.

Treatment. Tetracycline (500 mg. four times daily for 10 days) has been found to be an effective remedy. Metronidazole (750 mg. three times daily for 5 days) & Iodoquinol (650 mg. three times daily for 20 days) are alternative drugs.

Prophylaxis. This consists of protection against contamination of food and drink with faeces containing cysts of *B. coli* either of a pig or of man.

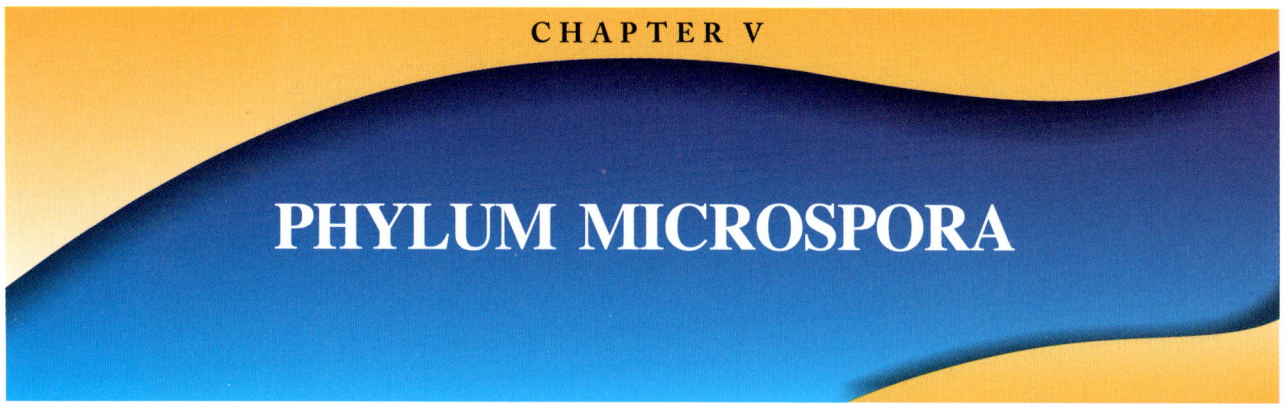

CHAPTER V

PHYLUM MICROSPORA

Microsporidia belongs to the phylum Microspora. Seven genera (Enterocytozoon, Encephalitozoon, Nosema, Pleistophora, Thelohanea, Trachipleistophora and Vittaforma) have been reported to cause the disease, microsporidiosis, particularly in AIDS patients and some genera can infect immunocompetent human in privileged sites (Vittaforma cornea). *Enterocytozoon bieneusi, Encephalitozoon intestinalis* frequently infect intestinal cells causing chronic diarrhoea, abdominal cramps, nausea, malabsorption in AIDS patients. Microsporidia are minute unicellular obligate intracellular spore-forming protozoa.

Life cycle has not been fully worked out. They have two stages of development inside a host's cell (i) schizogony, and (ii) sporogony.

The size of spore (which is the infective stage) varies with species and usually less than 10 μm in length. It rarely causes the disease microsporidiosis in immunocompetent person and it is potential opportunistic pathogen in patient with AIDS. Microsporodia can cause persistent diarrhoea, involvement of eyes, muscles, liver, central nervous system and kidney.

Enterocytozoon bieneusi: Since 1985 several human cases have been reported. The infection is acquired by ingestion of spore which in the intestine, due to high intracellular pressure, extrudes polar tube through which sporoplasm (infective material) is passed and penetrates the enterocytes. Successive cycles of merogony followed by sporogony occur and several spores are produced. These spores infect other cells.

The spore is oval or cylindrical in shape and measures 0.5 μm by 4 μm in size having thick double-layered wall. Within the cytoplasm spore possesses a coiled polar tube. Spore is passed with the faeces. It causes intestinal microsporidiosis in AIDS patients (persistent diarrhoea, nausea, enoroxia, abdominal pain etc.).

Diagnosis is done by detection of spore by electron microscopic or by light microscopic examination of small intestinal biopsy material. Detection of spore in stool, in duodenal and jejunal contents, after appropriate staining, is also helpful in diagnosis of disease. Immunodiagnosis by either indirect immunofluorescent antibody test or western blot technique is most sensitive diagnostic test. No effective treatment has been developed, against *E. bieneusi*.

Enterocytozoon hellam infection can cause disease involving cornea (keratoconjunctivitis), lung, kidney, muscle (myositis), liver, peritoneum (peritonitis) but not gastrointestinal disease in patients with AIDS.

Encephalitozoon cuniculi: It does not cause enteropathy as it lies within parasitophorous vacuole. Cases with neurological disorder, liver disorder and peritoneal involvement in patients with AIDS have been reported.

Encephalitozoon intestinalis or *Sepatata intestinalis:* The name itself suggests its development within parasitophorous vacuole which is septated. It invades intestinal villi causing persistent diarrhoea, gall bladder, kidney causing interstitial nephritis. The spores are shed in urine. Albendazole in dose of 400 mg twice daily for four weeks and fumagillim are effective drugs against encephalitozoon infection.

SECTION II

HELMINTHOLOGY

HELMINTHOLOGY

The helminthic parasites are multicellular, bilaterally symmetrical animals having three germ layers (triploblastic metazoa). The helminths of importance to human beings are divided into two main groups showing the following peculiarities.

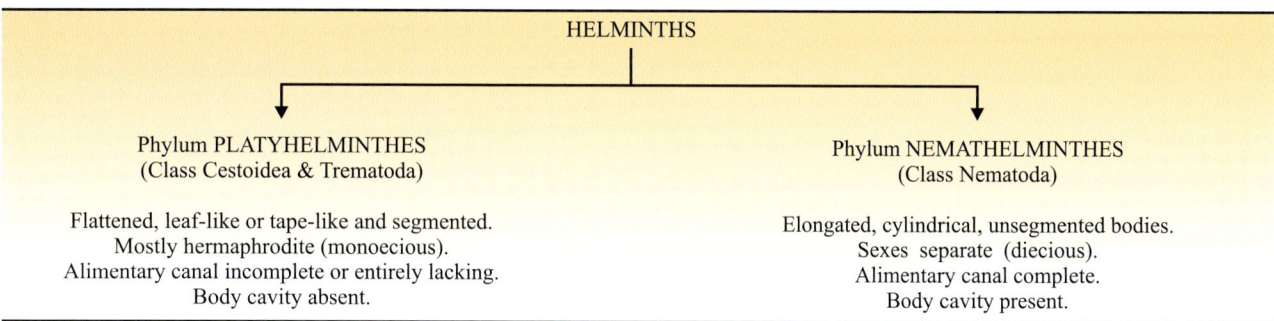

HELMINTHS

Phylum PLATYHELMINTHES
(Class Cestoidea & Trematoda)

Flattened, leaf-like or tape-like and segmented.
Mostly hermaphrodite (monoecious).
Alimentary canal incomplete or entirely lacking.
Body cavity absent.

Phylum NEMATHELMINTHES
(Class Nematoda)

Elongated, cylindrical, unsegmented bodies.
Sexes separate (diecious).
Alimentary canal complete.
Body cavity present.

Table showing the differences between Cestodes, Trematodes and Nematodes			
	CESTODE	**TREMATODE**	**NEMATODE**
Shape:	Tape-like; segmented.	Leaf-like; unsegmented.	Elongated, cylindrical; unsegmented.
Sexes:	Not separate, i.e., hermaphrodite (monoecious).	Not separate (monoecious), except Schistosomes which are diecious.	Separate (diecious).
"Head" End:	Suckers, often with hooks.	Suckers, no hooks.	No suckers, no hooks. Well-developed buccal capsule in some species.
Alimentary Canal:	Absent.	Present but incomplete; no anus.	Present and complete; anus present.
Body Cavity :	Absent.	Absent.	Present.

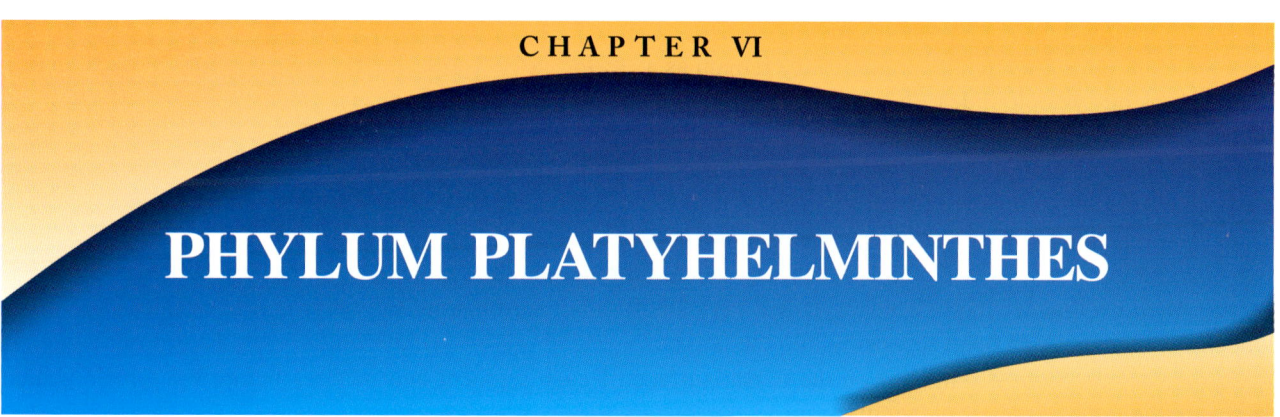

CHAPTER VI

PHYLUM PLATYHELMINTHES

Class CESTOIDEA: Subclass CESTODA

Order I Pseudophyllidea: Order II Cyclophyllidea

General Characters of Cestodes

1. The majority of cestodes are long, segmented and tape-like, hence called tapeworms. They are flattened dorsoventrally.
2. Sizes vary from a few millimetres to several metres.

3. Adult worms are found in the intestinal canal of man and animal.

4. "Head" is provided with suckers (slit-like or cup-like) and sometimes with hooks which serve as organs of attachment.

5. There are three regions in an adult worm: (i) a "head" (scolex), (ii) a "neck" and (iii) a strobila (a body or trunk) consisting of a series of segments (proglottides).

6. Sexes are not separate, i.e., each individual worm is a hermaphrodite.

7. Body cavity is absent.

8. Alimentary canal is entirely absent.

9. Excretory and nervous systems are present.

10. Reproductive system is highly developed and complete in each segment. According to the maturity of reproductive organs three types of segments of the strobila can be recognised from the front backwards:

Immature: Male and female organs not differentiated.

Mature: Male and female organs have become differentiated (male organs appear first).

Gravid: Uteri are filled with eggs (other organs atrophied or disappeared).

Reproductive System (Fig. 103)

FEMALE GENITAL SYSTEM. This lies on the ventral surface of each segment and comprises the following:

(i) *Ovary.* It may be single or paired. It is usually a bilobed organ lying behind the equatorial plane of each segment. It discharges ova into a minute duct, the oviduct, which connects the spermatic duct with the oötype.

(ii) *Vagina.* This extends from the genital pore to the oötype and is meant for the entrance of sperms. It contains at its inner end, an elongated chamber, the *seminal receptacle* for the storage of sperms, followed by a constricted tubule, the *spermatic duct.*

(iii) *Uterus.* This is a straight tube which arises from the oötype and when gravid, becomes filled with eggs. It may be open as in Pseudophyllidea, or it may remain as a blind sac, as in Cyclophyllidea.

(iv) *Oötype.* It is a chamber where the ovum is fertilised and all the components of the egg are collected. It is situated posteriorly in the middle of each segment.

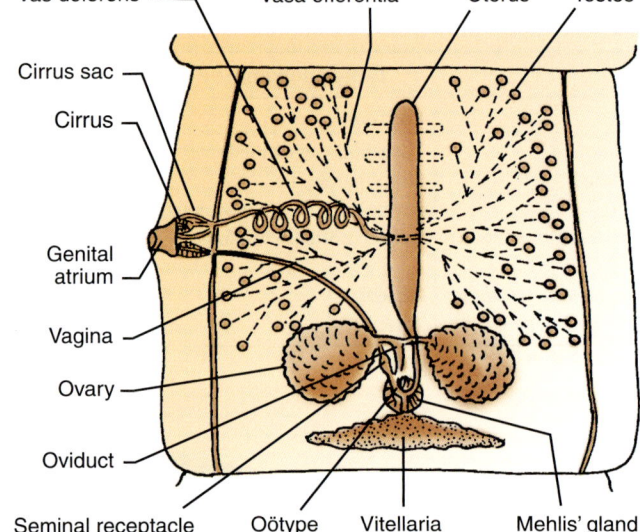

Fig. 103—**Reproductive system of cestodes.**
(A Cyclophyllidean cestode)

(v) *Vitelline Glands.* They may remain as a single mass lying behind the ovary, as in Cyclophyllidea, or scattered throughout the segment, as in Pseudophyllidea.

(vi) *Mehlis' Gland* ("Shell Glands"). It is a very small organ surrounding the oötype. It is composed of many unicellular glands which open separately into the oötype.

MALE GENITAL SYSTEM. This lies on the dorsal surface of each segment and matures before the female genital system. It comprises of the following:

(i) *Testes.* These are usually multiple follicles, except in Hymenolepis and are scattered throughout the parenchyma. They are connected by minute tubes (*Vasa efferentia*) with the vas deferens.

(ii) *Vas Deferens.* This is a thick, usually convoluted tube. It begins in the centre of each segment and in Cyclophyllidea, passes to the lateral margin to open in the genital atrium (the common genital pore). At its commencement it may be enlarged for the storage of sperms, the *seminal vesicle*. In Pseudophyllidea, it ascends upwards as a convoluted tube to open in the common genital pore.

(iii) *Cirrus Sac.* A sac at the end of vas deferens containing a coiled-up muscular organ which is called cirrus (penis). The cirrus and vagina open into a commoh cup-shaped chamber (common genital pore) either on the lateral border, as in Cyclophyllidea or on the mid-ventral surface, as in Pseudophyllidea.

FERTILISATION. This takes place between the segments; it may be a self-fertilisation or a cross-fertilisation between segments of the same or other worm.

DEVELOPMENT OF EGGS. The eggs are formed in the oötype where they are surrounded by protective coverings.

In Pseudophyllidean cestodes, the egg is operculated and has a single covering. The egg when first laid, does not contain an embryo. The membrane covering the embryo (which is formed outside) has a ciliated epithelium.

In Cyclophyllidean cestodes, the egg (Fig. 104) is not operculated and has two coverings. The outer cover is called the egg-shell and the inner one surrounding the embryo is called the embryophore. The egg, when first laid, contains an embryo which has no ciliated epithelium. The formed embryo is a six-hooked (hexacanth) sphere, called oncosphere. The space between the embryophore and the egg-shell is taken up by the yolk material. In some cases, the egg-shell is so thin that it is lost before the egg reaches the exterior along with the faeces. In such cases, the embryophore becomes thick and radially striated for the protection of the contained embryo, as in Taenia.

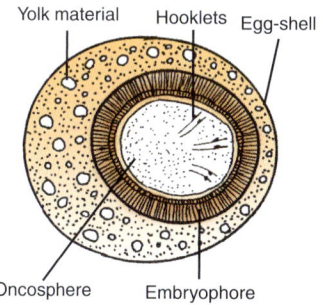

Fig. 104—Egg of a Cyclophyllidean cestode of the family Taeniidae.

LARVAL DEVELOPMENT. Two types of development are seen (see also p. 115).

In Pseudophyllidea—Solid larval forms, known as procercoid and plerocercoid.

In Cyclophyllidea—Larval forms are transformed into bladders (bladder-worm).

Terms Used in the Description of the Tapeworm (Cestode)

Strobila. The body or trunk of the adult worm (some authors use it for the entire worm—scolex, neck and body).

Scolex. Commonly called "head"; carries the organs of attachment or suckers.

"Neck". The region of growth behind the "head".

Proglottid. An individual segment comprising the complete unit of a tapeworm. According to its sexual maturity, a segment may be immature (reproductive organs not differentiated), mature (reproductive organs appeared) or gravid (uterus filled with eggs).

Rostellum. A beak-like projection on the "head" which carries hooklets in the armed species. It may remain invaginated between the suckers. The rostellar hooklets have characteristic shape in each Family.

Oncosphere. A six-hooked (hexacanth) embryo inside the egg.

Embryophore. The enveloping membrane surrounding the oncosphere.

Egg-shell. The outer membrane enclosing the oncosphere with the embryophore and containing the yolk materials.

Cysticercus. It is the resting stage of the larva in the intermediate host where it develops into a "bladder-worm". It consists of a hollow vesicle with the invaginated scolex on its wall and a central cavity containing a little fluid.

Cysticercoid. A small bladder containing the invaginated "head" proximally and a solid, elongated portion as a caudal appendage.

Coenurus. A larval stage in the form of "bladder-worm" containing many invaginated scolices.

Hydatid Cyst. The larval stage of the genus Echinococcus.

Coracidium. A ciliated oncosphere of Diphyllobothrium.

Procercoid. The first larval stage of Diphyllobothnum found in Cyclops. It is a spindle-like solid body with cephalic invagination and a caudal spherical appendage (cercomer) containing embryonal hooklets.

Plerocercoid. The second larval stage of Diphyllobothrium. The caudal appendage is solid, elongated and the "head" is invaginated in the "neck".

Sparganum. Applied to plerocercoid larva infecting man.

Sparganosis. Means infection by sparganum.

Classification of Cestodes Infecting Man

(A) According to Habitat

I. PSEUDOPHYLLIDEAN CESTODES: Possessing false or slit-like grooves (*bothria).*

  (1) ADULT WORMS IN INTESTINE

      GENUS DIPHYLLOBOTHRIUM: *D. latum* (fish tapeworm).

  (2) LARVAL STAGES (PLEROCERCOID) IN MAN

    (i) *Sparganum mansoni.*

    (ii) *Sparganum proliferum.*

II. CYCLOPHYLLIDEAN CESTODES: Possessing cup-like and round suckers (*acetabula).*

  (1) ADULT WORMS IN INTESTINE

    (i) Genus Taenia: *T. saginata* (beef tapeworm), *T. solium* (pork tapeworm).

    (ii) Genus Hymenolepis: *H. nana* (dwarf tapeworm), *H. diminuta* (rat tapeworm).

    (iii) Genus Dipylidium: *D. caninum* (double-pored dog tapeworm).

  (2) LARVAL STAGES IN MAN

    (i) Genus Echinococcus: Hydatid cyst of *E. granulosus* (dog tapeworm), *E. multilocularis.*

    (ii) Genus Taenia: *Cysticercus cellulosae* of *T. solium.*

    (iii) Genus Multiceps: *Coenurus cerebralis* of *M. multiceps, Coenurus glomeratus* of *M. glomeratus* and *Coenurus serialis* of *M. Serialis*

(B) Systematic Classification

Genus	Species	Definitive Host	Intermediate Host	Stage found in Man
ORDER I PSEUDOPHYLLIDEA: SUPERFAMILY BOTHRIOCEPHALOIDEA, FAMILY DIPHYLLOBOTHRIIDAE				
DIPHYLLOBOTHRIUM	D. latum	Man, Dog, Cat	Cyclops and Fish	Adult worm
SPIROMETRA	S. mansoni	Dog, Cat	Frog, Snake, Man	Larval stage
	S. proliferum			
ORDER II CYCLOPHYLLIDEA: SUPERFAMILY TAENIOIDEA, FAMILY TAENIIDAE				
TAENIA	T. saginata	Man	Cow	Adult worm
	T. solium	Man	Pig, Man	Adult; larval stage occasionally
MULTICEPS	M. multiceps	Dog	Sheep, Goat, Cattle, Man	Larval stage
ECHINOCOCCUS	E. granulosus	Dog, Wolf, Jackal	Sheep, Cattle, Pig, Man	Larval stage
	E. multilocularis	Fox, Dingo, Dog, Wolf	Field mouse, Tundra vole, Man	Larval stage
ORDER II CYCLOPHYLLIDEA: SUPERFAMILY TAENIOIDEA, FAMILY HYMENOLEPIDIDAE				
HYMENOLEPIS	H. nana	Man, Rat	Not required	Adult and larval stages in intestine
	H. diminuta	Rat (Man)	Rat flea	Adult worm
ORDER II CYCLOPHYLLIDEA: SUPERFAMILY TAENIOIDEA, FAMILY DILEPIDIDAE				
DIPYLIDIUM	D. caninum	Dog, Cat (Man)	Dog flea	Adult worm

Differences between a Pseudophyllidean Cestode and a Cyclophyllidean Cestode		
	PSEUDOPHYLLIDEAN CESTODE	CYOLOPHYLLIDEAN CESTODE
"Head":	Bears 2 slit-like grooves.	Bears 4 cup-like suckers.
Uterus:	No branching; the convoluted uterine tube assumes the form of a rosette.	Branching may or may not be present.
Uterine Pore:	Present.	Absent.
Common Genital Pore:	Ventral, in the middle line.	Lateral.
Eggs:	Operculated; give rise to ciliated larvae.	Not operculated; do not give rise to ciliated larvae.

Order I PSEUDOPHYLLIDEA

Superfamily BOTHRIOCEPHALOIDEA : Family DIPHYLLOBOTHRIIDAE Genus DIPHYLLOBOTHRIUM

General Characters of Pseudophyllidean Cestodes

1. Large worms consisting of a long chain of segments.

2. "Head" has in place of Suckers two slit-like sucking grooves called *bothria*.

3. Vitelline glands are scattered widely in the parenchyma and consist of many acini.

4. Genital pores are on the ventral surface of the segment and not marginal. There are three genital orifices in each segment, one male orifice (the opening of vas deferens) and two female orifices (the openings of the vagina and the uterus).

5. Uterus opens to the exterior through which eggs come out.

6. Eggs are operculated and can develop only in water. They are immature when oviposited. The oncosphere gives rise to ciliated embryo.

7. Larval development proceeds in two intermediate hosts. The first larval stage is called *procercoid* and the second larval stage is called *plerocercoid*.

Diphyllobothrium latum (Linnaeus, 1758) Lühe, 1910

Common Names: The fish tapeworm; the broad tapeworm (Russian).

Geographical Distribution. Central Europe, America, Japan and Central Africa. It has not yet been reported from India.

Habitat. Adult worm lives in the small intestine (ileum) of man; also in dog, cat, fox and other fish-eating mammals.

Morphology. The adult worm is yellowish-grey in colour with dark central markings caused by the egg-filled uterus. It measures 3 to 10 metres in length. The individual worm may live for a period of 5 to 13 years.

The *scolex* ("head") is elongated and spoon-shaped and measures 2 to 3 mm in length by 1 mm in breadth. It bears two slit-like grooves (bothria) situated on the dorsal and ventral surfaces respectively. There are no rostellum and no hooklets.

The "neck" is thin and unsegmented and is much longer than the "head".

Proglottides (Segments). These are 3,000 to 4,000 in number. The segments are greater in breadth than in length. A mature segment measures 2 to 4 mm in length by 10 to 20 mm in breadth and is practically filled with male and female reproductive organs. The terminal segments are apt to be shrunken and empty owing to the constant discharge of eggs through the uterine pore. Later the dried-up segments break off from the body, not singly but in chains, and are passed in the host's faeces. There are three genital pores comprising of the openings of vas deferens, vagina and uterus, lying close to one another in that order from the front, on the ventral surface in the middle line of each segment. The ovary is bilobed. The uterus is large and remains coiled in the centre of each segment in the form of a rosette (Fig. 105).

EGGS. These are passed out in the host's faeces in large numbers. The characteristics of the egg are as follows:

(i) Oval and brown in colour (bile-stained).

(ii) Measures 70 μm in length by 45 μm in breadth.

(iii) Contains abundant yolk granules and an unsegmented ovum.

(iv) There is an inconspicuous operculum at one end with a small knob at the other end.

(v) Does not float in saturated solution of common salt.

The eggs are not infective to man.

LARVAL STAGES. These are passed first in water and then in the respective intermediate hosts. There are three stages of larval development.

(i) The *first-stage larva* is known as *coracidium* which develops from egg in water.

(ii) The *second-stage larva* is known as *procercoid* and is found inside the cyclops, the first intermediate host.

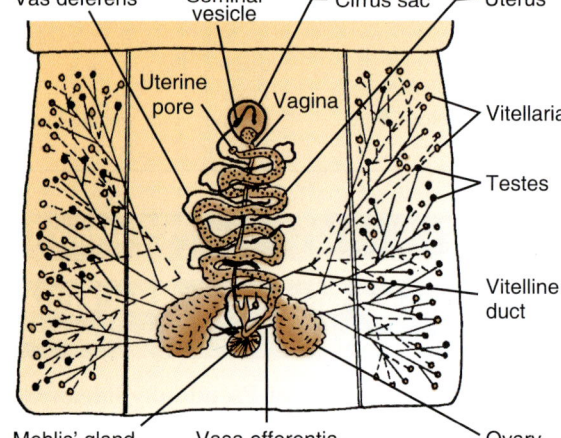

Fig. 105—The genital system of *D. latum*.

(iii) The *third-stage larva* is known as *plerocercoid* and is found in a fresh-water fish, the second intermediate host.

Note: A single egg gives rise to a single larva.

Life Cycle. The worm passes its life cycle (Fig. 106) in one definitive host and two intermediate hosts.

Definitive Hosts. Man, dog and cat; man is the optimum host. The adult worms are found in the small intestine.

Intermediate Hosts. Aquatic animals, where the larval stages are passed:

(i) The FIRST INTERMEDIATE HOST is a fresh-water crustacean, a cyclops or a diaptomus.

(ii) The SECOND INTERMEDIATE HOST is a fresh-water fish, pike, trout, salmon, perch and other fish.

DEVELOPMENT OF EGG IN WATER AND LIBERATION OF A CORACIDIUM. The operculated eggs are liberated through the faeces of definitive hosts in water. A spherical ciliated embryo containing 3 pairs of hooklets, called *coracidium*, develops within each egg-shell in the course of 1 to 2 weeks. The mature coracidium (40 to 55 μm in diameter) escapes into the water and is ingested by a cyclops.

LARVAL DEVELOPMENT INSIDE CYCLOPS. Inside the intestine of cyclops, the coracidium loses its cilia and the supporting cubical cells. It then penetrates through the intestinal wall and comes to rest inside its body cavity wherein about 3 weeks' time it is transformed into an elongated solid body with a caudal spherical appendage containing the six, now useless hooks, known as *procercoid larva*. The cyclops, containing the developing larvae (not more than two are present) is in its turn devoured by the second intermediate host, a fresh-water fish.

LARVAL DEVELOPMENT INSIDE FISH. In the intestine of fish, the procercoid larva (550 μm in length) after freeing itself, passes through the gut-wall and rests into the liver, muscles or voluminous fat in the mesentery and proceeds to develop further. In 1 to 3 weeks, the procercoid larva changes into a *"sparganum"* or *plerocercoid larva*. It has now lost its spherical caudal appendage and there is a depression at the anterior end representing the withdrawn and inverted "head" of the future adult worm. The body of the larva is white, somewhat flattened and marked by irregular unsegmented wrinkles. The smaller bodies (6 mm in length) lie straight in the flesh, but the larger ones (2 cm in length) remain bent and twisted.

INFECTION OF MAN AND DEVELOPMENT OF ADULT WORM. The plerocercoid larva is infective to man. It is not destroyed by ordinary salting, pickling or smoking and therefore with the eating of these insufficiently cooked fish or raw roe man is infected. Inside the intestine of man, the plerocercoid larva develops into an adult worm and after having attained sexual maturity in about 5 to 6 weeks, starts discharging eggs which are passed along with the faeces. The cycle is thus repeated.

Pathogenicity. *Mode of infection.* By ingestion of imperfectly cooked infected fish or roe containing plerocercoid larvae.

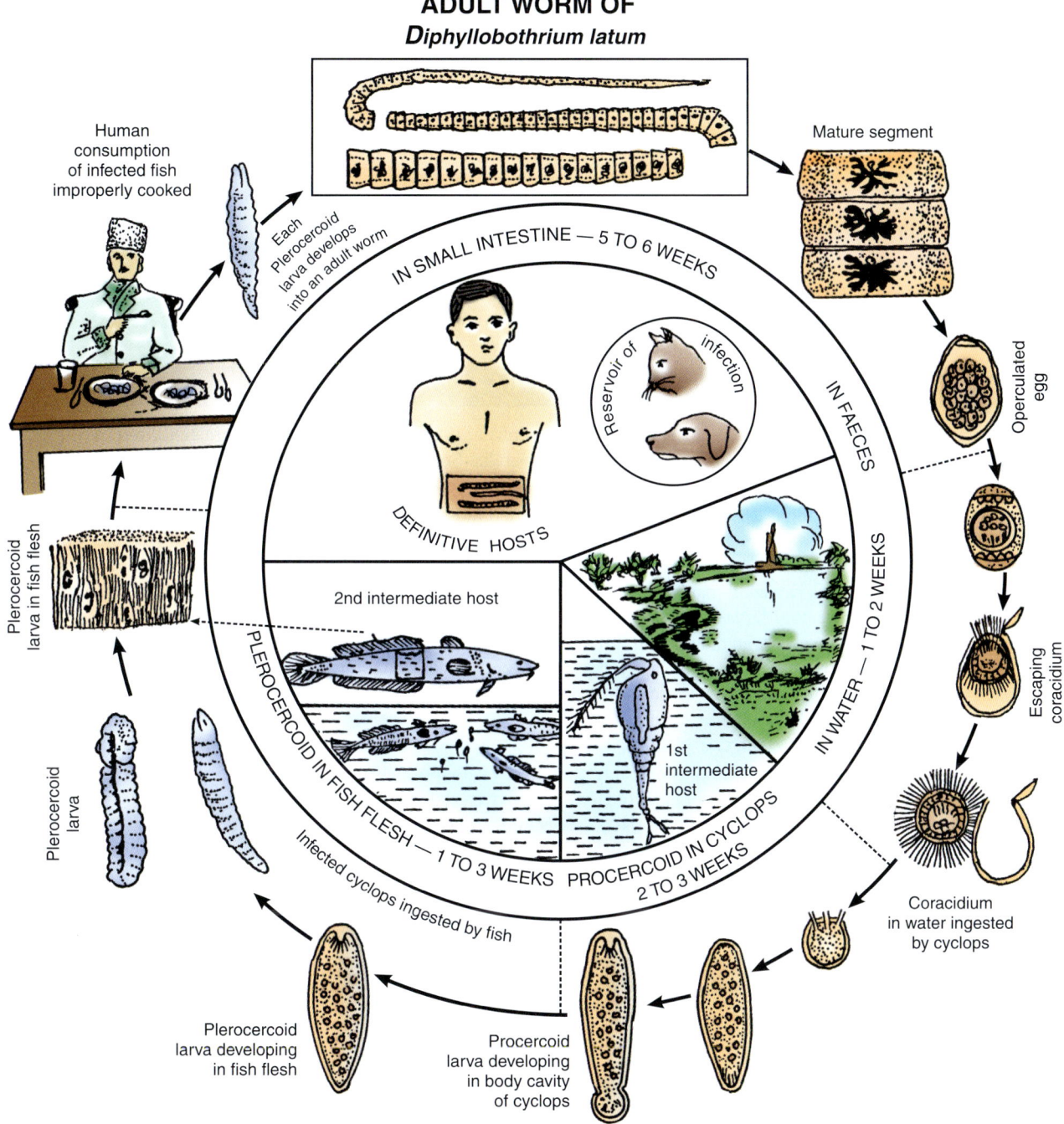

ADULT WORM OF
Diphyllobothrium latum

Human consumption of infected fish improperly cooked

Each Plerocercoid larva develops into an adult worm

Mature segment

IN SMALL INTESTINE — 5 TO 6 WEEKS

Reservoir of infection

IN FAECES

Operculated egg

DEFINITIVE HOSTS

Escaping coracidium

Plerocercoid larva in fish flesh

IN WATER — 1 TO 2 WEEKS

2nd intermediate host

PLEROCERCOID IN FISH FLESH — 1 TO 3 WEEKS

1st intermediate host

PROCERCOID IN CYCLOPS 2 TO 3 WEEKS

Coracidium in water ingested by cyclops

Plerocercoid larva

Infected cyclops ingested by fish

Plerocercoid larva developing in fish flesh

Procercoid larva developing in body cavity of cyclops

Fig. 106—Life cycle of *Diphyllobothrium latum.*

The infection of *D. latum* in man is known as *diphyllobothriasis*. The symptoms are gastrointestinal disturbances and anaemia. In persons having a hereditary, or racial tendency *D. latum* infection precipitates Addisonian anaemia (macrocytic). There is an early eosinophilia.

Bothriocephalus anaemia. The following views are held:

(i) The unsaturated fatty acids liberated by *D. latum* may cause interference with the intrinsic factor of Castle, giving rise to pernicious type of anaemia (Wardle and Green, 1941).

(ii) It has been shown that *D. latum* (when located in the proximal part of the jejunum) contains considerable amount of vitamin B_{12} and thus, may deprive the host of this essential nutritional component, causing pernicious anaemia (von Bonsdorff, 1956).

Diagnosis. This is established by a microscopical examination of faeces for the characteristic operculated eggs. Segments passed with the faeces may be recognised by the character of the uterus and the position of the genital pores. Many immunodiagnostic tests have been developed.

Treatment. Specific anthelmintic is praziquantel in a single dose of 10 mg/kg. Niclosamide in a dose of 1 gm in the morning followed by 1 gm after one hour was used for the treatment, in the past.

Prophylaxis. Preventive measures include the following:

1. Prevention of pollution of water: Efficient disposal of sewage.
2. Personal prophylaxis in endemic area: The fish should be cooked thoroughly before eating.
3. In endemic areas, the infection is maintained by dogs and cats fed on the offals of fish. This practice should be stopped.

Genus SPIROMETRA Müller, 1937

The term sparganum was applied to plerocercoid larvae of genus *Spirometra* and the disease sparganosis has been reported from Southeast Asia and Japan, less often from America and Australia. Some cases have also been reported from India. Genus Spirometra includes following species:

Spirometra mansoni (Cobbold, 1882). Cases have been reported mostly from the Far East. The adult worm has been found in the intestine of dogs, cats and other carnivorous animals. The procercoid stage is passed in cyclops and the plerocercoid stage in a species of frog or snake. Man obtains the infection by swallowing the procercoid stage in the cyclops along with drinking water and plerocercoid stage is passed in man which then forms the second intermediate host. Man thus takes the place of a frog or snake. In man, the plerocercoid larva has been found in the muscles and subcutaneous tissues. Infection has also occurred amongst the Chinese due to their custom of applying split raw frogs as poultices to hand or eye sores. The larva migrates from the frog into the tissues of the wound. Human infection can also occur by consumption of pork containing plerocercoid larvae. Diagnosis is usually possible by biopsy which reveals typical worm structure. No drug therapy is effective and excision of parasite wherever situated is the treatment of choice.

Spirometra proliferum (Ijima, 1905). Cases have been reported mainly from Japan. Nothing is known about the adult stage of the parasite and its life cycle. The infection is probably obtained by eating raw fish. The spargana occur in large numbers in the subcutaneous tissues, muscles and internal organs. In Ijima's case over 10,000 were found in the left thigh. The sparganum is found inside the cyst and often proliferates giving rise to supernumerary buds which eventually detach themselves and develop into larvae. Diagnosis can be made by biopsy which shows typical worm structure. No drug has been shown to be beneficial and excision of parasite is the only effective treatment.

Order II CYCLOPHYLLIDEA

Superfamily TAENIOIDEA: Family TAENIIDAE, HYMENOLEPIDIDAE, DILEPIDIDAE

General Characters of Cyclophyllidean Cestodes

1. Large or small worms consisting of chains of segments.
2. "Head" is quadrate in outline with four cup-like round suckers at each of the four angles. An apical rostellum in the centre armed with hooklets may be present.
3. Vitelline glands are concentrated into a single mass behind the ovary near the posterior margin of each segment.
4. The common genital pore is marginal, i.e., on the lateral side of each segment.
5. There is no uterine opening for the exit of eggs from the gravid uterus. The eggs can only escape by the disintegration or rupture of ripe segments. In Taeniidae, Dilepididae ripe segments are detached from the main body and passed in the faeces.
6. Eggs are not operculated and can develop only in the intermediate host. They are fully embryonated when detached from the segment. The oncosphere is never a ciliated embryo.
7. Larval development proceeds in one intermediate host.

Larval Development of Cyclophyllidean Cestodes (Fig. 107)

1. CYSTICERCOID. The entire larva is solid and only its proximal portion is vesicular containing the invaginated scolex. Such larval development is characteristic of tapeworms which have insects as intermediate host. The only exception is *H. nana*, where the cysticercoid stage of larval development is passed in a vertebrate host, either man or rat.

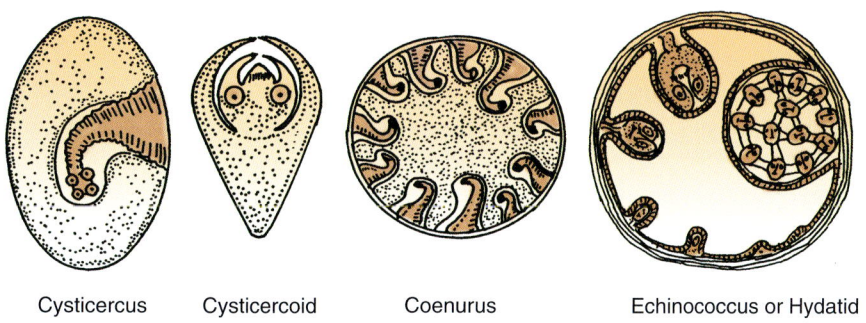

Cysticercus   Cysticercoid   Coenurus   Echinococcus or Hydatid

Fig. 107—Larval forms of Cyclophyllidean cestodes.

2. CYSTICERCUS (TRUE BLADDER-WORM) . The entire larva is transformed into a bladder from which the scolex, or "head" of the future adult worm sprouts. It may be divided as follows:

(a) *Cysticercus proper*. This consists of a bladder with one scolex, as in *T. saginata* and *T. solium*. The scolex remains invaginated within the cyst-wall and can be seen with the naked eyes as a milk-white spot about the size of a pin-head.

(b) *Coenurus*. A bladder with many scolices, as in the genus Multiceps.

(c) *Echinococcus (Hydatid)*. A bladder which multiplies by budding and forms many daughter and grand-daughter bladders. On the wall of these cysts, brood capsules are produced, inside which lie scolices, as in *E. granulosus*.

Note: Each scolex is capable of giving rise to one adult worm from larval cysts swallowed by the definitive host.

Family TAENIIDAE: Genus TAENIA

Taenia saginata Goeze, 1782

Common Names: The beef tapeworm; the unarmed tapeworm of man.

Geographical Distribution. World-wide. In India, it is particularly prevalent amongst Mohammedans but is not generally found amongst Hindu community who do not as a rule eat beef.

Habitat. Adult worm lives in the small intestine (upper jejunum) of man and moves against the peristaltic movement in the host's intestine.

Morphology. Adult Worm. It is white and semi-transparent; measuring 5 to 10 metres in length, but it may be up to 24 metres.

The *scolex* ("head") measures 1 to 2 mm in diameter, is quadrate in outline and has 4 circular suckers (may be pigmented). The "head" is not provided with any rostellum or hooklets and moves against the peristaltic movement in the host's intestine.

The "neck" is fairly long and narrow (about 0.5 mm in width); it is fragile.

Proglottides (Segments). The number varies from 1,000 to 2,000. The length of a gravid segment is 3 to 4 times its breadth. When relaxed, the terminal gravid segment measures about 2 cm in length by 0.5 cm in breadth. The common genital pore is situated marginally near the posterior end of each segment and alternates irregularly between the right and left margins. The vagina is provided with a sphincter muscle. The gravid uterus consists of a central longitudinal stem with 15 to 30 lateral branches on each side; these in turn sub-branch leaving practically no space in between. The gravid segments are expelled singly and may force their way through the anal sphincter often showing great activity outside. The free gravid proglottid while crawling out of the anal orifice oviposits in the perianal skin (Rupstra *et al*, 1961).

Life span of the adult worm is considerable; it may live for upwards of 10 years.

EGGS. As there is no uterine opening, the eggs are liberated by the rupture of ripe proglottides. The characteristics of the egg are as follows:

(i) Spherical and brown in colour (bile-stained).
(ii) Measure 31 to 43 μm in diameter.
(iii) The thin, outer transparent shell, when present, represents the remnant of the yolk mass; it causes the eggs to clump together.
(iv) The inner embryophore is brown, thick-walled and radially striated.
(v) Contains an oncosphere (14 to 20 μm in diameter) with 3 pairs of hooklets.
(vi) Does not float in saturated solution of common salt.
(vii) Eggs are resistant and may remain viable for 8 weeks.
(viii) Infective only to cattle.

Taenia solium Linnaeus, 1758

Common Names: The pork tapeworm; the armed tapeworm of man.

The rostellum resembles the conventional figures of the Sun, hence the name *"solium"*.

Geographical Distribution. World-wide. The infection is common amongst those eating raw or insufficiently cooked "measly" pork. It is uncommon in Jews and Mohammedans who are not generally pork-eaters.

Habitat. Adult worm lives in the small intestine (upper jejunum) of man.

Morphology. ADULT WORM. It measures about 2 to 3 metres in length.

The *scolex* ("head") measures 1 mm in diameter (about the size of a pin-head), is globular in outline and has 4 circular suckers. The "head" is provided with a rostellum armed with a double row of alternating large and small hooklets. The rostellar hooklets are shaped like daggers or Arabian poniards.

The "neck" is short, measuring from 5 to 10 mm in length.

Proglottides (Segments). The total number is less than a thousand (800 to 900). A gravid segment measures 12 mm by 6 mm. The common genital pore is marginal, thick-lipped and is situated near the middle of the lateral margin of each segment, alternating irregularly between the right and left margins. The vaginal opening is not guarded by a muscular sphincter. The gravid uterus consists of a median longitudinal stem with 5 to 10 compound lateral branches on each side. The gravid segments are expelled passively, in chains of 5 to 6 at a time, and not singly.

The worm has a *life span* of as much as 25 years.

EGGS. The characteristics are the same as those for *T. saginata*. The eggs are infective to pig as well as to man.

Adult Worms of *T. saginata* **and** *T. solium*		
	T. saginata	*T. solium*
LENGTH:	5 to 10 metres.	2 to 3 metres.
"HEAD":	Large, quadrate; without rostellum and hooks; suckers may be pigmented.	Small, globular; with rostellum and hooks; suckers not pigmented.
PROGLOTTIDES (Segments):		
NUMBER:	1000 to 2000.	Below 1000.
EXPULSION:	Expelled singly and may force anal sphincter.	Expelled passively in chains of 5 or 6.
UTERUS:	Lateral branches 15 to 30 on each side; thin and dichotomous.	Lateral branches 5 to 10 on each side; thick and dendritic.
VAGINA:	Vaginal sphincter present.	Vaginal sphincter absent.
OVARIES:	2 in number, without any accessory lobe.	2 in number, with an accessory lobe.
TESTES:	300 to 400 follicles.	150 to 200 follicles.

Life Cycle of *T. saginata.* The worm passes its life cycle (Fig. 108) in two hosts:

1. *The Definitive Host:* Man; harbours the adult worm.
2. *The Intermediate Host:* Cattle (cow or buffalo); harbours the larval stage.

The adult worm lives in the small intestine of man. The eggs or gravid segments are passed out with the faeces on the ground. The animals (cow or buffalo) swallow these eggs while grazing in the field. On reaching the alimentary canal of the intermediate host, the radially striated walls of the eggs rupture and oncospheres are liberated. These

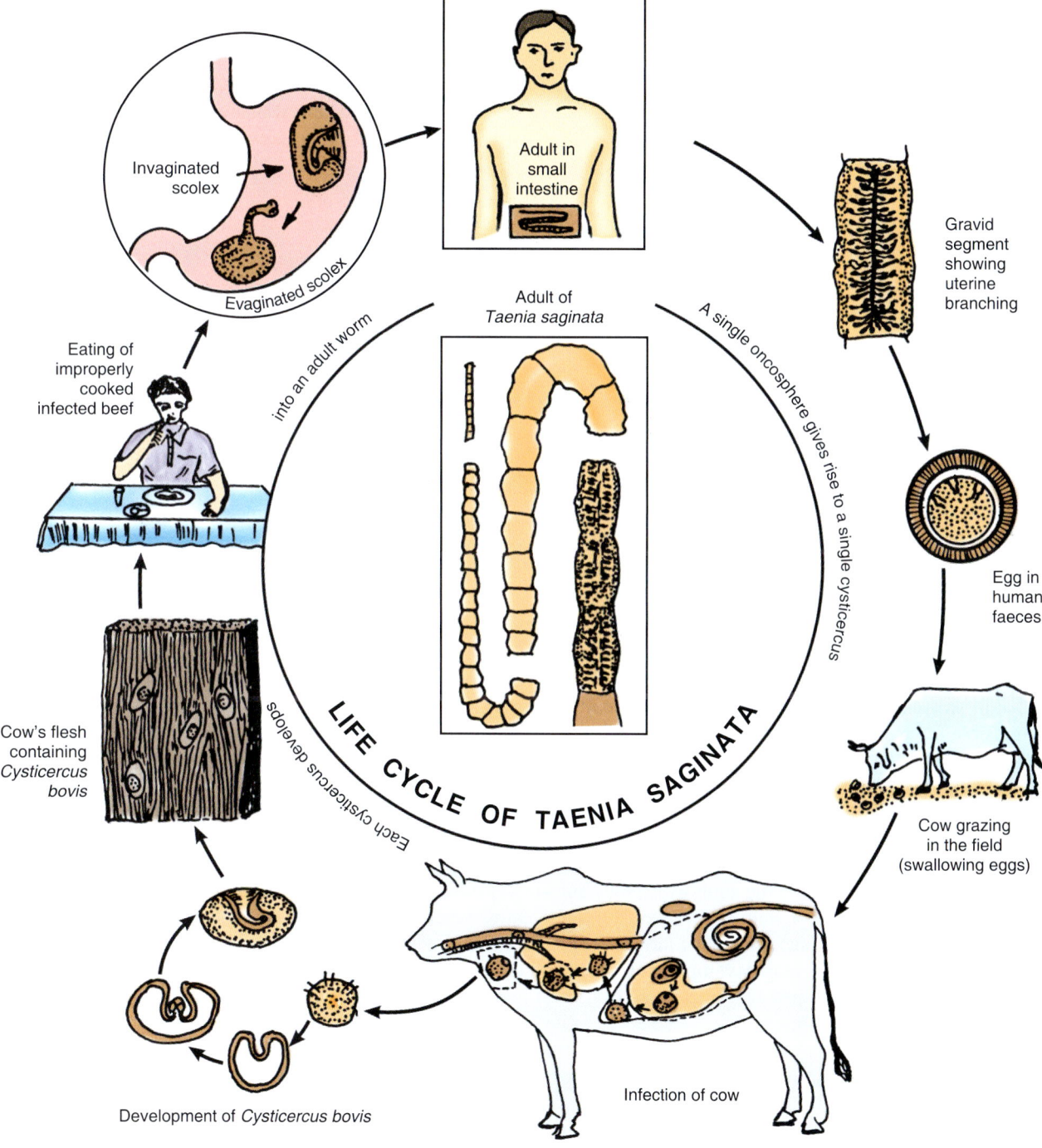

Fig. 108

penetrate the gut-wall with the aid of their hooks and gain entrance into the portal vessels or mesenteric lymphatics, finally reaching the systemic circulation. Usually, they travel *via* the portal vein and successively reach the following organs: the liver, the right side of the heart, lungs, the left side of the heart and the systemic circulation. The naked oncospheres are filtered out from the circulating blood into the muscular tissues where they ultimately settle down and undergo further development. The muscles most commonly selected are those of the tongue, neck, shoulder and ham; the cardiac muscle is also involved. The oncospheres lose their hooks on reaching their destination, the cells in the centre are liquefied and in about 8 days after infection each oncosphere forms an oval vesicle gradually increasing in size, containing at its bottom, the larva (the scolex or the future "head" of the adult worm)—referred to as *cysticercus*. It takes about 60 to 70 days for the oncospheres to metamorphose into the cysticercus stage. Human beings are infected through the eating of undercooked beef containing the cysticerci ("measly" beef). Inside the alimentary canal of man, the scolex, on coming in contact with the bile, exvaginates and anchors to the gut-wall by means of its suckers and develops into an adult worm by gradual strobilisation. The worm grows to sexual maturity in 2 to 3 months and starts producing eggs which are in their turn passed in the faeces along with the gravid segments, thereby repeating the cycle.

Life cycle of *T. solium* (Fig. 109). The life cycle is the same as described for *T. saginata*. The intermediate host is the pig. Human beings are infected through the eating of undercooked pork, containing the cysticerci ("measly" pork).

LARVAL DEVELOPMENT OF *T. saginata* AND *T. solium*

Cysticercus bovis. This is the larval stage of *T. saginata* developing in the muscles of a cow or a buffalo. It measures 5 to 10 mm in breadth by 3 to 4 mm in length and contains an unarmed scolex ("head" of the adult worm) invaginated at one side. It can live for about 8 months in the flesh of cattle and can only develop further when ingested by man, its definitive host. *Cysticercus bovis* does not occur in man.

Cysticercus cellulosae (Fig. 110). This is the larval stage of *T. solium* developing in the muscles of the pig. A mature cyst is an opalescent ellipsoidal body and measures 8 to 10 mm in width by 5 mm in length. The long axis of the cyst lies parallel with the muscle fibre. There is a dense milk-white spot at the side, where the scolex with its hooks and suckers remains invaginated. The cyst contains a fluid rich in salt and albuminous material. It can live for about 8 months in the flesh of pig and can only develop further when ingested by man, its definitive host.

Cysticercus cellulosae has also been found in man (*vide infra*).

Pathogenicity of Tapeworms and Clinical Features (*T. saginata* and *T. solium*)

MODE OF INFECTION. By ingestion of undercooked meat of the intermediate hosts:

(a) In *T. saginata*—Beef, containing *Cysticercus bovis*.

(b) In *T. solium*—Pork, containing *Cysticercus cellulosae*.

Adult worms while living in the intestine usually do not give rise to any symptom. Occasionally, they may be responsible for vague abdominal discomfort, chronic indigestion, anaemia and intestinal disorders, such as diarrhoea alternating with constipation. It is possible for the patient to detect the segments of the tapeworm in the faeces or on his own body or on his clothings.

Larval worms of *T. saginata* are not found in man but those of *T. solium* may occasionally be found.

Cysticercus cellulosae. Man, occasionally serving as the larval host of *T. solium*, becomes infected in the same way as the pig, i.e., either by drinking contaminated water or by eating uncooked vegetables infected with eggs. Besides this, a man harbouring the adult worm may auto-infect himself either due to unclean and unhygienic personal habits, or by a reversal of peristaltic movements of the intestine whereby the gravid segments are thrown back to the stomach, equivalent to the swallowing of thousands of eggs. These cysticerci are usually found in tens of thousands but sometimes singly. They may develop in any organ and the effect produced depends entirely on the location of the cysticerci in the body. The distribution of these cysticerci is usually in the subcutaneous tissues and muscles causing palpable or visible nodules but may be found in the brain leading to epileptic attacks. The clinical features of cysticercus cellulosae infection may vary. It may be asymptomatic or symptomatic.

Neurocysticercosis is now diagnosed by serodiagnosis (ELISA test—more than 80% sensitivity), CT scan of brain or MRI scan of brain.

Cysticercus cellulosae in the eye is easily diagnosed by ophthalmoscopic examination; due to the absence of fibrous encapsulation evagination of scolex can be visualised. They have a tendency to become calcified and obsolete in the course of 5 to 6 years.

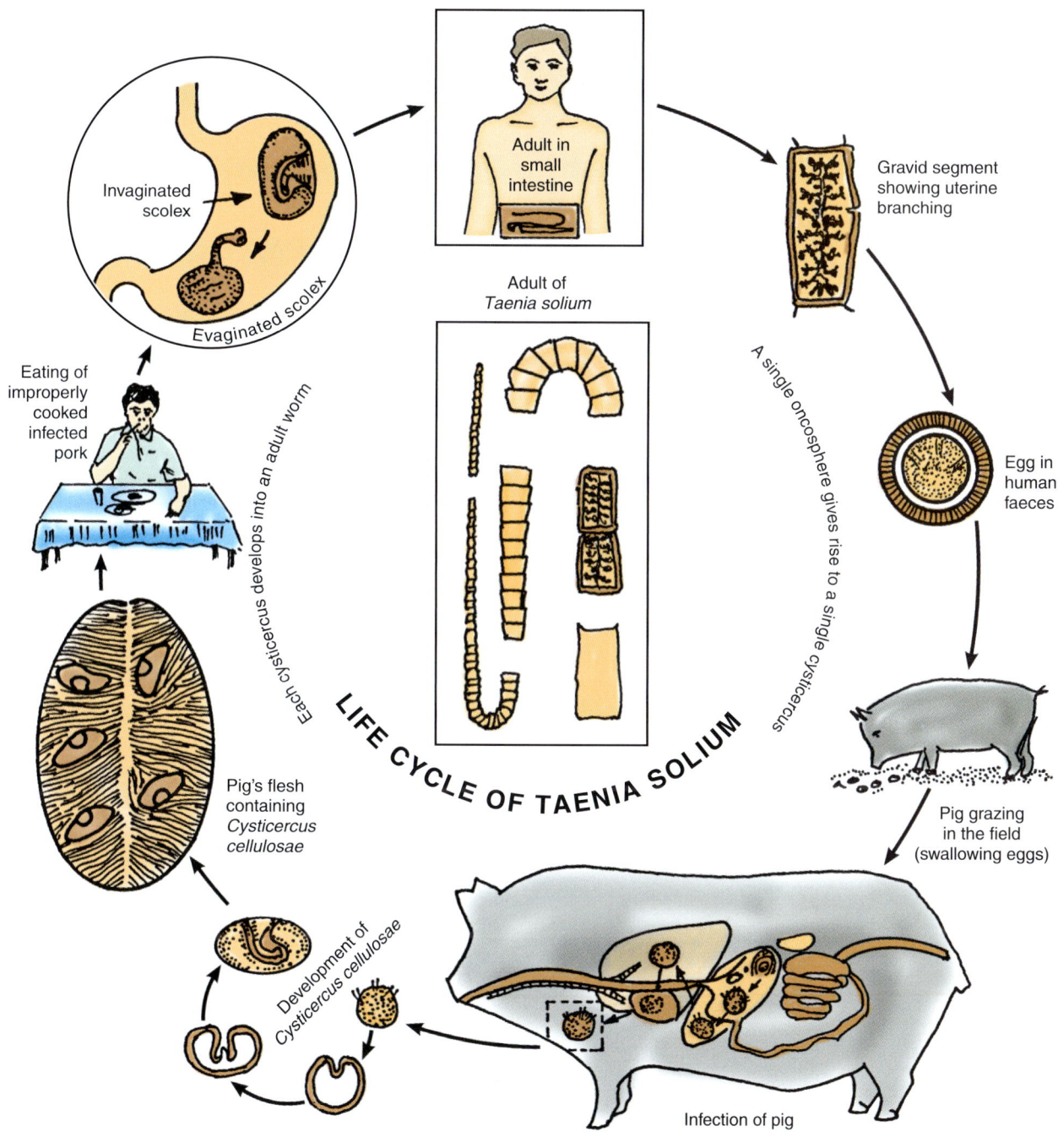

Fig. 109

Diagnosis of Tapeworm Infection. This is carried out by an examination of stool. At first, a naked eye examination of the specimen should be made for segments which, if found, should be collected for future study of the genital apparatus. The whitish segments can easily be recognised against the dark yellow mass of the faeces (Fig. 111). If the specimen is obtained after an anthelmintic, the sample of faeces may be screened and examined macroscopically for the "head" (scolex).

A microscopical examination of the stool for the eggs of the adult worm is carried out by (i) a direct smear preparation of the sample of faeces, or (ii) a smear preparation made from the sample after concentrating in one of the low density solutions.

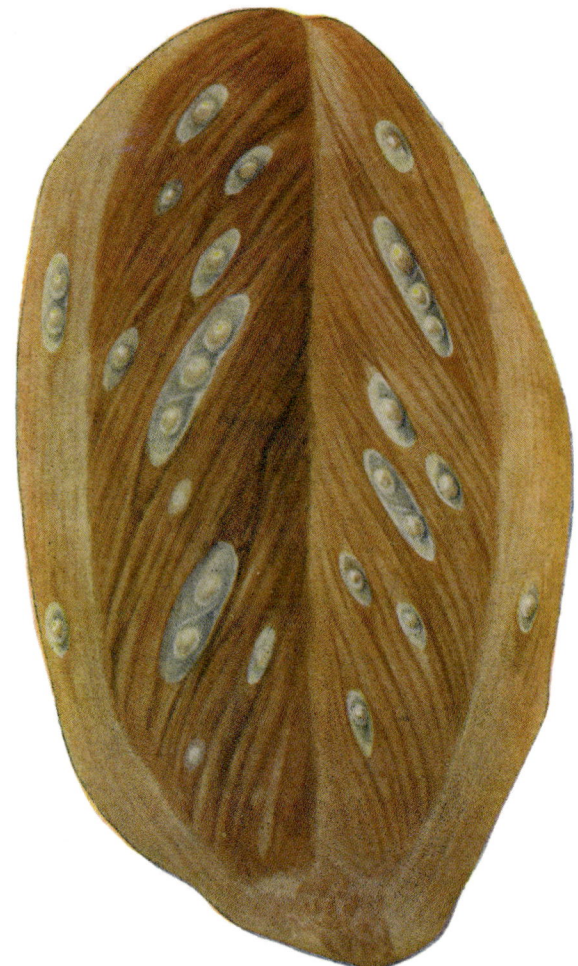

Fig. 110—*Cysticercus cellulosae* **in pig's muscle.**

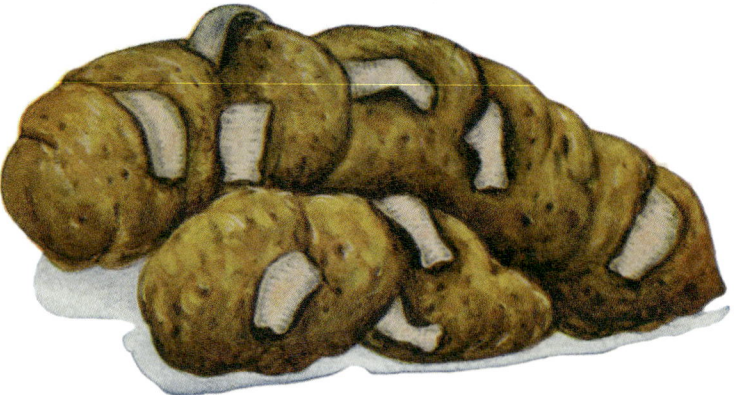

Fig. 111—**Tapeworm segments** (*T. saginata*) **in the faecal mass.**

A perianal swab (NIH swab) for the demonstration of eggs, as in enterobiasis, may sometimes be helpful in the diagnosis of *T. saginata* infection.

SPECIES DIAGNOSIS. As the eggs of *T. saginata* cannot be differentiated from those of *T. solium*, finding of tapeworm eggs is of no material help for a species diagnosis. The "head" and the gravid segment, when available, are the only means of establishing a species diagnosis (Figs. 112, 113, 114, 115 & 116).

"Head" and gravid segments of *T. solium* **and** *T. saginata.*
(Stained with acetic acid-alum-carmine solution.)

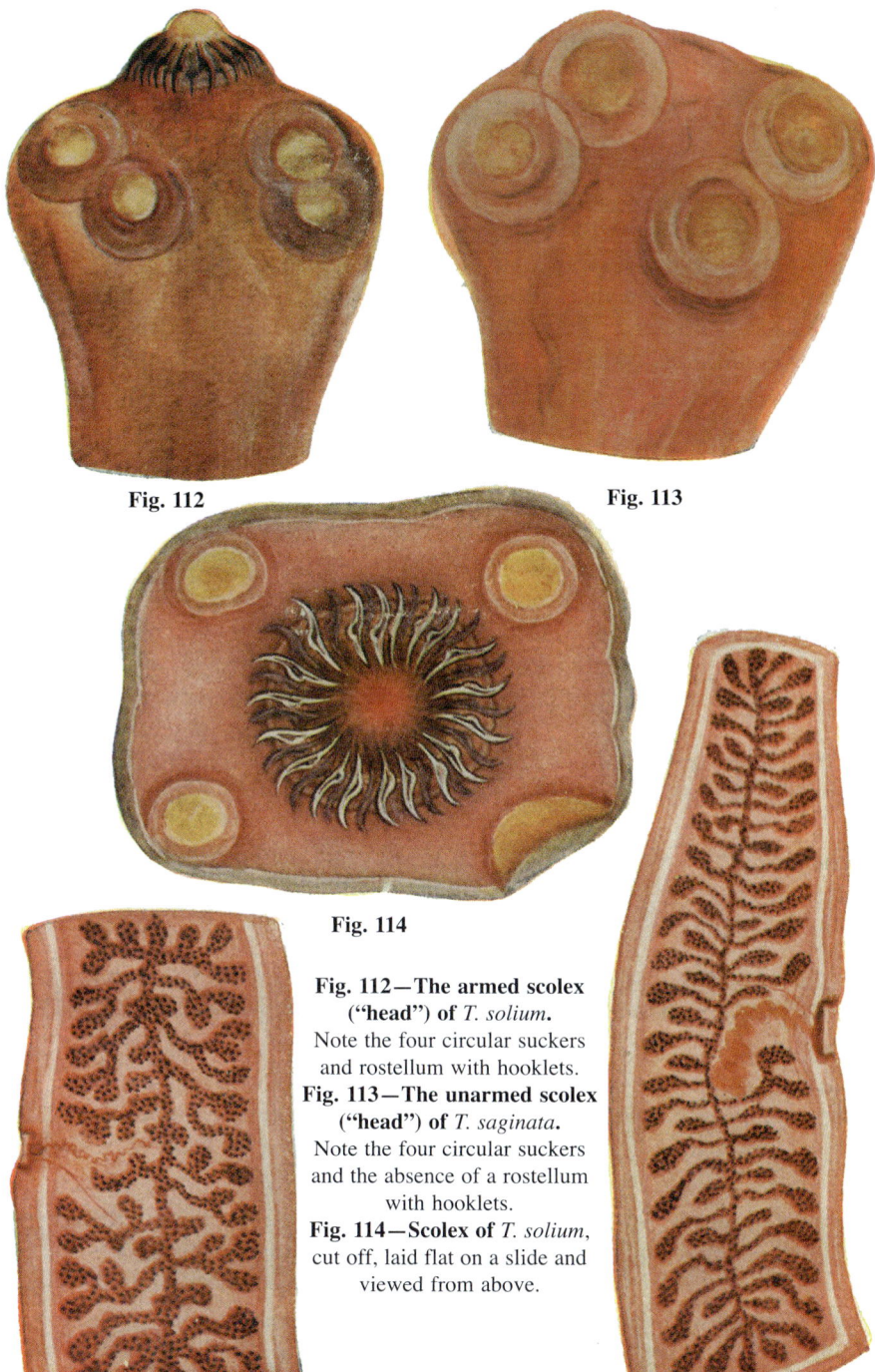

Fig. 112   **Fig. 113**

Fig. 114

**Fig. 112—The armed scolex
("head") of** *T. solium.*
Note the four circular suckers
and rostellum with hooklets.
**Fig. 113—The unarmed scolex
("head") of** *T. saginata.*
Note the four circular suckers
and the absence of a rostellum
with hooklets.
Fig. 114—Scolex of *T. solium*,
cut off, laid flat on a slide and
viewed from above.

Fig. 115—A gravid segment of *T. solium.*
The uterus is filled with eggs; other reproductive
organs are atrophied. Note the central longitudinal
stem of the uterus with 5 to 10 lateral branches.

Fig. 116—A gravid segment of *T. saginata.*
The uterus is filled with eggs; other reproductive
organs are atrophied. Note the central longitudinal
stem of the uterus with 15 to 30 lateral branches.

[*Drawn with the assistance of Dr. N. V. Bhaduri.*]

Molecular methods such as DNA probes and PCR have been developed to find out the differences between eggs of *T. solium* and *T. saginata* in faeces.

DIAGNOSIS OF CYSTICERCOSIS. This is based on the following:

(i) Biopsy examination of a subcutaneous nodule containing cysticerci.

(ii) Roentgenograms of skull and soft tissues (buttocks and thighs) may reveal calcified cysticerci.

(iii) CT scan of brain of affected oragan is used to detect calcified cystecerci or small hypodense lesion (ring or disc-like enhancing lesion) or small hypodense lesion with a bright central spot.

(iv) MRI scan of brain is more helpful in detection of ventricular cysticercosis.

(v) Myelography demonstrates spinal cysticerci.

(vi) Eosinophilia may occur in the invasive stage.

(vii) A positive indirect haemagglutination test using antigen from pig's cysticerci, IFA and ELISA tests are now widely used for detection of antibodies.

(viii) Antigen can be detected in serum and CSF by ELISA test.

(ix) A history of intestinal taeniasis often helps in the diagnosis.

Treatment of Tapeworm Infection. The drug of choice is praziquantel (5-10 mg/kg as a single dose after breakfast) for the treatment of *T. solium* and *T. saginata*. It is effective against adult tape worm in a single dose and it kills cysticerci in high dose (50-100 mg/kg/day in divided doses for one month). Other anthelmintic drug, effective in expelling the adult worm, is niclosamide (2 gm as a single dose in the morning in the empty stomach). For cerebral cysticercosis praziquantel in a dose of 50 mg/kg/day in three divided doses for one month and albendazole in a dose of 400 mg twice daily for 30 days may be administered but excision is the best method of treatment where possible.

Prophylaxis. The preventive measures include the following:

1. Individual prophylaxis consists of avoidance of eating raw or undercooked meat of the intermediate hosts.

2. Adequate meat inspection in the slaughterhouse.

3. Proper sanitary control of sewage disposal and effective treatment of infected individual to prevent infection of the intermediate hosts.

Owing to the risk of acquiring cysticercosis (*T. solium*), either from auto-infection, or from others infected with adult worm, care should be taken regarding personal hygiene as well as the effective treatment of all cases harbouring the adult worm.

Taenia saginata asiatica: It was discovered in 1993 and morphologically identical to *T. saginata*. It is found in Indonesia, Thailand, Taiwan, Korea, Myanmar and Philippines. Intermediate host is pig and location of cysticerci is in the liver of pig. The scolex is larger.

Genus MULTICEPS

Genus Multiceps includes three species: *M. multiceps, M. glomeratus* and *M. serialis*. These tapeworms are natural parasites of dog and other canine animals. Sheep, goat, cattle, horse and other herbivorous animals are natural intermediate hosts in which coenurus (larval stage) develops. Sometime man acts as an intermediate host and the condition is known as "coenurosis". Infections have been reported in man from England, USA, Brazil and Africa.

Multiceps multiceps (Leske, 1780) Hall, 1910
Syn. *Taenia multiceps* Leske, 1780

Common Name: The gid worm or the "gid" tapeworm.

The parasite causing cerebral coenuriasis in sheep and man.

The generic name is derived from many headed larval stage (from L. *multi*, many; *caput*, head).

The adult worm lives in the intestinal canal of dogs, foxes and incidentally in wolves. It measures 40 to 60 cm in length and has a scolex with an armed rostellum. The anatomy of the mature segment resembles closely that of *T. saginata*. The gravid uterus has 18 to 26 slightly branched lateral arms on each side of the main stem. The eggs measure about 36 microns in diameter. Man is infected by ingestion of food and water contaminated with dog's faeces containing eggs of parasite.

Life cycle: It was first worked by Kuchenmeister in 1853. The larval stage is passed in herbivorous animals such as sheep, goats, cattle and horse. These intermediate hosts are infected by swallowing eggs passed in the dog's faeces. The oncosphere, which hatches out in the intestine, penetrates its wall and lodges in various tissues of the animals, specially in the brain and spinal cord. Here the larva metamorphoses into coenurus, a bladder-worm with multiple scolices (heads). Each of these scolices is capable of developing into a complete adult worm in the dog in case it devours the brain of a sheep which has died of the infection. In the sheep the common clinical manifestation is "gid" (giddiness or vertigo) hence the name "gid worm".

The first human case recorded was that of a Paris locksmith (1911). That patient had clinical manifestation of a brain tumour, nausea, vomiting, headache, aphasia, epilepsy and paraplegia. Sites of affected part are brain, orbit and subcutenuous tissue. Diagnaosis is made by CT scan and MRI scan of brain. The prognosis of cerebral coenuriasis is always serious. Surgical removal of cyst is preferable. The diagnosis is confirmed by histological recognition of coenurus.

Multiceps glomeratus **Railliet and Henry, 1915**
Syn. Coenurus glomeratus (Railliet and Henry, 1915) Turner and Leiper, 1919

The larval stage (coenurus) was primarily recovered from gerbile by Railliet & Henry (1915). The first human infection was reported by Turner and Leiper (1919) in the cyst excised from the intercostals muscle of a native of Northern Nigeria. *M. glomeratus* and *M. brauni* are same. The adult worm possesses a scolex armed with thirty rostellar hooks. The coenurus of *Multiceps glomeratus* differs from that of *Multiceps multiceps* by its larger hooks.

Multiceps serialis **(Gervais, 1845) Stiles and Stevenson, 1905**
Syn. Coenurus serialis Gervais, 1845.

The adult worm is an intestinal parasite of dog; the larval stage (coenurus) is found in the intermuscular connective tissues of some rodents. A very small number of human cases of larval infection with this species has been reported. There are 32 hooklets arranged in two rows in each scolex.

Family TAENIIDAE: Genus ECHINOCOCCUS

Echinococcus granulosus (Batsch, 1786) Rudolphi, 1805

Syn. *Taenia echinococcus*

Common Names: The dog tapeworm; the hydatid worm.

The adult worm was discovered by Hartmann (1695) and the larval form by Goeze (1782).

Geographical Distribution. Although the hydatid disease is world-wide in distribution, it is most commonly found in those countries where sheep and cattle-raising constitutes an important industry and consequently, there is a close association between man, sheep and dog. It is more a disease of temperate climates than of tropical areas.

Habitat. Man harbours the larval form and *not the adult worm* which is however found in the small intestine of dog and other canine animals.

Morphology. ADULT WORM (Fig. 117). It is a small tapeworm, measuring 3 to 6 mm in length. It comprises of a *scolex* ("head"), "*neck*" and *strobila* consisting of 3 *segments* (occasionally 4). The first segment is immature, the second one is mature and the last one (as well as the fourth one, when present) is gravid. The terminal segment is by far the biggest, measuring 2 to 3 mm in length by 0.6 mm in breadth. The *scolex* bears four suckers and a protrusible rostellum with two circular rows of hooks. The "*neck*" is short and thick.

EGG. It is ovoid in shape and resembles other eggs of Taenia. It measures 32 to 36 μm in length by 25 to 32 μm in breadth and contains a hexacanth embryo with 3 pairs of hooks. The egg is infective to man, cattle, sheep and other herbivorous animals.

LARVAL FORM (Figs. 118 & 119). This is found within the hydatid cyst developing inside the intermediate hosts. It represents the structure of the *scolex* of the future adult worm and remains invaginated within a vesicular body. On entering the definitive host, the *scolex* with four suckers and rostellar hooklets, becomes evaginated and develops into an adult worm.

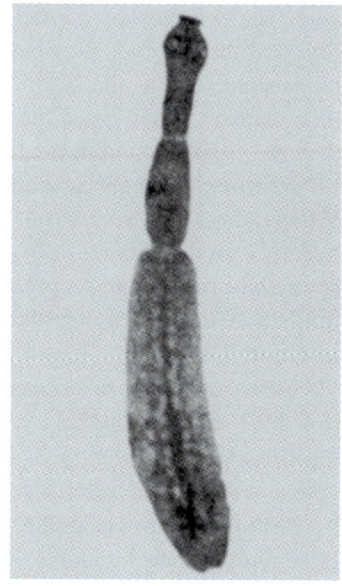

Fig. 117–*Echinococcus granulosus.* Adult worm from the small intestine of dog showing scolex with hooklets and suckers and entire strobila.

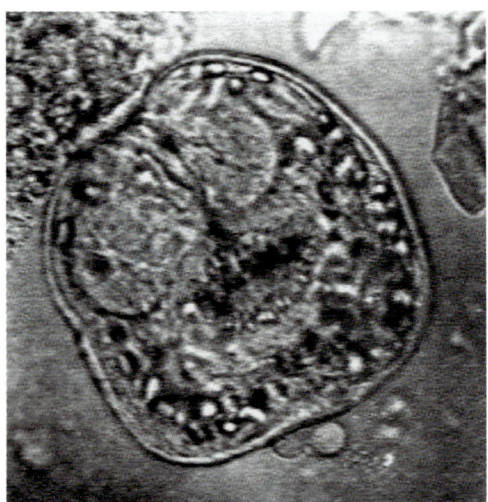

Fig. 118—Scolex from hydatid cyst.
Hooklets and suckers invaginated within a vesicle.

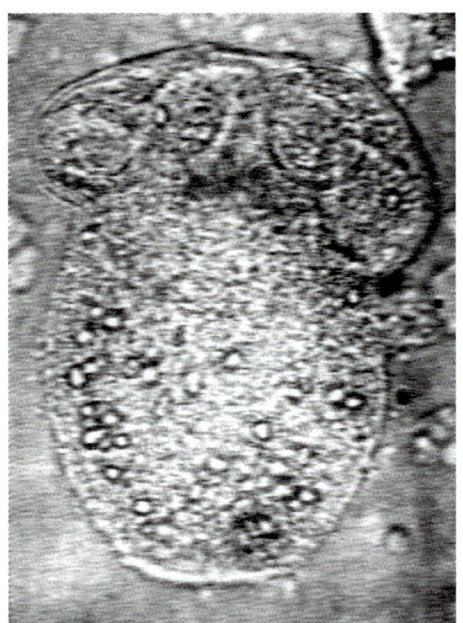

Fig. 119—Scolex from hydatid cyst.
Hooklets and suckers evaginating from the vesicle.

Life Cycle. The worm passes its life cycle (Fig. 120) in two hosts.

1. *Definitive Hosts.* Dog, wolf, fox and jackal. The adult worm lives in the small intestine of these animals who discharge a large number of eggs in their faeces. The dog is the optimum definitive host.

2. *Intermediate Hosts.* Sheep, pig, cattle, horse, goat and man. The larval stage is passed in these animals and man, giving rise to hydatid cyst. The sheep appears to be the optimum intermediate host.

The eggs are discharged with the faeces of the definitive hosts (dog and allied animals). These are swallowed by the intermediate hosts, sheep and other domestic animals while grazing in the field, and also by man (particularly children) due to intimate handling of infected dogs. In the duodenum, the hexacanth embryos are hatched out. About eight hours after ingestion, the embryos bore their way through the intestinal wall and enter the radicles of the portal vein. The embryos are carried to the liver to be arrested in the sinusoidal capillaries (the liver acts as the first filter). Some of the embryos may pass through the hepatic capillaries, enter the pulmonary circulation and filter out in the lungs (lungs act as the second filter). A few of the embryos may pass the pulmonary capillaries, enter the general blood stream and lodge in the various organs. Practically, all the organs of the domestic animals may be invaded but they are chiefly found in the liver and lungs.

Wherever the embryo settles, it forms a hydatid cyst, the young larva being transformed into a hollow bladder (G. *hydatis*, drop of water). From the inner side of the cyst, brood capsules with a number of scolices are developed. A hydatid cyst developing from a single egg (oncosphere) may contain thousands of scolices. A fully developed scolex is an end-product and its presence inside the hydatid cyst is a sign of "a complete biological development". These fertile hydatids, when ingested by the dog, are capable of growing into adult worms in about 6 to 7 weeks' time in the intestine. Thus, the cycle is repeated.

As the dogs have no access to the hydatid cyst developed in the viscera of man, the life cycle of the parasite comes to a dead-end. The natural cycle is thus maintained by dog and sheep.

Life span of the adult worm in the canine host is short (about 6 months). *Life span of the larval worm* is considerable and it may continue to develop for many years.

Pathogenicity. The adult worms of *E. granulosus* in dogs do not cause much inconvenience. They are found in large numbers (by hundreds or even thousands) in the small intestine of an infected dog where they lie embedded in the mucous membrane and appear on postmortem as small white specks on the reddish mucous surfaces (owing to the minuteness of size, they are often overlooked).

The larval worm of *E. granulosus* in man causes unilocular hydatid disease.

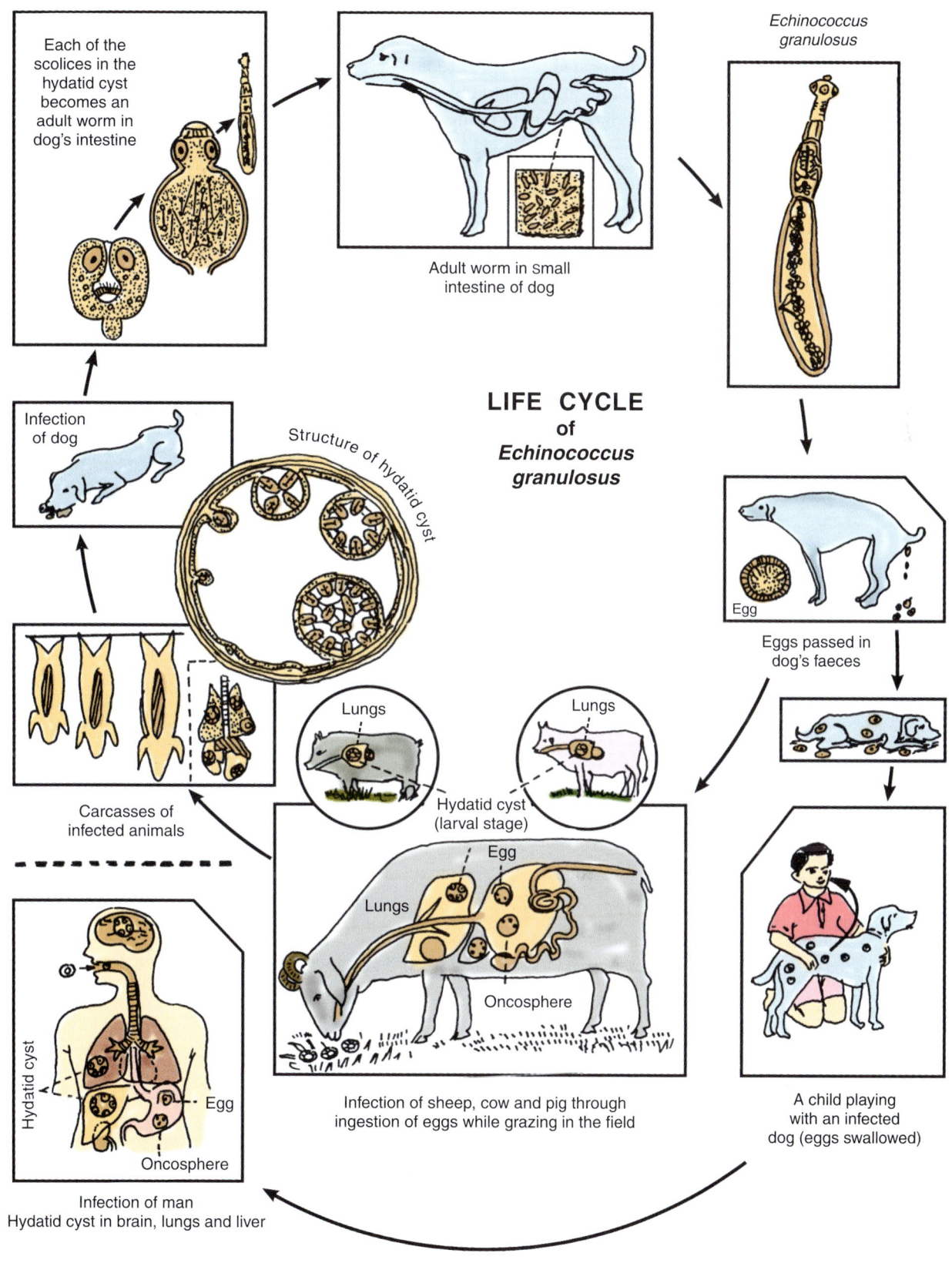

Each of the scolices in the hydatid cyst becomes an adult worm in dog's intestine

Adult worm in small intestine of dog

Echinococcus granulosus

Infection of dog

Structure of hydatid cyst

LIFE CYCLE
of
Echinococcus granulosus

Egg

Eggs passed in dog's faeces

Carcasses of infected animals

Lungs

Lungs

Hydatid cyst (larval stage)

Egg

Lungs

Oncosphere

Infection of sheep, cow and pig through ingestion of eggs while grazing in the field

A child playing with an infected dog (eggs swallowed)

Hydatid cyst

Egg

Oncosphere

Infection of man
Hydatid cyst in brain, lungs and liver

Fig. 120

MODE OF INFECTION. The eggs in the dog's faeces are ingested by man. This occurs in the following ways: (i) by a direct contact (handling and fondling) with infected dogs, (ii) by allowing the dog to feed from the same dish, and (iii) by taking uncooked vegetables contaminated with infected canine faeces. Infection through contaminated water is not common as the eggs being heavier sink to the bottom.

Infection is generally acquired in childhood (due to intimate association with dogs) though the disease dose not become manifest before adult life.

Infecting Agent—Eggs, in dog's faeces.

Portal of Entry—Alimentary tract.

Sites of Localisation—Viscera (liver, lungs and other organs).

EVOLUTION (PATHOGENESIS) OF HYDATID CYST. The cyst-wall secreted by the embryo consists of 2 layers:

(1) *Outer Cuticular Layer (Ectocyst).* It is a laminated hyaline membrane (Fig. 121) having a thickness up to 1 mm. To the naked eye, the ectocyst has the appearance of the white of a hard-boiled egg. It is elastic and when incised or ruptured curls on itself exposing the inner layer containing the brood capsules and daughter cysts.

(2) *Inner or Germinal Layer (Endocyst).* It is cellular and consists of a number of nuclei embedded in a protoplasmic mass (Fig. 122). It is very thin and measures about 22 to 25 µm in thickness. It is the vital layer of the cyst and (a) gives rise to brood capsules with scolices, (b) secretes the specific hydatid fluid, and (c) forms the outer layer.

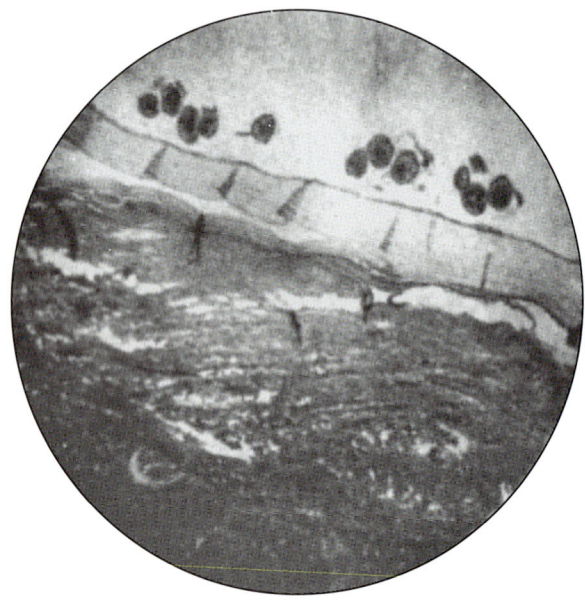

Fig. 121—Hydatid cyst of the liver.
(Seen under low power of microscope.)
Showing pericyst, ectocyst (laminated outer layer),
endocyst (granular germinal layer) and a few brood capsules.

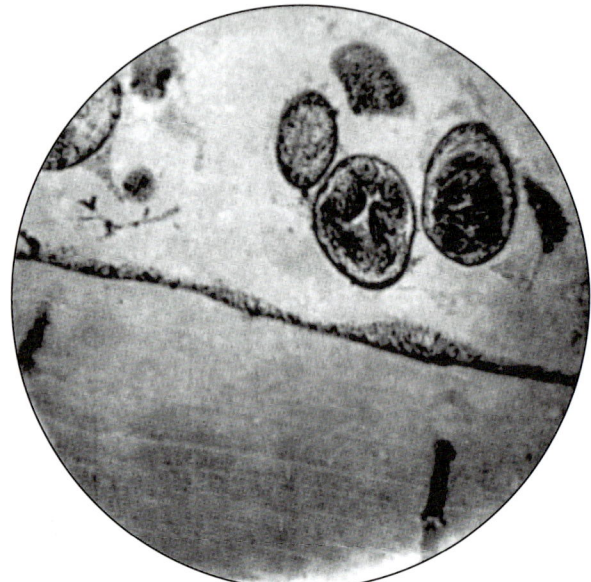

Fig. 122—The wall of the hydatid cyst.
(Higher magnification.)
Showing the laminated hyaline membrane, granular germinal
layer and free brood capsules.

Composition and Character of Hydatid Fluid:

  (i) Clear colourless fluid (may be pale yellow in colour).

 (ii) Specific gravity low, 1.005 to 1.010.

(iii) Reaction slightly acid, *p*H 6.7.

(iv) Contains sodium chloride, sodium sulphate, sodium phosphate and sodium and calcium salts of succinic acid (a Fehling reducing substance).

 (v) Antigenic, being used for immunological tests.

(vi) Highly toxic, when absorbed gives rise to anaphylactic symptoms.

(vii) Hydatid sand—A granular deposit found to settle at the bottom. It consists of liberated brood capsules, free scolices and loose hooklets.

Acephalocysts. Sometimes brood capsules are not developed and if developed, are without any scolices; these cysts are sterile and called *acephalocysts*. These sterile hydatid cysts are found in large numbers in cattle.

Endogenous daughter cyst formation in hydatid cysts is the result of growth over many years and is therefore particularly seen in man. The daughter cysts develop inside the mother cyst and may arise from the detached fragment of the germinal layer or from regressive changes of the young brood capsule and scolex bud. The daughter cyst also consists of an outer protective layer and an inner germinative layer from which brood capsules and scolices arise and even grand-daughter cysts may develop.

It is to be observed that "transformation of scolex into a daughter cyst" within the same host, without passing through the adult stage in the definitive host (a phenomenon observed by Naunyn as early as 1862), is against the "law of migration of the cestodes" enunciated by Van Beneden. A fully developed scolex is an end-product and is unable to undergo regressive changes and develop into a cyst. Experimental work has confirmed that *E. granulosus* does not follow the general biological laws and Deve (1925) confirmed that regressive metamorphosis could occur with hydatid scolices.

There is another type of development known as *exogenous cyst formation* which is found in the bone hydatid where the growth continues to take place in an outward direction. The high intracystic pressure causes herniation, or rupture of both the germinal and laminated layers through some weakened part of the adventitia, resulting in the formation of these exogenous cysts.

DEVELOPMENT OF BROOD CAPSULES AND SCOLICES. Brood capsules sprout from the germinal layer. It is at first spherical, but soon becomes vacuolated and transformed into a vesicle. The scolices, numbering 5 to 20 or more, develop within these brood capsules. A fully developed scolex represents the future "head" of the adult worm with suckers and a circle of hooklets invaginated inside the scolex.

In a growing hydatid cyst all the stages of development of a scolex may be found, beginning from the undifferentiated cellular bud to the fully developed stage with suckers and hooklets. The scolices may remain attached to the wall by means of pedicles, or may remain free inside the cavity of the cyst and form the grains of "hydatid sand" previously referred to.

REACTION OF THE HOST. Wherever the embryo settles an active cellular reaction consisting of monocytes (macrophages), giant cells and eosinophils takes place around the parasite. This is a defensive reaction on the part of the host and a large number of the parasites may be destroyed by the phagocytic activity of these cells. Some of the embryos, however, escape destruction and develop into hydatid cysts. The cellular reaction in these cases gradually disappears, followed by the appearance of fibroblasts, and the formation of new blood vessels which are ultimately transformed into fibrous tissue. This forms an enveloping fibrous layer around the growing embryo and is known as *pericyst*. It does not form any organic part of the true cyst but merges gradually into the surrounding healthy tissue and the parasite derives its nourishment through it. In an old cyst, the pericyst may become sclerosed or calcified and the parasite within it may die or degenerate owing to lack of nutrition.

RATE OF GROWTH OF HYDATID CYST. The development of hydatid cyst in man is very slow. At the end of a year, it is approximately 4 cm in diameter and the brood capsules and scolices begin to appear.

DISTRIBUTION OF HYDATID CYST. This is shown in the adjoining diagram (Fig. 123A). The organ most commonly involved is the liver, because it acts as the first filter and the next organ involved is the lung which forms the second filter. After it enters the systemic circulation, it may be distributed in various organs.*

Clinical Features. The chief clinical manifestations are entirely dependent upon local signs and if the cyst is situated superficially, it may cause a visible swelling. In the majority of cases, the disease remains latent (symptomless) for many years and its presence is only detected at autopsy or by its pressure-effects on the surrounding tissues or when the cyst ruptures or suppurates. The pressure symptoms will vary according to the site of the cyst. Rupture of a hydatid cyst is associated with anaphylactic symptoms and formation of localised or generalised secondary echinococcosis.

Laboratory Diagnosis. This consists of the following:

1. *Casoni's Reaction.* An immediate hypersensitivity skin test introduced by Casoni in 1911. Intradermal injection of 0.2 ml of a fresh sterile hydatid fluid (sterilised by Seitz filter) produces within half an hour, in all positive cases, a large wheal (5 cm in diameter) with multiple pseudopodia; it fades in an hour. Sterile normal saline, 0.2 ml, is injected in the other arm for control. Hydatid fluid from human cases (removed by operation) or from animals (obtained from slaughterhouse) is used as antigen.

---

* *Hydatid Cyst of the Orbit.* Although rare, two cases have been reported so far from India (Roy *et al*, 1967).

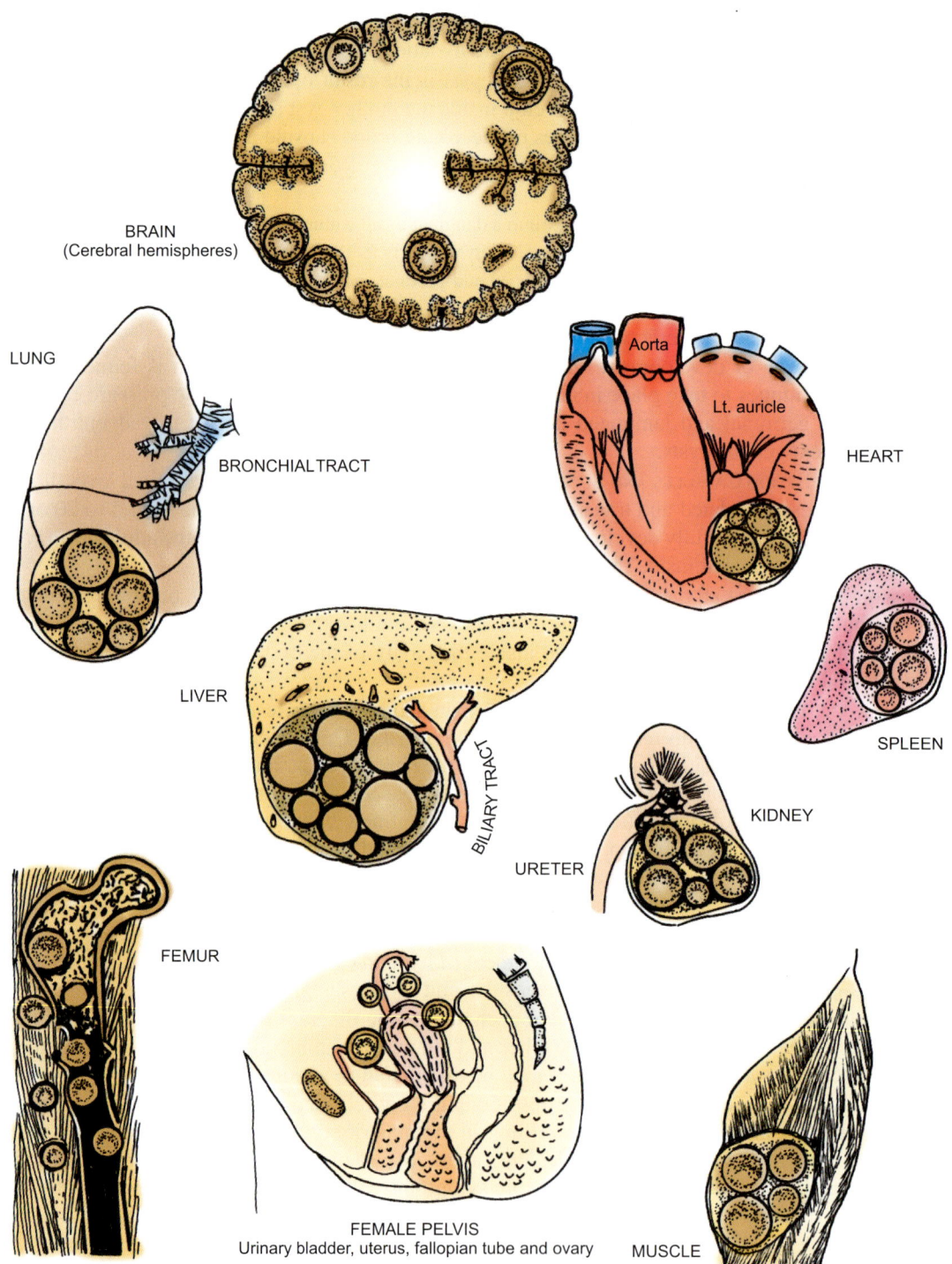

Fig. 123A—Hydatid cyst in different organs.

2. *Blood examination* may reveal a generalised eosinophilia of 20 to 25 per cent.

3. *Serological tests* (precipitin reaction and complement fixation test) carried out with hydatid antigen (fluid) have also been found to be positive. False positive reaction of CFT is seen in other condition and it is not a sensitive test.

IHAT, ELISA using *E. granulosis* hydatid fluid antigen are diagnostically 25-98% sensitive for hepatic cases, 50-60% sensitive for pulmonary cases and 50-60% sensitive for other multiple organs localisation cases.

Other tests introduced for serological diagnosis include:

(a) *Haemagglutination test* using fresh or formalinised sheep red cells sensitised with tannic acid and coated with echinococcus antigen (Boyden, 1951; Allain & Kagan, 1961).

(b) *Flocculation tests,* using bentonite particles or polystyrene latex particles coated with hydatid cyst fluid as antigen.

Bentonite flocculation test (Norman, Sadun and Allain, 1959). The antigen is first adsorbed onto standardised bentonite particles (1 to 2 μm). On a wax-ringed slide 0.1 ml of bentonite-antigen suspension is added to 0.1 ml of a serial dilution of serum (diluted with saline as 1 : 5, 1 : 10, 1 : 20). The slide is mechanically rotated for 15 minutes, after which the readings are taken. The dilution of the serum in which more than half of the particles are aggregated into floccules is considered positive. In a positive case, the serum is titrated to an end-point.

Latex test (Fischmar, 1960). The antigen used is polystyrene latex suspension of particles 0.81 μm diameter, sensitised with a pooled hydatid fluid. The diluted serum (double dilutions) is mixed with the antigen and the mixture is incubated in a water-bath at 37°C for 90 minutes and then kept over-night at 4°C, after which the reading is taken. A positive result is recorded, if there is a heavy precipitate.

(c) *Indirect fluorescent antibody test* (IFA) has also been found to be of great promise.

(d) *Immunoelectrophoresis (Arc 5).* It is now well accepted.

Immunoblotting for a relatively specific 8 KDa/12 KDa hydatid fluid polypeptide antigen is available now for diagnosis of disease.

(e) Molecular methods such as DNA probe and PCR have been developed but their applications are of limited value because of their technical complexity.

Note: Commonly ELISA test for IgG detection, IHAT and LAT with crude parasite antigen either alone or with combination are used for primary diagnosis of disease.

4. *Exploratory Cyst Puncture.* Though an accurate diagnosis may be made by withdrawing a few millilitres of the hydatid fluid and examining it under the microscope for scolices or hooklets, yet it is often attended with serious results and is therefore not advised.

5. *Radiological.* This is often helpful in the diagnosis of hydatid cysts of lungs and liver. Owing to the saline contents, the cyst is relatively opaque and casts a characteristic circular shadow with a sharp outline (Fig. 123B). In cases where the long bones are involved a mottled appearance is seen in the skiagram.

6. IV pyelogram is helpful for detection of renal hydatid cyst.

Ultrasonography of whole abdomen is useful in locating the site of hydatid cyst of the abdominal organs. CT scan is more helpful than MRI scan in the diagnosis of diseases of different organs.

Treatment. Mebendazole and preferably albendazole (400-800 mg twice daily for 1-6 months) are used for treatment of the disease. Surgical removal of the cyst where possible is best method of treatment. Recurrences are common. Postoperative chemotherapy with praziquantel and albendazole for 2 years may be given.

Prophylaxis. This consists of the following: (1) Prevention of infection of dogs and the deworming of dogs (with specific anthelmintics) in endemic areas and (2) personal prophylaxis (cleaning of hands before eating). Laboratory workers should guard against pollution of fingers while examining dog's faeces.

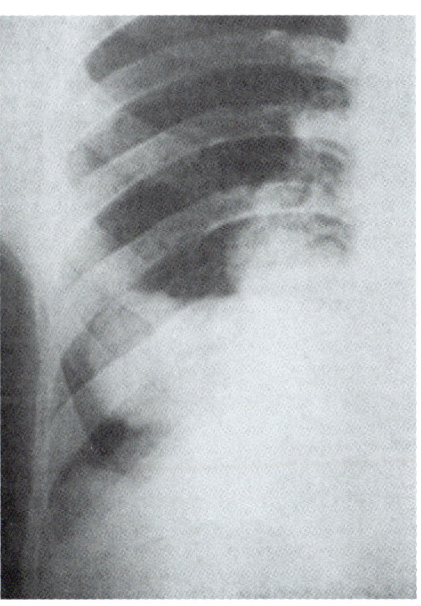

Fig. 123B—Skiagram showing multiple hydatid cysts (4 in number) in the lower lobe of the right lung.

Echinococcus multilocularis (Leuckart, 1863) Vogel, 1955

The larval worm causes alveolar or multilocular hydatid disease in man.

The definitive (adult) hosts are dogs, foxes and wolves, and the intermediate (larval) hosts are field mice and tundra voles. The size of the adult worm is 1.2 to 3.7 mm being much smaller than *E. granulosus*. Immunological and allergic tests are positive with the antigen derived from alveolar hydatid. The disease is prevalent in certain parts of Europe. The organ most commonly involved is the liver. Central necrosis and cavitation are the common findings. The cavity contains little or no fluid. Formation of hyaline layer is less conspicuous; the germinal layer is often hyperplastic and folded on itself and there is a tendency of persistent cellular reaction by eosinophil and endothelial cells in the surrounding tissue. The chief character of the lesion is its tendency to proliferate, thereby resembling a neoplasm. Most of the alveolar hydatid cysts (multilocular hydatid cysts) are sterile. The prognosis is grave and surgery is the only solution. The prognosis is grave and surgery is the only solution. Postoperative chemotherapy similar to that of hydatid disease caused by *E. granulosis*.

Family HYMENOLEPIDIDAE: Genus HYMENOLEPIS

The generic name is derived from the membranous character of the egg-shell (from G. *hymen*, membrane; *lepis*, rind or shell).

The characteristics of the genus Hymenolepis are as follows: there are three testes in each mature segment; the uterus is sac-like and transverse; the individual segment is greater in breadth than in length; the egg possesses two membranes, the outer one (egg-shell) is thin and transparent; the larval stage is cysticercoid. The following two species have been reported from man:

1. *Hymenolepis nana*. The common intestinal cestode of man and rodents.
2. *Hymenolepis diminuta*. An intestinal cestode found abundantly in rodents but relatively rare in man.

Hymenolepis nana (v. Siebold, 1852) Blanchard, 1891
Common Name: The dwarf tapeworm.

Geographical Distribution. Cosmopolitan.

Habitat. The abode of the adult worm is the small intestine (distal portion of the ileum) of man. It is also found in rodents, especially in mice and rats.

Morphology. ADULT WORM. *H. nana* is one of the small intestinal cestodes infecting man. It is small and thread-like, measuring 1 to 4 cm in length with a maximum diameter of 1 mm. The worms may be present in large numbers (from 1,000 to a maximum of 8,000). *Life span* of the adult worm is short (about 2 weeks).

The *scolex* ("head") is globular, has 4 suckers and is provided with a short retractile rostellum armed with a single row of hooklets numbering 20 to 30. The rostellum remains invaginated in the apex of the organ (Fig. 124). The rostellar hooklets are shaped like tuning forks. The "neck" is long.

Proglottides (Segments). The number of segments is about 200. A mature segment measures 0.3 mm in length by 0.9 mm in breadth. Genital pores are marginal and are situated on the same side. The uterus is a transverse sac with lobulated walls while there are three testes.

EGGS. These are liberated in the faeces by gradual disintegration of the terminal segments. The characteristics of the egg (Fig. 125) are as follows:

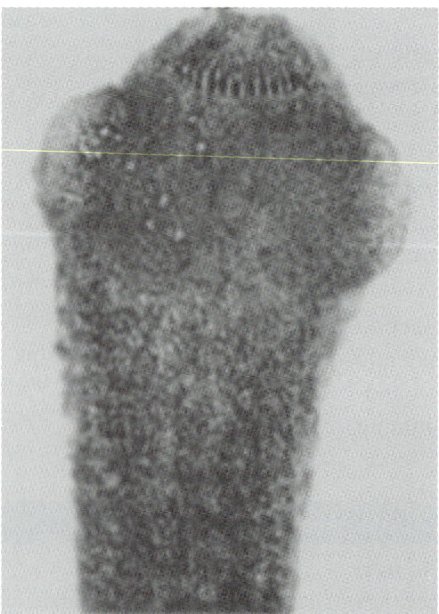

Fig. 124—The "head" of *H. nana*.
Note the suckers and crown of hooklets in the invaginated rostellum.

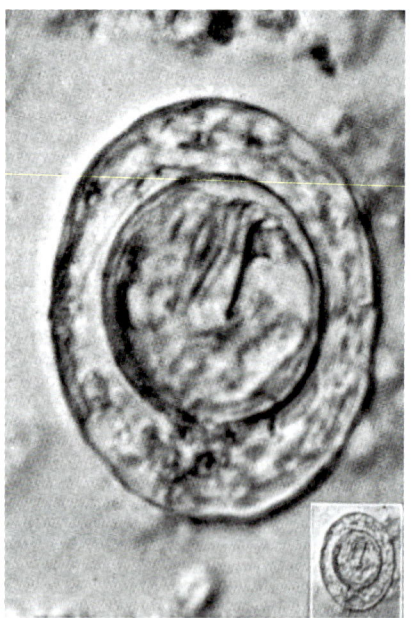

Fig. 125—Eggs of *H. nana*.
Inset: Size under high power with 5 ocular.

(i) Spherical or oval in shape, measuring 30 to 45 µm in diameter.
(ii) There are two distinct membranes: (a) The outer membrane is thin and colourless, and (b) the inner embryophore encloses an oncosphere with three pairs of lancet-shaped hooklets.
(iii) The space between the two membranes is filled with yolk granules and polar filaments (4 to 8) emanating from little knobs at either end of embryophore.
(iv) Floats in saturated solution of common salt.

Life Cycle. No intermediate host is required and the entire development from the larval to the adult stage takes place in one host (Fig. 126). *H. nana* is one of the exceptions to the general rule that the *helminths do not multiply inside the body of the definitive host.*

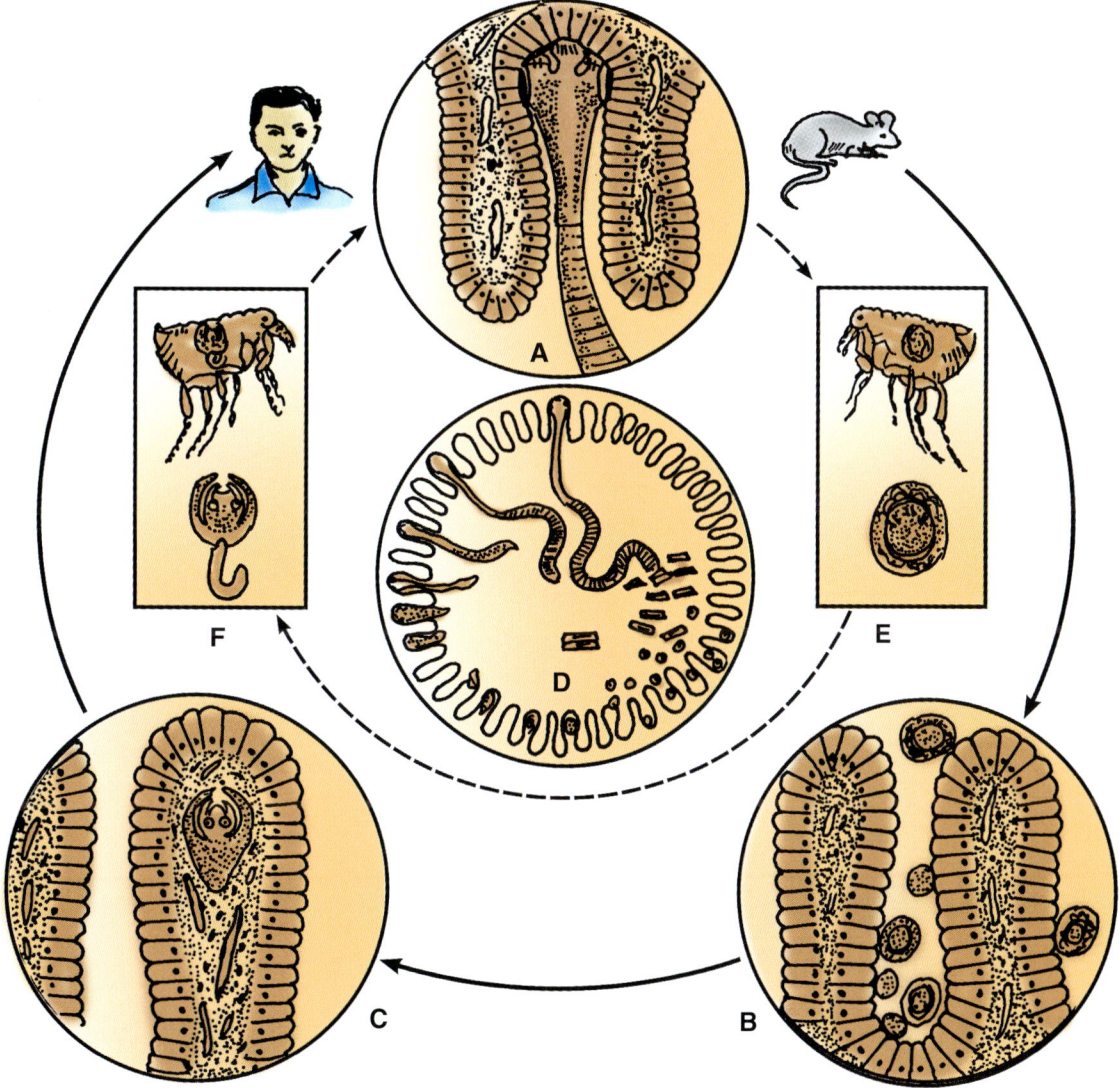

Fig. 126—Life cycle of *Hymenolepis nana.*
A, B, C, D direct cycle. A, E, F indirect cycle. A, head of the adult worm attached to the mucosa of the small intestine; B, oncosphere penetrating intestinal villi; C, cysticercoid in an intestinal villus; E, eggs in human faeces ingested by the rat flea; F, cysticercoid in the haemal cavity of the rat flea (ingestion of these fleas causes infection). D, stages of the evolution in the same host.

With the ingestion of a fully embryonated egg, a hexacanth embryo is liberated. It burrows into the villi of the anterior part of the small intestine and develops in about 4 days' time into a typical larval stage called "cysticercoid". After reaching maturity, the villus ruptures and the larva (scolex) re-enters the lumen of the small intestine. Later, it attaches to another villus further down and in the course of a fortnight develops into an adult worm. Strobilisation is rapid and in about 30 days after the infection, the eggs begin to appear in the faeces. Some of the eggs remaining in the bowel can start the cycle over again.

Besides the direct cycle, referred to above, an indirect cycle has been demonstrated. Certain rat fleas and beetles act as intermediate hosts and transmit murine infection to man (children); this is particularly true in Argentina.

Pathogenicity. MODE OF INFECTION. The first infection occurs through ingestion of food contaminated with eggs of *H. nana* liberated along with the faeces of an infected man or rodents. Afterwards, auto-infection increases the number of parasites.

There are usually no symptoms but with heavy infection, there is abdominal pain and diarrhoea.

Diagnosis. This is based on the finding of characteristic eggs in a microscopical examination of a sample of faeces. Concentration methods such as salt floatation technique and formal ether method may be used for demonstration of eggs. ELISA test has been developed with 80% sensivity.

Treatment. Niclosomide in a dose of 60-80 mg/kg for 5-7 days (maximum dose 2 gm/day) is used effectively. Praziquantel in a single dose of 25 mg/kg is highly effective. Mebendazole cures 50% cases only.

Hymenolepis diminuta (Rudolphi, 1819) Blanchard, 1891

It is a common parasite of rats and mice. It measures 20 to 60 cm in length. The unarmed "head" has four suckers. The proglottides number about 800 to 1000. The mature proglottides (segments) are much broader than long (2.5 mm by 0.75 mm) and the internal structures are the same as those of *H. nana* (Fig. 127). The egg is larger than that of *H. nana*. The outer shell is yellowish in colour and the inner embryophore has two knob-like thickenings; there are no polar filaments (Fig. 128). Life cycle is passed in two hosts; the larval stage (cysticercoid) is passed in fleas; the adult stage in rats and mice, and occasionally in man (children). Human beings are infected by the accidental swallowing of infected fleas. The cysticercoids, thus liberated, develop into adult worms. Human infection is asymptomatic. These parasites are easily expelled by anthelmintics, niclosamide and praziquantel.

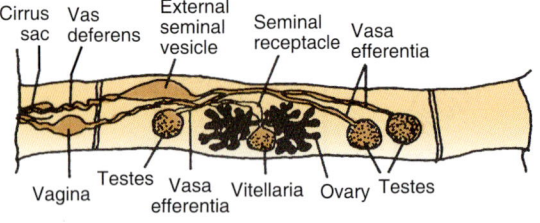

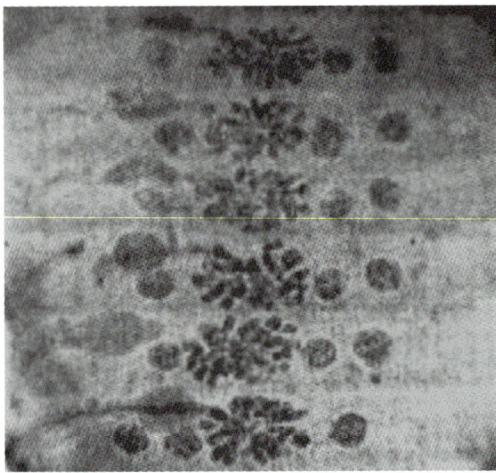

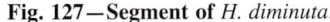

Fig. 127—Segment of *H. diminuta.*

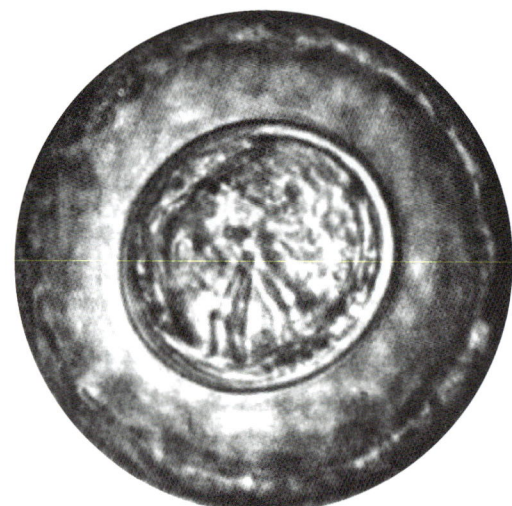

Fig. 128—Egg of *H. diminuta.*

Family DILEPIDIDAE: Genus DIPYLIDIUM

Dipylidium caninum (Linnaeus, 1758) Ralliet, 1892
(The double-pored dog tapeworm)

The generic name is derived from the presence of bilateral genital pores in each segment (from G. *dis*, two; *pylis*, gate; *dipylidium*, meaning having two entrances).

Morphology. It is a common intestinal tapeworm of dog and cat. The adult worm (Fig 129) measures 15 to 40 cm in length. The *head* is provided with a retractile rostellum, armed with 3 or 4 rows of hooks shaped like rose-thorns. There are 4 elliptical

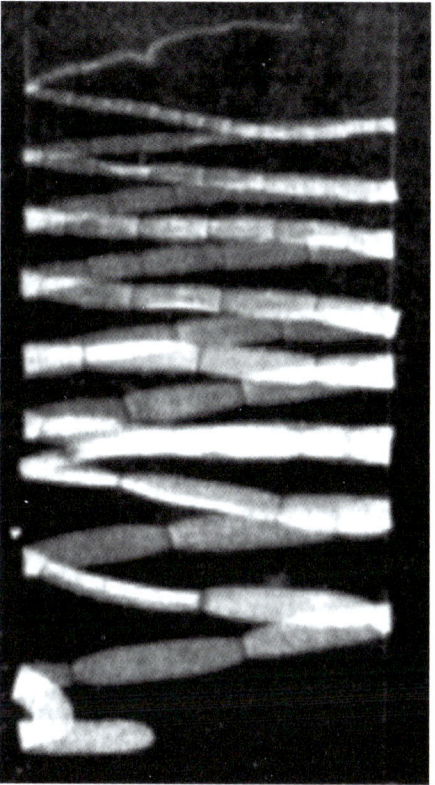

Fig. 129—Adult worm of *D. caninum.*

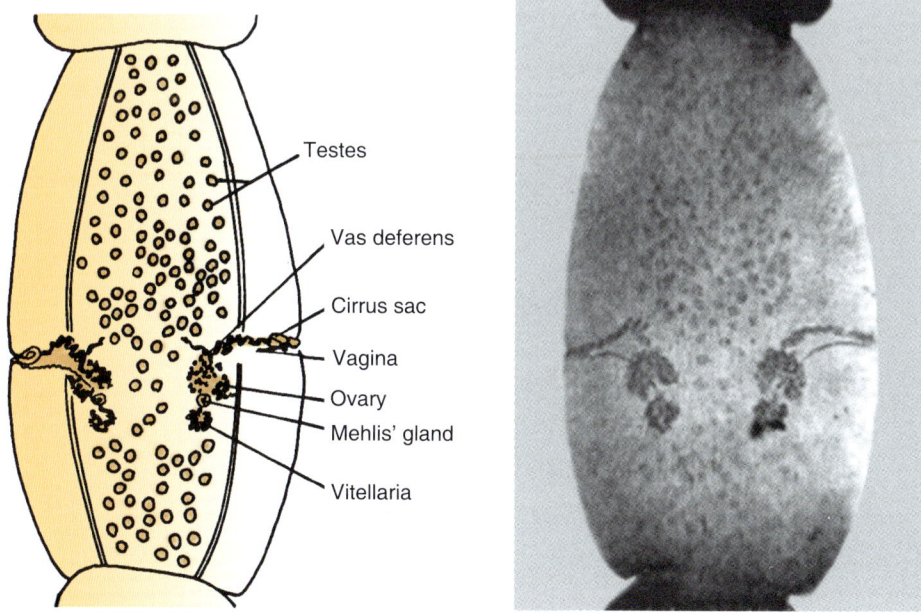

Testes

Vas deferens

Cirrus sac

Vagina

Ovary

Mehlis' gland

Vitellaria

Fig. 130—Segments of *D. caninum.*

suckers. The *neck* is short and thin. The *strobila* consists of about 200 proglottides which have the appearance of melon seeds. Each *segment* (Fig. 130) is provided with a double set of reproductive organs with genital pores situated at the lateral margins. The uterus is sac-like and when gravid, breaks up into a number of egg-capsules containing 8 to 16 eggs in each. The eggs (Fig. 131) are passed in the faeces along with the proglottides which may be disintegrated either in the bowel or later, after evacuation.

Life Cycle. The eggs with the segments are ingested by the fleas (dog flea, cat flea or human flea) or dog lice in whose intestinal tract, the oncospheres are liberated. They then migrate into the body cavity where they develop into cysticercoid larvae. When these insects are ingested by a mammalian host (dog or cat), the larvae develop into adult worms which become sexually mature in about 20 days. Many fleas die as a result of this infection. It has been observed that the eggs of *D. caninum* were devoured by the larval flea and not by the adult and the development is delayed until it passes through the pupal stage and is transformed into an adult.

Pathogenicity. Cases of human infection have been reported, mostly in children, the infection resulting from accidental ingestion of infected fleas (insect hosts) while fondling cats and dogs. Usually, there is not more than a single worm and the only clinical manifestation is a slight gastro-intestinal disturbance. Most of the cases have occurred in European countries. Chowdhury and Bandyopadhyaya (1962) from India (Calcutta) reported a case in a child from whom 2 adult worms were recovered (*J. I. Ped. Soc*, **1**, p.26). Human infection is generally asymptomatic.

Diagnosis. Based on finding the characteristic eggs in the faeces which are voided with the proglottides.

Treatment. This consists of administration of the same drugs (praziquantel and niclosamide) as used for other tapeworm infections.

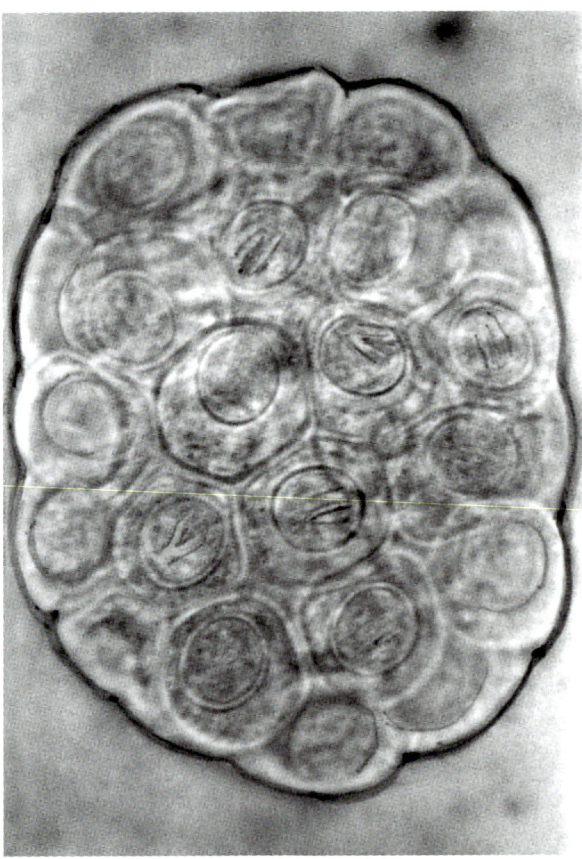

Fig. 131—Egg of *D. caninum.*

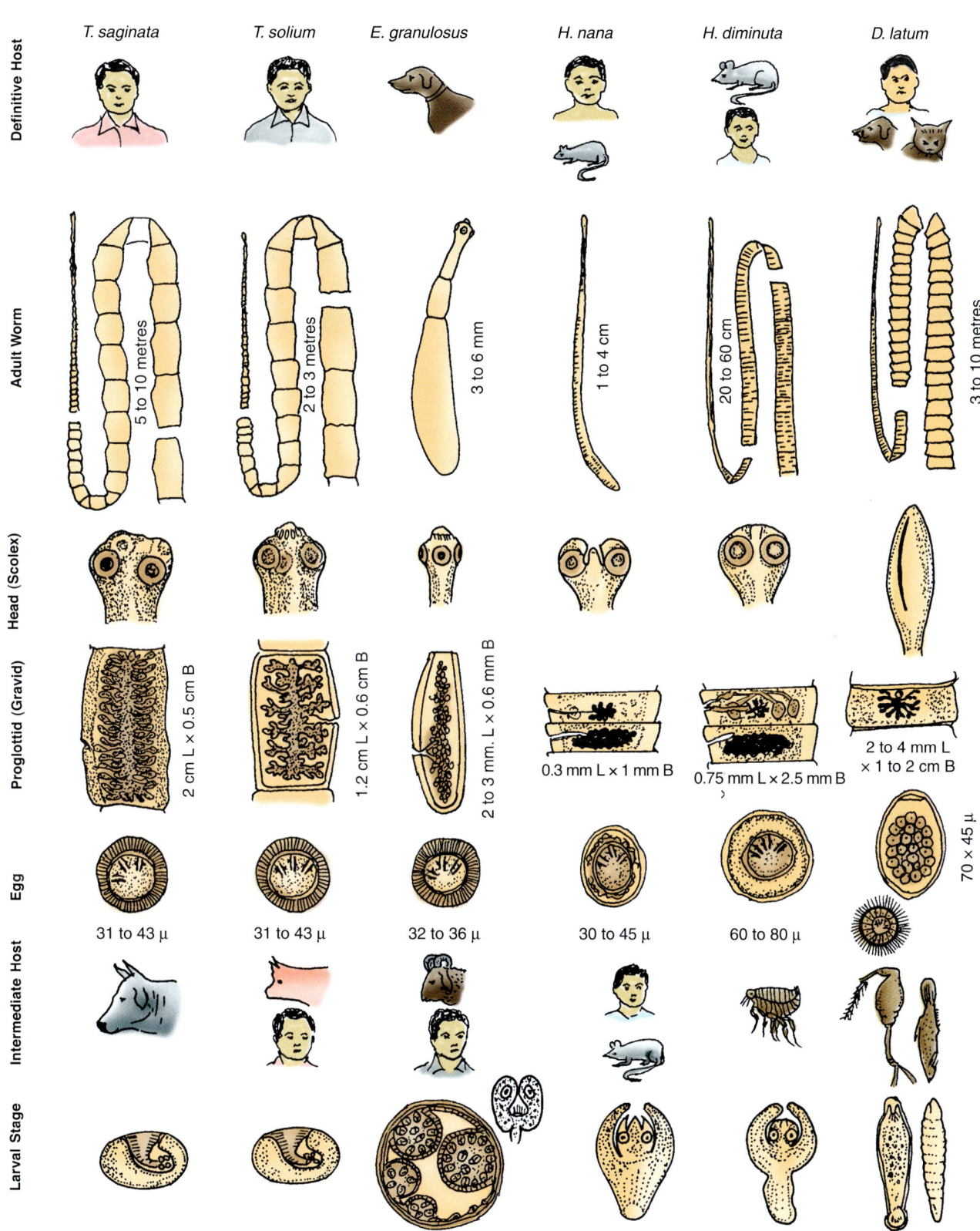

Fig. 132—Differentiating characters of important cestodes infecting man.

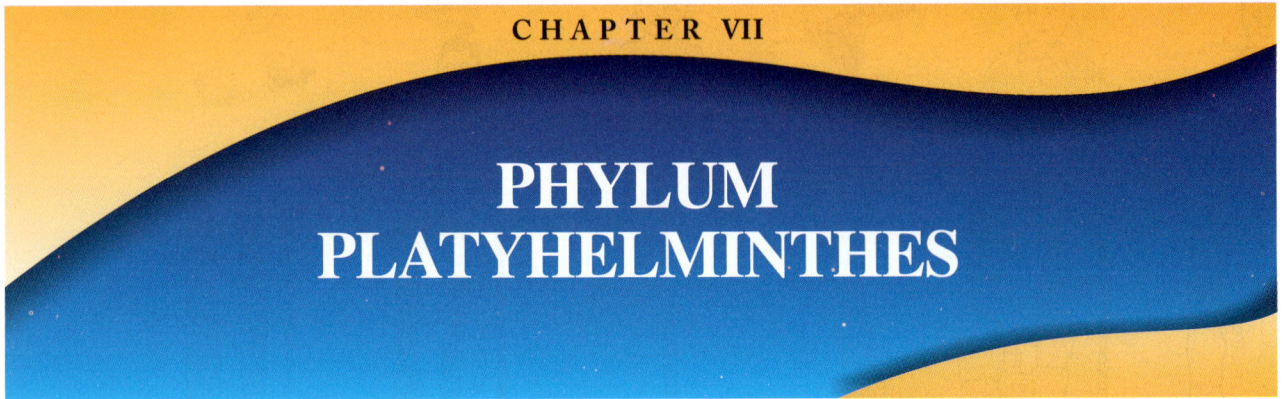

CHAPTER VII

PHYLUM PLATYHELMINTHES

Class TREMATODA: Subclass DIGENEA

The trematodes are so named on account of their conspicuous suckers (G. *trematos*, pierced with holes). The species parasitising man belong to the digenetic trematodes.

General Characters of Trematodes (Digenetic)

1. These are leaf-shaped unsegmented flat worms, called flukes.
2. Size varies from 1 mm to several centimetres in length.
3. The organs of attachment are two strong muscular cup-shaped depressions, called *suckers*. The one, surrounding the mouth is called the *oral sucker* and the other, on the ventral surface of the body, is called the *ventral sucker* (acetabulum).
4. Sexes are not separate, i.e., each individual worm is a hermaphrodite (monoecious) except the Schistosomes which are unisexual.
5. Body cavity is absent.
6. The alimentary canal is present but incomplete. The anus is absent. The oesophagus bifurcates in front of the ventral sucker into a pair of blind intestinal caeca or crura which may be simple (as in *C. sinensis*) or branched (as in *F. hepatica*) or may reunite to form a single caecum (as in *Schistosomes*).
7. Excretory and nervous systems are present. Excretory system consists of "flame cells" and collecting tubules which open posteriorly, into the excretory pore. The pattern of flame cells provides the basis for species identification.
8. Reproductive system is highly developed and complete in each individual. The genital organs lie between the two branches of the intestine.
9. The worm is oviparous, since eggs are liberated.
10. Eggs are all operculated (except those of *Schistosomes*) and can develop only in water. In a majority of cases they are immature when oviposited. Trematode eggs do not float in saturated solution of common salt.

Reproductive System (Fig. 133)

MALE GENITAL SYSTEM. This consists of the following: two *testes* (except in *Schistosomes*) in the posterior region of the body, two *vasa efferentia* and one *vas deferens*; the latter is dilated into a *seminal vesicle* followed by a constriction (ejaculatory duct) before opening into the genital atrium. The terminal part of the vas deferens is modified into a muscular *cirrus* which serves as the organs of copulation. The *prostate gland* surrounds the constricted portion of the vas deferens. The seminal vesicle, cirrus organ and the prostate gland are enclosed in a pouch, the *cirrus sac*.

FEMALE GENITAL SYSTEM. This consists of the following: a single ovary and its ducts, two vitellaria (yolk glands) and their ducts on either side, a vestigial vagina (Laurer's canal), seminal receptacle, uterus, oötype and Mehlis' gland.

The *ovary* usually lies in front of the testes.

The *uterus* emanates from the oötype and after a tortuous course terminates in the genital atrium; the terminal part is often called *metraterm* which, in the absence of the opening of Laurer's canal, acts as a vagina.

The *oötype* is the fertilising chamber where the ovum is fertilised by the spermatozoon and where all the components of the egg are collected. The oötype is joined with the uterus at one end and the oviduct at the other end; the oviduct, in turn, is joined by the common vitelline duct and the *seminal receptacle*.

The two *vitelline ducts* from each side join to form the common vitelline duct which opens in the oötype.

The *Laurer's canal* represents the rudimentary

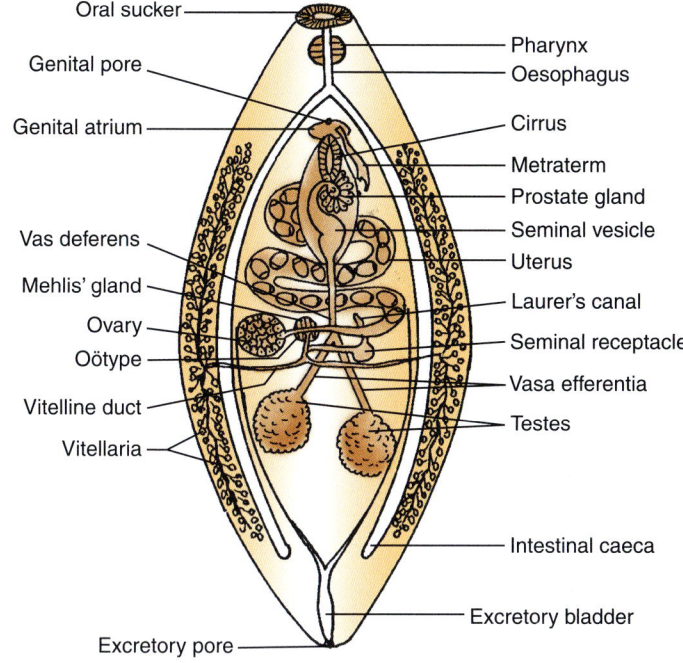

Fig. 133—**Reproductive System of a Trematode.**

vagina and appears as a dorsal outgrowth of the seminal receptacle. It may or may not open on the dorsal surface; an opening, if present, acts as a vagina for the entrance of sperms and helps in cross-fertilisation.

The *Mehlis' gland* surrounds the oötype.

The *genital atrium* opens on the ventral surface near the acetabulum.

Life Cycle of Trematodes (Digenetic). These worms pass their life cycle in two different hosts:

(1)   *Definitive Host:* Generally man. Harbours the adult worm.

(2)   *Intermediate Host:* A fresh-water snail or mollusc for larval development. A second intermediate host (fish or crab) is required for encystment in some trematodes.

The *eggs* liberated by the definitive host gain access into the water. A free-swimming ciliated embryo, *miracidium* develops and hatches out of the egg. The miracidium gains access to its proper intermediate host (snail or mollusc) and localises in the liver or lymph spaces for further development.

LARVAL DEVELOPMENT IN THE SNAIL

(i)   The miracidium is transformed into a sac-like structure called *sporocyst*. It contains a number of germ cells. Asexual multiplication does not occur at this stage except in Schistosomes where a *second generation of sporocyst* is formed.

(ii)   The sporocyst changes into a *redia*, having the following structural characters: an oral sucker, a pharynx, a sac-like intestine and a birth-pore through which the next generation escapes. Inside the redia a new crop of germ cells is produced, which develop either into daughter rediae (*a second generation rediae*) or into the next stage, *cercariae*. It is to be noted that asexual multiplication occurs at this stage in all trematodes. In Schistosomes, however, there is no stage of redia formation.

(iii)   The *cercaria* represents the final stage of larval development in the snail and is infective to man. The cercaria is provided with suckers and has an intestine like that of the adult worm. It possesses a tail by means of which it propels itself in water.

When mature, the cercariae escape from the snail into the water and may remain free in water or encyst (*metacercaria or adolescaria*) either in water-plants or in another intermediate host, a fresh-water fish or a crab.

Note: From a single miracidium a large number of cercariae are developed.

Man is infected either by drinking contaminated water or by ingesting encysted cercariae in the water-plant, fish, or crab. Free cercariae, in some cases, can enter directly through the skin. On entering the definitive host, the young worms proceed to their sites of localisation to grow into adult worms, become sexually mature and repeat the cycle.

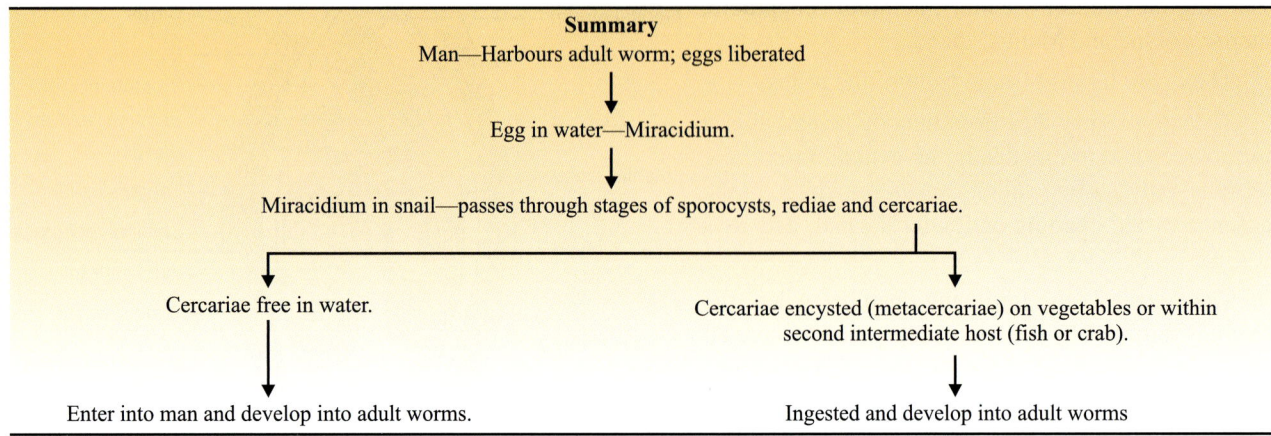

Mode of Infection. Trematode infection may occur in the following ways:

1. By ingestion of encysted cercariae in—
   (a) Vegetables, as in *F. hepatica, F. buski, W. watsoni.*
   (b) Fish, as in *C. sinensis, H. heterophyes, M. yokogawai.*
   (c) Flesh of crab or crayfish, as in *P. westermani.*
2. Free cercariae penetrating directly through the skin, as in *S. haematobium, S. mansoni, S. japonicum.*

Terms Used in the Description of Trematodes

Monogenetic (from G. *monos*, single; *genesis*, generation). A single generation completing the life cycle.

Digenetic (from G. *di*, two; *genesis*, generation). Two generations, a sexual and an asexual, completing the life cycle. In digenetic tremau Jes asexual multiplication occurs in the larval stages (in sporocyst or redia stage).

Distomata (from G. *di*, two; *stoma*, mouth). Possessing two suckers.

Acetabulum (from L., a shallow vinegar vessel or cup). A muscular organ of attachment, commonly called "sucker".

Gynaecophoric canal. A channel formed by the infolding of the lateral margins of the body of the male behind the ventral sucker for holding the female during copulation.

Miracidium (from G. "a little boy"). The first larval stage coming out of the Trematode egg in water; infective to mollusc only.

Sporocyst (from G. *sporos*, seed; *kystis*, cell or bladder). The second larval stage of the Trematode occurring in the mollusc. Asexual multiplication occurs at this stage only in Schistosomes.

Redia (named after Francesco Redi, Italian naturalist). The third larval stage of the Trematode occurring in the mollusc. Asexual multiplication at this stage occurs in all Trematodes except in Schistosomes where there is no stage of redia formation.

Cercaria (G. *kerkos*, tail). The final stage of larval development of Trematodes in the mollusc, possessing a body and tail. It escapes into the surrounding water and may remain either free or encysted on vegetables or in other animals. According to the nature of the tail of the cercaria, different names are given.

Furcocercus Cercaria. Fork-tailed (as in Schistosomes).

Microcercus Cercaria. Small, stumpy tail (as in Paragonimus).

Lophocercus Cercaria. Large fluted tail (as in Metagonimus, Clonorchis and Heterophyes).

Pleurolophocercus Cercaria. Long powerful tail with a pair of fin-folds (as in Opisthorchis).

Metacercaria or Adolescaria. The encysted cercaria without a tail; infective to definitive hosts.

Schistosomulum. Immature or growing worm of Schistosomes in the definitive host.

Classification of Trematodes (Digenetic). Following zoological nomenclature, the trematodes infecting man may be classified as follows:

A. Systematic Classification of Trematodes

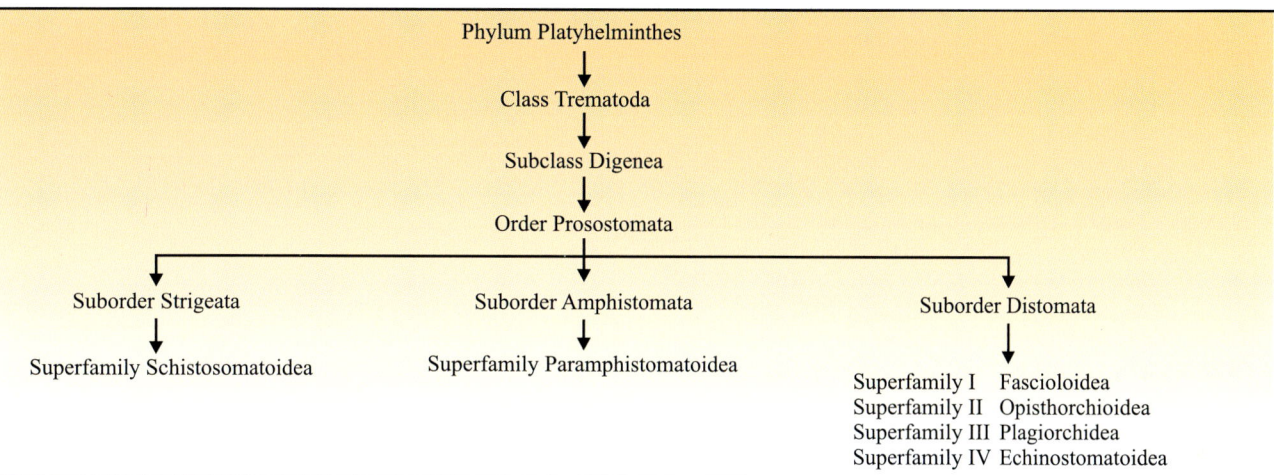

Phylum Platyhelminthes

Class Trematoda

Subclass Digenea

Order Prosostomata

Suborder Strigeata — Suborder Amphistomata — Suborder Distomata

Superfamily Schistosomatoidea

Superfamily Paramphistomatoidea

Superfamily I Fascioloidea
Superfamily II Opisthorchioidea
Superfamily III Plagiorchidea
Superfamily IV Echinostomatoidea

SUPERFAMILY	GENUS	SPECIES	HABITAT	CLINICAL MANIFESTATION
SCHISTOSOMATOIDEA	Schistosoma	S. haematobium	Blood	Haematuria
		S. mansoni	Blood	Dysentery
		S. japonicum	Blood	Dysentery and Cirrhosis liver
		S. intercalatum	Blood	Dysentery
		S. mekongi	Blood	Dysentery
PARAMPHISTOMATOIDEA	Gastrodiscoides	G. hominis	Large intestine	Mucous diarrhoea
	Watsonius	W. watsoni	Small intestine	Diarrhoea
FASCIOLOIDEA	Fasciola	F. hepatica	Liver of sheep and man	Biliary colic
	Fasciolopsis	F. buski	Small intestine	Diarrhoea
PLAGIORCHIDEA	Paragonimus	P. westermani	Lungs	Haemoptysis
OPISTHORCHIOIDEA				
Family OPISTHORCHIDAE	Clonorchis	C. sinensis	Liver	Jaundice
	Opisthorchis	O. felineus	Liver of cat, also man	Jaundice
Family HETEROPHYIDAE	Heterophyes	H. heterophyes	Small intestine	Diarrhoea
	Metagonimus	M. yokogawai	Small intestine	Diarrhoea
ECHINOSTOMATOIDEA	Echinostoma	E. ilocanum	Small intestine	Diarrhoea
	Paryphostomin	P. supraryfex	Small intestine	Diarrhoea

B. According to the Habitat of Trematodes (Flukes)

1. INTESTINAL TREMATODES (Intestinal flukes)
   (a) Small Intestine—*F. buski, H. heterophyes, M. yokogawai, W. watsoni, E. ilocanum, P. supraryfex.*
   (b) Large Intestine—*G. hominis.*
2. HEPATIC TREMATODES (Liver flukes)—*C. sinensis, O. felineus, F. hepatica.*
3. LUNG TREMATODES (Lung flukes)—*P. westermani.*
4. BLOOD TREMATODES (Blood flukes)
   (a) In the vesical venous plexus—*S. haematobium.*
   (b) In the rectal venous plexus and portal venous system—S. *mansoni, S. japonicum.*

Suborder STRIGEATA   Superfamily SCHISTOSOMATOIDEA

General Characters of Schistosomes:
1. The schistosomes are diecious trematodes, i.e., the sexes are separate.
2. Males are shorter and stouter than females; lateral margins of males are folded ventrally to form a *gynaecophoric canal* in which the females are received.

3. Suckers are armed with delicate spines.
4. The muscular pharynx is lacking.
5. Intestinal caeca reunite behind the ventral sucker to form a single canal; the length of the reunited intestine varies in different species.
6. The number of testes in the male varies from 4 to 8.
7. Laurer's canal is absent in the female.
8. Eggs are non-operculated and when laid are fully embryonated (containing a ciliated embryo, *miracidium*).
9. Cercariae have bifid tails and penetrate into the definitive host through the unbroken skin. There is no encysted meta-cercarial stage.
10. Adult worms live in the lumen of the portal vein and its radicles.

Species Infecting Man: (1) *S. haematobium*, (2) *S. mansoni*, (3) *S. japonicum*, (4) *S. intercalatum*, and (5) *S. mekongi*. Infections in man have also been reported with the followings:

1. *Schistosoma bovis*—(Sonsino 1876) Blanchard 1895
2. *Schistosoma mattheei*—Vaglia & Le Roux 1929
3. *Schistosoma curassoni*—Brumpt 1931
4. *Schistosoma malayensi*—Greer O.W. Yang & Hoi-Sen Yong 1988

Landmarks in the Evolution of the Knowledge of Schistosomes. A study of the mummies of ancient Egypt has shown that Schistosomiasis had been in existence since the earliest times. Schistosome eggs were found by Ruffer (1910) in the renal pelvis of a mummy of the twentieth dynasty (1250-1000 B.C.).

1847—Fujii mentioned about the "Katayama disease" (Schistosomiasis japonica) occurring in Japan.

1851—Bilharz discovered the adult worm of *S. haematobium* from the mesenteric vein of a native of Cairo; lateral-spined eggs were also observed by him.

1903—Manson observed lateral-spined eggs in the faeces of a patient who had no haematuria.

1904—Fujinami recovered an adult female of *S.japonicum* in the portal vein of a man at autopsy.

1904—Katsurada observed the eggs of *S. japonicum* in the human faeces.

1907—Sambon pointed out that the lateral-spined egg belonged to a separate species, *S. mansoni*.

1913-1914—Miyairi and Suzuki worked out the life cycle of *S. japonicum*.

1915—Leiper worked out the life cycle of *S. haematobium* in Bulinus in Egypt; also demonstrated by experimental work that *S. mansoni* is a distinct species.

1918—McDonagh advocated the use of tartar emetic in the treatment of vesical schistosomiasis.

Immunology. The antigen of living adult schistosome worm provides the major stimulus for provoking acquired immunity. In experimental animals a partial acquired immunity can be produced and in man a similar phenomenon can occur. In endemic areas schistosomiasis is mainly a disease of the young and the immunity develops gradually, taking several years to become pronounced (immunity is slight with a single infection). With advancing age the resistance develops and there is decreased passage of eggs with lessening of associated symptoms. The host thus acquires some degree of resistance against reinfection, but is unable to kill off the established population of the worms from primary infection (adult Schistosomes are long-lived worms). It is also known that the developing schistosmulae of a challenge infection are more susceptible to the immune response and death of the worm is found to be due to the destruction of the tegument of the worm.

The existence of immunity in the presence of an active adult infection is considered by Smithers and Terry (1969)* to be an example of *concomitant immunity*. The adult worms which provoke immunity are not themselves affected, because the worms living in the host incorporate host's material (antigen) into their cuticular tissues which are not attacked by host's antibodies. This might explain the mechanism of concomitant immunity by which the worm avoids destruction by the host, but through the agency of host's immunity creates barrier against continuous reinfection that might otherwise lead to overcrowding and death of the host (Smithers, 1972)**. A heterologous immunity develops in schistosomiasis and infection with "animal" schistosomes acts as a natural zooprophylaxis in human infection.

Schistosoma haematobium (Bilharz, 1852) Weinland, 1858

Common Name: The vesical blood fluke.

Geographical Distribution. Various parts of Africa and Middle East.

Gadgil and Shah (1952) reported a few cases from India (Ratnagiri in Maharashtra State).

Habitat. Adult worms live, *in copula*, in the pelvic venous plexus—vesical, prostatic and uterine plexuses of veins.

---

  * Smithers, S. R. and Terry, R. J. (1969). *Ann. N. Y. Acad. Sci.*, **160**, 826.
** Smithers, S. R. (1972). *British Medical Bulletin*. **28**, 49-54.

Morphology. In general, the three species of adult worms resemble each other closely; the peculiarities and differentiating features are however shown in the table on p. 138. Schistosomes are long-lived worms, having a *life span* of 20 to 30 years.

MECHANISM OF EGG-LAYING AND EGG-EXPULSION. Oviposition usually occurs in the small venules of vesical plexus. The female, held in the gynaecophoric canal of the male, extends its anterior end far into the smallest venules and deposits the eggs longitudinally, one at a time. Each time an egg is laid, the worm withdraws a short distance and lays another egg immediately behind the first. In this way, the venules are filled with eggs pointing backwards; the worms *in copula* migrate to an adjacent venule. The eggs are held in position by the spines and by the contraction of vessels resulting the withdrawal of the parent worm. The eggs then work their way through the vessels and the mucosa of the urinary bladder, enter into the cavity and escape with the urine, usually at the end of the micturition.

Differentiating Features of Schistosomes			
	S. haematobium	**S. mansoni**	**S. japonicum**
MALE:			
Size:	1 to 1.5 cm by 1 mm.	1 cm by 1 mm.	1.2 to 2 cm by 0.5 mm.
Cuticula:	Finely tuberculated.	Grossly tuberculated.	Non-tubercular.
Testes:	4 to 5; in groups.	8 to 9; in a zigzag row.	6 to 7; in a single file.
FEMALE:			
Size:	2 cm by 0.25 mm.	1.4 cm by 0.25 mm.	2.6 cm by 0.3 mm.
Ovary:	Behind the middle of the body.	Anterior to the middle of the body.	In the middle of the body.
Uterus:	Contains 20 to 30 eggs.	Contains 1 to 3 eggs (usually 1)	Contains 50 or more eggs.
REUNITED INTESTINE:	Long (reuniting about the middle of the body).	Longest (reuniting in the anterior half of the body).	Short (reuniting in the posterior fourth of the body).
EGG:	150 by 50 μm; terminal spine.	150 by 60 μm; lateral spine.	100 by 65 μm; lateral knob.
CERCARIAE: (Cephalic Glands)	2 pairs oxypilic and 3 pairs basophilic.	2 pairs oxyphilic and 4 pairs basophilic.	5 pairs oxyphilic (no basophilic).
INTERMEDIATE SNAIL HOST:	Bulinus (Physopsis) and Planorbarius.	Biomphalaria and Australorbis.	Oncomelania.
DEFINITIVE HOST:	Man.	Man.	Man and domestic animals.
GEOGRAPHICAL DISTRIBUTION:	Africa, Near East and Middle East.	Africa and South America.	Far East (Oriental).
HABITAT:	Vesical and prostatic venous plexus.	Mesenteric plexus of sigmoido-rectal area (inferior mesenteric vein and its radicles).	Mesenteric plexus of ileocaecal area (superior mesenteric vein and its radicles).

Life Cycle. *S. haematobium* passes its life cycle (Fig. 134) in two hosts.

Definitive Host. Man. Adult worm living in vesical and prostatic venous plexus.

Intermediate Host. Fresh-water snails (*Bulinus truncatus* and other species throughout Africa, *Planorbarius metidjensis* in Morocco and Portugal, and *Ferrissia tenuis* in India).

The embryonated eggs are passed with the urine of the definitive host and gain access to water. Ciliated larvae (miracidia), hatched out of the eggs, move freely in water in search of their intermediate host. The miracidium on entering its proper larval host, penetrates into the soft tissues of the snail and ultimately makes its way into the liver. Here it loses its cilia and other organs and in the course of 4 to 8 weeks undergoes developmental changes. The miracidium is transformed into a tubular sporocyst; the latter multiplies and forms a second generation of sporocysts. Several weeks after the infection, when no further multiplication occurs, the daughter-sporocysts give rise to the final larval forms, the fork-tailed cercariae which are infective to man. The cercariae break off from the sporocyst and escape from the snail into water.

Infection results when human beings bathing or wading in this water are infected, the cercariae penetrating the unbroken skin directly. On entry the cercariae cast off their tails (now known as schistosomulae) and gain access to a peripheral venule. From here, they are carried through the right heart into the pulmonary capillaries. It requires some days for the larvae to pass through the capillary bed in the lungs, whence they are carried through the left heart into the systemic circulation. The majority are shunted in the abdominal aorta and gain access to the mesenteric artery, pass

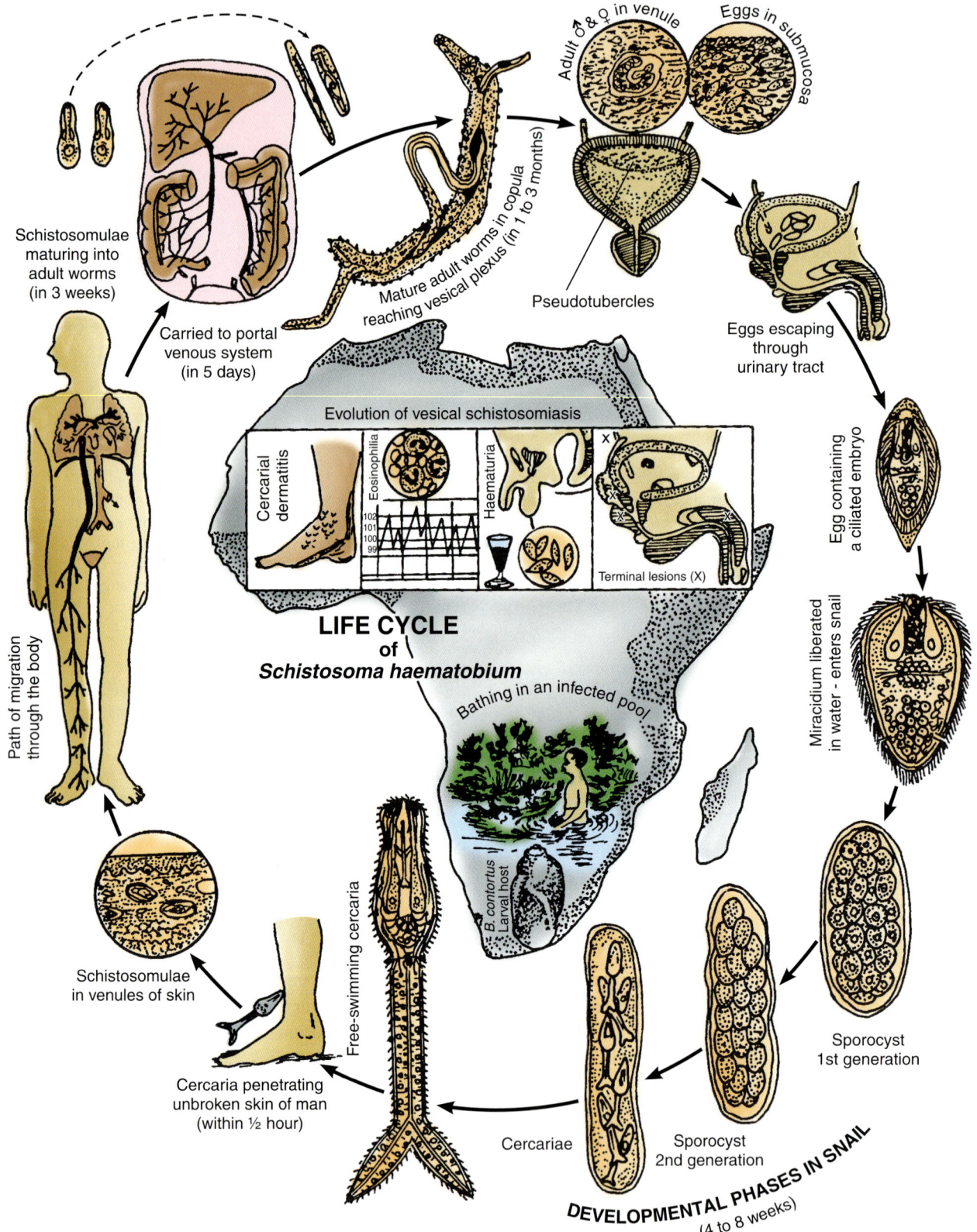

Schistosomulae maturing into adult worms (in 3 weeks)

Carried to portal venous system (in 5 days)

Path of migration through the body

Adult ♂ & ♀ in venule

Eggs in submucosa

Mature adult worms in copula reaching vesical plexus (in 1 to 3 months)

Pseudotubercles

Eggs escaping through urinary tract

Evolution of vesical schistosomiasis

Cercarial dermatitis

Eosinophilia

Haematuria

Terminal lesions (X)

LIFE CYCLE
of
Schistosoma haematobium

Bathing in an infected pool

Egg containing a ciliated embryo

Miracidium liberated in water - enters snail

B. contortus Larval host

Sporocyst 1st generation

Schistosomulae in venules of skin

Free-swimming cercaria

Cercaria penetrating unbroken skin of man (within ½ hour)

Cercariae

Sporocyst 2nd generation

DEVELOPMENTAL PHASES IN SNAIL
(4 to 8 weeks)

(Morphology after Looss, Cort & Others)

Fig. 134

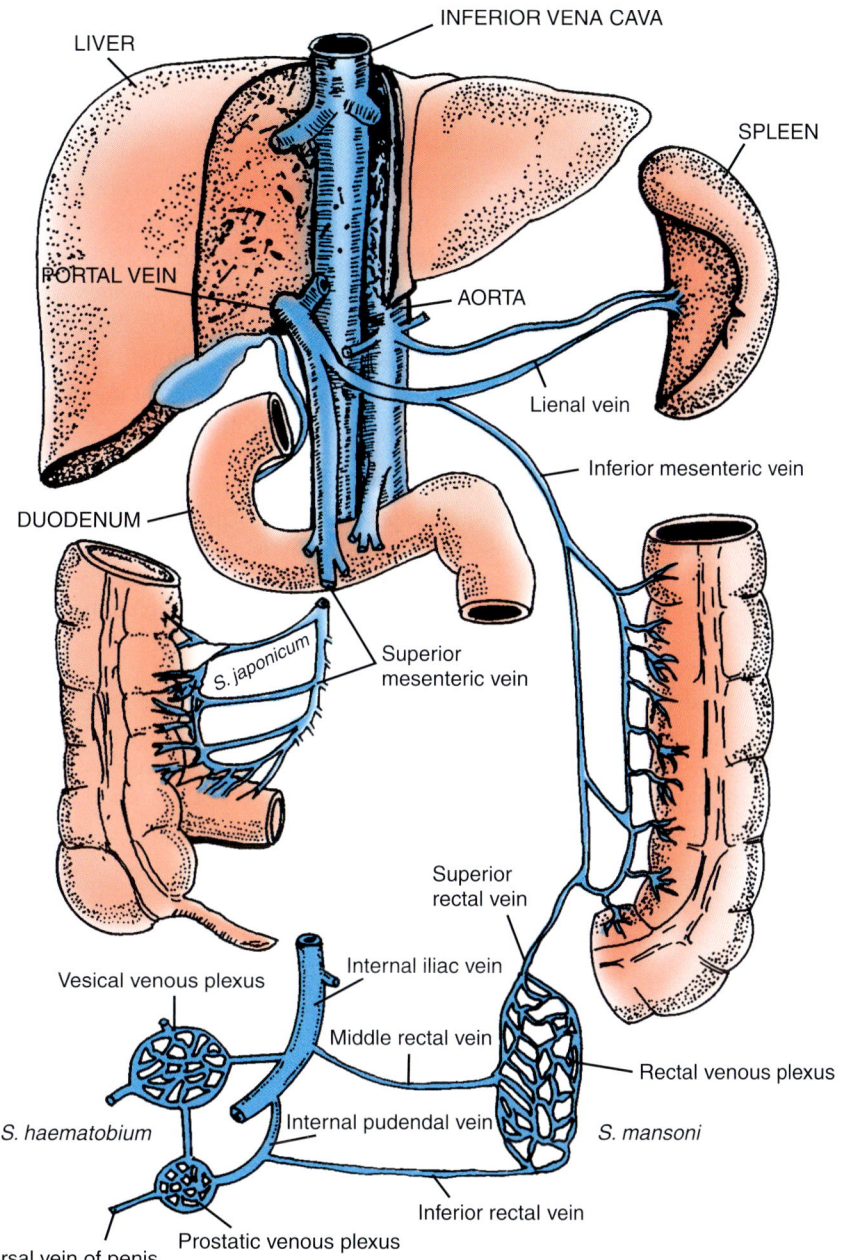

Fig. 135—Portal venous system and its connections.
Route through which adult Schistosomes migrate to their sites of location.

through the capillary bed in the intestine and enter portal circulation (taking 5 days to reach the liver). In the intrahepatic portion of the portal blood stream, the larvae grow into adults (maturing in 3 weeks from the time of entry). After becoming sexually differentiated, they move out of the liver against the blood current, migrating into the inferior mesenteric vein, rectal venous plexus, pelvic veins, and eventually enter the vesical plexus of veins (Fig. 135). It takes about 1 to 3 months for the worms to reach the vesical and pelvic plexuses of veins after the initial exposure of the skin. When the worms are sexually mature, they copulate (the females are enclosed in the males) and the fertilised females lay eggs which are ultimately voided with the urine. The cycle is thus repeated.

Note: Schistosomes are the single exception amongst the digenetic trematodes, where rediae are not produced, asexual multiplication taking place only in the sporocyst stage.

Pathogenicity. An individual bathing in an infected pool or coming in contact with contaminated water is liable to be infected. The cercariae stick to the surface of the skin of the swimmer or bather, by means of their ventral suckers (acetabula) and as the water begins to evaporate, penetrate the skin.

Infecting Agent—Cercariae. These have a free-swimming existence and can live in this state for a maximum period of 3 days.

Portal of Entry—Skin.   *Site of Localisation*—Vesical plexus of veins (urinary bladder).

PATHOGENESIS. The terminal-spined eggs of *S. haematobium* may erode blood vessels and cause *haemorrhages*. Schistosome eggs, deposited in the tissues, act like foreign protein and have an irritative effect leading to round cell infiltration and connective tissue hyperplasia. The tissue reaction in these cases produces what is known as formation of a "*pseudotubercle*" around each egg (egg-granuloma). The early nodules are highly cellular and are composed of eosinophils, giant cells, monocytes and lymphocytes; later on, the cellular reaction tends to disappear and is replaced by a whorl of fibrous tissue, in the centre of which degenerated and calcified eggs may be found. Large and progressive granulomas are found only around the eggs and may cause a diffuse fibrosis.

Schistosome granuloma. The Schistosome eggs secrete soluble substances which pass through the pores of the egg-shell and provoke a granulomatous reaction, a manifestation of cell-mediated delayed hypersensitivity. In sensitised individuals, granulomatous reaction becomes accelerated and enhanced on second exposure to eggs. The host-reaction is thus an immunological one and the sensitisation can be transferred by lymphoid cells and inhibited by immuno-suppressive agents (Warren, 1972)*.

The immunological reaction to Schistosome eggs plays a defensive as well as a destructive role, because (i) it can sequesterate antigen *in situ* and potentiate antigen catabolism and (ii) it can synthesise antibody locally in the cells that surround the mature granuloma.

* Warren, K. S. (1972). *Trans. Roy. Soc. Trap. Med. & Hyg.*, **66**, 417-32.

Clinical Features. The disease caused by infection with *S. haematobium* is referred to as schistosomiasis haematobia (urinary schistosomiasis or bilharziasis; endemic haematuria). Evolution of the disease passes through 3 phases:

(i) By the cercariae at the site of entrance: Local reaction (dermatitis). This is particularly seen with the cercariae of non-human schistosomes (adult worms in birds or small mammals).

(ii) By the toxic metabolites liberated during the growth of schistosomulae in the portal blood of the liver: General anaphylactic reaction characterised by fever, urticaria, eosinophilic leucocytosis, enlarged tender liver and palpable spleen. The symptoms appear between the 4th and the 5th week of the infection (k.a. Katayama fever in Japan). It is commonly seen in infection with *S. japonicum* and rarely with *S. haematobium*.

(iii) At the time of laying eggs: This may be regarded as a localising symptom, generally occurring within 3 to 9 months of the infection. The characteristic manifestation is a painless terminal haematuria. In course of time, the adjacent structures of uro-genital apparatus are involved, at first by the reversible granulomatous inflammatory reaction to eggs and later by the irreversible fibrosis and calcification.

It has been observed that a close relationship exists between vesical schistosomiasis and vesical carcinoma, particularly in areas where the infection is highly endemic.

ECTOPIC LESIONS. These are the result of an overflow phenomenon due to heavy infection. The eggs and worms escape into the pelvic veins and are carried to the lungs where the eggs excite a granulomatous reaction leading to fibrosis, pulmonary endarteritis, obstruction to pulmonary blood flow, pulmonary hypertension and finally chronic cor pulmonale. Eggs and adult worms have also been carried from the portacaval system into the distant parts of the body causing lesions in the brain (a space-occupying lesion, common in *S. japonicum*) and the spinal cord (transverse myelitis-like syndrome, common in *S. haematobium* and *S. mansoni*).

Diagnosis. This is based on the demonstration of eggs of *S. haematobium* in:

(a) A microscopical examination of urine (centrifuged deposit). Now-a-days sophisticated filtration techniques give quantitative estimation of egg excretion.

(b) Examination of stool: Direct smear of the stool is not sensitive. Concentration methods (Keto thick smear or its modified method) may detect the eggs of schistosoma species.

(c) A piece of vesical mucosa is removed by cystoscopic biopsy. The excised tissue is divided into two pieces. One piece is compressed between two slides and examined for eggs under the low power of the microscope. The other piece is placed in a fixative for histological examination.

OTHER TESTS: (i) *Blood Examination*. This should include:

(a) Eosinophilic Count—Increased in early cases.

(b) Aldehyde Test—Often positive (due to high globulin value).

(c) Complement Fixation Test—Sera of patients react positively with cercarial antigen obtained from infected snail's liver.

(ii) *Intradermal Skin Test*, with cercarial antigen (Fairley's Test). This is an allergic reaction, positive in all the varieties of schistosomiasis.

(iii) *Immunological Tests in Schistosomiasis*. Besides complement fixation test, sera of patients may be used for the demonstration of (*i*) precipitin formation around schistosome eggs—circumoval precipitin (COP) test of Oliver-Gonzalez (1954), (*ii*) miracidial immobilisation test of Senterft (1953) and (*iii*) development of pericercarial membranes around *Schistosoma* cercariae—"Cercarienhullen reaktion" (CHR) of Vogel and Mining (1949).

A fluorescent antibody technique (FAT) has been employed for the serological diagnosis of schistosomiasis, using both cercariae and miracidia as antigens. It is true antigen-antibody reaction and becomes positive in early stages of infection (Sadun, 1963).

Immunological tests in Schistosomiasis are group-specific and non-human species of *schistosoma* may be used as a satisfactory antigen. Highly specific and sensitive, ELISA, GPT, LAT, IHA, COPT, IFAT and RIA are also available and have superseded CFT and CHR tests.

(iv) X-ray examination can show calcified eggs in the urinary bladder. Cystoscopy, IVP, USG, CT and isotope renography are also useful in indirect diagnosis of disease.

Treatment. The drugs having specific actions on the schistosomes are praziquantel (40 mg/kg/day in two divided doses for 1 day) and metrifonate (Single dose of 7.5 mg to 10 mg/kg body weight, weekly for 3 weeks). Praziquantel is more effective drug than metrifonate.

Prophylaxis. The preventive measures include the following: (*i*) eradication of the disease in man, (*ii*) prevention of pollution of water with human excreta, (*iii*) destruction of the snail vector in endemic areas and (iv) avoidance of swimming, bathing, wading or washing in infected water.

Schistosoma mansoni Sambon, 1907
Common Name: Manson's blood fluke.

Geographical Distribution. Various parts of Africa and South America.

Habitat. Adult worms in the mesenteric veins of the sigmoido-rectal area; also in the branches of the portal vein in the liver.

Morphology. See page 177.

Life Cycle. Same as that *of S. haematobium.*

Definitive Host. Man.

Intermediate Host. Fresh-water snails (*Biomphalaria alexendrina* in Africa and *Australorbis glabratus* in South America).

The cycle is from man to snail *via* water and from snail to man again via water.

Like *S. haematobium* the schistosomulae are carried to the liver (the route taken being the same) where they feed upon portal blood and develop into adult worms. Their subsequent behaviour differs and they migrate against the blood stream into the inferior mesenteric vein to reach the capillaries of the sigmoido-rectal area where the eggs are laid. These finally escape through the faeces (Fig. 136).

Pathogenicity. The disease caused by *S. mansoni* is designated as schistosomiasis mansoni; also known as intestinal bilharziasis, schistosomal dysentery. The visceral form is known as visceral schistosomiasis or Egyptian splenomegaly.

The pathogenic effects are the same as in *S. haematobium* and are characterised by the usual 3 phases. The localising symptom is chiefly intestinal, involving the sigmoido-rectal area and manifested by dysenteric attack.

The ectopic lesions include hepatomegaly, periportal cirrhosis, portal hypertension (splenomegaly and haematemesis), cor pulmonale and myelitis.

Diagnosis. This is settled by demonstrating the eggs of *S. mansoni* in:

(i) A microscopical examination of faeces.

(ii) A piece of rectal tissue removed by rectal biopsy. The excised tissue is examined for eggs, in the same way as for *S. haematobium*. Rectal biopsy is a simple diagnostic technique and provides an effective way of visualisation of eggs. Schistosoma ova are often found in other locations and examination of biopsy materials of such sites is frequently needed for diagnosis of disease.

OTHER TESTS—Same as those for *S. haematobium (vide supra).*

VISCERAL SCHISTOSOMIASIS—Tissues removed from the liver and lungs are digested with potash solution. The excised tissue is examined for eggs.

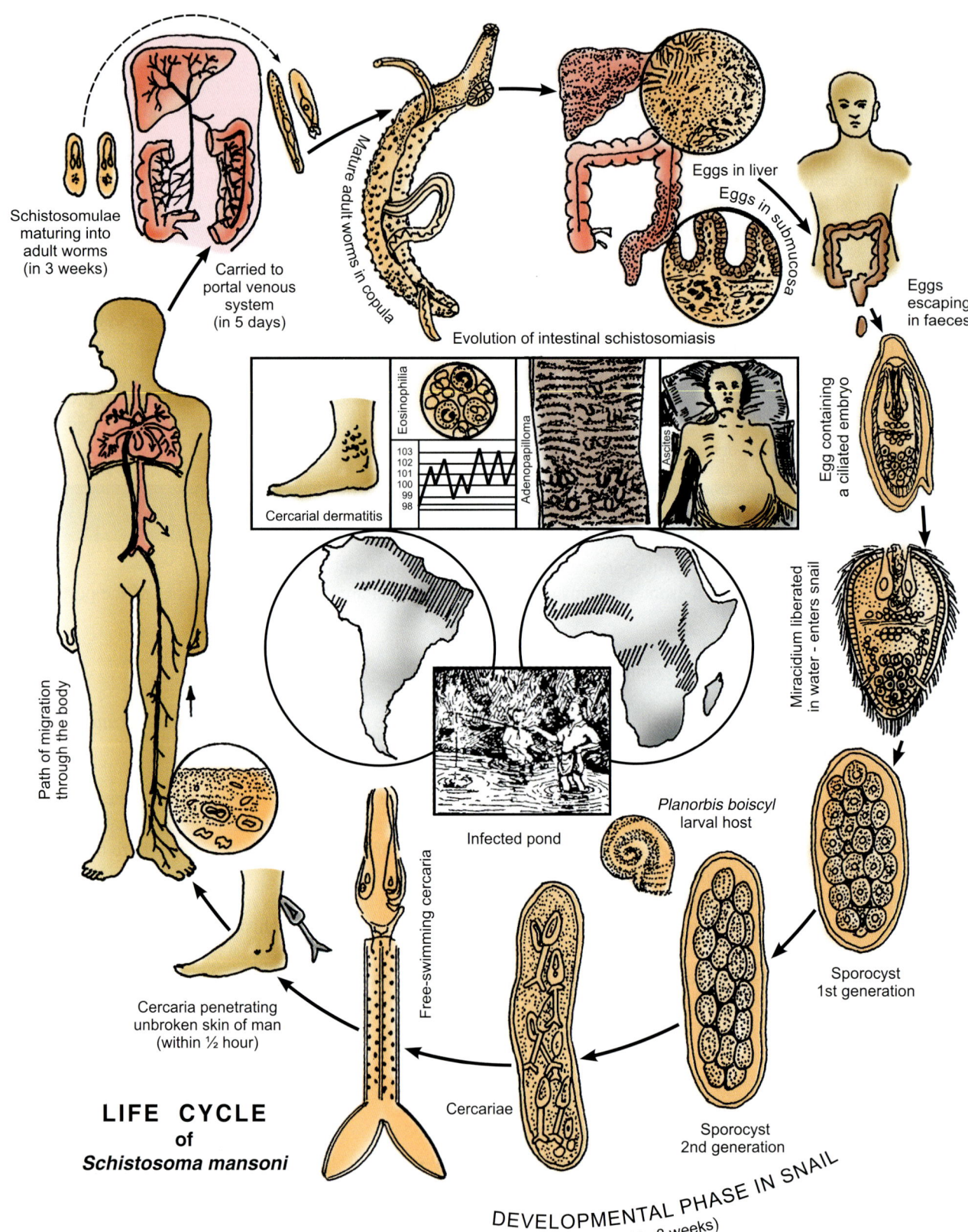

Schistosomulae maturing into adult worms (in 3 weeks)

Carried to portal venous system (in 5 days)

Mature adult worms in copula

Evolution of intestinal schistosomiasis

Eggs in liver

Eggs in submucosa

Eggs escaping in faeces

Egg containing a ciliated embryo

Miracidium liberated in water - enters snail

Eosinophilia

Cercarial dermatitis

103
102
101
100
99
98

Adenopapilloma

Ascites

Infected pond

Planorbis boiscyl larval host

Sporocyst 1st generation

Sporocyst 2nd generation

Path of migration through the body

Free-swimming cercaria

Cercariae

Cercaria penetrating unbroken skin of man (within ½ hour)

LIFE CYCLE of *Schistosoma mansoni*

DEVELOPMENTAL PHASE IN SNAIL (4 to 8 weeks)

Fig. 136

Treatment and Prophylaxis. Same as for *S. haematobium. See Appendix II.*

Besides praziquantel (40 mg/kg/day in two divided doses for one day), oxamniquine (15-20 mg/kg as a single dose) is also effective in the treatment of *S. mansoni.*

Schistosoma japonicum Katsurada, 1904
Common Name: The Oriental blood fluke.

Geographical Distribution. A parasite of the Far East—being found in China, Japan, Southern Formosa, Philippines, Celebes and Shan States of Burma.

Habitat. Adult worms are found in the following places:
 (i) Intrahepatic portion of the portal venous system.
 (ii) Mesenteric veins draining the ileo-caecal region.
(iii) Rectal (haemorrhoidal) plexus of veins.

Morphology. See page 177.

Life Cycle. Same as that of *S. haematobium.*

Definitive Host. Man. Domestic animals (cat, dog, pig and cattle) and field mice serve as reservoirs of infection.

Intermediate Host. Fresh-water snail of the genus *Oncomelania (Katayama or Blanfordia).*

The schistosomulae of *S. japonicum* are carried to the liver exactly in the same way as those of *S. haematobium.* They grow into adult worms and become sexually mature inside the intra-hepatic portion of the portal venous system but subsequently migrate against the blood stream into the superior mesenteric vein, down to the capillaries of the last part of the ileum, caecum and ascending colon. The eggs finally escape through the faeces (Fig. 137).

Pathogenicity and Clinical Features. The disease caused by *S. japonicum* is designated as schistosomiasis japonica or intestinal and hepatic schistosomiasis of the Orient; also known as Katayama disease.

Description: Follows the same general lines as mentioned under *S. haematobium.*

Note: The lesions produced in schistosomiasis japonica are much more pronounced than in schistosomiasis mansoni, because of the larger output of eggs. The localising symptom is chiefly intestinal, involving the ileo-caecal region and is manifested by dysenteric attacks. Further, on account of the proximity of its location to the liver, the chances of the liver being involved are greater.

LIVER. Periportal cirrhosis* ("clay pipe-stem cirrhosis" of Symmer). It is a granulomatous fibrosis pylephlebitis with terminal scarring developing round the eggs (not the dead adult worms) which lodge in the smallest portal venules. As a rule, the liver lobules are not affected and there is no nodular regeneration of the liver cells. A characteristic feature is the intense new formation of blood vessels in the portal field giving an "angiomatoid" appearance (capillary telangiectasis). Pigmentation due to deposition of haematin pigment, similar to malarial pigment, inside the Kupffer's cells may be found. Haematin pigment is regurgitated by the parent worm after digestion of blood in its alimentary canal, because the intestine terminates blindly.

Schistosomal Hepatic Fibrosis. Chronic hepatic lesions in schistosomiasis is not a true portal cirrhosis and is thus, different from that of Laënnec's cirrhosis or other types of cirrhosis. It is a confluent progressive fibrosis which is the outcome of sclerosis of many egg-granulomas. These are prominent along the portal ramifications. The eggs of *S. mansoni* and *S. japonicum* can induce a diffuse fibrosis in the liver, but the liver functions remain unimpaired due to compensatory increase in hepatic artery blood flow.

SPLEEN. Enlargement of the spleen is due to mechanical factor and results from pre-sinusoidal portal hypertension through intrahepatic block of small portal venules by fibrosis. Schistosomal lesion (egg-granulomas) are not found in the spleen.

OESOPHAGEAL VARICES. A consequence of portal hypertension; rupture leads to massive haematemesis.

BRAIN (space-occupying lesion) and Lungs (cor pulmonale) may also be involved.

Diagnosis. Same as described for schistosomiasis mansoni. Portal venography, USG and computed tomography are helpful in indirect disgnosis of disease.

Treatment and Prophylaxis. Same as described for *S. haematobium. See Appendix. II.*

---

*Cameron, G. R. and Ganguly, N. G. (1964). An experimental study of the pathogenesis and reversibility of schistosomal hepatic fibrosis, *J. Path. & Bact.*, 87, 2, 217-237.

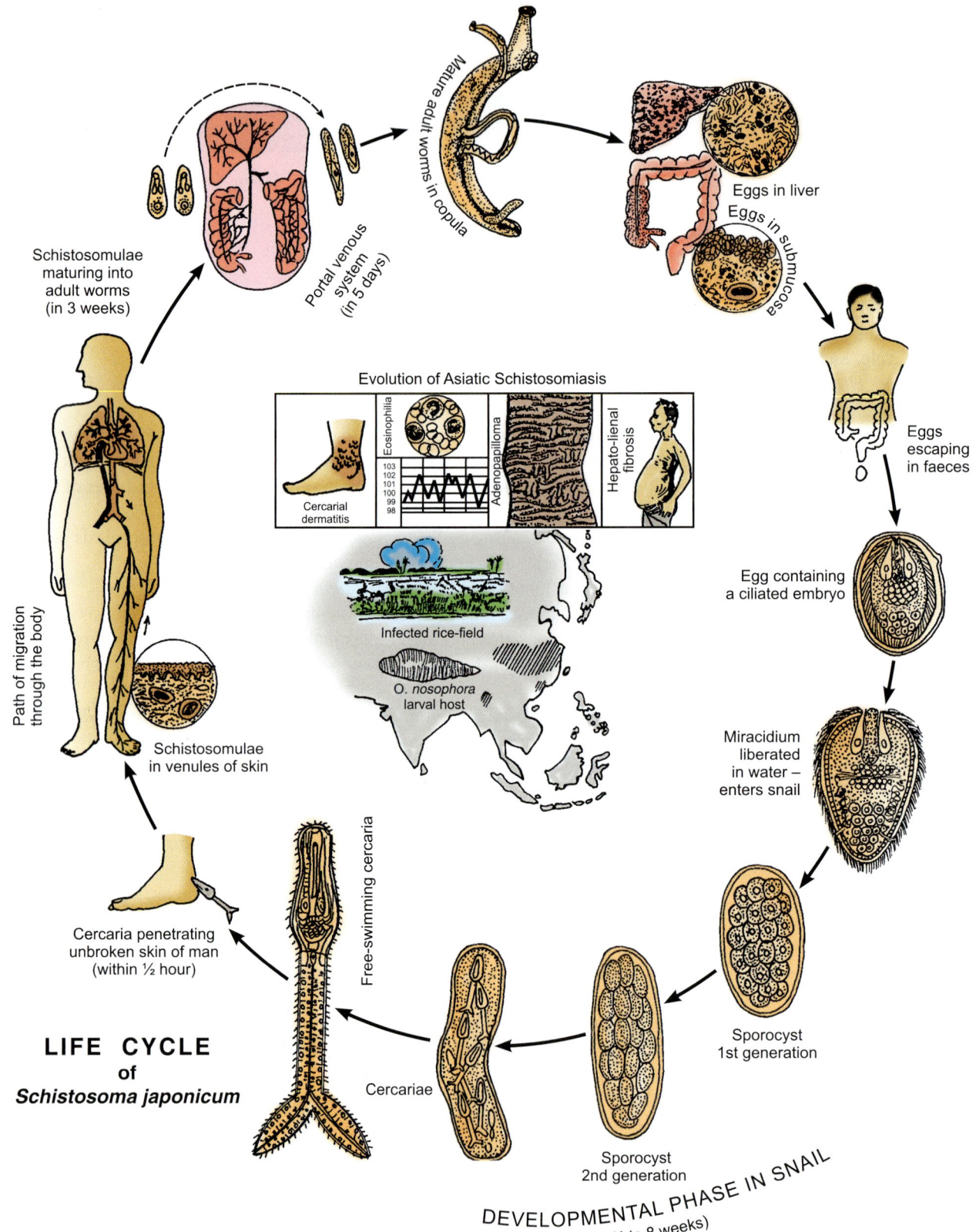

Mature adult worms in copula

Portal venous system (in 5 days)

Schistosomulae maturing into adult worms (in 3 weeks)

Eggs in liver

Eggs in submucosa

Eggs escaping in faeces

Egg containing a ciliated embryo

Miracidium liberated in water – enters snail

Path of migration through the body

Schistosomulae in venules of skin

Evolution of Asiatic Schistosomiasis

Cercarial dermatitis

Eosinophilia

103 102 101 100 99 98

Adenopapilloma

Hepato-lienal fibrosis

Infected rice-field

O. nosophora larval host

Cercaria penetrating unbroken skin of man (within ½ hour)

Free-swimming cercaria

Cercariae

Sporocyst 1st generation

Sporocyst 2nd generation

LIFE CYCLE
of
Schistosoma japonicum

DEVELOPMENTAL PHASE IN SNAIL
(4 to 8 weeks)

Fig. 137

Schistosoma intercalatum (Fisher, 1934).

Schistosoma intercalatum was first recognised in 1934 and occurs in humans in Western and Central Africa. The eggs have terminal spine, like *S. haematobium*, having a slight bend and egg shell is Ziehl-Neelsen positive. The disease is usually benign and the hapatomegaly usually is not marked. Digestive disturbance with abdominal pain and blood in stool are often the associated features.This is a haematobium-like worm, the terminal-spined eggs of which were recovered from the faeces of man in the Congo basin (egg measuring 175 μm by 60 μm and a longer terminal spine, up to 20 μm). The adult worms are found in the intestinal venous plexuses of man but not in the vesical venous plexus. The snail hosts are *Bulinus africanus* and *B. globosus*. Praziquantel in a single dose of 40 mg/kg is the drug of choice.

Schistosoma mekongi

Schistosoma mekongi was first recognised in 1978 and is endemic in Khong Island in the Mekong River in Southern Laos and Northern Cambodia and also common among people living in floating villages of raft houses in the Mekong River, South of Khong Island. Natural infection has been detected in humans and dogs. The eggs have close similarity with that of *S. japonicum*, being smaller and less elongated, having a size range of 30-35 μm by 50-65 μm. Prepatent period is longer than that of *S. japonicum*. Snail host (*Trienla aperta*) is aquatic (in *S. japonicum*—amphibious). In experimental infection in mouse and hamster, this is relatively more pathogenic than *S. japonicum*. The adults are normally found in mesenteric veins. In *S. mekongi*, as in *S. japonicum*, hepatomegaly, splenomegaly, ascites, dilated superficial abdominal veins are the common clinical findings.One day oral treatment by praziquantel in a dose of 60 mg/kg in 3 divided doses is found to be effective.

Suborder AMPHISTOMATA
Superfamily PARAMPHISTOMATOIDEA

The acetabulum is large, highly developed and occupies a position behind the reproductive organs and there is often a ventral pouch or disc. These are parasites of herbivorous animals living in the stomach or intestine. The species infecting man are included in two genera.
1. Genus GASTRODISCOIDES Leiper, 1913. Species *G. hominis*.
2. Genus WATSONIUS Stiles and Goldberger, 1910. Species *W. watsoni*.

Gastrodiscoides hominis (Lewis and McConnell, 1876) Leiper, 1913

Synonym—*Amphistomum hominis* Lewis and McConnell 1876)

Geographical Distribution. India (Bengal and Assam), Cochin-China, Malaya and Indian immigrants to British Guiana.
Habitat. Adult worm in the large intestine of definitive host. Pig is the common reservoir.
Morphology. The parasite is pyriform in shape. It measures 5 to 10 mm in length by 4 to 6 mm in breadth at its widest part. The body is divided into two parts: an anterior conical and a posterior hemispherical portion which is hollowed out ventrally to form a concave disc. The acetabulum is postero-terminal and is situated ventrally. There is a notch at the posterior end. The internal structure follows the same general pattern of Trematodes. The eggs are ovoid, operculated and measure 130 μm by 60 μm at their widest parts and are immature when oviposited.
Life Cycle. The eggs are passed with faeces and contaminate water. Eggs hatch and release miracidum, which invade the tissues of the intermidiate host, aquatic molluscan. Within mollusc, the miracidum develops into sporocyst, first and second generation rediae and finally into cercariae. After release from mollusc cercariae forms metacercarial cysts on fresh water plants. Man and other mammalian hosts are infected by ingestion of these plants.
Pathogenicity. Mucous diarrhoea.
Diagnosis. Characteristic eggs in stool.
Treatment. Praziquantel easily expels the worms.
Prophylaxis. Avoidance of consumption of raw or undercooked water plants is a useful prophylaxis measure.

Watsonius watsoni (Conyngham, 1904) Stiles and Goldberger, 1910

This fluke was recovered from man (at the autopsy of a negro from Nigeria) in 1904.

The normal host is the monkey and the parasite is found in Asia, Africa, Malaysia and Japan. It is pear-shaped, flattened dorso-ventrally and measures 8 to 10 mm in length by 4 to 5 mm in breadth. Near the posterior sucker, the body is ventrally concave. The eggs are similar to those of *G. hominis* but smaller in size. The diagnosis is based on the finding of eggs in the faeces. The worm is easily expelled by drugs used for other intestinal trematodes. Prophylaxis has not been studied.

Suborder DISTOMATA
Superfamily FASCIOLOIDEA

Adults are found in the intestine and biliary passages of herbivorous animals and man. Eggs are large, operculated and immature when laid, each containing a conspicuous unsegmented ovum. The miracidium develops within the eggs in water and has *x*-type of pigmented eye spots. Intermediate hosts are fresh-water molluscs where the miracidium passes through the stages of sporocyst and two or more generations of rediae. Cercariae encyst on vegetation and in fish which are the sources of infection to the definitive or final host. Those infecting man consist of two genera:

1. Genus FASCIOLA Linnaeus, 1758. Species *F. hepatica*.
2. Genus FASCIOLOPSIS Looss, 1899. Species *F. buski*.

Fasciola hepatica Linnaeus, 1758

Common Names: The sheep liver fluke; the common liver fluke.

Amongst the trematodes, this was the first to be discovered by Jehan de Brie in 1379,

Geographical Distribution. Cosmopolitan.

Habitat. A parasite of herbivorous animals (sheep, goat and cattle), living in the biliary passages of the liver. It is occasionally found in man.

Morphology. Adult Worm. It is a large leaf-shaped fluke, measuring 3 cm in length by 1.5 cm in breadth and brown to pale grey in colour. There are two suckers, the oral sucker is smaller. The anterior end bearing the oral sucker forms a conical projection. The posterior end is rounded. The acetabulum is situated in a line with the two shoulders formed by the broadening of the conical projection posteriorly. Both the intestinal caeca bear a number of lateral compound branches. The genital system follows the same general pattern of Trematodes.

Life span of the adult worm in sheep is 5 years and in man 9 to 13 years.

EGGS. The characteristics of the egg are as follows:

(i) Large, operculated, ovoid in shape, brownish yellow in colour (bile-stained).

(ii) Size 140 μm by 80 μm.

(iii) Contains a large unsegmented ovum in a mass of yolk cells.

(iv) Excreted with the bile into the duodenum and then passed out along with the faeces.

(v) Does not float in saturated solution of common salt.

(vi) Can develop only in water.

Life Cycle. *F. hepatica* passes its life cycle (Fig. 138) in two different hosts.

Definitive Hosts. Sheep, goat, cattle or man. Adult worm in the biliary passages of the liver. Reservoir host is primarily the sheep.

Intermediate Host. Snails of the genus *Lymnaea*. Larval development proceeds in this snail.

The eggs passed out in the faeces of definitive hosts, mature in water; inside each egg, a ciliated miracidium is developed in the course of 2 to 3 weeks' time. On escaping from the egg, the miracidium finds its way to its suitably intermediate host. Inside the lymph spaces of the molluscan host, the miracidium passes through the stages of sporocyst, two generations of rediae and finally to the stage of cercariae; the whole cycle takes a period of 30 to 60 days. The mature cercariae escape from the snail into the water and encyst (metacercariae) in blades of grass or water-cress. The encysted cercariae are swallowed along with the grass or water-cress by herbivorous animals (their final hosts) and occasionally by man. On entering the digestive tract, the metacercariae excyst in the duodenum, migrate through the intestinal wall into the peritoneal cavity, penetrate the capsule of the liver, traverse its parenchyma and ultimately settle in the biliary passages (taking about a month to migrate) and grow to sexual maturity. The eggs are liberated in the faeces through the bile in about 3 to 4 months after infection. The cycle is then repeated.

Pathogenicity and Clinical Features. Human infection is not exceptional and the symptoms of fascioliasis include biliary colic with vomiting, persistent diarrhoea, jaundice, ascites and a tender hepatomegaly with peripheral eosinophilia (40-85%). It is most common in sheep- and cattle-raising countries. In Britain, an outbreak* occurred in Hampshire in 1960. During migration through peritoneal cavity, the larvae may lodge in ectopic locations and may form abscess there.

---

*Facey, R. V. and Marsden, P. V. *Br. Med. J.*, **ii**, 619; 1960.

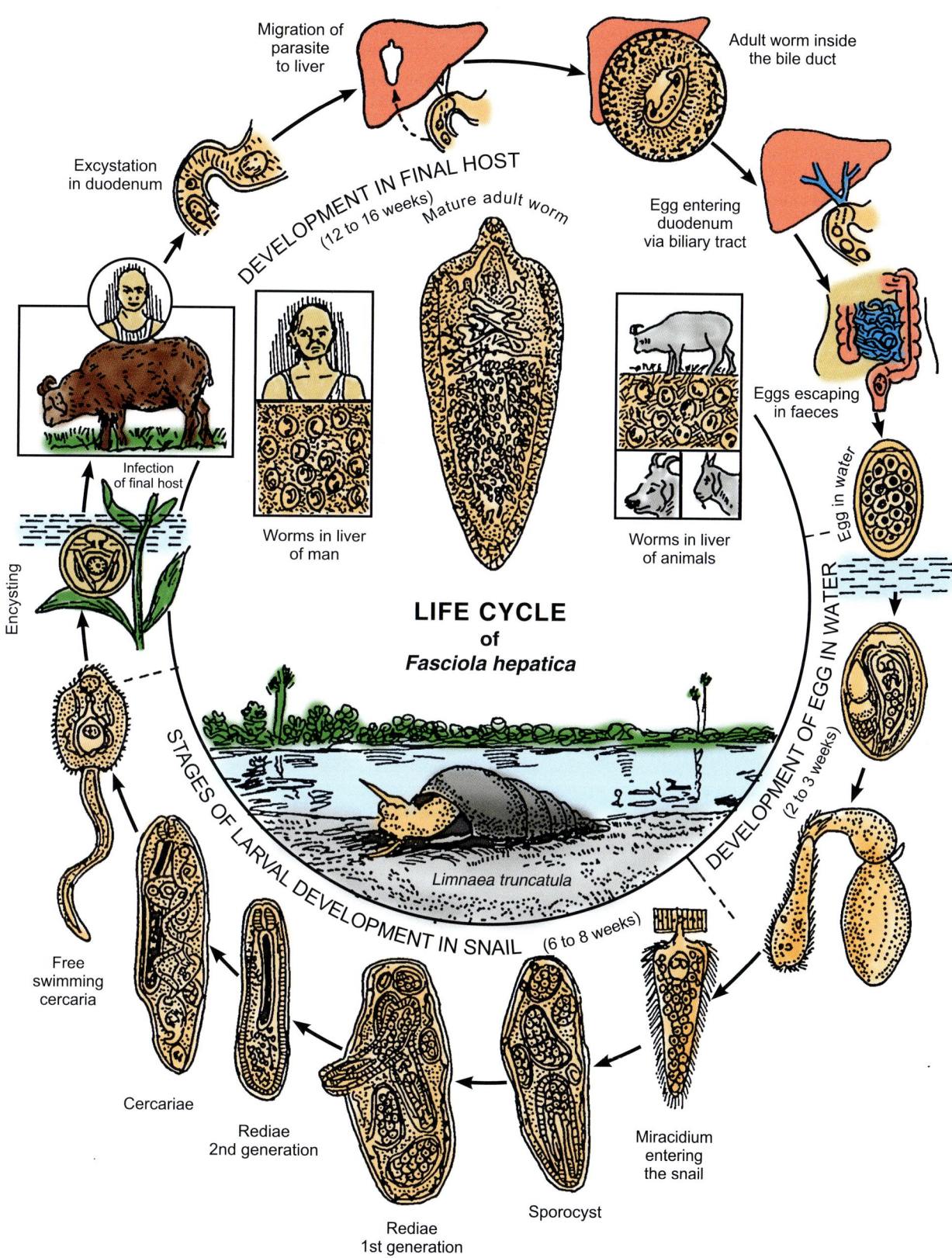

Migration of parasite to liver

Adult worm inside the bile duct

Excystation in duodenum

DEVELOPMENT IN FINAL HOST
(12 to 16 weeks)

Mature adult worm

Egg entering duodenum via biliary tract

Eggs escaping in faeces

Worms in liver of man

Worms in liver of animals

Infection of final host

Egg in water

Encysting

DEVELOPMENT OF EGG IN WATER
(2 to 3 weeks)

LIFE CYCLE
of
Fasciola hepatica

Limnaea truncatula

STAGES OF LARVAL DEVELOPMENT IN SNAIL (6 to 8 weeks)

Free swimming cercaria

Cercariae

Rediae 2nd generation

Rediae 1st generation

Sporocyst

Miracidium entering the snail

Fig. 138

"Halzoun", an acute dysphagia and laryngeal obstruction occurring in people of certain parts of Syria (Lebanon) who eat raw liver of sacrificial goats was formerly attributed to invasion by immature *F. hepatica* and was known as pharyngeal fascioliasis but is now considered to be due to the ingestion of nymphs of *Linguatula serrata*.

F. hepatica is primarily responsible for producing a disease in the animals, known as "liver rot". During migration of the young worms (metacercariae or adolescariae) and their localisation in the biliary passages, they cause extensive damage to the liver tissue and in heavy infections, may lead to portal cirrhosis. While in the biliary passages, they may interfere with normal flow of bile, causing obstructive jaundice. The mature worms cause marked pathological changes in the biliary tract by mechanical irritation as well as by their toxic secretion. They produce cystic dilatation of the bile ducts, the walls of which become greatly thickened by the development of fibrous tissue. The biliary epithelium proliferates, giving rise to adenomata.

Diagnosis. This is based on the finding of eggs in stool or in bile obtained by duodenal intubation. The eggs of *F. hepatica* and *F. buski* are indistinguishable. Eggs are not found in faeces in case of presence of worms in ectopic foci.

High to moderate eosinophilia and elevated liver function tests' levels are associated constant finding. Serological tests such as C.F.T., haemoagglutanation tests, immunofluorescence assay, immunodiffusion, immunoelectrophoresis and CCIE (sensitive test) may be helpful in diagnosis of the disease.

For immuno-diagnosis antigen from adult worm is used for complement fixation test and skin test.

Ultrasonography, ERCP and percutaneous cholangiography may be helpful in diagnosis of disease.

Treatment. In acute human infection, emetine injection has been attended with beneficial results. Bithionol (30–50 mg/kg for 10–15 days) and triclabendazole (10 mg/kg as a single dose) are now used. praziquantel is not effective drug. Nitazoxanide is another effective drug. Prednisolone at a dose of 10-20 mg/day is used to tackle toxoaemia. Antibiotics are recommended to control secondary bacterial infection.

Prophylaxis. Human infection can be prevented by the eradication of the disease in animals. The measures consist of treatment of infected animals and destruction of molluscan hosts.

Other Species:

Fasciola gigantica Cobbold 1856 (The giant liver fluke)

It is a parasite of herbivorus animals and human cases have been reported from Africa, Russia and Far East. The life cycle, pathogenicity and clinical features are similar to those of *F. hepatica* but intermediate hosts are different snails. The fluke is larger than *F. hepatica*. It lives in the biliary passage of its host. It is difficult to make difference of eggs from *F. hepatica*, *F. gigantica*, *F. buski* and *Echinostomes*.

Fasciolopsis buski (Lankester, 1857) Odhner, 1902

Common Name: The large or giant intestinal fluke.

Geographical Distribution. It is an Asiatic trematode and has been reported from China, Thailand and Malaysia, Bengal, Assam and other Oriental regions.

Habitat. The adult worm lives in the small intestine of man and pig. The normal host is the pig which serves as the reservoir of infection for man.

Morphology. Adult Worm. It is the largest trematode (Fig. 139) parasitising man and measures 2 to 7.5 cm in length, 8 to 20 mm in breadth and 0.5 to 3 mm in thickness. It is elongated and oval in shape, the anterior being narrower than the posterior. The acetabulum is large and lies close to the oral sucker. In general appearance, the worm resembles *F. hepatica* but it does not possess any cephalic cone and the two intestinal caeca do not bear any lateral branches. The genital system (Fig. 140) follows the same general pattern of Trematodes.

Life span of the adult worm is short (not more than 6 months).

Eggs. Same as that of *F. hepatica*. Each worm lays 25,000 eggs per day.

Life Cycle. Two different hosts are required (Fig. 141).

Definitive Hosts. Man and pig. Adult worms are found in the small intestine.

Intermediate Host. Small flatly coiled aquatic snails of the genus *Segmentina*.

The life cycle is the same as that described for *F. hepatica*.

The cercariae, on coming out of the snail, encyst on fresh-water plants, especially seed pods of water-caltrop, the bulb of water-chestnut and other aquatic vegetations which are fertilised with night-soil and are grown in shallow ponds where the snails abound. On being swallowed, the metacercariae excyst in the duodenum and the liberated

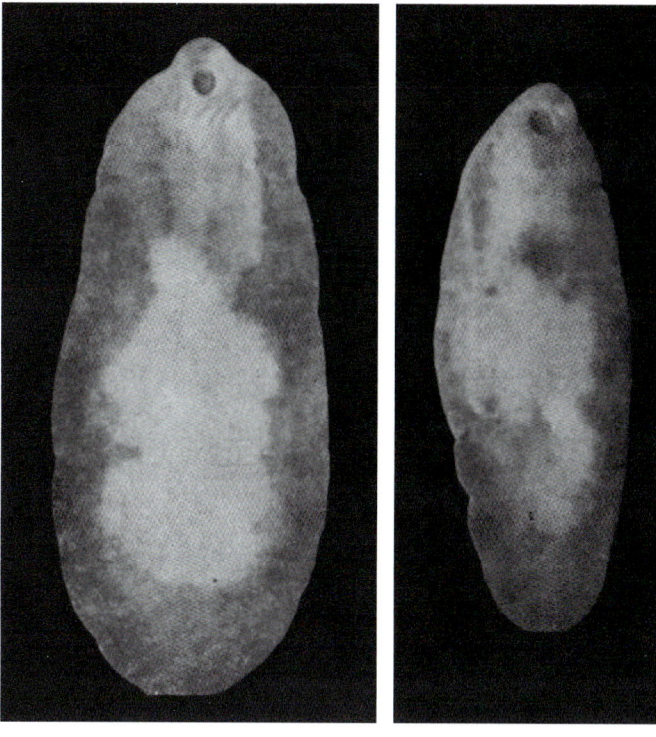

Fig. 139—Two adult specimens of *Fasciolopsis buski*.
(Twice enlarged, actual sizes are 4.2 cm × 18 mm and 3.7 cm × 15 mm)

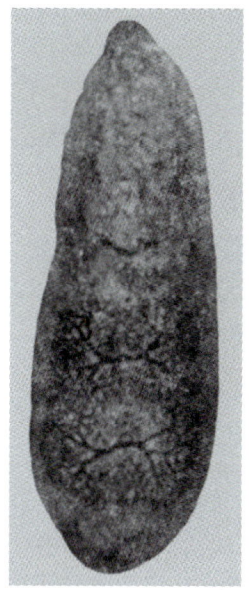

Fig. 140—*Fasciolopsis buski*.
Showing the internal anatomy of
the adult worm.

young worms attach themselves to the intestinal wall, developing into adult worms in about 3 months' time. The eggs are then liberated and the cycle is repeated.

Pathogenicity

Mode of Infection. Eating infected plants as raw foodstuff (peeling it with the teeth).

Portal of Entry. Alimentary canal.

Infecting Agent. Encysted cercariae (metacercariae).

Site of Localisation. Small intestine (duodenum and jejunum).

Infection with *F. buski* is known as fasciolopsiasis. The disease is characterised by asthenia, mild anaemia and chronic diarrhoea. In heavy infections, anaemia becomes more intense and absorption of by-products of the worm leads to oedema and eosinophilia. Paralytic ileus is a rare complication.

Diagnosis. This is based on the history of residence in endemic areas and on the finding of eggs in stool by microscopic examination. The eggs of *F. buski* and *F. hepatica* are indistinguishable. Adult worms may be recovered after a purgative or an anthelmintic.

Eosinophilia is often present. Serodiagnosis is of no value.

Treatment. Specific anthelmintic drugs include praziquantel (single dose of 75 mg/kg/day in three divided doses for one day).

Prophylaxis. This consists of the following: (i) sterilisation of the night-soil before being used as a fertiliser, (ii) destruction of molluscan hosts by copper sulphate solution (1 in 50,000 strength) and (iii) avoidance of eating raw vegetables (water-caltrop and water-chestnut) or before consumption these "should be cooked or immersed in boiling water for a few minutes.

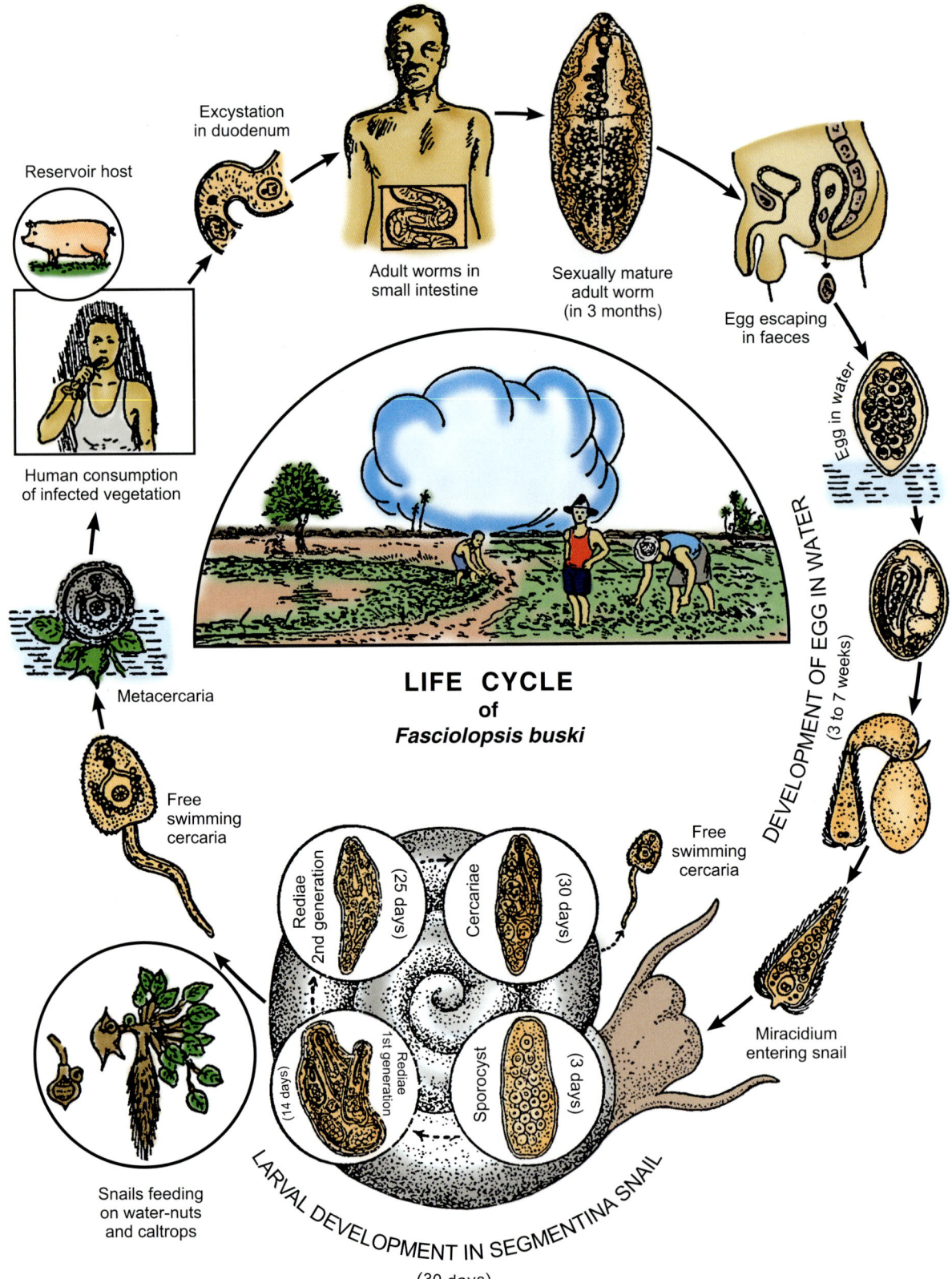

Reservoir host

Excystation
in duodenum

Adult worms in
small intestine

Sexually mature
adult worm
(in 3 months)

Egg escaping
in faeces

Human consumption
of infected vegetation

Metacercaria

Free
swimming
cercaria

DEVELOPMENT OF EGG IN WATER
(3 to 7 weeks)

Egg in water

LIFE CYCLE
of
Fasciolopsis buski

Rediae
2nd generation
(25 days)

Cercariae
(30 days)

Free
swimming
cercaria

Rediae
1st generation
(14 days)

Sporocyst
(3 days)

Miracidium
entering snail

Snails feeding
on water-nuts
and caltrops

LARVAL DEVELOPMENT IN SEGMENTINA SNAIL

(30 days)

(Morphology after Barlow)

Fig. 141

Suborder DISTOMATA: Superfamily ECHINOSTOMATOIDEA

Adults live in the intestinal tract of vertebrates. The anterior end of the worm is surrounded by a collar of large spines (circumoral spines). The eggs are large having small opercula. The miracidium has a median eye spot and passes through the stages of one or two generations of rediae and cercariae (no sporocyst-stage). Metacercariae may be found in the same species of molluscan host or other species in fish or on vegetation.

Human representatives are in two genera:

(a) Genus ECHINOSTOMA Species *E. ilocanum*.

(b) Genus PARYPHOSTOMUM Species *P. supraryfex*.

The various species of echinostomes have been reported from man and are regarded only as incidental parasitism the infection being obtained by the eating of raw fish or molluscan host or vegetation. The infection of man is confined to oriental countries and U.S.S.R.

Echinostoma ilocanum (Garrison, 1908) Odhner, 1911

(Garrison's fluke)

Garrison (1907) first discovered the eggs of the fluke in a native prisoner in Manila and obtained the adult worms after the administration of drug filix mas.

E. ilocanum is a small spinose trematode parasitising dogs of China and rats of the Philippines (Manila). Human cases are chiefly reported from ilocanan population of Luzon Province, the Philippines, Japan, China, Indonesia, Taiwan and India (Assam). The adult worm lives in the small intestine of the definitive host. The word 'echinostoma' means 'spiny mouth' which is characteristic feature of the worm. It is about 20 mm long and 2 mm wide. The larval stages are passed in two molluscan hosts; the cercariae liberated from the first host encyst in the second host. Eggs are similar to those of *F. buski* but smaller in size. Operculated eggs are 90 to 125 μm in length and 55 to 75 μm in breadth. Man is infected by ingesting metacercariae along with the second molluscan host. Definitive hosts are pigs, rats and other mammals and man. *Snails* and fresh water molluscs are two intermediate host. Mild infection in man is usually asymptomatic but heavy infection causes nausea, severe diarrhoea, abdominal pain, distension of abdomen. Diagnosis is done by detection of eggs in faeces. The distinctive features of eggs are dark brown colour and very immature larvae, even uncleaved zygotes that are unlike those of other intestinal trematodes. Paziquantel, albendazole, mebendazole, bithionol, hexylresorcinol, niclosamide easily cured the disease. Adult worms are recovered from faeces after treatment.

Other Species:

Echinostoma malayanum (Leiper, 1911): It is a common intestinal parasite of tribes living in the Sino-Tibetian frontier (Bare, 1930). It was first reported from Singapore and Kuala Lumpur, hence it is commonly called "Malayan Fluke".

Echinostoma revolutum (Forhlich, 1802): A parasite of ducks, geese and fowls (human infections are accidental) and *Emelis* (the Roumanian fluke).

Paryphostomum supraryfex (Lane, 1915) Bhalerao, 1931

(Lane's fluke)

It is an intestinal parasite of pigs in India, belonging to the family Echinostomatidae. Some cases have been reported from man in India. The clinical picture closely resembles that of fasciolopsiasis.

Suborder DISTOMATA: Superfamily OPISTHORCHIOIDEA

Eggs are very small, thick-shelled, operculated and when oviposited contain a fully developed miracidium which does not hatch in water but only after ingestion by the appropriate molluscan host which belongs to the genus Melania and Bythinia. Metacercariae in fish are the source of infection for the final host. It contains 2 families: (1) Family Opisthorchiidae and (2) Family Heterophyidae.

Family OPISTHORCHIIDAE

These are flat, transparent, medium-sized worms living in the biliary passages of fish-eating animals. Species infecting man are included in two genera:

1. Genus CLONORCHIS Looss, 1907. Species *C. sinensis*.
2. Genus OPISTHORCHIS Blanchard, 1895. Species *O. felineus*.

Clonorchis sinensis (Cobbold, 1875) Looss, 1907

Common Names: The Chinese liver fluke; Oriental liver fluke; "Distome of China".

McConnell (1875) discovered this parasite from the autopsy of a Chinese carpenter in the Calcutta Medical College Hospital. Details of the life cycle were worked out by Faust and Khaw (1927).

Geographical Distribution. A parasite of the Far East. The endemic areas include Japan, Korea, Formosa, Southern China, South Vietnam and North Vietnam.

Habitat. A common parasite of dog, cat, pig, rat and man. The adult worm lives in the biliary tract of the liver. Man is the principal defenetive host. Dog, cat, rat, pig are intermediate host & act as a reservoir of infection (Zoonotic aspect).

Morphology. Adult Worm. It is a narrow, oblong, flat worm with a somewhat pointed anterior. Its size varies greatly, measuring 10 to 25 mm in length by 2 to 3 mm in breadth. The oral sucker is slightly larger than the ventral sucker; the latter is at the junction of the anterior and the middle-third of the body. The blind intestinal caeca are simple and extend to the caudal region. The genital apparatus is the same as that of other Trematodes. The two testes are large, deeply branches and lie in the posterior third of the body, one behind the other.

Life span of the adult worm is 20 to 30 years.

EGGS. The characteristics of the *egg* are as follows:

  (i) Yellowish brown in colour (bile-stained), flask-shaped and operculated.
 (ii) Possesses a terminal hook-like spine (resembling an electric bulb).
(iii) Small in size, measuring 35 μm by 20 μm.
 (iv) When oviposited, it contains a ciliated embryo (miracidium).
  (v) Does not hatch in water but is ingested by its molluscan host.
 (vi) Does not float in saturated solution of common salt.
(vii) Infective to snails only.

Life Cycle. *C. sinensis* passes its life cycle (Fig. 142) in three hosts—one definitive host and two intermediate hosts.

Definitive Hosts. Man, dog, cat, pig. Adult worms in the biliary tract of the liver.

Intermediate Host. Where the larval development proceeds.

FIRST INTERMEDIATE HOST. A snail of the subfamily *Buliminae (Bithyniinae)*.

SECOND INTERMEDIATE HOST. A cyprinoid fish.

Eggs containing miracidia are passed with the faeces of definitive hosts and on entering into water, are ingested by the appropriate molluscan host. The miracidium hatches out in the mid-gut of the snail, penetrates its intestinal wall and enters the vascular spaces where it passes through the stages of sporocyst, redia and cercaria, the complete development taking about three weeks' time. The mature cercariae escape from the snail into water and after a brief period of free-swimming existence, attack certain fresh-water fish of the family *Cyprinidae*. The cercariae cast off their tails and encyst in the scale or in the flesh of the fish. These encysted eercariae (metacercariae or adolescariae) when ingested by definitive hosts, excyst in the duodenum. They then attach themselves to the mucosa in the region of the common bile duct, make their way through the ampulla of Vater and migrate to the distal biliary passages of the liver where they settle down and attain maturity in about one month's time.

Pathogenicity. MODE OF INFECTION. Man acquires the infection by eating raw, inadequately cooked, dried, salted or pickled fresh-water fish, harbouring the metacercariae (adolescariae) of *C. sinensis*. It causes the disease clonorchiasis.

Infecting Agent—Metacercariae in fish flesh.

Portal of Entry—Alimentary canal.

Site of Localisation—Biliary tract of the liver.

The immature worm while travelling upwards along the bile duct with the help of the suckers, often causes trauma to the bile duct epithelium. The main pathological changes are therefore confined to the wall of the bile duct and consist of the following:

 (1) Epithelial hyperplasia followed by adenomatous tissue formation. In chronic infection there is less adenomatous tissue but marked connective tissue formation.
 (2) Blood vessels of peribiliary plexus are increased in number and congested.

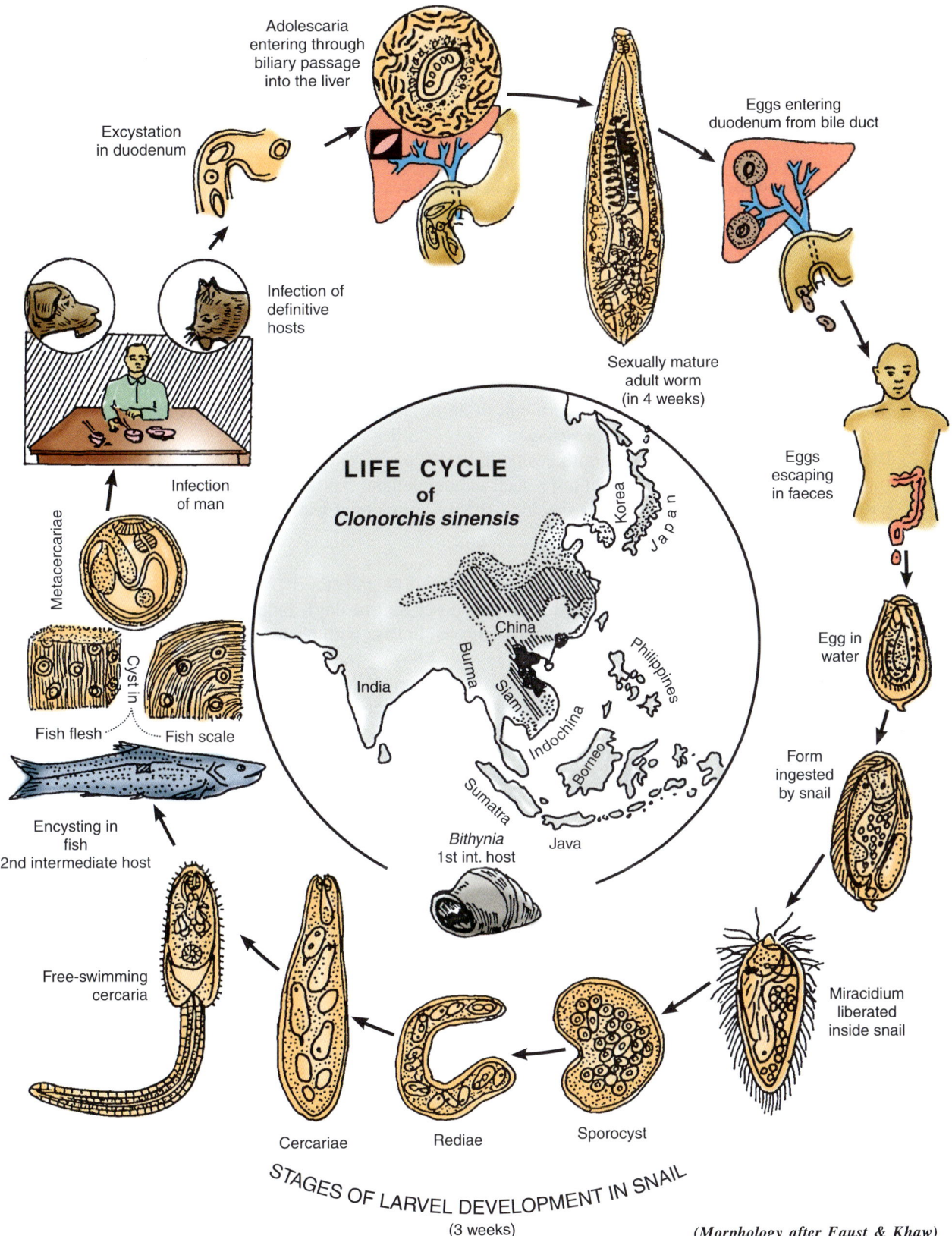

Adolescaria
entering through
biliary passage
into the liver

Excystation
in duodenum

Eggs entering
duodenum from bile duct

Sexually mature
adult worm
(in 4 weeks)

Infection of
definitive
hosts

Infection
of man

Eggs
escaping
in faeces

Metacercariae

Egg in
water

Cyst in

Fish flesh   Fish scale

Form
ingested
by snail

Encysting in
fish
2nd intermediate host

Free-swimming
cercaria

Miracidium
liberated
inside snail

Cercariae   Rediae   Sporocyst

**LIFE CYCLE
of
Clonorchis sinensis**

Korea

Japan

China

Burma

India

Siam

Indochina

Philippines

Borneo

Sumatra   Java

Bithynia
1st int. host

STAGES OF LARVEL DEVELOPMENT IN SNAIL

(3 weeks)

(Morphology after Faust & Khaw)

Fig. 142

(3) In uncomplicated cases there is no cellular infiltration.

(4) The adjacent liver tissue does not show any significant change and Hou Pao-chang* (1955) basing his observation on 500 necropsy cases stated that there was no direct relationship between *Clonorchis sinensis* infection and multilobular cirrhosis of the liver.

The worm lives on protein and glucose of blood in peribiliary plexus and on mucus secreted by the epithelial cells of the bile duct. Hence, the above changes help the worm to receive its nutrition from the host.

Adult worm cannot reach the gall bladder unless the cystic duct is dilated, but once it enters the gall bladder, it cannot survive. Live worms have however been found in the pancreatic duct.

With heavy infection, the disease is characterised by chronic diarrhoea, pain in right hypochondrium, hepatomegaly and recurring attacks of jaundice. The worms cause blocking of the biliary passage leading to stagnation of bile which favours bacterial infection and ultimately causes death of the worm. Complications that may develop during the course of the disease are infection (cholangitis), intra-hepatic calculi formation and cholangiocarcinoma or anaplastic carcinoma, resembling a primary liver cell carcinoma.

Diagnosis. This is based on the following:

1. Demonstration of eggs by a microscopical examination of faeces or aspirated bile. Keto thick smear, Stoll's dilution or quantitative formalin ether acetate concentration technique are used to detect moderate to heavy infections. The eggs of *C. sinensis* are difficult to be differentiated from those of *Heterophyes heterophyes*, *Metagonimus yokagawai* and *Opisthorchis* species.
2. Blood examination—Leucocytosis with eosinophilia (40 p.c).
3. Immunodiagnosis. (a) By serological tests, such as complement fixation test, gel precipitation tests, indirect haemagglutination test (sensitive and specific), (b) By intradermal test, an immediate hypersensitivity type of reaction.
4. Faecal antigen detection by ELISA.
5. Ultrasonography reveals enlarged gall bladder with sludge or gall stone.

Treatment. Praziquantel (75 mg/kg/day in three divided doses for one day), and albendazole (10 mg/kg/day for 7 days) have been found to be effective remedy for clonorchiasis. In case with obstructive jaundice, surgical intervention may be necessary.

Prophylaxis. The measures include (i) prevention of pollution of water with human night-soil and faeces of reservoir hosts (dog and cat), (ii) eradication of snail hosts, and (iii) checking the habit of eating raw fish.

Opisthorchis felineus (Rivolta, 1884) Blanchard, 1895
(The cat liver fluke)

The internal structure of the parasite is the same as that of Clonorchis except that the testes are not branched. The parasite inhabits the biliary and pancreatic passages of its host. The reservoir hosts are cat, dog, fox and pig (zoonotic aspect). It is a common fluke infection of man in Prussia, Poland and Siberia; it has also been reported from Japan, but not from endemic areas of Clonorchis infection. Chandler found that 60 per cent of cats in Calcutta (India) were infected with the parasite and human cases have also been reported from India. The life cycle and other features are the same as those of *C. sinensis*. Praziquantel (75 mg/kg/day in three divided doses for one day orally) and other drug albendazole (100 mg/kg in two divided doses for three days orally) are used for the treatment of the disease.

Other species:

(i) *Opisthorchis viverrini* (Poirier, 1886) Stiles and Hassall, 1896. This is an important human infection in Thailand. The normal host is the civet cat (*Felis viverrus*). It is distinguished from *O. felineus* by the greater proximity of its ovary and testis and few clusters of "*Vitellaria*". During early phase of heavy infection, diarrhoea, pain in the right hypochondrium and mild jaundice may be encountered. Periportal fibrosis of liver, inflammation of biliary canaliculi with epithelial hyperplasia develop in chronic stage of illness. *O. viverrini* has been linked to bile duct carcinoma.

(ii) *Opisthorchis noverca* Braun, 1902. This has been recovered from Pariah dog and pig in India as also from man.

Family HETEROPHYIDAE

These are small egg-shaped flukes which are normally parasite in the intestinal tract of fish-eating animals (man, cats and dogs). Species infecting man are included in two genera:

---

*Hou Pao-chang (1955). *J. Path. & Bact.,* **70**, 53-64.

1. Genus HETEROPHYES Cobbold, 1866. Species *H. heterophyes*.
2. Genus METAGONIMUS Katsurada, 1912. Species *M. yokogawai*.

Because of their similarity, the species of Heterophyes, Metagonimus, Haplorchis and Carneophallus have been grouped under the term "Heterophyids" and they may cause disease in man.

Heterophyes heterophyes (Siebold, 1855) Stiles and Hassall, 1900
Common Name: Von Siebold's fluke.

Geographical Distribution. A common parasite of Egypt. It is also found in Palestine and in the Far East.

Habitat. The adult worm lives in the middle of the small intestine of definitive hosts.

Morphology. It is the smallest fluke, measuring less than 2 mm in length by 0.3 to 0.4 mm in breadth. It is flattened dorso-ventrally with a narrow anterior and a rounded posterior. A sucker surrounds the genital pore which opens postero-laterally near the acetabulum. Eggs are minute (30 μm by 16 μm) operculated bodies, oval and coloured light-brown; when oviposited each of them contains a fully developed miracidium. The *life span* of the adult worm is about 2 months.

Life Cycle. The *definitive hosts* are cat, dog, wolf, fox and man. The *molluscan host* in Egypt is a marine and brackish-water snail, *Pirenella conica*. The miracidium passes through the sporocysts and one or two generations in the rediae stage from which ultimately the cercariae are developed. These cercariae encyst under the scales and in the flesh of mullets (*Mugil cephalus*), the *second intermediate host*. On ingestion of these raw mullets, definitive hosts become infected.

Pathogenicity and Clinical Features. Infection with *H. heterophyes* causes a disease in man called heterophyiasis. The worm lives in the intestinal canal (lying on the surface of the mucous membrane) and may give rise to colicky pains and mucous diarrhoea. At times, the worm invades the tissues and may remain imprisoned. The eggs in these cases do not come out in the faeces but are carried by the lymphatics or blood vessels to distant organs (cardiac valves and brain) giving rise to unusual manifestations.

Diagnosis. This is based on the finding of eggs in the stool. The differentiation between the species of heterophyes, clonorchis and opisthorchis by egg is extremely difficult.

Treatment. Drug used is praziquantel (20 mg/kg/day for 3 days).

Prophylaxis. Avoidance of eating of raw or uncooked fish (mullets) in endemic areas.

Metagonimus yokogawai Katsurada, 1912
Common Name: Yokogawa's fluke.

Geographical Distribution. Far East (Korea, Formosa, Japan and China), Siberia, Balkan States and Egypt.

Habitat. The adult worm lives in the small intestine of the definitive host.

Morphology. It is a very minute worm, measuring 2 mm in length by 0.5 mm in breadth. The acetabulum is displaced laterally to the right side of the middle line. The common genital pore lies in a pit anterior to the acetabulum. The eggs are indistinguishable from those of *H. heterophyes*.

Life Cycle. The *definitive hosts* are man, pig, dog, cat and the pelican. The snails serving as the *first intermediate host* are species of *Melania* in which the miracidium passes through the stages of sporocyst and two generations of rediae from which lophocercus cercariae emerge. The *second intermediate host* is a fresh-water fish, *Plectoglossus altivelis* in whose flesh cercariae become encysted. Infection of the definitive hosts results from the ingestion of raw flesh of these fish.

Pathogenicity and Clinical Features. The parasite causes in man the disease called metagonimiasis. The usual clinical manifestation is a mild diarrhoea.

Diagnosis. Based on the finding of characteristic eggs in stools. Species diagnosis can only be made, if the adult worms are obtained, after treatment.

Treatment and Prophylaxis. Same as that of *H. heterophyes*.

Suborder DISTOMATA
Superfamily PLAGIORCHIDEA

Adults are parasitic in carnivorous animals and reside in the lungs. The worm possesses integumentary spines and an excretory vesicle which is tubular or Y-shaped. The genital pore lies behind the acetabulum and the cirrus sac is absent. The vitellaria are highly developed and occupy the whole of the lateral fields. The miracidia are without eye spots. Larval development occurs in two intermediate hosts, the first a snail and the second, a crustacean. Cercariae have knob-like tails and oral stylets.

GENUS PARAGONIMUS Braun, 1899. Species *P. westermani*.

Paragonimus westermani (Kerbert, 1878) Braun, 1899

Common Names: The Oriental lung fluke, the lung distome.

Geographical Distribution. Far East, especially in Japan, Korea, Formosa and China; in India, reported from Bengal, Assam and South India. Also reported from Nepal and some parts of Africa and South America. There are two types of *Paragonimus westermani* in Asia today. One is with triploid chromosomes and other is diploid chromosomes. The former distributes mainly in Japan and Formosa and latter is found in other parts of Asia.

Habitat. Adult worms live in the respiratory tract (lungs) of man.

Morphology. ADULT WORM. It is thick, fleshy and egg-shaped. Its anterior end is slightly broader than the posterior end. It measures 8 to 12 mm in length by 4 to 6 mm in breadth and 3 to 5 mm in thickness. The ventral sucker is situated near about the middle of the body. The excretory vesicle is large and extends from the posterior extremity to the anterior region, dividing the body into two equal halves. The two blind intestinal caeca are unbranched and extend to the caudal region. The genital apparatus follows the same general pattern of Trematodes.

Life span of the adult worm is about 6 to 7 years.

EGGS. These are golden brown in colour, oval in shape and are provided with flattened opercula. They measure 80 μm by 55 μm and each egg contains an unsegmented ovum surrounded by yolk cells.

Life Cycle. *P. westermani* passes its life cycle (Fig. 143) in three hosts—one definitive host and two intermediate hosts.

Definitive Hosts. Man and domestic animals. Usual hosts in Asia are the tiger and the leopard. Feline hosts serve as reservoirs of infection.

Intermediate Hosts. FIRST HOST. A fresh-water snail of the genus *Melania**

SECOND HOST. A fresh-water crayfish or a crab.

The adult worms live in the respiratory tract of definitive hosts. The eggs generally escape in the sputum and some are eliminated in the faeces. In water, a ciliated embryo (miracidium) develops inside the egg in 2 to 7 weeks' time. On attaining maturity, the miracidium escapes into water and swims about in search of its snail host, a species of the genus *Melania*. Inside the soft tissue of the snail, the miracidium casts off its tail and passes through the stages of sporocyst and two generations of rediae being finally transformed into cercariae, the whole cycle taking about 10 to 12 weeks. The mature cercariae escape from the snail into water and enter into its second intermediate host, a fresh-water crab or a crayfish. Inside the crustacean host, they become encysted in the viscera, muscles and gills.

When the raw flesh of an infected crab or crayfish is eaten by man and other susceptible hosts, the cyst-wall is dissolved by the gastric juice and the adolescaria is released in the duodenum. These young worms penetrate the wall of the small intestine and enter the abdominal cavity. Later, they migrate upwards, piercing through the diaphragm and the two layers of the pleura, to gain entrance into the lungs where they finally settle and grow to sexual maturity (taking a period of two weeks for such migration). Eggs are discharged into a bronchiole and are coughed out with the sputum. The cycle is thus repeated.

Pathogenicity and Clinical Features. Infection with *P. westermani* is known as paragonimiasis.

MODE OF INFECTION. Eating of raw or improperly cooked flesh of an infected crab or crayfish. Strips of raw crab meat soaked in alcohol, k.a., "drunken crab" is a popular delicacy in China.

Infecting Agent—Metacercaria or adolescaria inside a cyst.

Portal of Entry—Digestive tract.

Site of Localisation—Lungs.

Pathology. The adult worm, as it moves around, causes lesions (worm cysts and "burrows") by mechanical damage. The eggs also excite a foreign body granulomatous reaction which may soften to form cavities, the wall of which is composed of fibrous granulation tissue (epitheloid cells, lymphocytes, plasma cells, eosinophils, giant cells and fibroblasts).

Clinical manifestation. This may be divided into 2 groups: Pulmonary and Extrapulmonary paragonimiasis.

---

*The optimum snail host is *Semisulcospira libertina* (Syn. *Melania libertina*).

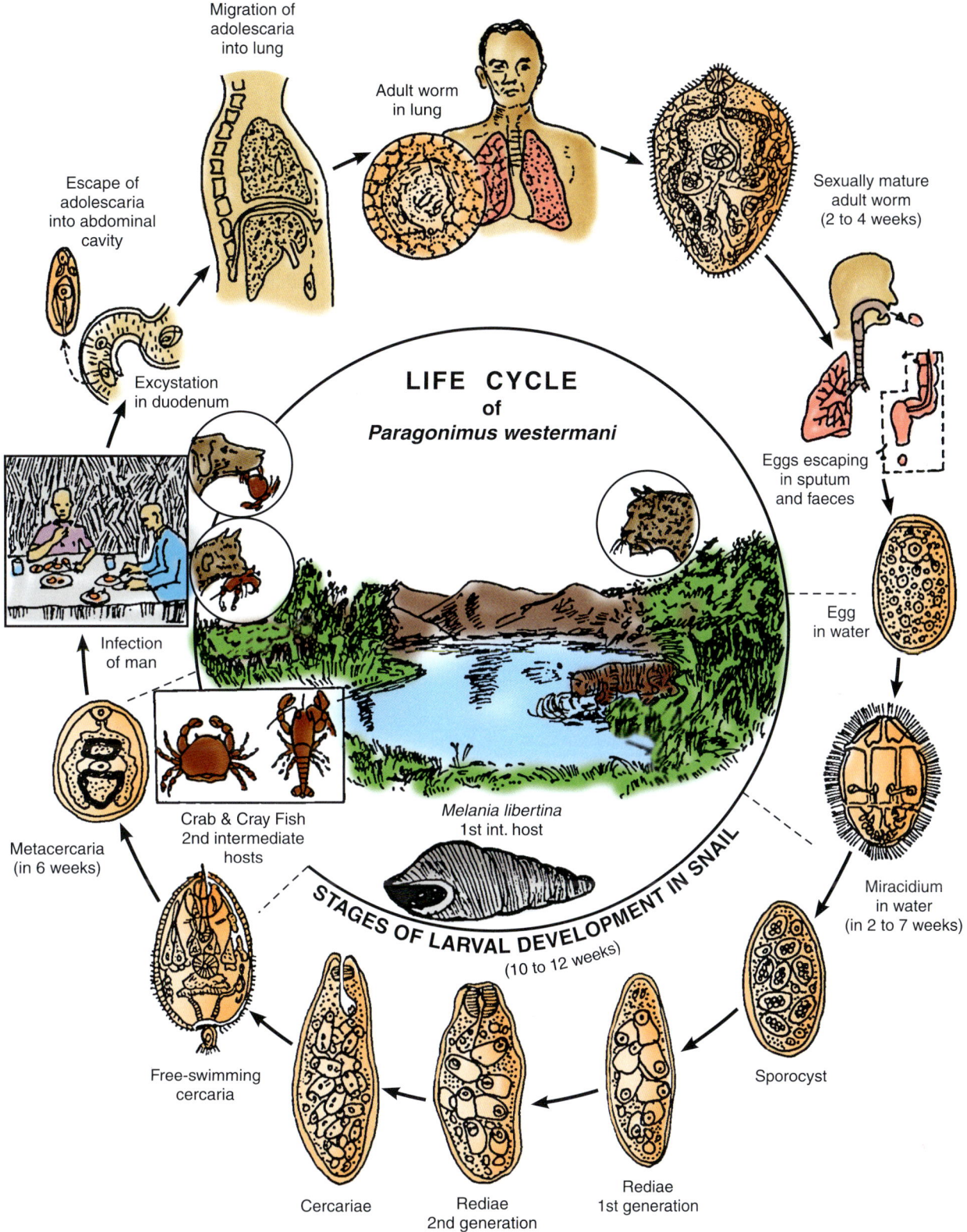

LIFE CYCLE
of
Paragonimus westermani

Migration of adolescaria into lung

Adult worm in lung

Sexually mature adult worm (2 to 4 weeks)

Escape of adolescaria into abdominal cavity

Excystation in duodenum

Eggs escaping in sputum and faeces

Egg in water

Infection of man

Miracidium in water (in 2 to 7 weeks)

Crab & Cray Fish 2nd intermediate hosts

Melania libertina 1st int. host

Metacercaria (in 6 weeks)

STAGES OF LARVAL DEVELOPMENT IN SNAIL (10 to 12 weeks)

Sporocyst

Free-swimming cercaria

Cercariae

Rediae 2nd generation

Rediae 1st generation

(Morphology after Looss, Belding & Cheng)

Fig. 143

The symptoms of pulmonary paragonimiasis are chronic cough with recurring attacks of haemoptysis, simulating a case of bronchiectasis or pulmonary tuberculosis.

Extrapulmonary paragonimiasis. Although the lung is the normal site of localisation for the young parasite, it can enter any organ of the body, such as liver, intestine, peritoneum and other organs. The clinical manifestations in these cases depend on the organs involved. In case of abdominal organs, the symptoms include pain in the abdomen, diarrhoea and enlargement of the liver. In cerebral infection, Jacksonian type of epilepsy and other symptoms, characteristic of brain tumour develop and may even terminate fatally. In generalised paragonimiasis, there is fever, generalised lymphadenitis and cutaneous ulceration.

Diagnosis. This is determined by the presence of the characteristic eggs in the sputum when examined under the microscope. Eggs have also been detected in the stool, gastric washing or tissue material.

Immunodiagnosis. An intradermal test carried out with a saline extract of adult *P. westermani* or other suitable antigen gives an immediate sensitivity reaction in infected persons. It remains positive long after recovery, thereby indicating past infection. A positive complement fixation test has also been used for the diagnosis and indicates an active infection.

IHA and ELISA tests (highly sensitive) are available. The tests become negative within 3-4 months after successful treatment.

Chest X-ray reveals abnormal shadows (nodular, cystic and infiltrative) in the middle and lower lung fields similar to pulmonary tuberculosis, whereas the presence of shadows of tunnels and "burrows" in the lung bases resemble bronchiectasis. CT scan of chest also helps in diagnosis of pulmonary lesions.

Treatment. Praziquantel (75 mg/kg/day in three divided doses for 2 days, orally) and niclofan (as a single oral dose of 2 mg/kg) have both been used for treatment of paragonimiasis. Bithionol, a dichlorophenol derivative (30-50 mg/kg on alternate day for 15 days has been found by Yokogawa and De Jongh (1961) to give encouraging results.

Prophylaxis. The measures include (i) disinfection of the sputum and faeces, (ii) eradication of molluscan host and (iii) avoidance of the consumption of raw, freshly salted or inadequately cooked crabs and crayfish as food.

CHAPTER VIII

PHYLUM NEMATHELMINTHES

Class NEMATODA

General Characters

1. The nematodes are unsegmented worms without any appendage. They are elongated and cylindrical or fili-form in appearance; both ends are often pointed.
2. The *sizes* show a great variation, the smallest (*T. spiralis* and *S. stercoralis*) measures less than 5 mm and the largest (*D. medinensis*) measures up to 1 metre.
3. The *body* is covered with a tough cuticle.
4. The worm possesses a *body cavity* in which the various organs, such as the digestive and genital systems, float. Excretory and nervous systems are rudimentary.
5. The *alimentary canal* is complete, consisting of an oral aperture, mouth cavity, oesophagus, intestine and a sub-terminal anus. The mouth cavity, when present, may have teeth or cutting plates; in other cases, where the mouth cavity is absent, the oral aperture is directly continuous with the oesophagus.
6. The nematodes of man are all diecious helminths, i.e., the sexes are separate. The male is generally smaller than the female and its posterior end is curved or coiled ventrally.

Reproductive System (Fig. 144)

The *male genital system* consists of a long convoluted tube which can be differentiated into testis, vas deferens, seminal vesicle and ejaculatory duct. The genital duct forms a common passage with the intestine and is known as cloaca. Accessory copulatory organs such as spicule and gubernaculum, are also present.

The *female genital system* consists of a single or double con-voluted tubes. Each part of the tube is differentiated into ovary, oviduct, seminal receptacle, uterus, vagina and vulva. The female genital pore opens either in the middle of the body or near

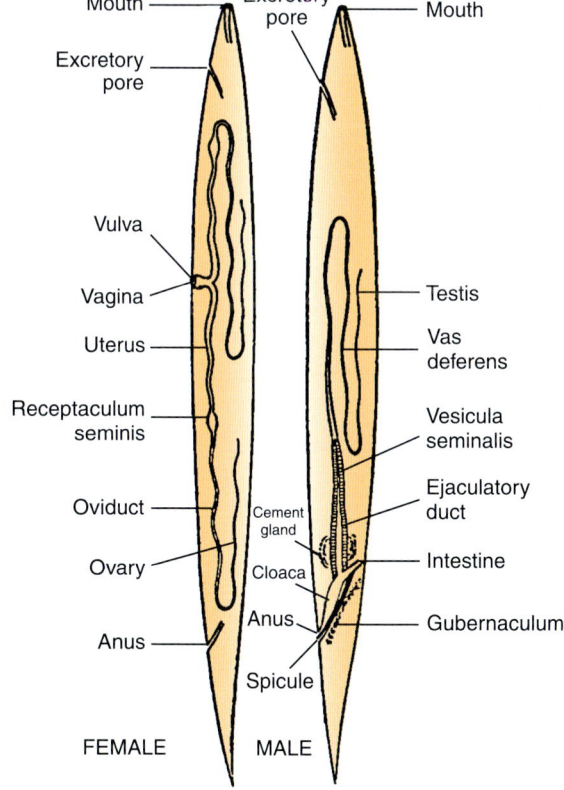

Fig. 144–Reproductive system of a Nematode.

the mouth. Where the female genital system has two tubes, the two unite into a common duct, vagina, before terminating in the genital pore.

The female nematodes may be divided as follows:

(1) *Viviparous,* giving birth to larvae; examples are *D. medinensis, W. bancrofti, B. malayi* and *T. spiralis.*

(2) *Oviparous,* laying eggs; examples are *A. lumbricoides, T. trichiura* (laying unsegmented eggs), *A. duodenale* and *N. americanus* (laying eggs with segmented ovum), *E. vermicularis* (laying eggs containing larvae).

(3) *Ovo-viviparous,* laying eggs containing larvae which are immediately hatched out; example is *S. stercoralis.*

Life Cycle. Man is the optimum host for all the nematode parasites. They pass their life cycle in one host except the superfamilies *Filarioidea* and *Dracunculoidea,* where two hosts are required. In *Filarioidea,* the second host is an insect vector in which the larval development takes place. In *Dracunculoidea,* cyclops constitutes the second host for the growth of its larva.

In cases where the nematodes choose one host, they localise in the intestinal tract and start developing. The eggs in these cases come out of the body and undergo certain developmental changes before they can enter a new host.

In the case of *T. spiralis,* pig is the optimum host and man represents the alternative host but the worm passes both its adult and larval stages in the same host.

Modes of Infection of Nematode Parasites

1. By ingestion of: (a) Embryonated *eggs* contaminating food and drink, as in *A. lumbricoides, E. vermicularis* and *T. trichiura.* (b) Growing embryos in an intermediate host (infected cyclops), as in *D. medinensis.* (c) Encysted embryos in infected pig's flesh, as in *T. spiralis.*

2. By penetration of the skin: The filariform larvae boring through the skin, as in *A. duodenale, N. americanus* and *S. stercoralis.*

3. By blood-sucking insects, as in the parasites belonging to the superfamily *Filarioidea.*

4. By inhalation of infected dust containing embryonated eggs, as in *A. lumbricoides* and *E. vermicularis.*

Larval Stages of Nematodes Normally Parasitic in Lower Animals Infecting Man

DEFINITIVE HOST	ADULT WORM	HABITAT	INFECTION	DISEASE
Hookworms of dogs and cats	*Ancylostoma braziliense* and *A. caninum*	Small intestine	Filariform larva entering skin	Custaneous larva migrans
Ascarids of dogs and cats	*Toxocara canis* and *T. cati*	Small intestine	Eggs ingested	Visceral larva migrans and granulomatous ophthalmitis
Ascarids of sea mammals	*Anisakis marina*	Small intestine	Ingestion of larva in marine fish	Eosinophilic granuloma of bowel
Rat lungworm	*Angiostrongylus cantonensis*	Pulmonary artery	Ingestion of 3rd stage larvae in molluscs or carrier hosts	Eosinophilic meningoencephalitis
Spiruroid worm of dogs and cats	*Gnathostoma spinigerum*	Tumour of the stomach wall	Ingestion of 3rd stage larvae in 2nd intermediate host, fish	Cutaneous larva migrans, cerebral and ocular gnathostomiasis
Filarial worms of dogs and cats	*Brugia pahangi*	Lymphatics	Bite of an infected insect vector	Tropical pulmonary eosinophilia

Classification of Nematodes

(A) According to Habitat of Adult Worms

I. INTESTINAL	II. SOMATIC (Inside the Tissues and Organs)	
Small Intestine Only	Lymphatic System	Mesentery
Ascaris lumbricoides (Common roundworm)	*Wuchereria bancrofti*	*Mansonella perstans*
Ancylostoma duodenale (The Old World hookworm)	*Brugia malayi*	*Mansonella ozzardi*
Necator americanus (American hookworm)	Subcutaneous Tissues	Conjunctiva
Strongyloides stercoralis	*Loa loa* (African eye worm)	*Loa loa.*
Trichinella spiralis (Trichina worm)	*Onchocerca volvulus*	
Capillaria philippinensis	*Dracunculus medinensis*	
Caecum and Vermiform Appendix	(Guinea worm)	
Enterobius vermicularis (Threadworm or pinworm)	Lungs	
Trichuris trichiura (Whipworm).	*Strongyloides stercoralis*	

(B) Systematic Classification of Nematodes

Class NEMATODA				
SUBCLASS	ORDER	SUPERFAMILY	GENUS	SPECIES
Aphasmidia (No caudal chemo-receptors)	Enoplida	Trichinelloidea	Trichinella Trichuris Capillaria	*T. spiralis* *T. trichiura* *C. philippinensis* *C. hepatica* *C. aerophilia*
Phasmidia (Having caudal chemo-receptors)	Rhabditida Strongylida	Rhabditoidea Strongyloidea	Strongyloides Ancylostoma Necator Oesophagostomum Ternidens	*S. stercoralis* *A. duodenale* *N. americanus* *O. apiostomum* *T. deminutus*
		Trichostrongyloidea Metastrongyloidea	Trichostrongylus Parastrongylus	*T. colubriformis* *P. cantonensis,* *P. costaricensis*
	Oxyurida Ascaridida	Oxyuroidea Ascaridoidea	Enterobius Ascaris Toxocara	*E. vermicularis* *A. lumbricoides* *T. canis* and *T. cati*
	Spirurida	Spirudoidea	Gnathostoma Anisakis	*G. spinigerum* *A. simplex*
		Filarioidea	Wuchereria Brugia	*W. bancrafti* *B. malayi* *B. timori*
			Onchocerca Mansonella	*O. volvulus* *M. perstans* *M. streptocerca* *M. ozzardi*
			Dirofilaria	*D. conjunctivae* *D. immitis*
			Loa	*L. loa*
		Dracunculoidea Spiruroidea	Dracunculus Thelazia	*D. medinensis* *T. cellipaeda*

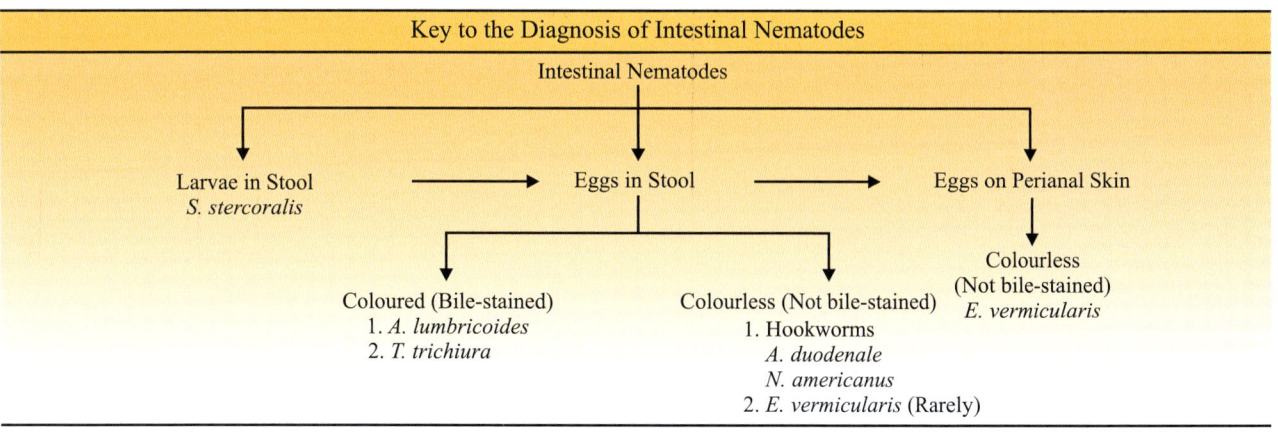

Key to the Diagnosis of Intestinal Nematodes

Intestinal Nematodes

Larvae in Stool → Eggs in Stool → Eggs on Perianal Skin
S. stercoralis

Coloured (Bile-stained)
1. *A. lumbricoides*
2. *T. trichiura*

Colourless (Not bile-stained)
1. Hookworms
   A. duodenale
   N. americanus
2. *E. vermicularis* (Rarely)

Colourless (Not bile-stained)
E. vermicularis

Terms Used in the Description of Nematodes

Cuticula. An outer hyaline, non-cellular layer forming the integument of nematodes.

Cervical Alae. Wing-like expansion of the cuticula near mouth.

Cervical Papillae. Protuberances of cuticula near oesophagus.

Buccal Capsule. When the oral aperture leads to a mouth cavity; it niay contain teeth or cutting organs.

Cloaca. A common passage in male nematodes where the rectum and the genital duct open.

Filariform Larva. The oesophagus is long compared to the length of the larva; its posterior end is not dilated like a bulb.

Rhabditiform Larva. The length of the oesophagus is short compared to the length of the larva and its posterior end is dilated like a bulb.

Gubernaculum. An elevation on the dorsal wall of cloaca which guides the spicule during copulation.

Spicule. Represents the accessory copulatory organ; it is rod-like and protrusible.

Copulatory Bursa (Bursa Copulatrix). An umbrella-like expansion of the cuticula surrounding the cloaca of the male nematode of certain species. It is supported by fleshy rays comparable with the ribs of umbrella.

Superfamily TRICHINELLOIDEA

The body of the worm is divided into two distinct parts, *viz.*, a hair-like or filiform anterior and a stout posterior. Oesophagus is more or less degenerate and consists of a narrow channel running through a column of large cells; intestine is cellular. The female possesses a single ovary. The superfamily contains three genera of medical importance.

1. Genus TRICHINELLA Railliet, 1895.   Species *T. spiralis.*
2. Genus TRICHURIS Roederer, 1761.   Species *T. trichiura.*
3. Genus CAPILLARIA Zeder, 1800.   Species *C. philippinensis.*

Trichinella spiralis (Owen, 1835) Railliet, 1895
Common Name: The trichina worm.

Geographical Distribution. Common in Europe and United States. Also reported from some parts of Africa, China and Syria. Natural human infection with this helminth has yet been reported from India*.

Habitat. It starts as an intestinal parasite, remaining buried in the duodenal or jejunal mucosa, where its adult life is passed but its stay there is relatively short. The fertilised female discharges embryos into the circulating blood which ultimately encyst in the striated muscles of the animal harbouring the adult worm, such as the pig, rat or man.

Morphology. ADULT WORM. It is one of the smallest nematodes infecting man. The *male* measures 1.4 to 1.6 mm in length with a diameter of 0.04 mm. The spicule and the copulatory sheath are lacking, but at the tail-end, there are two conspicuous conical papillae on either side. The *female* is much longer than the male, measuring 3 to 4 mm in length by 0.06 mm in breadth. The females are viviparous and discharge embryos instead of eggs.

LARVAE. These measure 100 µm by 6 µm. They remain encysted in the striated muscles (not cardiac or smooth muscle) of the host. Inside the cyst, the larva continues to develop up to the stage of sexual differentiation and when fully grown, it becomes ten times its original size, i.e., from 100 µm (0.1 mm) it increases to 1000 µm (1 mm) in length. The maximum size is attained by the 35th day. Usually, one larva is present in a single cyst.

Encapsulation of the larva begins about the 21st day and is completed within 3 months. A blunt ellipsoidal lemon-shaped sheath (0.4 by 0.25 mm) develops as a result of host-tissue reaction around the tightly coiled larva. The long axis of the capsule is parallel to that of the muscle fibre. Calcification occurs in course of 6 to 18 months, when it appears as a fine, opaque granule. The muscles heavily parasitised are diaphragm, intercostals, pectoralis major, deltoid, biceps and gastrocnemius. There may be a thousand trichinella larvae pey gramme of muscles.

Life span of the adult worm is very short. The male, after fertilising the female, dies, i.e., about one week after infection. The female also dies after about 16 weeks, the period required for discharging larvae. The majority of the larvae encysted in muscles die within 6 months but some may live for many years (10 to 31 years).

Life Cycle. The whole life cycle (Fig. 145A) is passed in one animal (pig, rat or man) but a transference of the host is required for the preservation of the species from extinction. Thus, although one individual animal serves both as definitive and intermediate host, two hosts are required to complete the life cycle. The parasite gaining entrance into

---

*The reports are available where trichinella larvae were found from animals in India (Maplestone & Bhaduri from Calcutta in 1942, Kalapasi & Rao from Bombay in 1966 and Schad & Chowdhury from Calcutta in 1965). In 1996, one human case has been reported from Punjab.

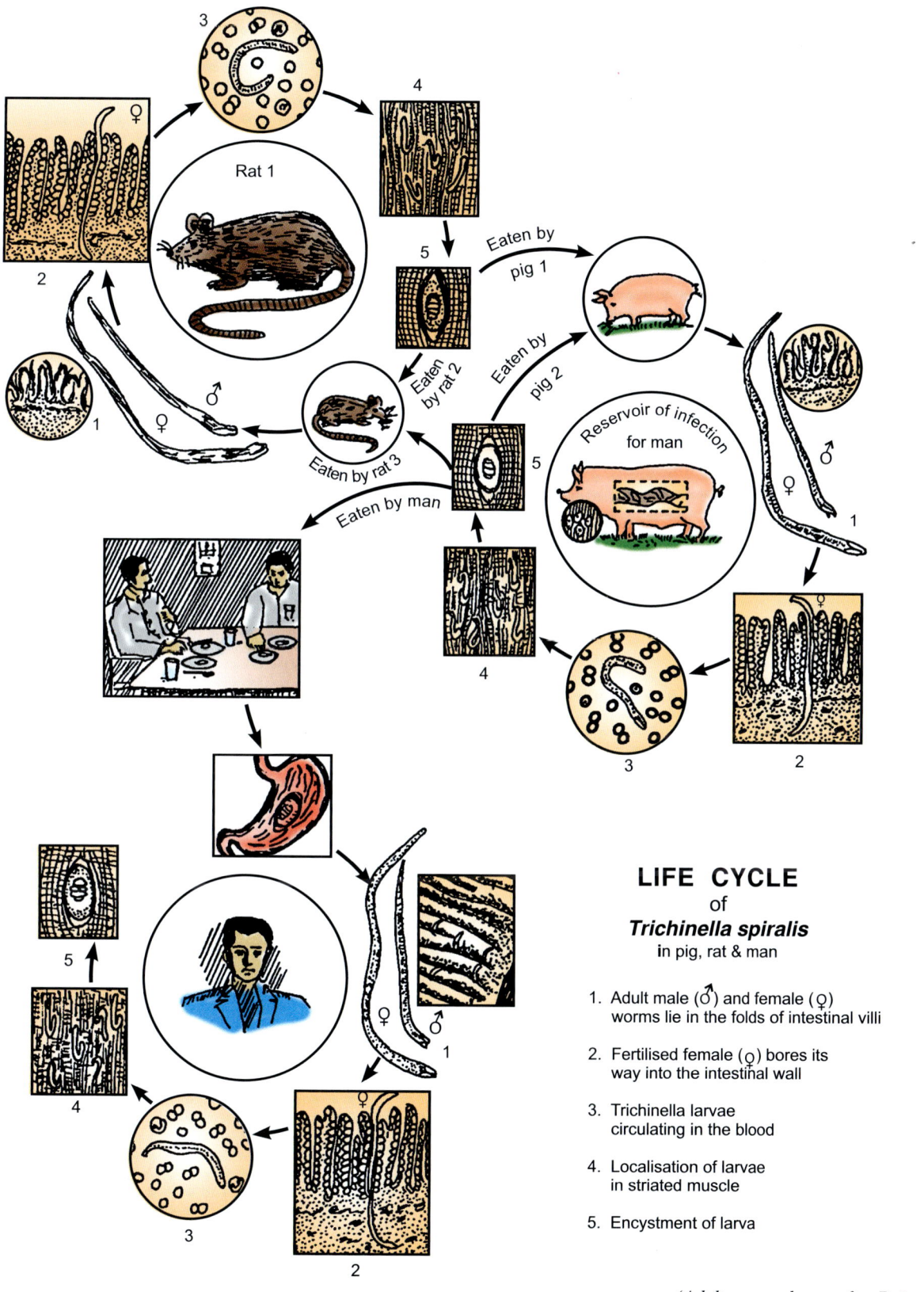

LIFE CYCLE
of
Trichinella spiralis
in pig, rat & man

1. Adult male (♂) and female (♀) worms lie in the folds of intestinal villi

2. Fertilised female (♀) bores its way into the intestinal wall

3. Trichinella larvae circulating in the blood

4. Localisation of larvae in striated muscle

5. Encystment of larva

(Adult worms drawn after Brümpt)

Fig. 145 A

man is unable to complete its life cycle. The continuance of the species, however, is maintained by other animals. The primary host of *T. spiralis* is the pig which serves as the reservoir host for man. Infection normally passes from pig to pig and rat, and from rat to rat. Infection of a new host is always brought about by ingestion of raw flesh of the trichinosed animal containing the viable encysted larvae. The course of development may be summarised as follows:

(a) Trichinella larvae remaining encysted in rat's muscle are eaten by a healthy rat.

(b) After ingestion, larvae (male and female) develop into adults in the intestine in a very short time (within 48 hours). Male and female worms become sexually mature. Fertilisation occurs and in another 24 hours larvae are liberated.

(c) Larvae gain entrance into the blood stream and encystment occurs in the muscles. They develop into adult worms only when they are taken up by another rat or a pig.

(d) When eaten by pigs, the same process of development occurs and larval encystment in muscle continues.

(e) Infected pig's muscle containing the larval trichinellae is eaten by man. The larvae, set free in the duodenum and jejunum, grow into adult worms and within 5 to 7 days become sexually mature. The male, after fertilising the female, dies. The fertilised female then burrows deeply into the mucosa of the intestine and discharges a large number of larvae (a total of about 1500) into the lymphatics or blood vessels; this process continues for a period of 4 to 16 weeks or as long as the mother worm is alive. The female dies after discharging her progeny. The larvae choose for their permanent abode the striated muscles where they undergo encystment. In man the cycle ends here.

Immunology. Two types of immunity, cellular and humoral, develop in trichinosis. Immunised mice when exposed to a challenging infection rapidly eliminate the adult worms by a process of cell-mediated immunity. Humoral antibodies developing in the course of infection are not protective but can be used for a serological diagnosis and for an immediate hypersensitive reaction of the skin to trichinella larvae (antigen). IgE fraction of serum gamma globulin is greatly increased.

Pathogenicity. MODE OF INFECTION. By ingestion of infected pig's flesh, raw or insufficiently cooked, containing the viable larvae.

Clinical Features. The clinical condition associated with *T. spiralis* infection in man is known as trichinelliasis (trichiniasis or trichinosis—Fig. 145B). The symptoms are grouped as follows:

1. *Stage of Intestinal Invasion* (Incubation). This is the period (5-7 days) during which the larvae grow into adult worms and the female begins to discharge larvae into the circulation. The symptoms are chiefly gastro-intestinal (nausea, vomiting, abdominal pain, loose motion or constipation).

2. *Stage of Larval Migration*. The invasion of muscles occurs from the 7th to the 10th day after infection, i.e., when the first batch of larvae are discharged and covers a period of 4 to 16 weeks. The manifestations are remittent temperature, urticarial rash, cutaneous symptom (sensation of worms crawling under the skin), subungual "splinter haemorrhages", oedema of the eyelids and face (Fig. 145B) myositis. There may be respiratory symptoms, bronchitis and bronchopneumonia, signs of myocarditis and protean neurological signs initiated by invading larvae. At this stage, there may be profound and at times fatal toxaemia.

3. *Stage of Encystation*. This occurs only in striated muscles while in other tissues they degenerate and are absorbed. The symptoms may clear up rapidly or disappear gradually as the larvae become encysted or may leave permanent injury.

Mortality rate is about 5%. Serous complication is granulomatous myocarditis which is manifested by congestive cardiac failure, and terminated by sudden death during 6th to 8th week of infection. Occasionally large arteries of brain or extremities are thrombosed.

Diagnosis. A correct diagnosis can only be achieved by demonstrating the trichinella larvae in the muscle obtained either from biopsy or autopsy. The following measures may be adopted:

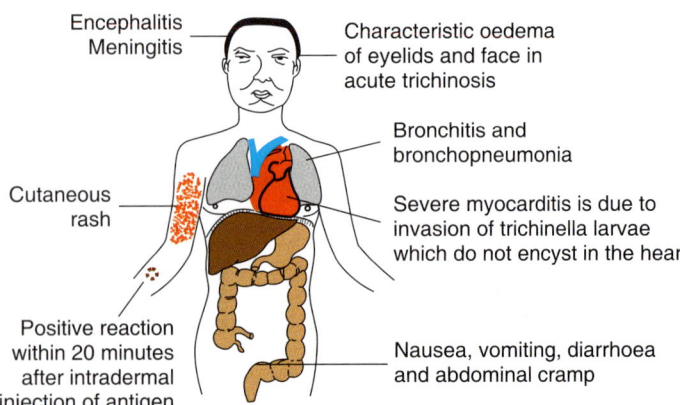

Fig. 145B—Features of trichinosis.

(i) *Stool* examination for adult worms or for larvae (rarely recovered).

(ii) *Blood* examination shows eosinophilic leucocytosis (eosinophils 15-50%).

(iii) Serological tests, such as complement fixation, precipitin and bentonite flocculation test. Recently an agglutination test with latex particles coated with *Trichinella* antigen has been introduced by Innella and Redner (1959). ELISA test is also available (by using antigen obtained from the infective stage larvae of *T. spiralis*). Bentonite flocculation test and complement fixation test become positive 3-4 week after infection.

A serological test based on staining with fluorescent antibody and using larvae from infected rats as antigens has been found to be specific for trichinosis. The reaction becomes positive about 48 days after infection (Sadun et al, 1962).

(iv) *Muscle Biopsy* (by 3rd or 4th week of infection). The excised tissue may be pressed flat between glass slides and examined under the low power of a microscope or the larvae may be demonstrated by digesting the excised muscle in artificial gastric juice. Suitable sites of biopsy are the tendinous insertions of deltoid or gastrocnemius muscle.

(v) *Xonodiagnosis*. Biopsy bits are fed to laboratory rat and killed after one month. The larvae can be demonstrated in the muscles of that killed rat.

(vi) *Skin Test*. Intradermal injection of 0.1 ml of 1 in 10,000 dilution of the Bachman's antigen (prepared from trichinella larvae obtained from infected rabbit's muscle) causes an immediate (within 15 to 20 minutes) erythematous patch. A positive test persists for 10-20 years.

(vii) *X-ray* examination may be of value if the cysts are calcified (represents old infection), but the worms are too small to be detected on an X-ray plate.

Treatment. Promising results have been obtained in the treatment of trichinosis by thiabendazole (in a dose of 25 mg/kg twice daily for one week) and alternative drug albendazole (400 mg twice daily for 8-15 days). Mebendazole (400 mg three times daily for two weeks) is also an effective drug. Corticosteroids have been found to be helpful in alleviating clinical symptoms.

Prophylaxis. The measures include (i) careful inspection of meat at slaughterhouse and (ii) avoidance of eating raw or imperfectly cooked pig's flesh.

Trichuris trichiura (Linnaeus, 1771) Stiles, 1901

Common Name: Whipworm.

Geographical Distribution. World-wide. Commoner in warm moist regions.

Habitat. The adult worm lives in the large intestine of man, particularly in the caecum; also in the vermiform appendix.

Morphology. ADULT WORM. In shape and general appearance the worm resembles a whip (Fig. 146), the anterior three-fifth is very thin and hair-like and the posterior two-fifth is thick and stout, resembling the handle of a whip. The worm lives in the large intestine (caecum) with the whole of its anterior portion embedded in the mucous membrane. The hair-like anterior extremity consists of a long oesophagus which is really a minute channel in a single column of large secretory cells. The thick posterior portion contains the intestine and sex organs. The adult worm may live in the human bowels for many years.

Male. It measures 3 to 4 cm in length. Its caudal extremity is coiled ventrally.

Female. It measures 4 to 5 cm in length. The caudal extremity is cither shaped like a "comma" or an arc. The worm is oviparous.

EGGS. The distinctive features (Fig. 147) of a *Trichuris* egg are as follows:

(i) Size about 50 μm in length by 25 μm in breadth.

(ii) Colour, brown (bile-stained); has a double shell, the outer one is bile-stained.

(iii) Barrel-shaped with a mucous plug at each pole.

(iv) Contains an unsegmented ovum when the egg leaves the human host.

(v) Floats in saturated solution of common salt.

The eggs when freshly passed are not infective to man.

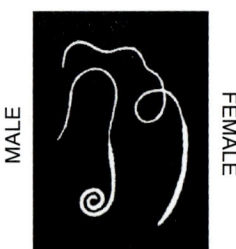

Fig. 146—*T. trichiura.*
(Natural size of adult worms)

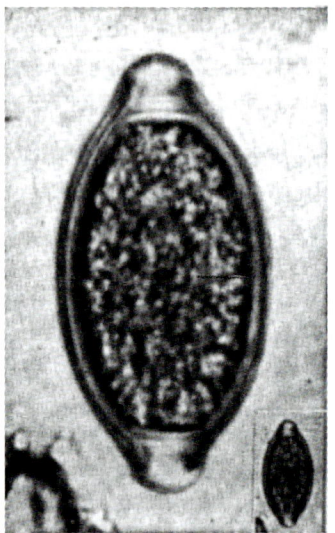

Fig. 147—**Eggs of** *T. trichiura.*
Inset : Size under high power

Life Cycle. No intermediate host is required. The worm passes its life cycle (Fig. 148) in one host, man. A change of host is necessary for the continuance of the species. The eggs come out of the human host with the faeces and the development proceeds slowly in water or damp earth, depending upon the environmental conditions. In tropical climates a rhabditiform larva develops within the egg in the course of 3 to 4 weeks. In temperate climates, the larva takes a long time (6 to 12 months) to complete its development. The embryonated eggs are infective to man.

Man is infected when the embryonated eggs are swallowed with food or water. The egg-shell is dissolved by the digestive juices and the larva emerges through one of the poles of the eggs. The liberated larvae pass down into the caecum, their site of localisation. They grow directly into adult worms and embed their anterior parts in the mucosa of the intestine. The worms become sexually mature within a month from the time of ingestion of the eggs and the gravid female begins to lay eggs. The cycle is then repeated.

Pathogenicity and Clinical Features. Infection with *T. trichiura* is known as trichuriasis. Usually the worms do not produce any pathogenic effect. The worms inhabiting the vermiform appendix may give rise to symptoms of acute appendicitis. In heavy infections the patient often complains of abdominal pain, mucous diarrhoea often with blood-streaked stool and loss of weight. Prolapse of rectum has occasionally been observed in massive trichuriasis.

Laboratory Diagnosis. This is established by the finding of characteristic eggs by a direct microscopical examination of a saline emulsion of the stool. Adult worms may occasionally be present in the stool. The degree of infection can be determined by egg count. Proctoscopy examination shows worm on the rectal mucosa in diarrhoea caused by parasite.

Treatment. The drugs at present available for the treatment of trichuriasis are thiabendazole and mebendazole (100 mg twice daily for 3 days). Albendazole (400 mg daily for three days) is also effective. Ivermectin (200 μg/kg) is also used in combination with albendazole (400 mg).

Prophylaxis. This includes (i) proper disposal of the night-soil and (ii) prevention of the consumption of un-cooked vegetables and fruits grown in native gardens.

Superfamily TRICHINELLOIDEA: Genus CAPILLARIA
Capillaria philippinensis (Chitwood et al, 1968)

The parasite was first discovered in 1963 from a fatal case in Philippines.

Geographical Distribution. It has been reported chiefly from the northern Philippines and the infection occurred in an epidemic form. The infection is now known to occur in Thailand, Indonesia, Japan, Iraq, Egypt and India.

Habitat. It is a nematode parasite inhabiting the mucosa of the small intestine, particularly jejunum.

Morphology. The adult worm measures 2 to 4 mm by 0.03 to 0.04 mm.

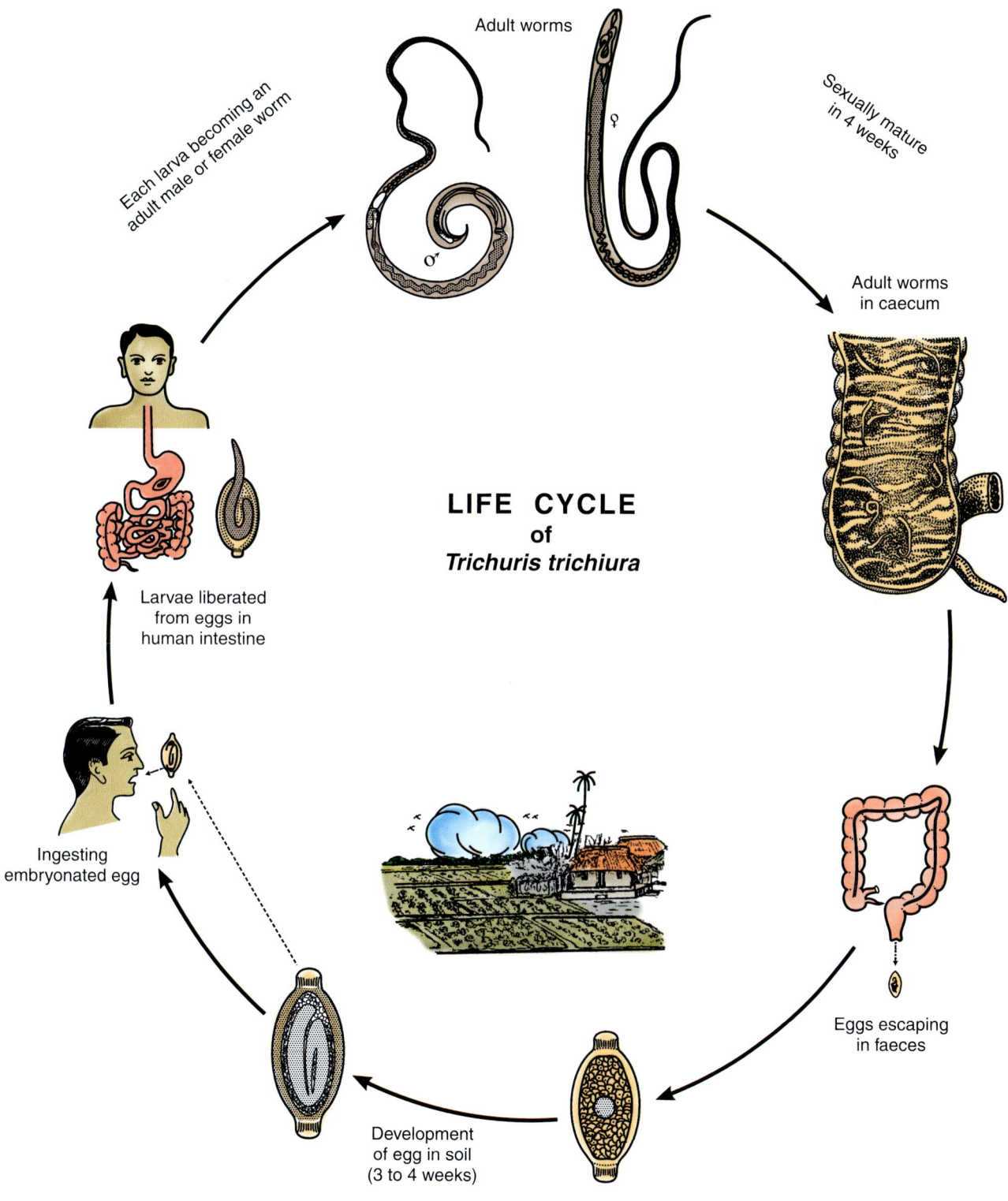

Adult worms

Each larva becoming an adult male or female worm

Sexually mature in 4 weeks

Adult worms in caecum

LIFE CYCLE
of
Trichuris trichiura

Larvae liberated from eggs in human intestine

Ingesting embryonated egg

Development of egg in soil (3 to 4 weeks)

Eggs escaping in faeces

Fig. 148

The eggs are similar to *Trichuris trichiura* but are smaller (45 × 21 μm), more oval with flattened and less prominent bipolar plugs. The differences between the eggs of *Capillaria philippinensis* and *Trichuris trichiura* are shown in the following table (Whalen *et al*, 1969; *Lancet*, **1**, 13).

Eggs	*C. philippinensis*	*T. trichiura*
Size	45 × 21 μm	52 × 26 μm
Shape	Peanut	Ellipse
Plugs	Bipolar, flattened	Bipolar, protuberant
Shell	Pitted	Smooth

Life Cycle. Auto-infection may be a part of the life cycle but how the man is originally infected remains unknown.

Pathogenesis. *Mode of Infection*. It is direct from man to man by the faecal-oral route. Crustaceans may act as paratenic or transport hosts.

Symptoms. The patient suffers from colicky abdominal pain, intestinal "gurgling" (borborygmi), chronic watery diarrhoea (8 to 10 voluminous watery stools), muscle wasting and oedema. These result from a protein-losing enteropathy and malabsorption of fats and sugars.

Tissue invasion similar to Strongyloides has been observed at post mortem examination.

The cause of malabsorption and protein-losing enteropathy may be related to the size of worm burden associated with derangement of intestinal function. Large numbers of organism attached to the mucosa derive nutrient from the interstitial fluid in the lamina propria and cause lymphatic obstruction.

Clinical Pathology. Fat analysis shows an increased excretion of fat (fatty acid). There is marked reduction of potassium and calcium level of the plasma.

Diagnosis. This is made by finding the characteristic eggs in the stool. The presence of Trichuris eggs may give a clue to detect Capillaria. The eggs of *Capillaria philippinensis* are similar to those of *Trichuris trichuria* but are smaller in size. Adults and larval forms are also found in the stool. Jejunal biopsy reveals adult worms embedded in the mucosa.

Treatment. The parasite may be eliminated with prolonged mebendazole (200 mg daily for 20 days) or albendazole (200 mg daily only for 10 days) therapy to prevent relapses.

Capillaria hepatica may infect man on rare occasions. It is recognised by finding the Trichuris-like eggs encapsulated in the liver. Cases have been reported from England, Nigeria and USA. First human case was reported in 1923 in a British soldier at autopsy in India.

Men are infected by ingestion of contaminated vegetables, fruits and water.

Diagnosis is made by demonstration of eggs in liver biopsy material.

Superfamily RHABDITOIDEA

A number of small worms with a peculiar life cycle, having parasitic and free-living existence. The oesophagus of parasitic female is a long cylindrical muscular tube with a posterior bulb containing valves; also possesses a prebulbar swelling. Females are ovo-viviparous.

Genus strongyloides Grassi, 1879. Species *S. stercoralis*.

Strongyloides stercoralis (Bavay, 1876) Stiles and Hassall, 1902

Geographical Distribution. World-wide. Common in Brazil, Far East (Cochin-China and Philippines) and Africa.

Habitat. The parasitic females live in the wall (mucous membrane) of the small intestine of man, especially in the duodenum and jejunum. They can be demonstrated post-mortem by examining scrapings of the mucosa, under low power of the microscope.

Morphology. Adult Worm. In the parasitic phase, the females are readily discovered but not the males.

The *parasitic females* are hardly visible to the naked eye; they measure 2.5 mm in length by 40 to 50 μm in breadth. The cylindrical muscular oesophagus extends through the anterior third of the body and the intestine extends through the posterior two-thirds. The anus opens mid-ventrally, a short distance in front of the caudal tip. The posterior extremity is pointed. The vulval opening is at the junction of the middle and posterior thirds of the body. The paired genitalia extend at right angles from the vulva, one set being disposed anteriorly and the other set posteriorly. The females are ovo-viviparous.

The *parasitic males*, as described by Kreis, are shorter and broader than the females. They resemble the males of free-living sexual generation, except for their conspicuous buccal cavity. They have no penetrating power and remain parasitic in the lumen of the bowel. The parasitic males were discovered only by Kreis (1932) but others have so far failed to demonstrate them.

Eggs. In the gravid female, the eggs are conspicuous within its body, lying antero-posteriorly in a single file (5 to 10 eggs in each uterus). The eggs measure about 55 μm in length by 30 μm in breadth; they are thin-shelled, transparent and oval. They contain larvae ready to hatch. As soon as the eggs are laid, the rhabditiform larvae start hatching and bore their way out of the mucous membrane into the lumen from where they are passed in the faeces. Hence, it is the larvae and not the eggs which are found in the human faeces.

Larvae. Two types of larvae are found:

(*a*) rhabditiform larvae and (*b*) filariform larvae.

Rhabditiform Larvae. These are developed directly from the gravid females and are found in the lumen of the bowel. They measure 200 to 250 μm in length by 16 μm in breadth; they have short mouth and double-bulb oesophagus. The course of development of these larvae are as follows:

(i) While in the lumen of the bowel, they are metamorphosed into filariform larvae (often facilitated by steroid therapy). These may penetrate the intestinal epithelium, thus providing internal reinfection. If the larvae are carried down the bowel, they may be voided with the faeces and during transit some may penetrate the perianal and perineal skin without leaving the host and going through a soil phase again, thus providing a source of auto-infection (hyperinfection). This explains the heavy worm loads in some individuals and also the persistence of infection (20 to 30 years) in persons who have left endemic areas.

(ii) The rhabditiform larvae may be voided with the faeces and may undergo development in the soil—Direct (host-soil-host) and Indirect cycle.

(a) Indirect (heterogenetic) Development. The rhabditiform larvae mature in course of 24 to 30 hours into free-living sexual generations, males (0.7 mm) and females (1 mm). Copulation between the sexes takes place, resulting in the production of a second batch of rhabditiform larvae which are indistinguishable from those produced by the parasitic females. In 3 to 4 days' time, they are transformed into filariform larvae. Each pair from the first batch of rhabditiform larvae gives rise to 30 filariform larvae.

(b) Direct Development. In this type, the rhabditiform larvae directly metamorphose, in 3 to 4 days' time, into filariform larvae, the sexual phase being omitted. In this cycle, each rhabditiform larva gives rise to only one filariform larva.

Filariform Larvae. These are longer and more slender than the rhabditiform larvae. They have short mouths and cylindrical oesophagus. They constitute the infective stage and enter the body of the human host through the skin, in the same manner as ancylostomes. As already stated they are developed in the following ways:

   (i) Metamorphosed in the human bowel from the first batch of rhabditiform larvae.

  (ii) Rhabditiform larvae voided with the faeces directly metamorphosed into filariform larvae in the soil. It occurs in temperate climates.

 (iii) Rhabditiform larvae voided with faeces pass a sexual phase in the soil, giving rise to a second batch of rhabditiform larvae from which filariform larvae are developed. It occurs in moist tropical climates.

Life Cycle. No intermediate host is required. The worm passes its life cycle (Fig. 149) in one host and unlike other nematodes, a change of host is not essential as it undergoes a hyperinfective form of development. Man is the optimum host.

Mode of Infection (Entrance into the Host). This occurs when a man walks bare-foot on the faecally contaminated soil. The filariform larvae penetrate directly through the skin coming in contact with the soil.

Infecting Agent—Filariform larvae.

Portal of Entry—Skin.

Site of Localisation—Lungs, intestine.

Migration and Localisation. The filariform larvae invade the tissues, penetrate into the venous circulation and are carried by the blood stream to the right heart and then to the lungs. They leave the pulmonary capillaries and enter the lung alveoli; they then migrate to the bronchi, trachea, larynx and epiglottis, are swallowed back and enter the intestinal tract. On arrival into the duodenum and jejunum, they develop into parasitic females and possibly males. The parasitic females then burrow into the mucous membrane and begin to oviposit in the tissues. The rhabditiform larvae hatch out immediately and enter into lumen of the bowel. Parasitic males do not invade the tissues and are therefore eliminated in the faeces. A parasitic female, before penetrating, may possibly be fertilised by a parasitic male but as there is no general agreement about the existence of parasitic males, the parasitic females are considered to be parthenogenetic.

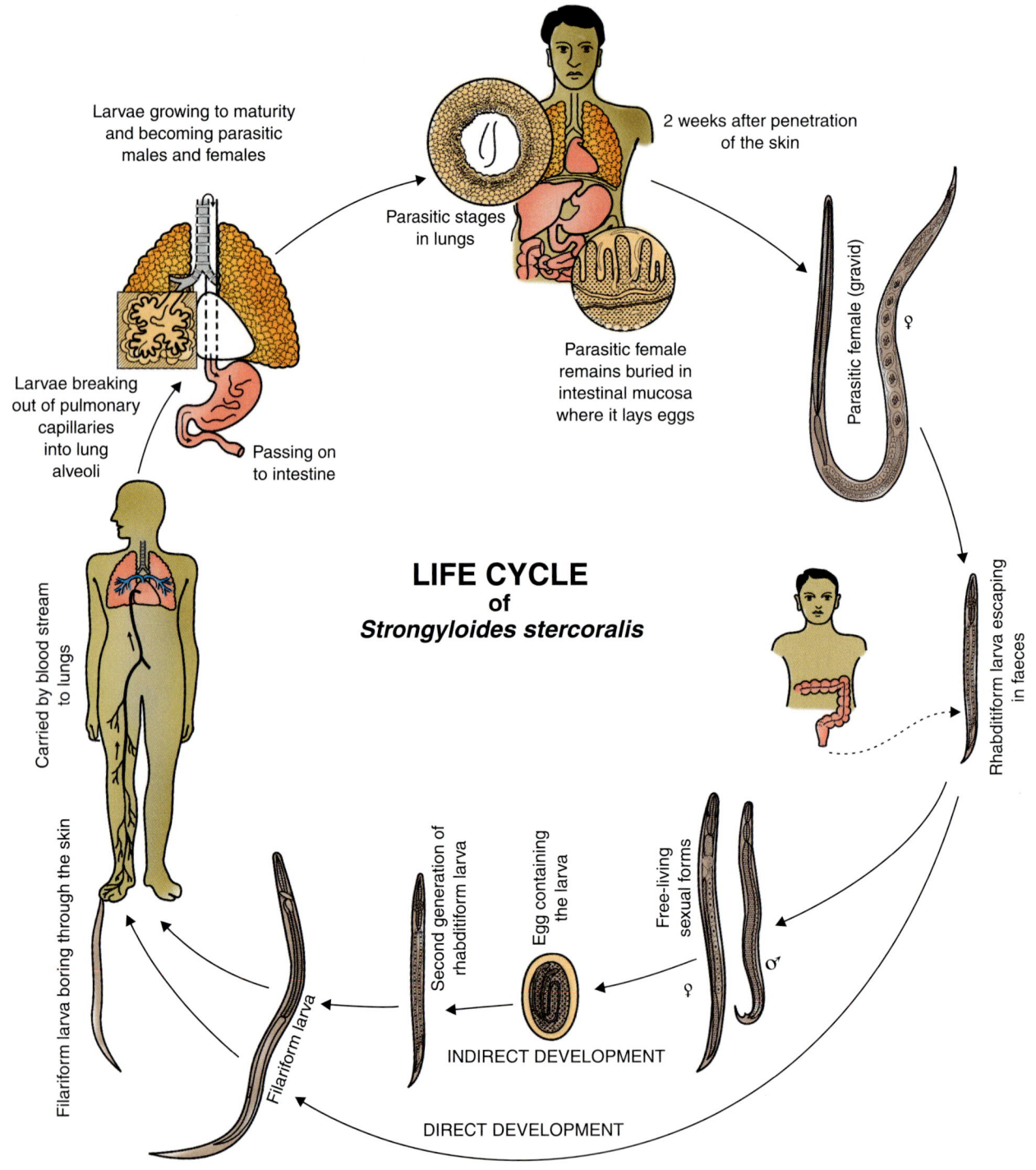

Larvae growing to maturity and becoming parasitic males and females

Parasitic stages in lungs

2 weeks after penetration of the skin

Parasitic female remains buried in intestinal mucosa where it lays eggs

Parasitic female (gravid) ♀

Larvae breaking out of pulmonary capillaries into lung alveoli

Passing on to intestine

LIFE CYCLE
of
Strongyloides stercoralis

Rhabditiform larva escaping in faeces

Carried by blood stream to lungs

Free-living sexual forms ♀ ♂

Filariform larva boring through the skin

Second generation of rhabditiform larva

Egg containing the larva

Filariform larva

INDIRECT DEVELOPMENT

DIRECT DEVELOPMENT

(Morphology after Looss)

Fig. 149

The developmental cycle of the worm is shown in the table below.

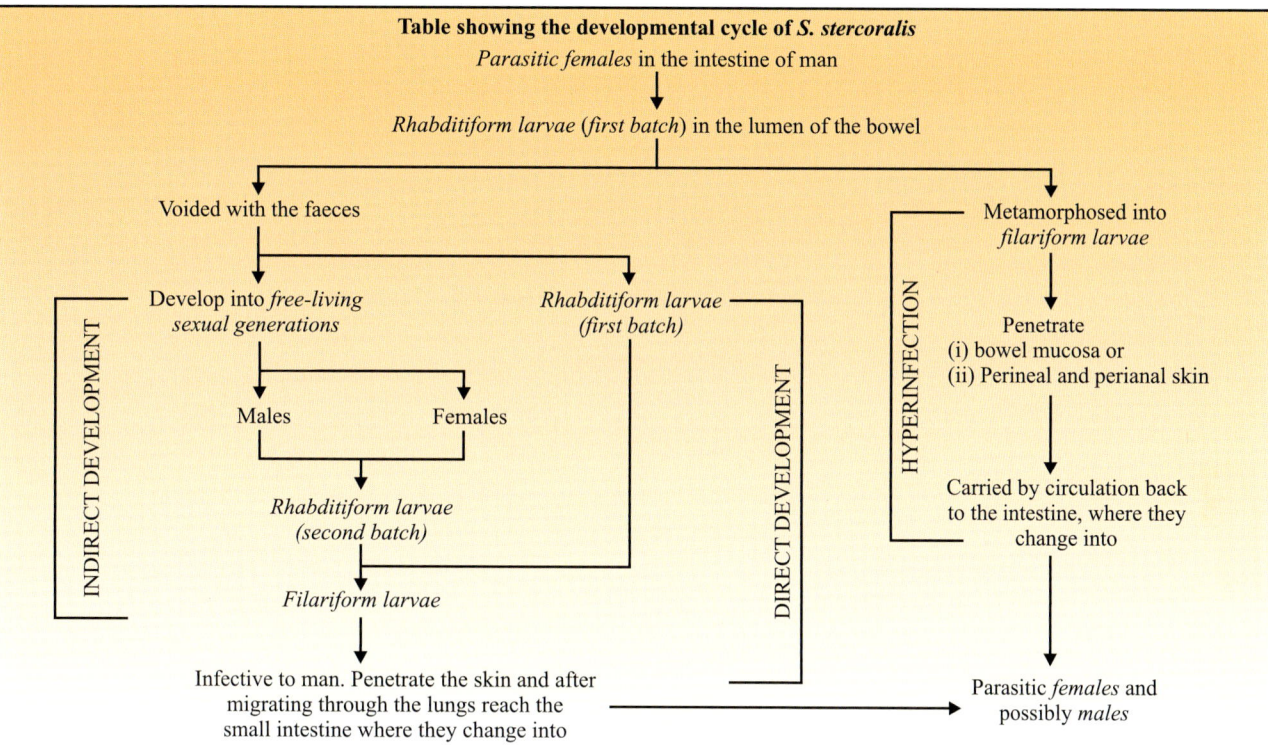

Table showing the developmental cycle of *S. stercoralis*

The females may at times enter the columnar epithelium of the bronchi, where they oviposit but the majority of the females passes up the respiratory tract. Fertilisation, if ever occurs, may also take place in the bronchi and trachea.

Immunology. After the first primary infection an immunity develops which prevents reinfection and the *Strongyloides* larvae and adult worms remain confined to the intestine and tissue invasion is prevented. The immunity may be diminished in immuno-suppressive states which reduce the resistance of the body, leading to an extensive tissue invasion by the adult worm. An infected individual when exposed to reinfection responds by tissue hypersensitivity with eosinophilia and giant urticaria. Serum antibody develops in strongyloidiasis and gives a cross reaction with filarial complement fixation test.

Pathogenicity. Infection with *S. stercoralis* is known as strongyloidiasis. The following lesions may be observed:

1. *Skin Lesions* (2 types). An urticarial rash at the site of entry and a linear, erythematous urticarial wheal around the anus caused by migrating filariform larvae.

2. *Pulmonary Lesions*. Haemorrhages in the lung alveoli and bronchopneumonia. These develop during migration of filariform larvae through the lungs and form an avenue of escape into the alveoli. These areas are often infiltrated with eosinophil cells.

3. *Intestinal Lesions*. Intractable diarrhoea with blood and mucus, produced by the mechanical movements of the female parasites. Microscopically small tunnels through which parasitic females have burrowed their ways may be seen; congestion haemorrhages, round cell infiltration and desquamation of epithelial cells are observed.

4. *Blood Changes*. A marked eosinophilia and a moderate leucocytosis during the invasive stage.

Note. Patients with *Strongyloides* infection when on steroids or in immunosuppressive states (in AIDS patients) may develop massive strongyloidiasis (*hyperinfective syndrome*) which then becomes a real danger. Severe diarrhoea, malabsorption, paralytic ileus, peritonitis, meningitis, brain abscess may occur in this hyperinfective condition. Excessive internal reinfection may lead to increase in number of worms in the intestine and lung and larvae in various tissues.

Filariform larvae may act as vehicles of microbial infection leading to Gram-negative bacteriaemia (Woodruff, 1968). Effective prompt management with albendazole and other measures may save the life of the patient.

Diagnosis. A specific diagnosis is based upon the finding of the typical rhabditiform larvae in freshly passed stool. A high eosinophilia is often a feature of strongyloidiasis. In pulmonary infection examination of the *sputum* will demonstrate the presence of rhabditiform larvae. In case of scanty larvae in faeces, culture of faeces is helpful.

Microscopical examination of duodenal washing and material obtained from jejunal biopsies may reveal larvae of *S. stercoralis*. C.F.T., I.H.A. & ELISA (75% positive) tests are used for diagnosis of the disease.

Treatment. The specific anthelmintics for strongyloidiasis are thiabendazole, albendazole, mebendazole and ivermectin.

Prophylaxis. Same as those for hookworm infection.

Superfamily STRONGYLOIDEA

The peculiarities are as follows:

  (i) Possesses a well developed mouth cavity (buccal capsule); may contain teeth or cutting organs.

 (ii) Male possesses a bursa (bursa copulatrix) which surrounds the cloaca.

(iii) Egg possesses a transparent shell and is hatched in a segmented condition. The larva develops in moist earth.

The superfamily Strongyloidea is divided as follows:

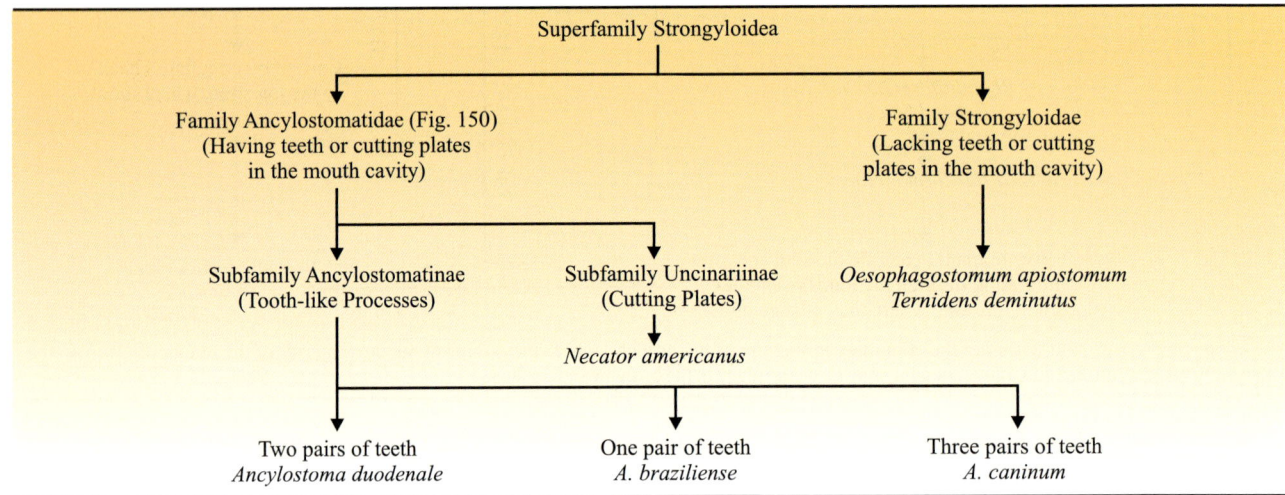

Superfamily Strongyloidea

Family Ancylostomatidae (Fig. 150)
(Having teeth or cutting plates
in the mouth cavity)

Family Strongyloidae
(Lacking teeth or cutting
plates in the mouth cavity)

Subfamily Ancylostomatinae
(Tooth-like Processes)

Subfamily Uncariinae
(Cutting Plates)

Oesophagostomum apiostomum
Ternidens deminutus

Necator americanus

Two pairs of teeth
Ancylostoma duodenale

One pair of teeth
A. braziliense

Three pairs of teeth
A. caninum

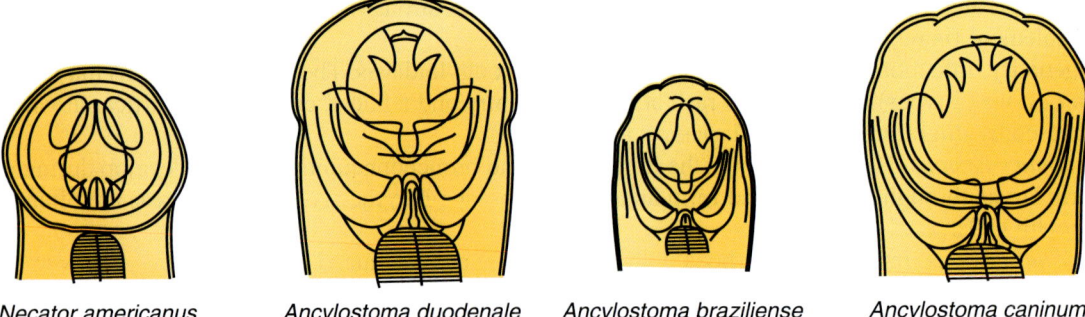

Necator americanus   Ancylostoma duodenale   Ancylostoma braziliense   Ancylostoma caninum

Fig. 150–Buccal capsules of hookworms of man and animals. (Magnification ×20)

Ancylostoma duodenale Dubini, 1843) Creplin, 1845

Common Name: The Old World hookworm.

The parasite was first discovered in 1838 by an Italian physician Angelo Dubini. The pathogenesis and mode of entrance of the larvae into man was worked out by Looss in 1898.

Geographical Distribution. It is widely distributed in all tropical and subtropical countries extending from parallel 36°N to parallel 30°S, occurring in places wherever humidity and temperature are favourable for the development of larvae in the soil. It is found in Europe, North Africa (specially prevalent in Egypt), India (Punjab and Uttar Pradesh), Sri Lanka, Central and North China, Pacific Islands and Southern States of America.

Habitat. The adult worm lives in the small intestine of man, particularly in the jejunum, less often in the duodenum and rarely in the ileum.

Morphology. ADULT WORM. It is small, greyish white, cylindrical worm. When freshly passed, the worm has a reddish brown colour due to the ingested blood in its intestinal tract. The anterior end of the worm is bent slightly dorsally, *hence the name hookworm*. This bend is in the same direction as the general body curvature. The oral aperture is not terminal but directed towards the dorsal surface. The large and conspicuous *buccal capsule* is lined with a hard substance and is provided with 6 teeth, 4 hook-like on the ventral surface and 2 knob-like (triangular plates) on the dorsal surface. There are five glands connected with the digestive system; one of them, called the oesophageal gland, secretes a ferment which prevents the clotting of blood.

The sexes are easily differentiated by their sizes, the shape of the tail (posterior end) and the position of the genital opening (*see* the table below). Owing to the position of the genital opening, the worm assumes a Y-shaped figure during copulation.

Copulatory bursa. This consists of 3 lobes: 1 dorsal and 2 lateral. Each lobe is supported by chitinous rays; the dorsal lobe contains 3 (1 single dorsal ray and 2 externodorsal rays); the two lateral lobes contain 10 (3 pairs of lateral rays and 2 pairs of ventral rays). Total number of rays are 13.

Male and Female of *A. duodenale*		
	MALE	**FEMALE**
Size:	Smaller; about 8 mm (1/3 in.) in length.	Longer than male; about 12.5 mm (1/2 in.) in length.
Posterior End:	Expanded in an umbrella-like fashion (copulatory bursa).	Tapering; no expanded bursa.
Genital Opening:	Posteriorly opens with the cloaca.	At the junction of posterior and middle third of the body.

Life span. The life span of the adult worm in the human intestine has been estimated to be about 3 to 4 years.

EGGS. The eggs are passed out with the faeces and the distinctive features of the egg (Fig. 151) are as follows:

(i) Oval or elliptical in shape, measuring 65 μm in length by 40 μm in breadth.

(ii) Colourless (not bile-stained).

(iii) Surrounded by a transparent hyaline shell-membrane.

(iv) Contains a segmented ovum usually with 4 blastomeres; has a clear space between the eggshell and the segmented ovum.

(v) Floats in saturated solution of common salt.

The eggs are first laid in an unsegmented stage and during their passage through the bowel, segmentation proceeds up to the 4-celled stage. The eggs, when passed out with the faeces, are not infective to man.

Immunology. In *A. caninum*, infections in dogs almost complete immunity may develop by small repeated infections. A similar phenomenon may also occur in human infections. In endemic areas most patients have minimal intestinal infection and no significant symptoms of anaemia and this may be attributed to the development of a partial immunity. Asymptomatic infections (worm burden small) outnumber symptomatic infections and they represent a carrier state in whom some degree of host resistance has been acquired. A heavy infection with symptoms of anaemia may result from the failure of development of immunity.

Life Cycle. No intermediate host is required and like other helminths, multiplication of worms does not occur inside the human body. Man is the only definitive host for *A. duodenale*. The following are the various stages of the life cycle (Fig. 152).

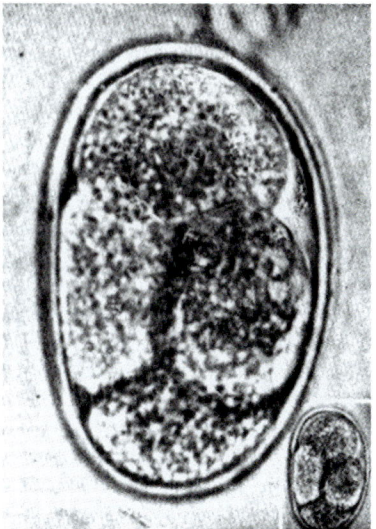

Fig. 151—Eggs of *A. duodenale*,
showing 4 blastomeres.
Inset: Shows the size under high power
with 10 ocular.

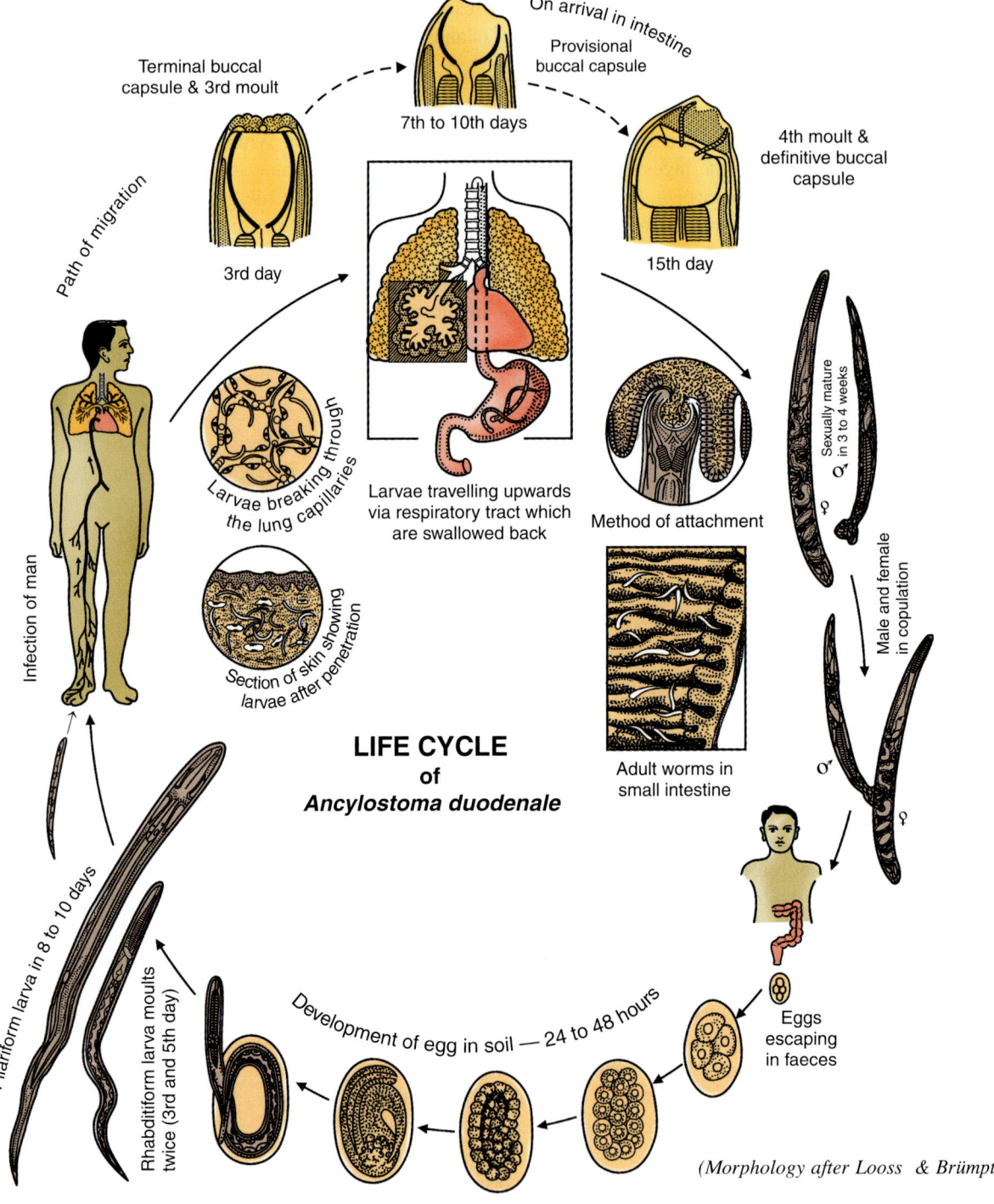

Terminal buccal
capsule & 3rd moult

On arrival in intestine

Provisional
buccal capsule

7th to 10th days

4th moult &
definitive buccal
capsule

Path of migration

3rd day

15th day

Sexually mature
in 3 to 4 weeks

Larvae breaking through
the lung capillaries

Larvae travelling upwards
via respiratory tract which
are swallowed back

Method of attachment

Male and female
in copulation

Infection of man

Section of skin showing
larvae after penetration

**LIFE CYCLE
of
*Ancylostoma duodenale***

Adult worms in
small intestine

Filariform larva in 8 to 10 days

Eggs
escaping
in faeces

Rhabditiform larva moults
twice (3rd and 5th day)

Development of egg in soil — 24 to 48 hours

(Morphology after Looss & Brümpt)

Fig. 152

STAGE 1. *Passage of Eggs from the Infected Host.* The eggs, containing segmented ova with 4 blastomeres, are passed out in the faeces of the human host.

STAGE 2. *Development in Soil.* From each egg a *rhabditiform larva* (250 μm in length) hatches out in the soil in about 48 hours. The rhabditiform larva moults twice, on the third day and the fifth day. It then develops into a *filariform larva* (500 to 600 μm in length), the infective stage of the parasite. The time taken for development from eggs to filariform larvae is on an average 8 to 10 days.

STAGE 3. *Entrance into a New Host.* The filariform larvae are infective to man. The larvae cast off their sheaths and gain entrance to the body by penetrating the skin.

STAGE 4. *Migration.* On reaching the subcutaneous tissues, the larvae enter into the lymphatics or small venules. They pass through the lymph-vascular system into the venous circulation and are carried *via* the right heart into the pulmonary capillaries, where they break through the capillary walls and enter into the alveolar spaces. They then migrate on to the bronchi, trachea and larynx, crawl over the epiglottis to the back of the pharynx and are ultimately swallowed. During migration or on entering the oesophagus, a third moulting takes place and a terminal buccal capsule is formed. The period taken for such migration is about 10 days.

STAGE 5. *Localisation and Laying of Eggs.* The growing larvae settle down in the small intestine, undergo a fourth moulting and develop into adolescent worms. At this stage, the provisional toothless buccal capsule, formed previously, is cast off and the definitive buccal capsule complete with teeth, is formed. In 3 to 4 weeks' time, they are sexually mature and the fertilised females begin to lay eggs in the faeces. The cycle is thus repeated. The interval between the time of skin infection and the first appearance of eggs in the faeces, is about 6 weeks.

Pathogenicity and Clinical Features. The worm causes hookworm disease or ancylostomiasis in man, characterised chiefly by anaemia.

MODE OF INFECTION. This occurs when man walks bare-foot on the faecally contaminated soil. The filariform larvae penetrate directly through the skin with which they come in contact. The most common sites of their entry are (*i*) the thin skin between the toes, (*ii*) the dorsum of the feet and (*iii*) the inner side of the soles. The larvae can penetrate any part of the skin which is sufficiently thin. In the case of gardeners and miners, the skin of the hands may be the portal of entry.

Infection may also occur by the accidental drinking* of water contaminated with filariform larvae. Infection by this method is not common.

Infecting Agent—Filariform larva.

Migration—Through lungs.

Portal of Entry—Skin.

Site of Location—Small intestine.

PATHOGENIC EFFECTS. These may be considered under two heads:

1. Those produced by the larval forms while entering the skin of the host and during migration through the lungs.
2. Those produced by the adult worms in the small intestine.

1. PATHOGENIC EFFECTS CAUSED BY ANCYLOSTOME LARVAE

(a) LESIONS IN THE SKIN: (i) Ancylostome dermatitis and (ii) Creeping eruption.

(i) ANCYLOSTOME DERMATITIS OR GROUND ITCH (Fig. 153) occurs at the site of entry. It is more commonly seen with *Necator* infection than with *Ancylostoma* and generally disappears in the course of one to two weeks' time. The skin lesion precedes the general symptoms of ancylostomiasis by 2 to 4 months.

(ii) CREEPING ERUPTION is a condition in which the filariform larvae wander about through the skin in an aimless manner for several weeks and months (up to 2 years), producing a reddish itchy papule along the path traversed by the larvae (termed "larva migrans"). This is particularly seen with those species of parasites (*A. braziliense* and *A. caninum*) which are not adapted to man and therefore after having penetrated the skin layers, cannot proceed to normal development in the small bowel. Maplestone (1933) had on occasions observed such lesion amongst the tea-garden coolies in India with the larvae of *N. americanus*.

The filariform larvae of non-human hookworms do not penetrate below the level of stratum germinativum of human skin. They remain in a tortuous and serpiginous tunnel, the roof being formed by the stratum granulosum and the floor by the corium. The larvae move in the tunnel and progress very slowly and irregularly at the rate of 1 to 2 cm per day. As the larva advances, the path left by it becomes dry and crusty. This migration persists for many months before the larva dies. The migrating filariform larva of *Strongyloides* moves rapidly in a short line at the rate of 3-4 cm in an hour, hence it is termed "larva currens". The form of "creeping eruption" caused by *Strongyloides* larvae lasts only for a few weeks; it results from autoinfection.

---

*Okamoto (1961) and Higo (1962) have demonstrated by experimental study that mature filariform larvae of *A. duodenale*, when swallowed, will develop into mature worms, without the lung passage.

(b) LESIONS IN THE LUNGS. *Bronchitis* and *broncho-pneumonia* may occur when the larvae break through the pulmonary capillaries and enter alveolar spaces (Fig. 154). A marked eosinophilia (Fig. 155) occurs at this stage.

2. PATHOGENIC EFFECTS CAUSED BY ADULT WORMS

The adult worms inhabit the small intestine (jejunum) of man, attaching themselves to the mucous membrane by means of their powerful buccal armature (Fig. 156). In course of time, a severe progressive anaemia of microcytic hypochromic type develops.

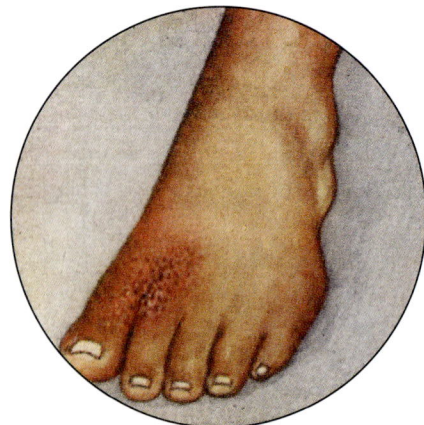

Fig. 153—Ancylostome dermatitis.

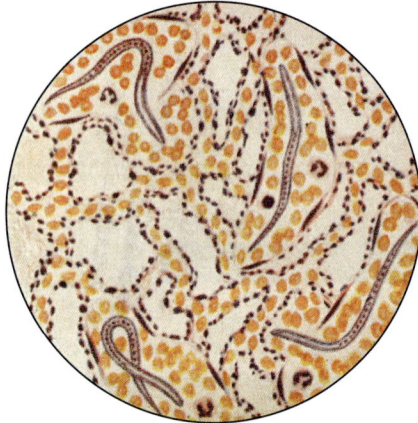

Fig. 154—Ancylostome pneumonia.

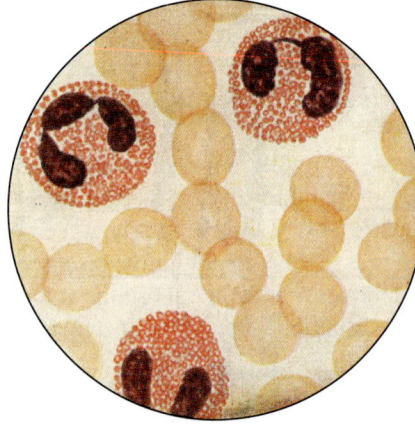

Fig. 155—Eosinophilia.
This is particularly seen during the invasive stage.

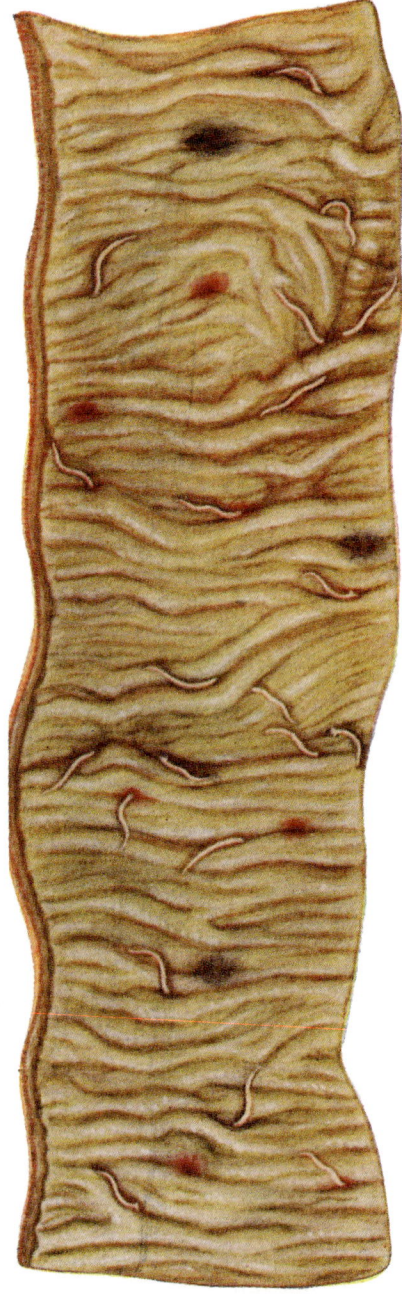

Fig. 156—Small intestine in ancylostomiasis.
Note the pigmented areas (the sites of old haemorrhages) and recent haemorrhagic areas. Some of the worms are still attached while others are free in the lumen.

Causes of Anaemia (Fig. 157). The worm, a habitual blood sucker, is primarily responsible but it appears that some other factors are to be taken into account to explain the development of anaemia. It may be ascribed to the following causes:

(i) CHRONIC BLOOD LOSS. This results from the withdrawal of blood by the (a) parasites for their food and (b) chronic haemorrhages from the punctured sites. It is known that each worm* is capable of drawing from 0.03 to 0.2 ml of

NORMAL IRON METABOLISM

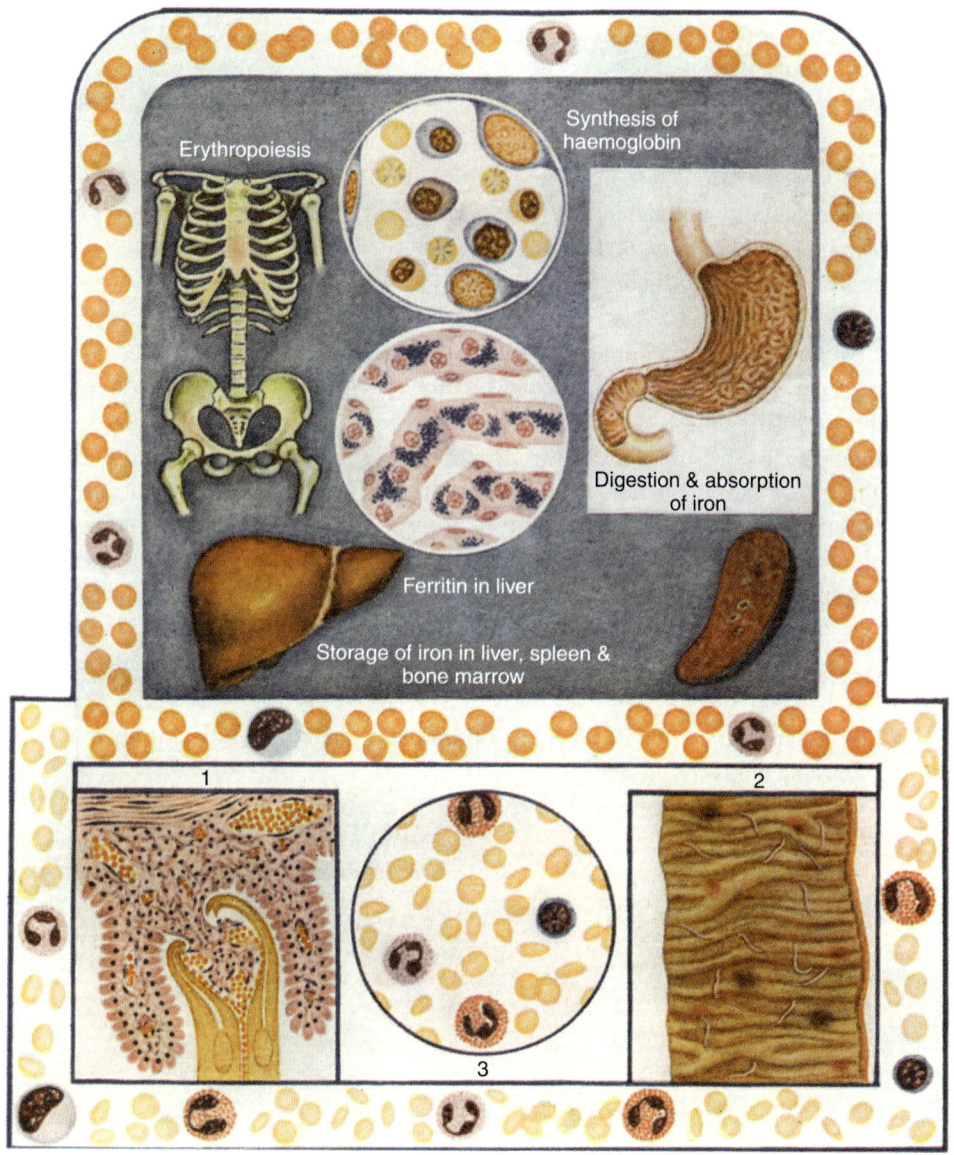

LOSS OF IRON THROUGH LOSS OF HAEMOGLOBIN

Fig. 157—Iron metabolism and hookworm anaemia.
1, *A. duodenale* sucking blood; 2, haemorrhages from the sites of attachment of the worms;
3, hypochromic microcytic anaemia.

---

*Roche *et al* (1957) estimated the average loss of blood by the host, per worm per day as follows: with *N. americanus* 0.03 ml and with *A. duodenale* 0.2 ml. It has been further observed that plasma forms the main source of nourishment and the red blood cells pass out from the worm practically unchanged into the lumen of host's intestine. The development of hookworm anaemia is also related to a certain extent on the amount of reabsorption of the iron in the lost blood from the intestinal tract.

blood, and in heavy infections such daily withdrawal of blood by a large number of parasites over a prolonged period would be sufficient to cause anaemia. Darling estimated the loss of haemoglobin for each 12 worms to be 1 per cent.

(ii) NUTRITIONAL DEFECTS. Some other contributory factors include deficiency of the available iron and other haemopoietic substances in the diet. It is apparent that a chronic blood loss cannot be fully compensated for in infected individuals with a faulty diet. Gases are on record where anaemia has been cured completely by iron treatment even without the use of any specific anthelmintic. Thus, depending upon the nature of the nutritional defect, the types of anaemia may vary. With iron deficiency, a *hypo-chromic microcytic* anaemia and with deficiency of folic acid and vitamin B_{12} (extrinsic factor of Castle), a *macrocytic* type of anaemia; deficiency of both iron and vitamin B_{12} or folic acid causes *dimorphic* anaemia.

Clinical Features of Hookworm Anaemia. These may be considered under two heads: Gastro-intestinal manifestations and Effects of anaemia.

1. *Gastrointestinal Manifestations.* There may be dyspeptic troubles associated with epigastric tenderness simulating duodenal ulcer. Occasionally, the patient may have an abnormal appetite showing a perverted taste for such things as earth, mud or lime (*pica or geophagy*). Analysis of gastric acid secretion showed varying grades of acidity; hypoacidity is more frequent than achlorhydria. It may be that iron deficiency anaemia may cause a low secretion of gastric acid.

Bowels are generally constipated. Sometimes, the patient complains of steatorrhorea (fatty diarrhoea), the pathogenesis of which is uncertain. It can neither be correlated with hookworm load nor with any mucosal abnormality as observed by jejunal biopsy.

2. *Effects of Anaemia.* The skin assumes a sallow appearance (light yellow colour) and the mucous membrane of the eyes, lips and tongue shows extreme pallor. The face appears puffy with the swelling of lower eyelids and there is oedema of the feet and ankle. Koilonychia is frequently observed. The general appearance of the patient is a pale plumpy individual with protuberant abdomen and dry lustreless hair. The effect of anaemia on cardiovascular system is manifested by a hyperkinetic circulatory state which may ultimately lead to circulatory failure. Growth and development in children may be retarded.

The clinical diagnosis of hookworm anaemia can only be confirmed by a microscopical examination of stool and other laboratory procedures (Fig. 158).

Blood Changes in Hookworm Infection. Typical haemograms of distinctive types of anaemia seen in hookworm infection are given in the table below.

	Hypochromic Anaemia	Macrocytic Anaemia	Dimorphic Anaemia	Normal Range	
Red blood cells in millions per mm³	2.9	0.73	1.3	4.8 to 5.5	For adult male
Haemoglobin in g per 100 ml of blood	4.6	3.48	3.77	15 to 17	
Packed cell volume (PCV) in per cent	21	10	16	43 to 47	
Mean corpuscular volume (MCV) in femtolitres (fl)	72	137	123	75 to 100	
Mean corpuscular haemoglobin (MCH) in picogram (pg)	16	47	24	24 to 33	
Mean corpuscular haemoglobin concentration (MCHC) in per cent	22	34	23	30 to 36	

Morbid Anatomy. This may be discussed under two heads:
 (1) The lesions produced by adult worms in the intestine.
 (2) The effects produced by anaemia.
 (1) *Intestinal Lesions by Adult Worms.* Areas of small extravasation of blood, some fresh and some old; the latter are indicated by pigmentation. If the examination is made within 3 hours after death, the worms may still be found attached to the centre of erosions in the mucosa. If the examination is delayed, the worms will be found free in the lumen of the bowel (see Fig. 156).

HOOKWORM ANAEMIA

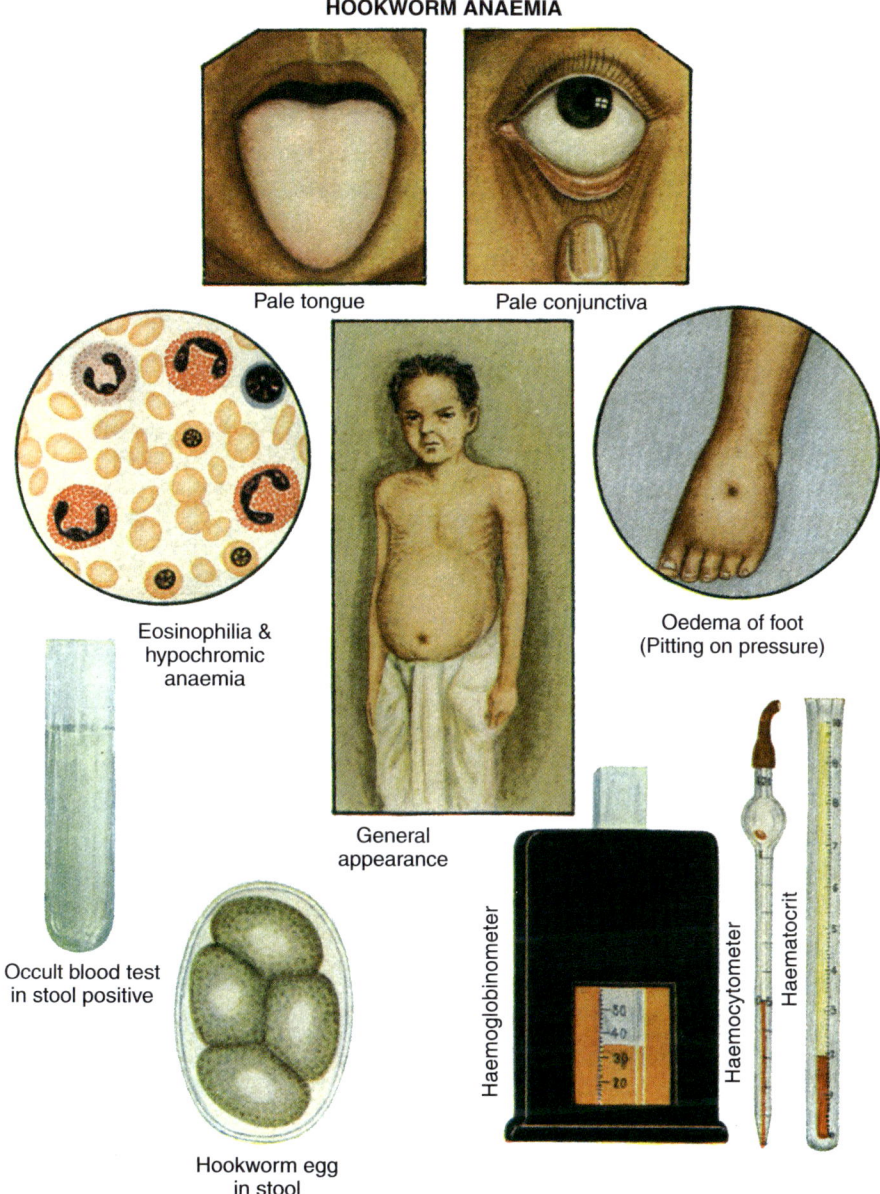

Fig. 158—Clinical and laboratory diagnosis of hookworm anaemia.

(2) *Effects of Anaemia*. In advanced cases, there is generalised oedema of the subcutaneous tissues with collection of fluid in the serous cavities (transudation of fluid results from lowering of colloid osmotic pressure of blood). Fatty changes in the liver and heart may be well marked in severe cases. Bone marrow often shows an erythroblastic reaction and the yellow marrow is transformed into a red formative marrow.

Laboratory Diagnosis. This consists of the following:

1. DIRECT METHODS

(i) *Examination of Stool*. A *macroscopic* examination of stool is necessary to find the adult worms which may be passed out spontaneously or after a vermifuge. A direct *microscopical* examination of stool may easily demonstrate the presence of characteristic hookworm eggs. Concentration method may be used.

For estimating the intensity of hookworm infection, the various egg-counting methods may be employed.

(ii) *Study of Duodenal Contents*. The material obtained by duodenal intubation (Ryle's tube) may sometimes reveal either eggs or the adult worms (*Necator* or *Ancylostoma* or both).

2. INDIRECT METHODS

(i) *Examination of Blood*. This is carried out to ascertain the nature of anaemia and the presence of eosinophilia.

(ii) *General Examination of Stool*. In a majority of cases of hookworm anaemia, test for occult blood in the stool gives a positive reaction. Charcot-Leyden crystals are often found in the stool.

SPECIFIC DIAGNOSIS. A specific diagnosis of hookworm anaemia whether due to *A. duodenale* or *N. americanus* cannot be made from the morphology of eggs discovered in an examination of the stool. Such a distinction can only be made by studying the morphology of adult worms or the mature infective filariform larvae.

Treatment. For the treatment of hookworm infection the following steps are to be taken: (a) Expulsion of worms by anthelmintic and (b) treatment of anaemia.

Specific anthelmintic treatment should not be started if the haemoglobin is below 30 per cent. In such a case, anaemia is to be treated first with iron and after the haemoglobin has come above 50 per cent, specific anthelmintic is to be administered.

For hookworm infection the anthelmintic drugs used are thiabendazole (25 mg/kg for two days), pyrantel pamoate (oral dose of 10 mg/kg for 3 days, maximum 1 gm), mebendazole (100 mg twice daily for 3 days or 500 mg once), and albendazole (400 mg once). Albendazole gives good results against *A. duodenale* and *N. americanus*. Thiabendazole is effective against migratory larvae and dormant larvae. Levamisol (4 mg/kg) is less effective against *N. americanus*.

Hookworm anaemia responds readily to oral iron (ferrous sulphate 200 or 400 mg thrice daily, according to the tolerance of the patient). Folic acid and vitamin B_{12} may be indicated in some cases.

Prophylaxis. The following measures may be adopted:

1. *Attack on Adult Parasite*. Treatment of carriers and diseased persons simultaneously with wholesale treatment of community (treatment *en masse*).
2. *Attack on Larvae*. Prevention of soil-pollution by proper control of sewage disposal. Disinfection of faeces or soil.
3. *Personal Protection*. Wearing of boots and gloves.

Necator americanus (Stiles, 1902) Stiles, 1903
Common Name: **The American hookworm or the New World hookworm.**

Geographical Distribution. It is the most common species in Sri Lanka and India (except in Punjab and Uttar Pradesh). Although first discovered in America, it is more likely of African origin. From its original focus (Tropical and South Africa), it has spread to India, Far East, Australia and America.

The life cycle, general morphology, pathogenicity, diagnosis and treatment are the same as described for *A. duodenale*. The differentiating features between the adult worms and filariform larvae of the two species are shown in the table below.

Differentiating Features of the Two Species		
	A. duodenale	*N. americanus*
ADULT WORMS		
SIZE:	Adult worms large and thicker.	Adult worms smaller and more slender.
ANTERIOR END: (Figs. 159 & 160)	Bends in the same direction as the body curvature.	Bends in the opposite direction to the body curvature.
BUCCAL CAPSULE: (Figs. 161 & 162)	6 teeth—4 hook-like teeth on ventral surface and 2 knob-like teeth on dorsal surface.	4 chitinous plates—2 on ventral surface and 2 on dorsal surface.
COPULATORY BURSA: (Figs. 163 & 164)	Dorsal ray is single. Total number of rays—13. Two spicules, separate.	Dorsal ray is split from the base. Total number of rays—14. Two spicules, fused at the tip.
POSTERIOR END OF FEMALE:	A spine is present.	There is no spine.
VULVAL OPENING:	Behind the middle of the body.	In front of the middle of the body.
PATHOGENICITY:	More pathogenic*.	Less pathogenic.

*Blood loss is higher in *A. duodenale* because (*i*) it is a larger worm, (*ii*) it is armed with teeth, and (*iii*) it is more migratory, leaving more bleeding points.

A. duodenale
(Adult worms)

Male

Female

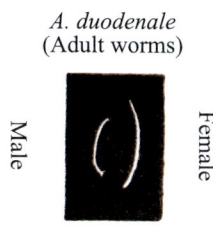

Fig. 159
(Natural sizes)

N. americanus
(Adult worms)

Male

Female

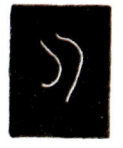

Fig. 160
(Natural sizes)

Buccal capsule and Copulatory bursa of

A. duodenale

N. americanus

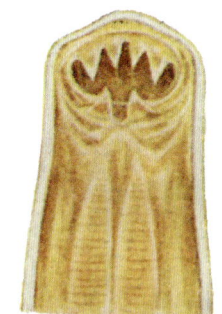

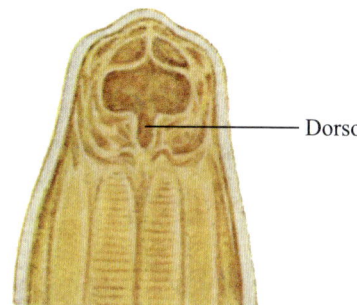

— Dorso median tooth

Fig. 161—Showing 4 hook-like ventral teeth on top and 2 knob-like dorsal teeth below.

Fig. 162—Showing 4 chitinous plates, 2 on ventral surface and 2 on dorsal surface.

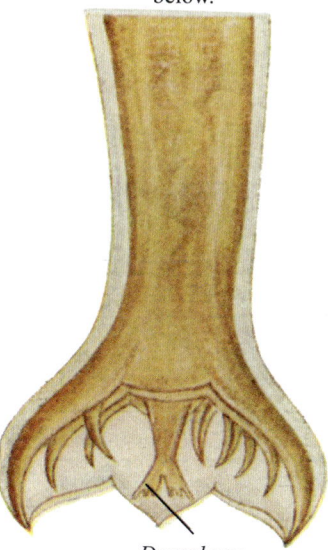

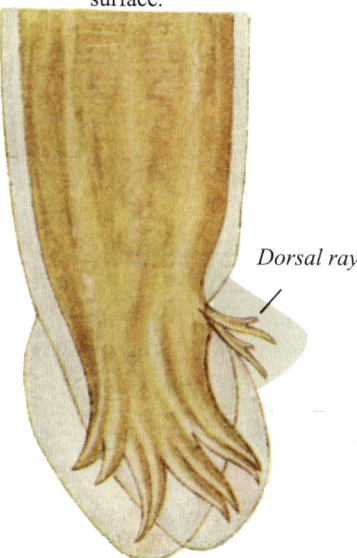

Dorsal ray

Dorsal ray

Fig. 163—Note the dorsal ray is single but partially divided at the tip and each division is tripartite. Total number of rays—13

Fig. 164—Note the dorsal ray is split from the base and each division is bipartite. Total number of rays—14.

[Drawn with the assistance of Dr. N.V. Bhaduri]

Filariform Larvae (Third-Stage Larvae)		
	A. duodenale	*N. americanus*
BUCCAL CAVITY: (Fig. 165)	Shorter 10 to 10-5 μ long. Lumen larger. Chitinous walls thinner; bounded by one line dorsally and two less prominent lines ventrally converge anteriorly. A fine line joins the oral depression and the anterior end of the buccal structure.	Larger 15 to 16 μ long. Lumen shorter. Chitinous walls thicker; dorsal and ventral walls are of equal thickness; diverge anteriorly. No line visible between the oral depression and the anterior end of buccal structure.
OESOPHAGO-INTESTINAL JUNCTION: (Fig. 166)	No gap between the oesophagus and the intestine. Anterior dilatation of intestinal lumen less prominent.	An apparent gap between the oesophagus and the intestine is present. Anterior dilatation of intestinal lumen more prominent.
POSTERIOR END OF THE INTESTINE: (Fig. 166)	A small refractive body (ampulliform dilatation) is present.	No refractile body (ampulliform dilatation).
POSITION OF THE GENITAL RUDIMENT (Fig. 166)	Behind the point mid-way between the end of the oesophagus and the anus.	In front of the point mid-way between the end of the oesophagus and the anus.
TRANSVERSE CUTICULAR STRIAE:	Less prominent.	More prominent.
SHAPE OF THE HEAD:	Slightly conical.	Rounded.

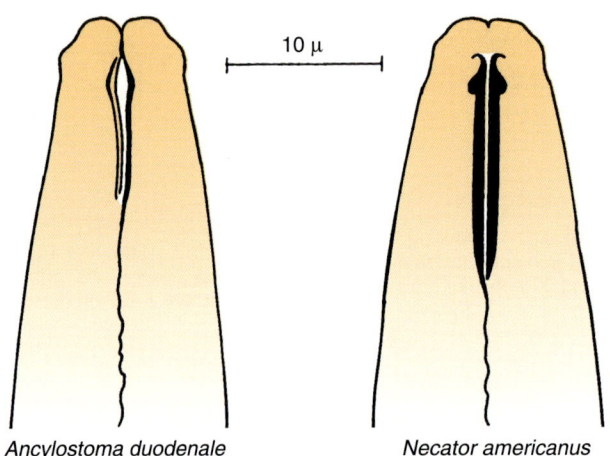

10 μ

Ancylostoma duodenale   *Necator americanus*

Fig. 165—Buccal cavity of filariform larvae of *Ancylostoma duodenale* **and** *Necator americanus*.

Ancylostoma duodenale

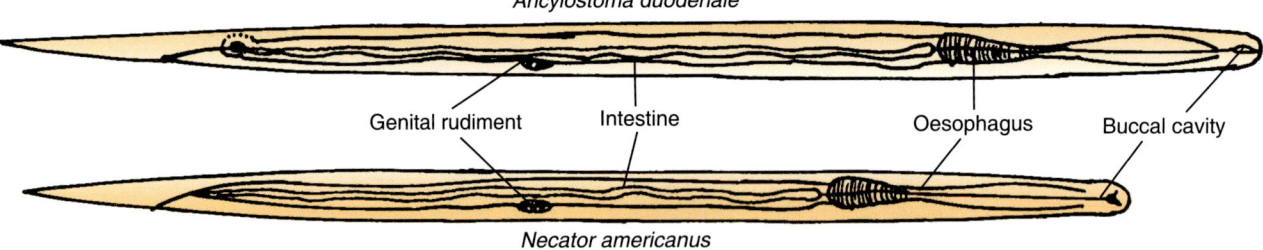

Genital rudiment   Intestine   Oesophagus   Buccal cavity

Necator americanus

Fig. 166—Filariform larvae of *Ancylostoma duodenale* **and** *Necator americanus*.
[*Figs.* 165 & 166 after *Heydon; Med. J. Australia*, Vol 1, 1927]

Ancylostoma braziliense Gomes de Faria, 1910

It is a parasite of dogs and cats in Brazil, India and Malaysia States. The adult worm is much smaller than *A. duodenale*. The buccal capsule has a small orifice and the ventral dental plate contains one pair of large teeth. The life cycle is the same as that of *A. duodenale*. Man is an unsuitable host and the filariform larvae penetrating the human skin cannot localise in the bowels and therefore wander in the skin, causing creeping eruption. Thiabendazole and albendazole are used for the treatment of creeping eruption.

Ancylostoma ceylanicum

This is found in the civet cat in Ceylon (Sri Lanka). *A. braziliense* and *A. ceylanicum* are considered by some to be one and the same species. *A. ceylanicum* however does not produce cutaneous larva migrans in man. Instances are on record where adult worms have been found in the intestine of man also and are regarded as biological variants (human strain, *A. braziliense* vel *ceylanicum*).

Ancylostoma caninum (Ercolani, 1859) Hall, 1913

This is a common parasite of dog, having a cosmopolitan distribution. The buccal capsule has the largest orifice; each of the paired ventral plates contains 3 teeth, the innermost being the smallest and the outermost the largest. The life cycle is the same as that of other Ancylostomes. Infective filariform larvae are capable of producing creeping eruption in man.

For "creeping eruption" caused by *A. caninum* and *A. braziliense* thiabendazole has been found to be an effective remedy. It has been observed that 99 per cent of all the larvae stopped activity on the first day of therapy (Stone and Mullins, 1965). A single dose of 400 mg oral albendazole or single dose oral 12 mg ivermectin gives good cure rates. A seven days treatment course of 400 mg oral albendazole daily prevents relapse. Tropical thiabendazole is also effective.

Genus OESOPHAGOSTOMUM
OESOPHAGOSTOMUM APIOSTOMUM (Willach, 1891) Railliet and Henry, 1905

The nodular worm of monkeys

Geographical Distribution. Africa, Philippines and China.

Habitat. It is parasitic in the walls of the large intestine of Africa apes and when the infection is severe, it causes dysenteric symptoms in these animals. It has also been recorded in men and it occurs as an accidental infection in man.

Morphology. The worm is very small and covered with a transversely striated cuticula which is dilated anteriorly to form an ovoid swelling. The mouth is surrounded by 6 circumoral papillae and a ring of setae. The *male* measures 8 to 10 mm in length and 0.35 mm in breadth. There is a campanulate bursa with supporting rays. The copulatory is long and curves posteriorly. The *female* measures 8.5 to 10.5 mm in length by 0.325 mm in breadth. The vulvar opening is situated just in front of the anus. The *eggs* measure 60 to 63 microns by 27 to 40 microns and are indistinguishable from those of hookworms (Ancylostoma and Necator).

Life Cycle. Life cycle is completed in a single host. The eggs develop in the soil and give rise to free-living larvae. They do not penetrate the skin but are swallowed with food or water and pass undigested through the stomach and small intestine. On arrival in the caecum, they leave their sheaths and invade the wall, where they cause formation of cystic nodules. Larval development is completed inside the cyst. On maturation, the larvae burst through these nodules and enter into the intestinal lumen. They attach to the mucosa and develop into adult worms.

Pathogenicity. It causes dysentery in apes and monkeys. Human infection is rare and occurs directly. It produces nodular cystic masses (*polyposis intestini*) both on the outer and inner side of the bowel wall, especially in the lower part of the ileum, caecum and colon. The worms lie within these cysts. A rupture of the cysts into the intestinal lumen will cause dysenteric symptoms, whereas a rupture outside, will cause peritonitis.

Diagnosis. This may be established by a microscopical examination of the stool for the presence of eggs. But such a diagnosis is not practicable during life as the eggs of these worms have a close similarity with those of hookworms and it is difficult to distinguish one from the other.

Treatment. Surgical intervention is sometimes necessary to relieve the mechanical pressure caused by cystic nodules.

OTHER SPECIES. *Oesophagostomum stephanostomum* var. thomasi (Railliet and Henry, 1909). It was reported by Thomas from Brazil where it was found to be parasitic in monkeys. Human infection has also been recorded.

Genus TERNIDENS
TERNIDENS DEMINUTUS Railliet and Henry, 1909

Geographical Distribution. South Africa and India. It is seen as an accidental infection in man.

Habitat. It inhabits the large intestine of monkeys. A rare parasite of man in Transvaal and Nyasaland.

Morphology. It closely resembles Ancylostoma. The buccal capsule is terminal, surrounded with a corona of two rows of stout bristle (setae). The entrance to the oesophagus is guarded by three serrated teeth. The *male* measures 9.5 mm in length and 0.56 mm in breadth. Copulatory rays of the bursa divide into two at their distal extremity, and the branches bifurcate. The *female* measures 14 to 16 mm in length and 0.75 mm in breadth. The vulvar opening is posterior and subterminal. The *eggs* are oval, measuring 84 microns in length by 40 microns in breadth. They are passed in advanced stage of development, usually in the 8-celled stage. They closely resemble those of *N. americanus* but are larger.

Life Cycle. The life cycle has not been completely worked out. The eggs develop into larvae in the soil. It follows the same course of development as the hookworm. The larvae can withstand desiccation for prolonged periods. They do not bore into the skin but cause infection when swallowed.

Pathogenicity. The worm is capable of producing considerable pathological damage by the formation of cystic nodules.

Diagnosis. This is based on discovery of eggs in the stool.

Treatment. The thiabendazole is the drug of choice.

Superfamily TRICHOSTRONGYLOIDEA Cram, 1927
Genus TRICHOSTRONGYLUS

Forms with reduced mouth; buccal capsule lacking or rudimentary. Body slender. Bursa copulatrix conspicuous. Development direct; requires only one host. Larval period free. Members of this group are commonly parasitic in the digestive tract of herbivorous animals; in man, infections are incidental.

Type-Species: 1. *Trichostrongylus colubriformis*

Other Species: 2. *Trichostrongylus orientalis* Jimbo, 1914. Confined to man, mostly among agricultural populations in Japan, Korea and Formosa. This is the only species of the genus first recovered from man and where man constitutes its natural host and other mammals its incidental host.

3. *Trichostrongylus probolurus* (Railliet, 1896) Looss, 1905. Human cases reported from Egypt.

4. *Trichostrongylus uitrinus* Looss, 1905. Human cases reported from Egypt.

TRICHOSTRONGYLUS COLUBRIFORMIS (Giles, 1892) Ransom, 1911

(Pseudohookworm disease)

Geographical Distribution. It occurs in India, Japan, Egypt and Central Africa, but more frequently in Japan and Korea. Chandler* has recorded it in 10 per cent of cases of hookworm infection in Assam. In sheep- and goat-raising localities, such as Kashmir, Chandler observed that 14 to 18 per cent of the people were infected. Maplestone and Bhaduri** (1940) found it in 6 per cent of the dogs in Calcutta.

Habitat. It is a parasite of sheep and goat. The worm is found as an occasional parasite in the upper part of the small intestine of man. As an accidental infection it occurs in man. The worm lives with its head embedded in the epithelium of the mucosa.

Morphology. It is a small slender worm of pale pink colour. The anterior extremity is thinned out. The mouth is unarmed. The *male* measures 4 to 5 mm in length and 0.07 mm in breadth in the region of the copulatory bursa. Its tail-end possesses a bilobed copulatory bursa and two spicules. The *female* is slightly longer (5 to 6 mm) than the male and 0.08 mm in breadth in the region of the vulva. The vulva is situated in the posterior quarter of the body. These worms penetrate the intestinal mucosa and may temporarily burrow it. They are known to suck blood at times. The *eggs* resemble those of hookworms and are often mistaken for them; hence the term *pseudohookworm* is often used in case of infection caused by this parasite. But they are somewhat larger (measuring 89 by 48 microns) and oval (often egg-shaped with one end pointed). The eggs are thin-shelled and are passed in a more segmented stage, containing a morula at oviposition.

Life Cycle. It completes the life cycle in a single host. Development of the eggs in the soil and it takes about 6 days' time for the infective filariform larvae to appear. The human infection is direct and the larvae gain entrance through the digestive tract. They pass to the intestine via oesophagus and stomach without migrating through the lungs. They become sexually mature adults in about 25 days.

Pathogenicity. Human infection occurs through ingestion of larvae on vegetation. It is usually non-pathogenic but may produce a severe anaemia of microcytic type. Faust*** is of the opinion that presence of several hundreds of worms are required to produce any manifest clinical symptom.

Diagnosis. This is based on the finding of the characteristic eggs in the faeces. Haroda-Mori method of culture of stool helps to differentiate between larvae of hookworm and pseudohookworm.

Treatment. Levamisole as single oral dose of 2.5 ml is the drug of choice for the treatment of disease. Thiabendazole is less effective.

Superfamily Metastrongyloidea
Genus Parastrongylus

The genus Parastrongylus (Angiostrongylus) includes many species and among them two species pathogenic to man are as follows: (1) *A. cantonensis* (causing eosinophilic meningoencephalitis) and (2) *A. costaricensis* (causing abdominal angiostrongyliasis).

---

*   Chandler A.C. (1949). Introduction to Human Parasitology, John Wiley & Sons, New York, London.
**   Maplestone P.A. and Bhaduri N.V. (1940). The helminthic parasites of dogs in Calcutta and their bearing on human parasitology. *Indian Journal Med. Res.*, 28: 595-604.
*** Faust E.C. (1949). Human Helminthology, 3rd edition. Henry Kimpton, London.

*Parastrongylus cantonensis** (Chen 1935) Dougherty, 1946 (*Angiostrongylus cantonensis*)

(The rat lungworm)
The parasite causing eosinophilic meningoencephalitis in man.

EOSINOPHILIC MENINGOENCEPHALITIS

The syndrome of meningoencephalitis caused by *A. cantonensis* is prevalent in several areas including the Pacific islands and South-East Asia. The parasite was first recovered in Formosa in 1944 by Nomura and Lin (1945) from the C.S.F. of a young man who had shown this manifestation. The second case was reported from Hawaii in 1961 by Rosen *et al* (1962). Some human cases have been reported from India.

A. cantonensis. It is a nematode which utilises molluscs as the intermediate host and rat as the final or definitive host. The habitat of the adult worms (both males and females) is in the two main branches of the pulmonary artery of the rat. The gravid female worms lay eggs into the blood stream and these are carried by the blood into the smaller vessels of the lungs where they lodge as emboli. The eggs become embryonated in about 6 days. The length of the adult worm varies from 17 to 25 mm.

Life Cycle:

The first stage larvae. These measure about 0.27 to 0.3 mm in length by 0.015 to 0.016 mm in breadth. They come out of the eggs, break through the alveolar walls, migrate up to the trachea and larynx to be swallowed back into the alimentary canal. They are finally eliminated with the faeces of the host. In fresh water or sea water, these larvae are able to live for about 6 days and 3 days respectively.

The intermediate host. These include terrestrial molluscs (land molluscs)—snails and slugs. The first stage larvae enter through the digestive tract of the mollusc or by active penetration of its cuticle. They undergo 2 moultings and become *third stage larvae* in about 2 weeks, measuring about 0.5 mm in length by 0.25 mm in breadth. They can survive in the body of the fresh-water snail for a period up to 12 months.

Development in the definitive host, rat. The rat is infected by eating the mollusc infested with the 3rd stage larvae or drinking the water contaminated with such larvae. The 3rd stage larvae on entering the alimentary canal pass through the stomach and the small intestine into the portal circulation and then via hepatic circulation are passively transferred to the lungs. They however do not lodge in the lung capillaries but enter the systemic circulation through which they are carried to the central nervous system for which they have a strong affinity.

Two additional moultings occur within the brain in the course of a fortnight, after which they are transformed into adult worms. They emerge on the surface of the brain and remain in the subarachnoid space for about 2 weeks. The juvenile worms measure about 11-12 mm in length, enter the wall of the cranial venules and then *via* right ventricle travel to the main branches of the pulmonary artery where they lodge. These become sexually mature in about one week's time and start laying eggs which require about 6 days to embryonate and hatch in the lung capillaries. The first stage larvae are usually found in the faeces of the rat 42-48 days after infection.

Human infection. This may occur in the following ways:

1. By ingestion of raw vegetables containing the 3rd stage larvae of *A. cantonensis* in hand planaria and molluscs or ingestion of tissues of improperly cooked infected intermediate hosts (amphibian snails) and carrier or paratenic hosts (crabs, prawns, pigs).
2. By drinking water contaminated with the infected larvae.

The 3rd stage larvae after entering the alimentary canal of man follow the same route, as in the rat, to reach the brain. They are unable to proceed further and die, exciting an inflammatory reaction in the brain and meninges. The eosinophilic response noted in the CSF of human cases has been suggested as being due to the metabolic products left behind by the parasite or resulting from the death of the parasite in the central nervous system. Larvae and adult worms may be found in CSF. Man behaves as a paratenic host in which the infection reaches a dead end. In the Pacific the disease is of short duration and often terminates spontaneously; only a minority may have a residual paralysis (commonly facial palsy). Immunity does not develop after recovery from infection and reinfection occur (2nd and 3rd attacks have been described).

Clinical features: Incubation period is 16 days. Clinical manifestations are symptoms and signs of eosinophilic meningitis (intense headache, fever, neck stiffness, convulsions and paralysis). Eye complications, optic neuritis is found in association with eosinophilic meningoencephalitis and the sixth cranial nerve palsy can also occur.

---

*Joseph E, Alicata. *Advances in Parasitology*, vol. 3, p. 223, 1965

A specific skin test can be performed with the help of a purified worm antigen. Various serological tests, used in diagnosis are IHA, ELISA, IFA, CIEP, but these are not very sensitive and specific. The disease is self-limiting and usually lasts for 3-6 weeks. The instances of fatalities have also been reported. Treatment of the disease by albendazole under cover of steroid has beneficial effects.

In the Pacific a patient who develops brain syndrome (headache, neck stiffness and paraesthesia in the limbs) with peripheral eosinophilia and the CSF showing eosinophilic pleocytosis (50-75%) should be suspected as a case of angiostrongyliasis. Other helminthic parasites which may cause this syndrome are cerebral gnathostomiasis, cerebral cysticercosis, cerebral echinococcosis, cerebral schistosomiasis, trichenelliasis, cerebral paragonimiasis, dirofilariasis and toxocara infection in young children. These should be considered in the differential diagnosis.

Parastrongylus costaricensis (Morena & Cespedes, 1971) (*Angiostrongylus costaricensis*)

The parasite causing abdominal angiostrongyliasis.

EOSINOPHILIC GASTROENTERITIS

Geographical Distribution. It is found in men in Costa Rica, Mexico, Central and South America.

Habitat. The adult worm lies in the mesenteric arteries of different rats and wild rodents.

Pathogenicity. Consumption of vegetables contaminated by third stage larvae causes infection in man. The third stage larvae lodged in mesenteric venules, cause thrombosis, infarction, ulceration of the intestine. Sometimes even peritonitis may develop.

Clinical Features. Pain in lower abdomen, vomiting and diarrhoea are the main clinical features which mimic appendicitis.

Diagnosis. It is made by histological examination of the lesion which shows eosinophilic granuloma. Eggs or larvae can also be found in the lesion.

Treatment. Surgical removal of the lesion is the only treatment of this disease.

Superfamily OXYUROIDEA

Small forms, more or less pin-shaped. The cuticula near the mouth forms wing-like expansion on each side. There is a globular enlargement at the posterior end of the oesophagus. The male possesses caudal papillae. The posterior extremity of the female is drawn out into a long, tapering and finely pointed tail which constitutes nearly one-third of the length of the worm.

GENUS ENTEROBIUS Leach, 1853. Species *E. vermicularis*

Enterobius vermicularis (Linnaeus, 1758) Leach, 1853

Common Names: Threadworm, pinworm, seatworm.

Leuckart (1865) first worked out its life cycle.

Geographical Distribution. It is cosmopolitan in distribution, being found all over the world.

Habitat. Adult worms (gravid females) live in the caecum and vermiform appendix of man, where they remain until the eggs are developed. They generally remain on the surface of the mucosa and may occasionally encyst in the submucosa.

Morphology. ADULT WORM. It is small (Fig. 167) and white in colour. It is more or less spindle-shaped and resembles a short piece of thread. In both male and female, a pair of *cervical alae* (wing-like expansions) is present at the anterior extremity (Fig. 168). There is no buccal cavity. The posterior end of the oesophagus is dilated into a conspicuous globular bulb (a double-bulb oesophagus), a characteristic feature of this nematode.

Male. It measures 2 to 4 mm in length and 0.1 to 0.2 mm across its girth. The posterior third of the body is curved and sharply truncated. It is rarely seen and is difficult to obtain except after a purge. It usually dies after fertilising the female.

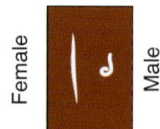

Fig. 167—*E. vermicularis.* (Natural sizes of adult worms.)

Female. It measures 8 to 12 mm in length and 0.3 to 0.5 mm across its thickest part. The posterior extremity is straight and drawn out into a long, tapering and finely pointed tail which is nearly one-third the length of the worm. The gravid female, after oviposition, dies within 2 to 3 weeks.

EGGS. The general characteristics of the *egg* (Fig. 169) are as follows:

 (i) Colourless, i.e., not bile-stained.
 (ii) Asymmetrical in shape, being plano-convex, i.e., flattened on one side (the ventral side) and convex on the other (the dorsal side).
 (iii) Measures 50 to 60 μm in length by 30 μm in breadth.
 (iv) Surrounded by a transparent shell.
 (v) Contains a coiled tadpole-like larva.
 (vi) Floats in saturated solution of common salt.

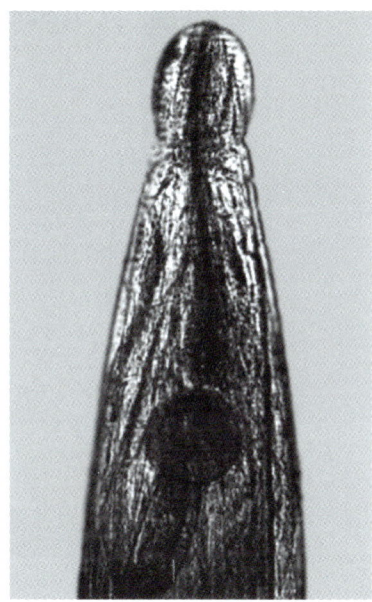

Fig. 168–Anterior end of *E. vermicularis.*
Note the cuticular cervical expansions (alae) and the double-bulb muscular oesophagus. (Similar in both sexes.)

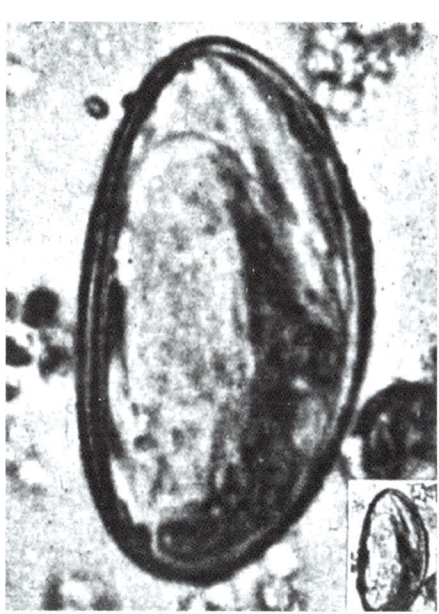

Fig. 169–Eggs of *E. vermicularis.*
Inset: Size under high power with 5 ocular.

Life Cycle. No intermediate host is required (Fig. 170). Each of the eggs, newly-laid on the perianal skin, containing a tadpole-like larva completes its development in 24 to 36 hours' time, in the presence of oxygen. Infection occurs by ingestion of these eggs. The egg-shells are dissolved by digestive juices and the larvae escape in the small intestine where they develop into adolescent worms. After the worms become sexually mature, the male fertilises the female and dies. The gravid female then migrates from the small intestine down to the caecum and colon (also the vermiform appendix) and remains there until the eggs develop. The fertilised female then wanders down the rectum and works its way out of the anus during the night (after the patient has retired to bed) to deposit eggs on the perianal skin. The cycle is then repeated. The whole life cycle is completed in 2 to 4 weeks' time.

Pathogenicity. Infection of *E. vermicularis* in man is known as enterobiasis.

MODE OF INFECTION. Children are the usual victims and familial infection is common. Transmission is effected from one person to another by the ingestion of eggs. The first infection is either contagious from close association or due to contaminated food and drink. Persons handling the night-clothes and bed linens of infected patients often contract the infection. There is also a possibility of the infection being air-borne, specially in an infected place.

Auto-infection. The movement of the worms at the time of egg-laying causes intense itching, inducing the patient to scratch the affected part and thereby carrying the eggs containing the infective larvae on their fingers. These eggs are subsequently transferred to food and swallowed by the patient himself or the infection may occur direct from anus-to-mouth, a very common habit with children.

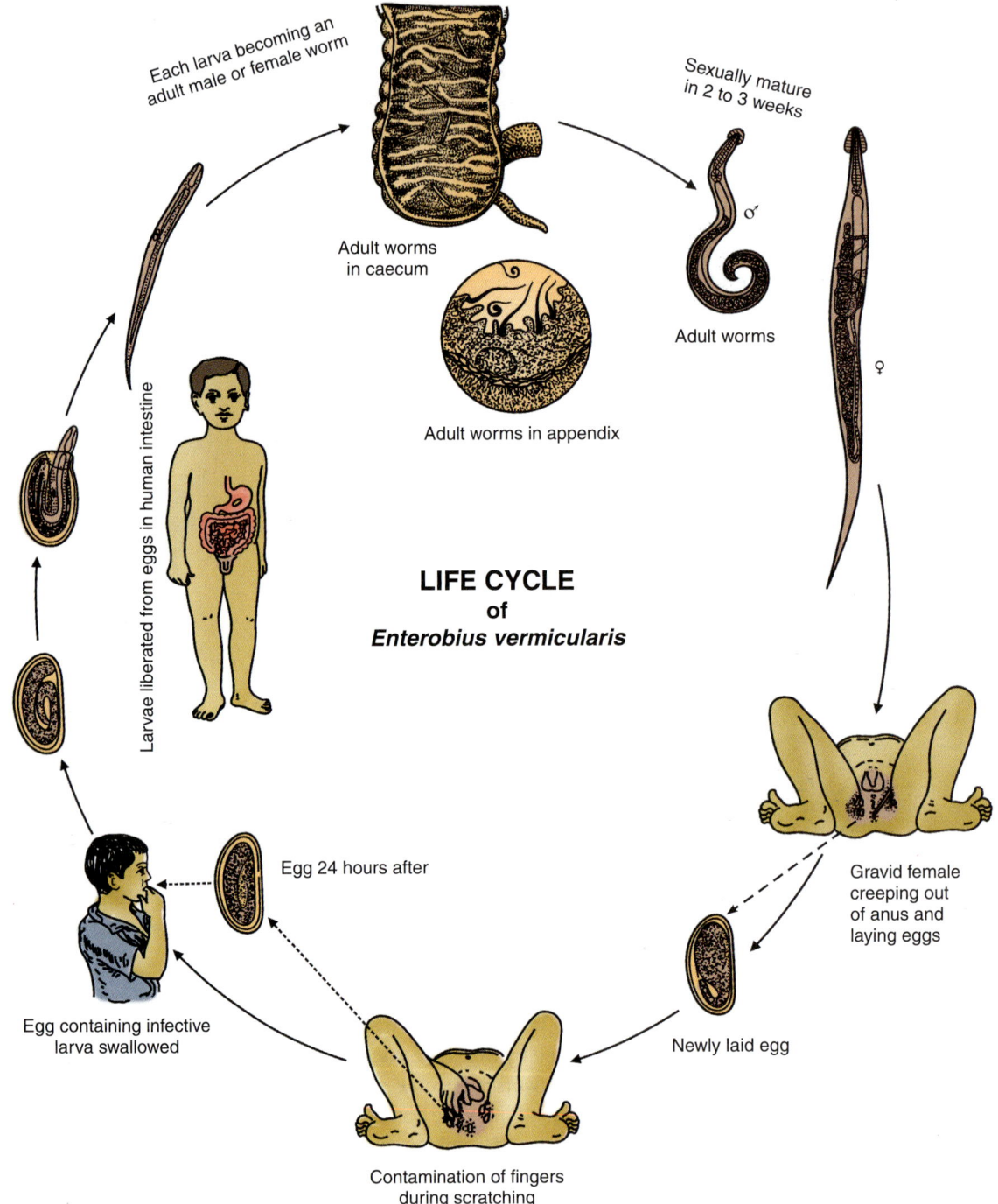

Each larva becoming an adult male or female worm

Sexually mature in 2 to 3 weeks

Adult worms in caecum

Adult worms in appendix

Adult worms

Larvae liberated from eggs in human intestine

LIFE CYCLE
of
Enterobius vermicularis

Gravid female creeping out of anus and laying eggs

Egg 24 hours after

Newly laid egg

Egg containing infective larva swallowed

Contamination of fingers during scratching

Fig. 170

Retrofection (Retrograde Infection). This is a process in which the eggs laid on the perianal skin immediately hatch into the infective-stage larvae and migrate through the anus to develop into adolescent forms in the colon.

PATHOGENESIS. The significant pathology is the irritation caused by the gravid females around the anus. The migrating females often enter into the female genital tract and female urethra, causing inflammation. These worms may even enter into the peritoneal cavity through the Fallopian tubes.

Clinical Features. The manifestations which are attributed to enterobiasis include the following: Pruritus periani et perinei and an eczematous condition round the anus and perineum, salpingitis, nocturnal enuresis (frequency of micturition) and sometimes (2 per cent of cases) inflammation of the vermiform appendix.

Laboratory Diagnosis. This depends upon (*i*) the finding of adult worm and (*ii*) demonstration of eggs.

DETECTION OF ADULT WORMS

(a) The worms are often discovered by the patient himself or by the parents of the children.

(b) If there is any history of passage of small whitish worms in the faeces, the patient should be instructed to bring such specimens preserved in alcohol, or 10 per cent formaldehyde, for examination.

(c) The adult worms may be recovered from stool after a purge or an enema.

(d) Inspection of the anal region at the time of commencement of itching may reveal the gravid females.

DEMONSTRATION OF EGGS. Although oviposition in the bowel is exceptional, microscopical examination of stool for eggs of *E. vermicularis* either by a direct smear examination or by concentration method may occasionally be successful. Eggs are generally demonstrated in the scrapings from the perianal skin by a NIH swab (Fig. 171); it is advisable to take the swab immediately after the patient wakes up in the morning. Eggs can also be recovered from under the finger-nails and the washings from garments.

Treatment. The specific anthelmintics for enterobiasis are pyrantel pamoate (10 mg/kg as a single dose), thiabendazole, mebendazole (100 mg as a single dose), albendazole (400 mg as a single dose). The treatment with any drug can be repeated at the interval of two weeks. Infection usually affects a group and treatment of whole family or group is advisable.

Prophylaxis. This includes (i) prevention of re-infection of the individual already infected and (ii) prevention of the infection by contact for which mass treatment of all infected cases may be required, along with other hygienic measures.

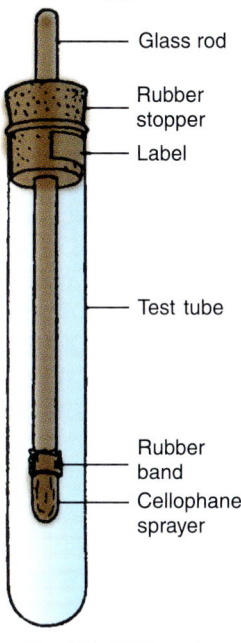

Labels: Glass rod, Rubber stopper, Label, Test tube, Rubber band, Cellophane sprayer

Fig. 171–NIH swab.

Superfamily ASCARIDOIDEA

Stout worms of fairly large size. The mouth is provided with three lips but lacks a buccal capsule. There is a simple digestive tube. The male has one or two copulatory spicules. The female is somewhat longer than the male.

Genus: ASCARIS Linnaeus, 1758. Species: *A. lumbricoides*.

Ascaris lumbricoides Linnaeus, 1758

(The common roundworm)

Details of the life cycle of the parasite were not known before 1916.

Geographical Distribution. It is cosmopolitan, having a world-wide distribution, being specially prevalent in the tropics, such as China, India and South-East Asia. It occurs in persons with unhygienic habits. It is present in about 25% human population. The calculated annual global mortality from ascariasis was about 20 thousand (mainly to intestinal complication) and morbidity about 10,00,000 cases (mainly to malnutrition and pulmonary complication).[*]

Habitat. The adult worm lives in the lumen of the small intestine (jejunum) of man and maintains its position by its muscle tone.

A species (*A. suum*) morphologically identical, though biologically separate, has been encountered in the pig and gorilla. Human infection with pig *Ascaris* is very rare. Crewe and Smith[**] (1971) reported a case in a child who passed a single adult worm. Examination of the teeth on the dentigerous ridges revealed it to be a pig *Ascaris*, because the teeth are typically triangular (in human *Ascaris*, the teeth have concave sides). This is the only way of distinguishing morphologically between human and pig strains of *Ascaris*, as described by Sprent[***] (1952).

Morphology. ADULT WORM. It resembles an ordinary earthworm and is the *largest intestinal nematode* parasitising man. When fresh from the intestine, it is light brown or pink in colour (*see* Fig. 172), but it gradually changes to white. In shape, it is rounded and tapers at both ends, the anterior end being thinner than the posterior. The mouth opens at the anterior end and possesses three finely toothed lips, one dorsal and two ventral (Fig. 173). The digestive and reproductive organs float inside the body cavity containing an irritating fluid. The irritant action is due to the presence

---

[*] Walsh & Warren, 1979

[**] *Annals of Trop. Med. & Parasit.*, **65**, p. 85.

[***] *Nature, Lond.*, **170**, p. 627.

of a substance, ascaron or ascarase which is probably of the nature of primary albumoses (proteose). Allergic manifestations seen in infected individuals and amongst laboratory workers dissecting the worms are due to this ascaron. The *life span* of the adult worm in the human host is less than a year.

Male. It measures about 15 to 25 cm in length with a maximum diameter of 3 to 4 mm. The tail-end of the male is curved ventrally in the form of a hook having a conical tip. The genital pore opens into the cloaca from which two curved copulatory spicules protrude (Fig. 174). The anus opens with the ejaculatory duct into the cloaca.

Female. It is longer stouter than the male and measures 25 to 40 cm in length with a maximum diameter of 5 mm. The posterior extremity is neither curved nor pointed but is conical and straight. The anus is subterminal and opens directly on the ventral aspect in the form of a transverse slit (Fig. 174). The vulva opens at the junction of the anterior and the middle-third of the body on the midventral aspect; this section of the worm is narrower and is called the vulvar waist (Fig. 172). The egg-laying capacity of a mature female Ascaris has been found to be enormous, liberating about 200,000 eggs daily.

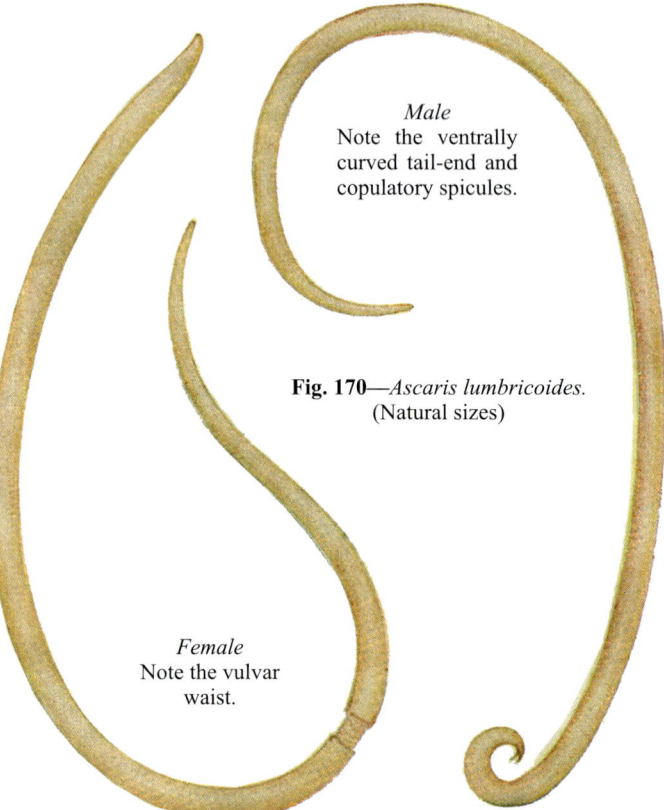

Male
Note the ventrally curved tail-end and copulatory spicules.

Fig. 170—*Ascaris lumbricoides.*
(Natural sizes)

Female
Note the vulvar waist.

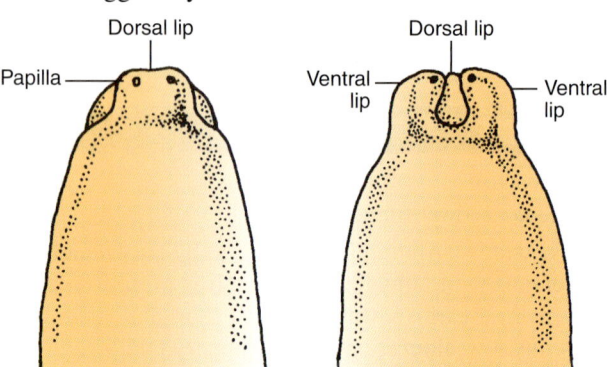

Fig. 173–Anterior ends of *A. lumbricoides.*
(Similar in both sexes)

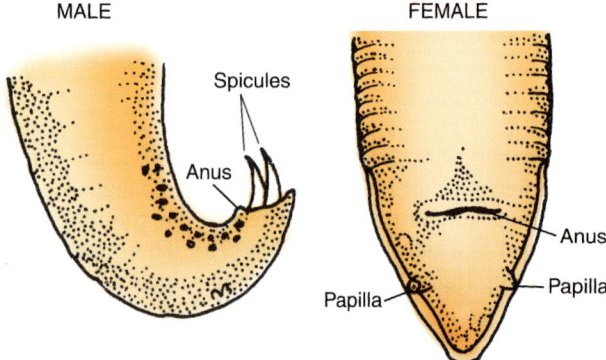

Fig. 174—Posterior ends of *A. lumbricoides.*

EGGS. The eggs liberated by a fertilised female pass out of the human host with the faeces. The characteristics of a fertilised egg (Fig. 175) are as follows:

(i) Round or oval in shape (60 to 75 mm in length by 40 to 50 mm in breadth). (ii) Always bile-stained and brownish (golden brown) in colour. (iii) Surrounded by a thick smooth translucent shell with an outer albuminous coat which is thrown into rugosities or mammillations; this outer coat is sometimes lost (decorticated egg). (iv) Contains a very large conspicuous, unsegmented ovum (the nucleus is concealed by a large amount of coarse yolk granules); there is a clear crescentic area at each pole. (v) Floats in saturated solution of common salt.

The female, even if not fertilised, is capable of liberating eggs. The characteristics of this *unfertilised egg* (Fig. 176) are as follows:

(i) Narrower, longer (80 mm in length by 55 mm in breadth) and more elliptical. (ii) Brownish in colour (bile-stained). (iii) Has a thinner shell with an irregular coating of albumin. (iv) Contains a small atrophied ovum with a mass of disorganised, highly refractile granules of various sizes. (v) Does not float in salt solution (heaviest of all helminthic eggs).

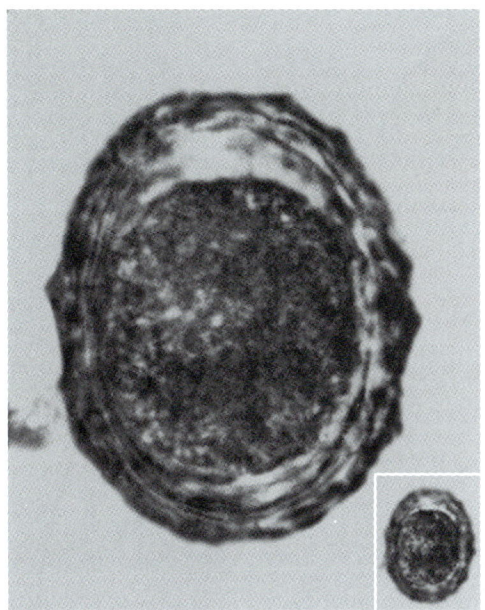

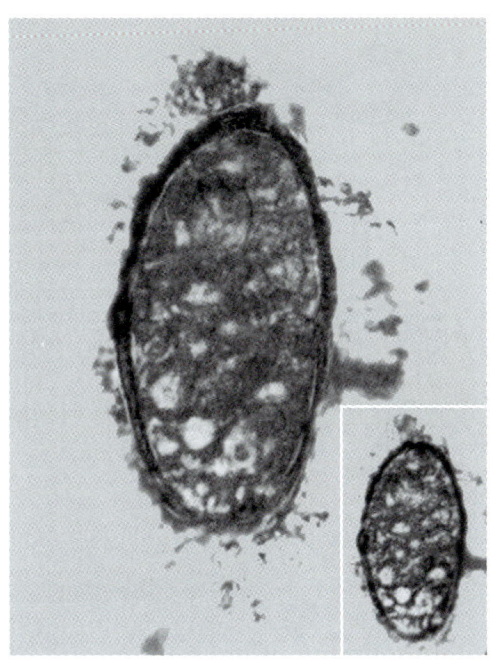

Fig. 175—Fertilised eggs of *A. lumbricoides.*   **Fig. 176—Unfertilised eggs of** *A. lumbricoides.*

Inset: Seen under high power with 5 ocular.

Both fertilised and unfertilised eggs may be found in a sample of stool but if a specimen shows only the unfertilised eggs, it signifies that the host is harbouring female Ascaris or mating between males and females has not occurred.

Life Cycle. The worm passes its life cycle in one host (Fig. 177) and no intermediate host is required. Continuance of the species is maintained by transference from one individual to another. Man is the only known definitive host of *A. lumbricoides.* The various stages in the life cycle are described below:

STAGE 1. *Eggs in Faeces.* Fertilised eggs containing the unsegmented ovum are passed with the faeces. They are not infective to man when freshly passed.

STAGE 2. *Development in Soil.* A rhabditiform larva is developed from the unsegmented ovum within the egg-shell in 10 to 40 days' time, depending on the atmospheric temperature and humidity. This takes place in the soil (that is outside the human host). The ripe egg containing the coiled-up embryo is infective to man. Before hatching, the larva undergoes a moulting. The second one, though commences in the egg, may be completed during early migration in the intestinal wall or in the liver of definitive host.*

STAGE 3. *Infection by Ingestion and Liberation of Larvae.* When ingested with food, drink or raw vegetables, the embryonated eggs pass down to the duodenum where the digestive juices weaken the egg-shell and stimulate the enclosed larvae into activity. Splitting of egg-shell occurs and the rhabditiform larvae measuring 0.25 mm in length by 14 µm in breadth are liberated in the upper part of the small intestine.

STAGE 4. *Migration through the Lungs.* The larvae liberated in the small intestine do not directly develop into mature worms. The newly hatched larvae burrow their way through the mucous membrane of the small intestine and are carried by the portal circulation to the liver; here, they live for a period of 3 to 4 days. Finally, they pass out of the liver and via right heart enter the pulmonary circulation. While in the lungs they grow much bigger and increase in length from 0.2 mm to 2 mm and moult twice (first, on the fifth or sixth day and the second, after the tenth day). Breaking through the capillary wall they reach the lung alveoli. The time taken for such migration is on an average 10 to 15 days.

STAGE 5. *Re-entry into the Stomach and the Small Intestine.* From the lung alveoli the larvae crawl up the bronchi and trachea, and aided by the current caused by the ciliated epithelium of the respiratory tract, they are propelled into the larynx and pharynx and are once more swallowed. The larvae pass down the oesophagus to the stomach and localise in the upper part of the small intestine, their normal abode. Another moulting occurs between the twenty-fifth and the twenty-ninth day of infection.

STAGE 6. *Sexual Maturity and Egg Liberation.* The larvae on reaching their habitat grow into adult worms and become sexually mature in about 6 to 10 weeks' time. The gravid females begin to discharge eggs in the stool within about two months from the time of infection. The cycle is again repeated.

---

*Mauug 1978

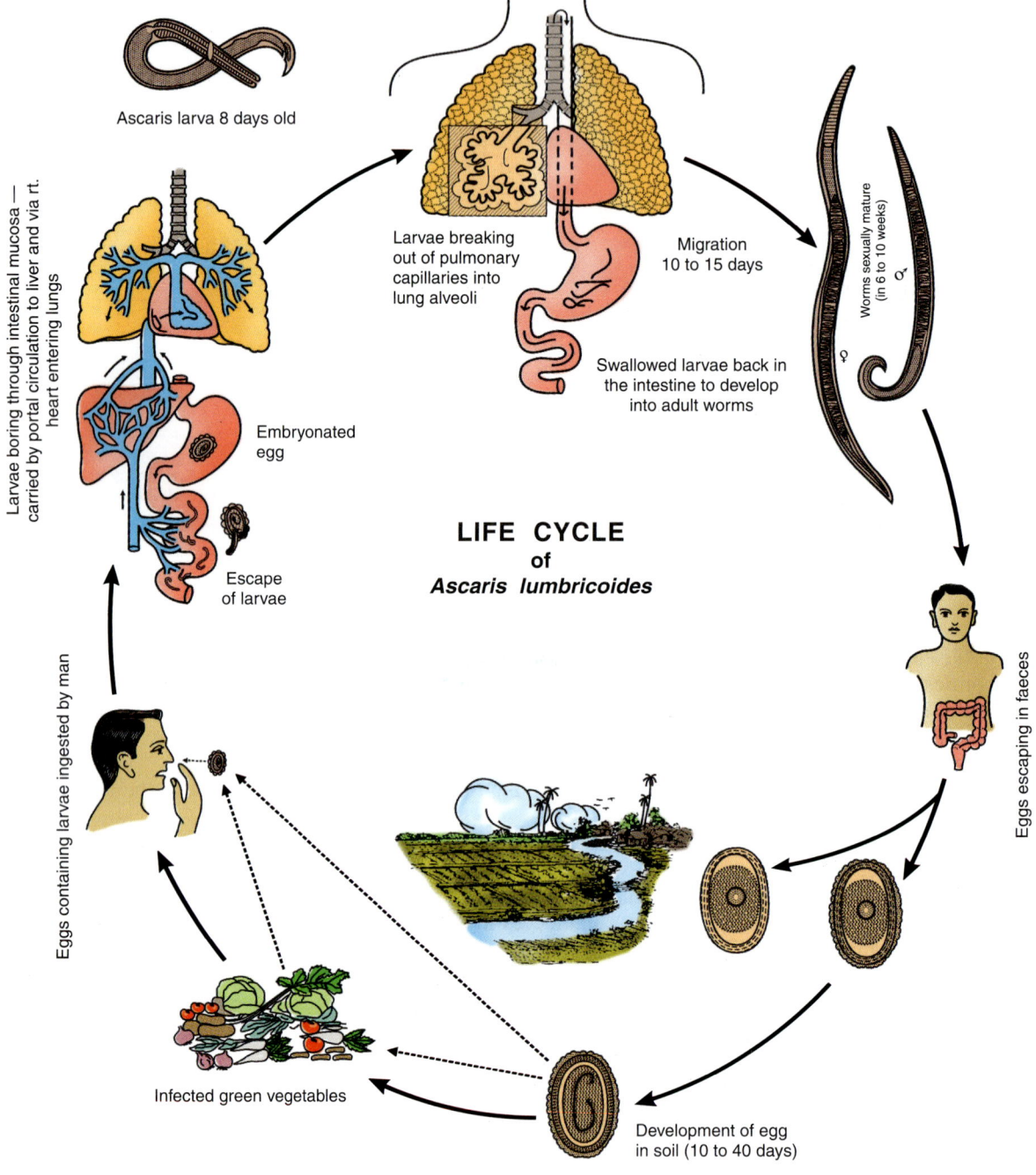

Ascaris larva 8 days old

Larvae breaking
out of pulmonary
capillaries into
lung alveoli

Migration
10 to 15 days

Swallowed larvae back in
the intestine to develop
into adult worms

Worms sexually mature
(in 6 to 10 weeks)

Larvae boring through intestinal mucosa —
carried by portal circulation to liver and via rt.
heart entering lungs

Embryonated
egg

Escape
of larvae

LIFE CYCLE
of
Ascaris lumbricoides

Eggs escaping in faeces

Eggs containing larvae ingested by man

Infected green vegetables

Development of egg
in soil (10 to 40 days)

Fig. 177

Note: Four moultings of the larva occur—one outside while within the egg-shell, two in the lungs and one in the intestine.

With massive infection some larvae may reach the general circulation to be filtered out in various organs and tissues. When they happen to lodge in such aberrant sites as kidneys, brain, spinal cord and other organs, they are unable to grow to maturity and perhaps most of them are destroyed. In a heavy infection, the larvae may even be excreted in the urine.

MODE OF INFECTION. Infection is effected by *swallowing* ripe Ascaris eggs (embryonated eggs) with raw vegetables cultivated on a soil fertilised by infected human excreta. Water-supplies may be contaminated and infection may occur by drinking such water. Where soil-pollution is common, the eggs may directly be conveyed to the mouth by dirty fingers.

Infection may also occur by *inhalation* of desiccated eggs in the dust reaching the pharynx and swallowed. The eggs, instead of being swallowed, may hatch on moist mucous surface of the upper air passage and the larvae may directly penetrate into the blood stream.

It may be remarked that porcine infection does not play any part in the etiology and epidemiology of human ascariasis. The infective-stage eggs are invariably obtained from human sources.

Infecting Agent—Embryonated egg.   *Migration of Larvae*—Through lungs.

Portal of Entry—Alimentary canal.   *Site of Location*—Small intestine.

Immunology. A partial immunity may be acquired by man, induced by the migrating larvae. Antigens are liberated during the moulting period of the larvae and produce protective antibodies which lower the worm burden and play a part in the immune response. A severe allergic reaction (urticaria and fall of blood pressure) occurs when the larvae reach the small intestine for the second time. Eosinophilic count is increased at the time of tissue invasion. Specific antibodies (complement-fixing and precipitating) can be demonstrated in Ascaris infection. Hypersensitivity to Ascaris is determined by skin test.

Pathogenicity and Clinical Features. Infection of *A. lumbricoides* in man is known as ascariasis. The symptoms attributed to Ascaris infection,may be divided into two groups: (a) those produced by the migrating larvae and (b) those produced by the adult worms.

SYMPTOMS DUE TO THE MIGRATING LARVAE

Larvae in the Lungs: Ascaris Pneumonia (Loeffler's Syndrome). In heavy infections typical symptoms of pneumonia such as fever, cough and dyspnoea may appear. Sputum which is often blood-tinged may contain Ascaris larvae. Urticarial rash and eosinophilia (20 per cent) are seen in such cases.

Larvae in General Circulation. If the Ascaris larvae pass beyond the pulmonary capillaries and reach the general circulation, they are filtered out to various organs where they may set up unusual clinical symptoms. Disturbances have been reported due to their presence in the brain, spinal cord, heart and kidneys.

Note. Micro-organism may be carried by the migrating larvae from the intestine to other tissues.

SYMPTOMS DUE TO THE ADULT WORMS

Incubation Period. In man it takes 60 to 75 days from the time of exposure to infection, for the mature female to lay eggs and that is the period when the symptoms are manifested.

Pathogenesis. As the worm inhabits the upper part of the small intestine, the symptoms are therefore mostly related to the gastro-intestinal tract. The adult worm may produce its pathogenic effects in the following ways:

(1) SPOLIATIVE ACTION: By robbing the host of its nutrition (protein and vitamin content of the worm is high). This effect is readily observed in hyperinfected children and may contribute to protein-energy malnutrition. Ascaris infection may cause vitamin A deficiency (night blindness). Antienzymes (antitryptic and antipeptic) liberated by Ascaris protect the worm from digestion by the host's intestinal ferments; they also help the development of malnutrition.

(2) "TOXIC" ACTION: The body fluid of Ascaris when absorbed is toxic and may give rise to typhoid-like fever; also responsible for various allergic manifestations such as urticaria, oedema of the face, conjunctivitis and irritation of the upper respiratory tract.

(3) MECHANICAL EFFECTS: (i) The presence of *A. lumbricoides* has led to the occurrence of intussusception (Fig. 178); (ii) it may penetrate through the ulcers of the alimentary canal (Figs. 179 & 180); (iii) a large number of Ascaris forming a bolus has been known to produce intestinal obstruction (Fig. 181), particularly in young children, because of relative small size of the intestinal lumen.

Ectopic Ascariasis. The worms frequently migrate and may enter the stomach and may be vomited out or may pass up through the oesophagus at night, coming out through the mouth or nose. Thus, during migration, Ascaris worms may accidentally enter into the respiratory passage causing suffocation by blocking the rima glottidis or may even enter into a bronchus.

Wandering Ascaris may enter the lumen of an appendix, causing appendicitis. Obstructive jaundice and acute haemorrhagic pancreatitis have been known to occur when the worm has entered into the biliary passage. At times, it penetrates high up in the liver causing one or more abscesses.

Laboratory Diagnosis. This may be described under two heads: Direct evidences and indirect evidences.

I. DIRECT EVIDENCES

(a) *Finding of Adult Worms*

(i) IN THE STOOL OR VOMIT. The adult worm may pass out spontaneously in the stool or *per anum* between stools, or be vomited or escape through nares. Administration of a specific anthelmintic may lead to the expulsion of worm and its detection.

(ii) X-RAY DIAGNOSIS. The presence of *A. lumbricoides* has been demonstrated by radiography with barium emulsion, which being ingested by the worm within 4 to 6 hours, casts an opaque shadow (string-like shadow).

SURGICAL ASPECTS OF ASCARIASIS

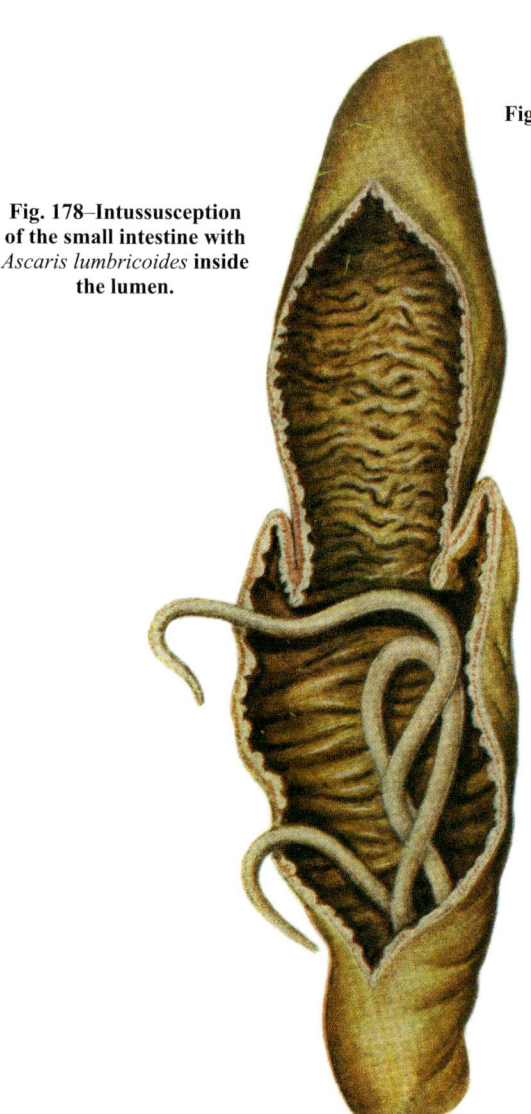

Fig. 178–Intussusception of the small intestine with *Ascaris lumbricoides* **inside the lumen.**

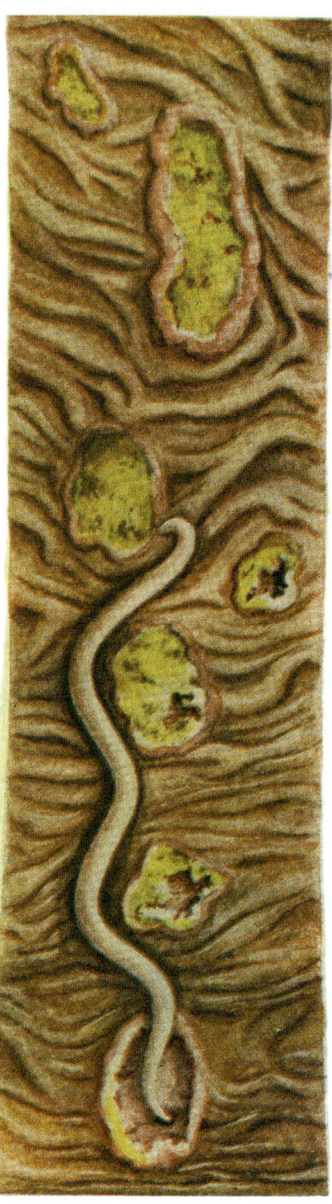

Fig. 179–*Ascaris lumbricoides* **perforating through a typhoid ulcer.**

(b) *Finding of Eggs*

(i) IN THE STOOL. As the Ascaris eggs are passed in the stool in enormous numbers, it should be easy to detect the infected persons by a *direct microscopical examination* of a saline emulsion of the stool. Concentration by *floatation method* may be employed for the detection of eggs in the stool. It is to be noted that unfertilised eggs do not float in salt solution. If the patient harbours a solitary male Ascaris, eggs are not found in the stool.

(ii) IN THE BILE. Microscopical examination of the bile obtained by duodenal intubation may reveal Ascaris eggs.

II. INDIRECT EVIDENCES

Blood Examination. Eosinophilia is present only at the early stage of invasion, but if present in the intestinal phase suggests associated strongyloidiasis or toxocariasis.

Dermal Reaction (Allergic). "Scratch test" with powdered Ascaris Antigen has often been found to be positive but the results are variable.

Serological tests are useful in diagnosis of extraintestinal ascariasis (Loeffler's syndrome).

Note: Larvae may be found in the sputum during the stage of migration.

SURGICAL ASPECTS OF ASCARIASIS

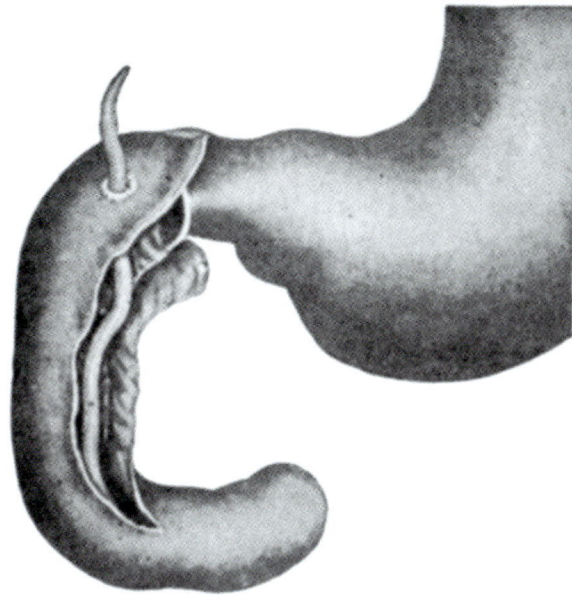

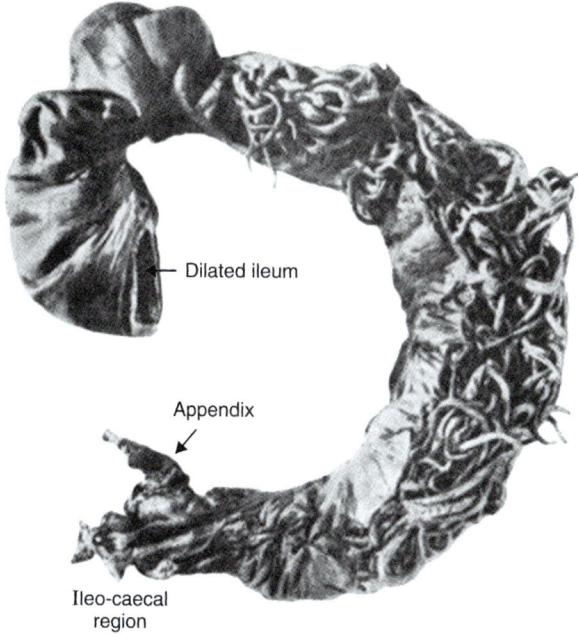

Fig. 180—*A. lumbricoides* **perforating through a duodenal ulcer.**

Fig. 181—**A large number of** *A. lumbricoides* **impacted in the ileum near the ileo-caecal junction caused fatal intestinal obstruction.**

Treatment. Drugs which are known to have specific action on Ascaris include the following: pyrantel pamoate (a single dose of 10 mg/kg, maximum 1 gm), thiabendazole and mebendazole (100 mg twice daily for three days), albendazole (a single dose of 400 mg).

Prophylaxis. The measures should consist of (i) proper disposal of human faeces, (ii) treatment of parasitised individuals, and (iii) education of children in schools on sanitary laws and hygiene.

Superfamily SPIRUROIDEA

Genus GNATHOSTOMA

Gnathostoma spinigerum (Owen, 1836). Adults (about 3 cm long) are normally found in the tumours of the stomach wall of the definitive hosts, dogs, cats, tigers and other animals. Eggs (oval with a mucous plug in one pole and unsegmented) are extruded from lesions of the stomach of definitive hosts and evacuated via faeces into water where they embryonate and hatch. The larvae are ingested by Cyclops, the first intermediate host and are metamorphosed into the 2nd stage larvae. These are then eaten by a fish, frog or snake, the second intermediate host and develop into the 3rd stage larvae in the flesh of these animals. The definitive hosts are infected by eating the 3rd stage larvae in the second intermediate host which develop into adult worms in the stomach wall in about 7 months.

Man becomes infected with the 3rd stage larvae of *G. spinigerum* by eating inadequately cooked infected flesh of the second intermediate host, but they are unable to grow up to the adult stage. The immature 3rd stage larva resembles the adult worm in morphology, having 4 to 8 rows of sharp recurved hooklets on the cephalic bulb. It migrates through the subcutaneous tissues, causing fugitive swelling and cutaneous larva migrans. It has been known to invade the brain and eyes. The diagnosis of Gnathostoma infection is established by finding the immature worm in the lesion and by an intradermal skin test with the larval or adult antigen. The worm may be treated with albendazole undercover of steroid and sometimes the worm is to be removed surgically. Infection can be avoided by sterilising the infected second intermediate host by boiling or immersing in strong vinegar for 5½ hours. Gnathostomiasis is commonest in Thailand but also reported from Vietnam, Malaysia and India.

G. hispidum Fedtschenka, 1873. The definitive host is a pig. Adult worms are larger and have 12 rows of hooklets on the cephalic bulb. A few cases of human infection have been reported from India, Canton and Japan.

Genus: ANISAKIS

Anisakiasis or Herring worm disease in a man

Anisakid nematodes belong to the family Anisakidae. Among several members of the genera, Anisakis and Phocanema are potential aetiological agents of human anisakiasis. The disease is common in Japan and other places where undertreated or raw infected fish is taken as food.

Anisakis simplex Rudolphi 1809. It is an ascarid parasite. The adult worm inhabits the intestine of large sea mammals (porpoises, dolphins, seals, whales). Its larval stage is found in the flesh of a variety of marine fish (cod, salmon and herring) and causes *amsakiasis* or herring-worm disease in man. The infection is acquired by consuming raw or inadequately pickled fish and is common in places where such food is considered a delicacy, as in some Scandinavian countries, Holland and Japan. The larva liberated from the digestion of flesh of fish enters the mucosa of stomach and intestine, producing an eosinophilic granulomatous tumour simulating malignancy. The patient may complain of colicky abdominal pain and symptoms of intestinal obstruction.

The eggs are passed in the host's faeces and in water, embryonation and larval differentiation within the eggs continues. The second stage larvae hatch out and remain free-swimming in water. They are ingested by the first intermediate host (shrimp like crustaceans) and develop into third stage larvae within body cavity or in the surrounding tissue, which are infected to fish and squid (the second intermediate host). Being ingested by variety of fish (cod, salmon and herring) and squid, the larvae migrate from the intestine to the tissues (like liver) or peritoneal cavity and grow to the size up to 3 cm or more in length and remain encysted. By predation these larvae can be transferred from fish to fish. When the infected fish is eaten by the definitive host (including human) the larvae penetrate the stomach and intestinal mucosa and live in clusters, develop into adult males and females and remain in position by embedding the anterior end of the body in crater-like tumour. The fertilized females lay eggs which are expelled with faeces of the definitive host.

Diagnosis: Indirect haemagglutination test with Anisakis antigen is positive. Diagnosis with fluorescent antibody can be done. Diagnosis is established by finding larvae in tissues removed by surgical resection.

Treatment: There is no effective treatment. Endoscopic removal of tumour is the only treatment.

Superfamily FILARIOIDEA

This superfamily includes nematodes inhabiting the blood vessels, lymphatic system, connective tissues and serous cavities of man and animals. The adult worms are slender and thread-like, usually measuring 2 to 10 cm in length (except females of *Onchocerca*); the females are much longer than the males. The worm has a simple lipless mouth, a cylindrical oesophagus without a bulb and a simple intestine which may be atrophied posteriorly. The caudal alae are often lacking and the copulatory spicules are unequal and dissimilar. The females are viviparous, giving birth to larva, known as *microfilaria*. The life cycle is passed in two hosts: man and a certain blood-sucking insect. Microfilaria completes its development in the insect host, giving rise to the infective form. Infection is transmitted to man by the bite of the insect by inoculation. Species-diagnosis is generally made from a study of larval forms; adult worms are rarely obtained.

The superfamily Filarioidea includes four families and the species parasitic to man belong to the family *Acanthocheilonematidae*. The family is divided as follows:

Superfamily FILARIOIDEA: Family ACANTHOCHEILONEMATIDAE				
SUBFAMILY	GENUS	SPECIES	HABITAT OF ADULT WORMS	MICROFILARIA IN
Acanthocheilo-nemantinae	Wuchereria	*W. bancrofti*	Lymphatic system	Blood
	Brugia	*B. malayi* and *B. timori*	Lymphatic system	Blood
	Onchocerca	*O. volvulus*	Connective tissues	Skin
		M. perstans	Connective tissues	Blood
		M. streptocerca	Connective tissues	Skin
	Mansonella	*M. ozzardi*	Mesentery	Blood, skin
Dirofilarinae	Dirofilaria	*D. conjunctivae* (*D. repens* and *D. tenuis*)	Connective tissues and eyelid	
		D. magalhaesi	Heart	
		D. immitis	Heart of dog	Blood
	Loa	*L. loa*	Connective tissues; conjunctiva	Blood

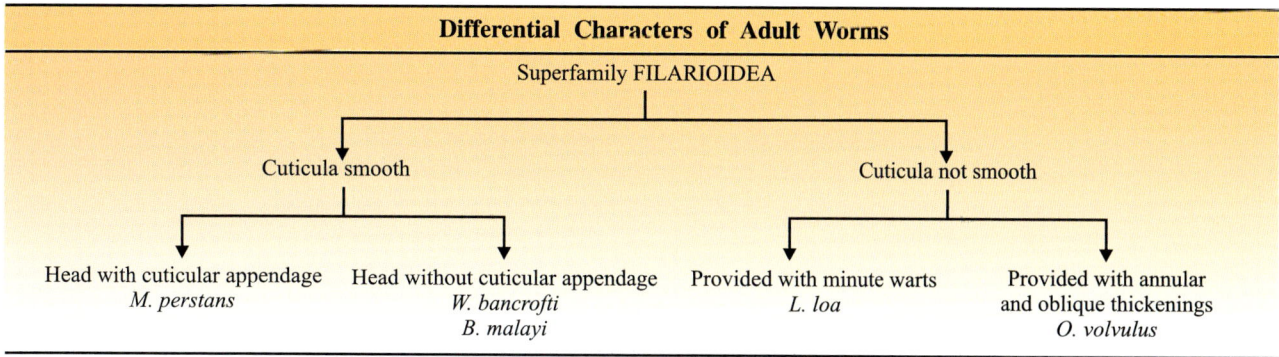

Differential Characters of Adult Worms

Superfamily FILARIOIDEA

Cuticula smooth

Head with cuticular appendage
M. perstans

Head without cuticular appendage
W. bancrofti
B. malayi

Cuticula not smooth

Provided with minute warts
L. loa

Provided with annular
and oblique thickenings
O. volvulus

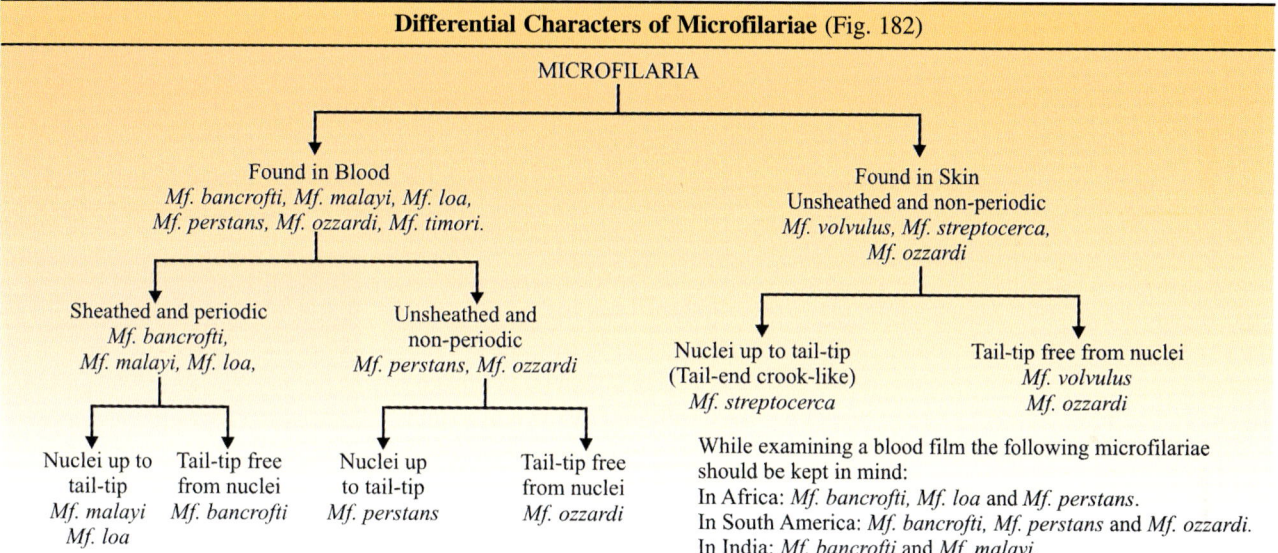

Differential Characters of Microfilariae (Fig. 182)

MICROFILARIA

Found in Blood
Mf. bancrofti, Mf. malayi, Mf. loa,
Mf. perstans, Mf. ozzardi, Mf. timori.

Found in Skin
Unsheathed and non-periodic
Mf. volvulus, Mf. streptocerca,
Mf. ozzardi

Sheathed and periodic
Mf. bancrofti,
Mf. malayi, Mf. loa,

Unsheathed and
non-periodic
Mf. perstans, Mf. ozzardi

Nuclei up to tail-tip
(Tail-end crook-like)
Mf. streptocerca

Tail-tip free from nuclei
Mf. volvulus
Mf. ozzardi

Nuclei up to
tail-tip
Mf. malayi
Mf. loa

Tail-tip free
from nuclei
Mf. bancrofti

Nuclei up
to tail-tip
Mf. perstans

Tail-tip free
from nuclei
Mf. ozzardi

While examining a blood film the following microfilariae
should be kept in mind:
In Africa: *Mf. bancrofti, Mf. loa* and *Mf. perstans.*
In South America: *Mf. bancrofti, Mf. perstans* and *Mf. ozzardi.*
In India: *Mf. bancrofti* and *Mf. malayi.*

Immunology. Living adult worms or microfilariae do not cause any reaction in a normal host. A marked immune response is observed against killed adult and larval worms. It is known that man develops a well-marked resistance to superinfection, except in onchocerciasis. The immune mechanism in wunchereriasis is both humoral and cellular and is effective only against microfilariae. This helps to lower the microfilarial density in man in the age group 15-20 years (in onchocerciasis the microfilaria rate does not decrease with age). A high level of serum antibody found in occult filariasis (tropical pulmonary eosinophilia) is related to the immune responses (may be genetically determined) developing against *W. bancrofti, B. malayi* or other animal filaria and prevents microfilariae in reaching the peripheral blood.

The humoral antibodies found in filarial infections are complement-fixing, haemagglutinating and fluorescent. The CF test is carried out with antigen from *D. immitis* (dog heartworm) and positive results are obtained in high per cent of cases of loiasis and onchocerciasis; it is universally positive in occult filariasis. Cross reactivity with CF test is seen in other helminthic infections, such as strongyloidiasis,

SHEATHED MICROFILARIAE

Mf. bancrofti   *Mf. malayi*   *Mf. loa*

UNSHEATHED MICROFILARIAE

Mf. perstans   *Mf. ozzardi*   *Mf. streptocerca*   *Mf. volvulus*

Fig. 182—Tail-ends of microfilariae found in man.

ascariasis and schistosomiasis. An immediate hypersensitivity type of humoral response against dead microfilaria forms the basis of intradermal test in onchocerciasis (Mazzotti's test) and wuchereriasis. A significant increase of serum IgM level is observed in wuchereriasis and serum IgE level in onchocerciasis.

Wuchereria bancrofti (Cobbold, 1877) Seurat, 1921

(SYNONYM: *Filaria bancrofti* Cobbold, 1877)

Common Name: **Bancroft's filaria.**

The larval forms of the parasite were first found by Demarquay (1863) in the hydrocele fluid of man. Later Wucherer (1866) found them in the chylous urine and Lewis (1872) found them in the human blood. Bancroft (1876) found the adult females, hence the specific name was given after the discoverer.

Geographical Distribution. The parasite is largely confined to the tropics and subtropics, occurring in India, the West Indies, Puerto Rico, Southern China, Japan, Pacific Islands, West and Central Africa and South America. In India, it is distributed chiefly along the sea-coast and along the banks of big rivers (except Indus); it has also been reported from Rajasthan, Punjab, Uttar Pradesh and Delhi.

Habitat. Adult worms are found in the lymphatic vessels and lymph nodes of man only. Bancroftian filariasis is not a zoonotic disease.

Morphology. ADULT WORMS. These are long hair-like (Fig. 183) transparent nematodes (often creamy-white in colour). They are filiform in shape and both ends are tapering, the headend terminating in a slightly rounded swelling. The *male* measures 2.5 to 4 cm in length by 0.1 mm in thickness. Its tail-end is curved ventrally and contains two spicules of unequal length. The *female* measures 8 to 10 cm in length by 0.2 to 0.3 mm in thickness. Its tail-end is narrow and abruptly pointed. The females, though liberating active embryos, are really ovo-viviparous (laying eggs with well developed embryos). Males and females remain coiled together and can only be separated with difficulty (females are usually more numer-

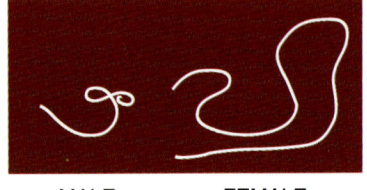

MALE   FEMALE

Fig. 183–Adult worms of *W. bancrofti* (natural sizes).

ous than males and the latter are difficult to find). The *life span* of the adult worms is long, probably several years (5 to 10 years).

EMBRYOS (MICROFILARIAE). Passing through the lymph nodes, these embryos find their way by the main lymphatic trunks into the circulating blood. They are very active in their habits and can move both with and against the blood stream. When *unstained*, they appear as colourless and transparent bodies with blunt heads and rather pointed tails. The embryo measures about 290 µm in length by 6 to 7 µm in breadth. When dead and *stained* with Romanowsky's stains, the embryo (Fig. 184) shows the following morphological peculiarities:

(i) *A Hyaline Sheath.* This is a structureless sac which is best seen where it projects slightly beyond the extremities of the embryo. The sheath is much longer (359 µm) than the larval body so that the larva can move forwards and backwards within it. The sheath represents the chorionic envelope of the egg; it remains as an investing membrane round the larva.

(ii) Cuticula is lined by *subcuticular cells* and is seen only with vital stains.

(iii) *Somatic Cells* or *Nuclei.* These appear as granules in the central axis of the body and extend from the head to the

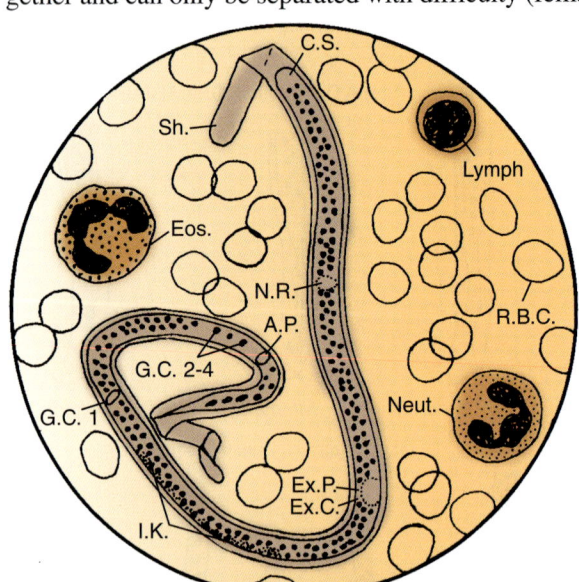

Fig. 184—Morphology of *Microfilaria bancrofti.*
Sh., Sheath; C.S., cephalic space; N.R., nerve ring; Ex. P. excretory pore; Ex. C, excretory cell; I.K., innenkörper; G.C., 1 & G.C. 2-4, G-cells (so called "genital cells"); A.P., anal pore; R.B.C., red blood cells; Neut., neutrophil; Eos., eosinophil; Lymph., lymphocytes.

tail-end. The granules do not extend up to the tip of the tail (terminal 5 per cent) and serve as a distinguishing feature of *Mf. bancrofti*. At the anterior end there is a space, also devoid of granules, called the *cephalic space* which is as long as it is broad. With vital stains the presence of a *stylet* is seen.

(iv) The granules *are broken at definite places* serving as the landmarks for identification of the species. They include the following: (a) Nerve ring, an oblique space, (b) anterior V-spot, represents the rudimentary excretory system, and (c) posterior V-spot or tail-spot, represents the terminal part of the alimentary canal (anus or cloaca).

(v) *A few G-cells* (the so-called "genital cells") posteriorly; while G-cells 2, 3 and 4 are just in front of the anal pore, G-cell 1 is situated further in front.

(vi) *Innenkörper of Fülleborn or Central (Internal) Body of Manson* extends from the anterior V-spot to the G-cell 1. It represents the rudimentary alimentary canal.

The larval forms do not undergo any further development in the human body unless they are taken up by their appropriate intermediate host (mosquito). If these microfilariae are not sucked up by the mosquito, they die in course of time. The *life span* of microfilariae in the human body has been found to be as long as 70 days (Rao, 1933).

Periodicity of Mf. bancrofti. The microfilariae of Oriental countries (India and China) are not constantly found in the peripheral blood but appear periodically at night mostly between 10 P.M. and 4 A.M., thus showing a nocturnal periodicity. It has been suggested that during daytime they retire principally inside the capillaries of lungs, kidneys (glomerular tufts), heart and the big arteries, such as the carotid. The mechanism of:this nocturnal periodicity is not yet clearly known but it is presumed to be in some way related with the night-feeding habit of its intermediate host, *Culex pipiens fatigans*.

Note: In Pacific Islands, *Mf. bancrofti* does not exhibit any periodicity, being found in the peripheral blood both during the day and at night, in equal numbers (non-periodic). In this case, however, the intermediate host is *Aedes polynesiensis* which feeds by day also.

Life Cycle. *W. bancrofti* passes its life cycle (Fig. 185) in two hosts: *man* and *mosquito.*

1. *The definitive host* is man, in whose lymphatic system the adult worms are harboured. Live embryos (microfilariae) are discharged which find their way into the blood stream. The embryos are capable of living in the peripheral blood for a considerable time without undergoing any developmental metamorphosis. They are subsequently taken up by the female culicine mosquitoes during their blood-meal.

2. *The intermediate host* is a mosquito, in which the microfilariae undergo further development, after which they become infective to man. A large number of species of mosquito belonging to the genus Gulex, Aedes and Anopheles act as intermediate hosts for *W. bancrofti*.

STAGES IN THE DEVELOPMENT OF MICROFILARIA IN THE MOSQUITO

(i) Sheathed microfilariae ingested by the mosquito during its blood-meal collect round the anterior end of the stomach. They cast off their sheaths quickly, penetrate the gut-wall within an hour or two and migrate to the thoracic muscles. Here they rest and begin to grow.

(ii) In the next 2 days, the slender, snake-like organism changes to a thick, short, sausage-shaped form with a short spiky tail, measuring 124 to 250 μm in length by 10 to 17 μm in breadth (the *first-stage larva*). It possesses a rudimentary digestive tract.

(iii) In 3 to 7 days' time, the larva grows rapidly, moults (sheds cuticle) once or twice and at the end of this stage measures 225 to 330 μm in length by 15 to 30 μm in breadth (the *second-stage larva*).

(iv) On the 10th or 11th day, the metamorphosis becomes complete: the tail atrophies to a mere stump and the digestive system, body cavity and genital organs are now fully developed. This is the *third-stage larva* which measures 1,500 to 2,000 μm in length by 18 to 23 μm in breadth and has 3 subterminal caudal papillae (*B. malayi* has 2). At this stage, it is infective to man and enters the proboscis sheath of the mosquito on or about the 14th day. It should be noted that one microfilaria gives rise to one infective larva in the proboscis sheath. There may be several larvae remaining coiled up, waiting for an opportunity to infect man while the mosquito is having its blood-meal.

Note: The time taken for the complete development of microfilaria in the mosquito varies from 10 to 20 days or more, depending however on the atmospheric temperature, humidity and also to a certain extent, on the species of the mosquito.

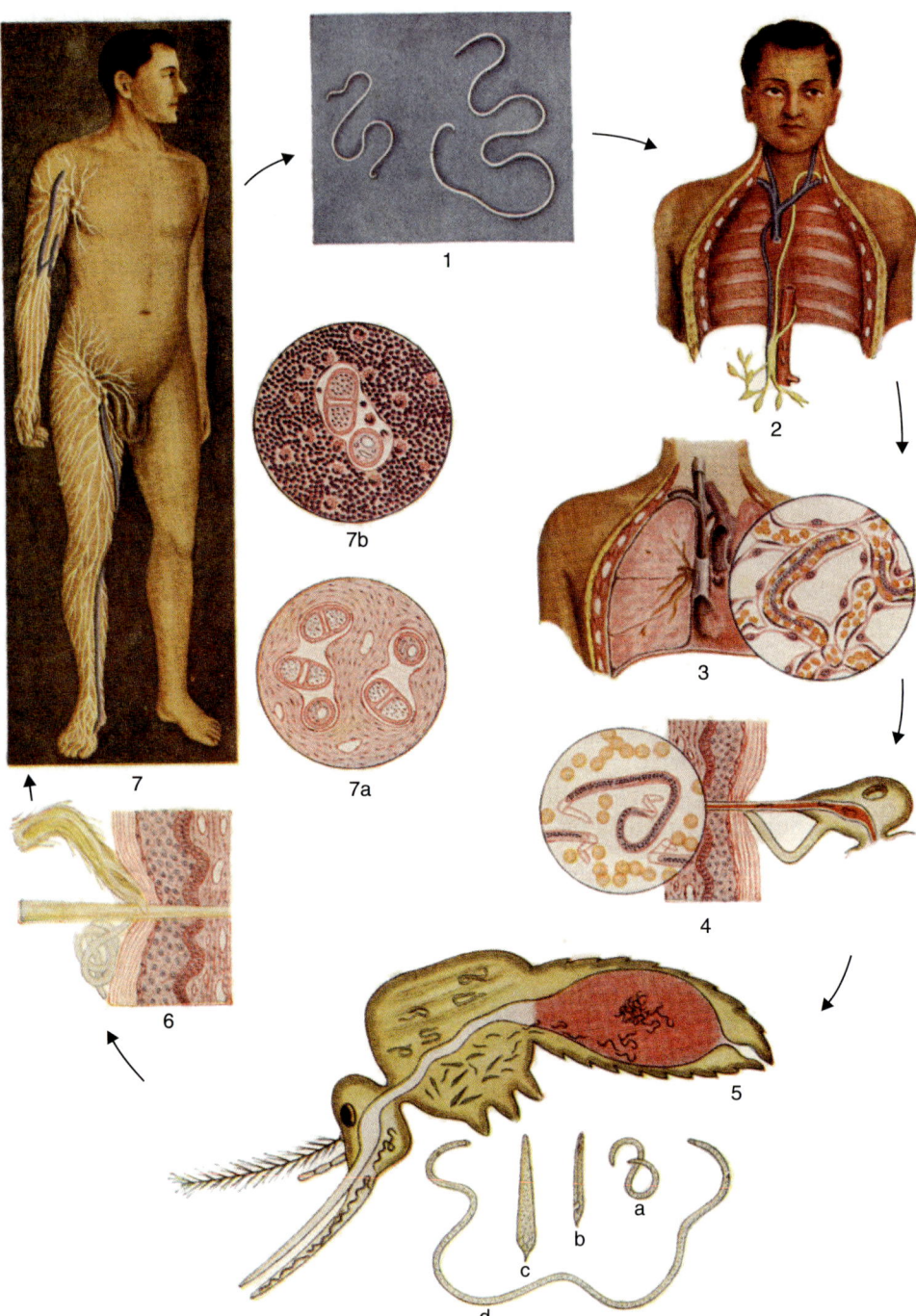

Fig. 185—Life cycle of *Wuchereria bancrofti*

1, Adult worms (male and female); 2, diagram showing the opening of the thoracic duct into the left subclavian vein (microfilariae discharged by adult wuchereiae in the lymphatic system enter into the venous circulation *via* the thoracic duct); 3, *Mf. bancrofti* in the pulmonary capillaries during daytime; 4, female mosquito (*Culex p. fatigans*) sucking microfilariae from peripheral blood at night; 5, stages in the development of *Mf. bancrofti* in the mosquito—(a) microfilariae without its sheath, (b) first-stage larva, (c) second-stage larva, (d) third-stage or mature infective larva; 6, the infective larvae are seen escaping from the proboscis sheath and entering through the skin, while the female mosquito is taking its blood-meal; 7, lymphatic system of superior and inferior extremities and external genitals (the habitat of adult worms); 7a, adult worms (male and female) inside the lymphatic vessels of the subcutaneous tissues; 7b, adult male and female inside the lymph node.

ENTRANCE INTO MAN AND DEVELOPMENT INTO ADULT WORMS

When the infected mosquito bites a human being, the *third-stage larvae* are not directly injected into the blood stream like malarial parasites but are deposited on the skin near the site of puncture. Later, attracted by the warmth of the skin, the larvae either enter through the puncture wound or penetrate through the skin on their own.

The *third-stage larvae* (infective larvae), having penetrated the skin, reach the lymphatic channels, settle down at some spot (inguinal, scrotal or abdominal lymphatics) and begin to grow into adult forms. In course of time, probably after a period of 5 to 18 months they become sexually mature. The male fertilises the female and the gravid females give birth to larvae. A new generation of microfilariae is emitted which passes either through the thoracic duct or the right lymphatic duct, to the venous system, and pulmonary capillaries and then to the peripheral circulation (capillaries of the systemic circulation), thus completing the cycle.

Pathogenicity and Clinical Features. The morbid change initiated by *W. bancrofti* is essentially confined to the lymphatic system. Infection with this parasite is called wuchereriasis (commonly called "filariasis").

Note: The term "filariasis" is commonly used to denote the morbid changes produced by the lymphatic-dwelling *Wuchereria* and *Brugia* but this is not at all a happy term, because it may mean infection with any member of the superfamily Filarioidea with or without any associated pathological change.

MODE OF INFECTION. Inoculative method, through the bite of mosquito.

Transmitting Agent—Female mosquitoes (Culex, Aédes or Anopheles).

In India and China: *Culex pipiens fatigans (C. p. quinquefasciatus).*

In Pacific Islands: In Melanesian Islands (except Fiji and New Caledonia), *Anopheles punctulatus* and in Polynesian Islands, *Aëdes polynesiensis.*

Infective Form—Third-stage larvae of developing *Mf. bancrofti.*

Portal of Entry—Skin.

Site of Localisation—Lymphatic system of superior or inferior extremities according to the site of bite, most commonly of the inguino-scrotal region.

Biological Incubation Period (Prepatent Period)—This lasts about 1 to 1½ years. During this period the third-stage infective larvae grow to adult forms which become sexually mature; mating subsequently occurs, the fertilised females begin to parturiate and the microfilariae appear in the peripheral blood (*patent period*).

Pathogenesis. The pathogenic effects seen in wuchereriasis (Bancroft's filariasis) are produced by the adult wuchereria, living or dead. Living microfilariae circulating in the blood are not known to produce any pathogenic effect, except in occult filariasis. The injurious influence excited by the adult worm and developing larva on its host is an inflammatory reaction of the lymphatic system, *lymphangitis* which forms the basic lesion in classical filariasis. Lesion in occult filariasis is caused by microfilariae and is found not only in the lymph nodes but also in the lungs, liver and spleen.

	Table Showing the Differences between Classical and Occult Filariasis	
	CLASSICAL FILARIASIS	OCCULT FILARIASIS
Cause	Developing worms and adults.	Microfilariae.
Basic lesions	Acute inflammation followed by an epitheloid granuloma surrounding the adult worm and a fibrous scar.	An eosinophilic granuloma (allergic or hyper-sensitivity reaction).
Organs involved	Lymphatic system (lymphatic vessels and lymph nodes).	Lymphatic system, lungs, liver and spleen.
Microfilaria	Present in blood.	Present in affected tissues but not in blood.
Therapeutic response	No response to any drug.	Responds to microfilaricidal drug, diethylcarbamazine.
Serological test	Complement fixation test not so sensitive.	Complement fixation test highly sensitive.

The metabolites of the growing larvae in highly reacting individuals (immigrants or unsuitable hosts) may give rise to allergic manifestations, such as urticaria, "fugitive swellings" (raised, painful, tender, red areas of the skin at the extremities) and lymphoedema. These symptoms may appear much earlier, within a few months (three and a half months) after the exposure. Examination of the peripheral blood fails to demonstrate any microfilaria at this stage, but biopsy of a regional lymph node may show the presence of mature or immature adult Wuchereria.

CAUSES OF LYMPHANGITIS. These may be discussed as follows:

(i) *Mechanical irritation* caused by the movement of the adult parasite inside the lymphatic system.

(ii) *Liberation of metabolites* of the growing larvae in highly reacting individuals and *secretion of some toxic fluid* by fertilised females at the time of parturition.

(iii) Absorption of *"toxic" products* liberated from dead worms undergoing disintegration.

Note: Factors (ii) and (iii) appear to be allergic.

(iv) *Bacterial Infection.* Adequate evidence that Streptococci play an etiological role is not forthcoming, but they may appear as secondary invaders and may supplement the wuchereriae in the production of the characteristic lesion.

CAUSES OF LYMPHATIC OBSTRUCTION. The following are the various factors which cause an obstruction to the lymph flow:

(i) *Mechanical blocking* of the lumen by dead worms (single or a bunch) which act as an embolus.

(ii) *Obliterative Endolymphangitis.* Endothelial proliferation and inflammatory thickening of the walls of lymphatic vessels.

(iii) Excessive *fibrosis of the lymphatic vessels* caused by recurrent and repeated attacks of lymphangitis.

(iv) *Fibrosis of afferent lymph nodes* draining a particular area.

EFFECTS OF LYMPHATIC OBSTRUCTION. Two types of conditions are produced:

(a) Lymph varix—Varicosity of lymphatic vessels.

(b) Elephantiasis—Hypertrophy of the affected part.

Wuchererial Infection and Immunity: Role of Reticulo-endothelial System. The lymphatic nodes are one of the essential elements of the reticulo-endothelial system in which the adult worm of *Wuchereria bancrofti* localises. The lymph of the lymph node provides the nutritive requirements of the worm and any factor which tends to obstruct the lymph flow may cause die death of the worm. In the earlier stages the worm provokes a cellular reaction, chiefly of eosinophilic granulocytes around its location (Fig. 186). This has been attributed to the action of metabolites of the growing worm (maturation of the infective larvae introduced by the mosquito) and also to the secretion of a "body fluid" ("helminthic toxin") by the gravid female, as in guinea worm, at the time of parturition. In highly reacting individuals, these excite a local allergic reaction, lymphangitis and lymphadenitis which tend to strangulate the worm. As a consequence, there is lymphoedema, presumably to provide nutrition for the growing parasite (Fig. 187). The littoral cells of the lymph sinuses may also show proliferation. With the growth of the parasite, these changes become more pronounced and there may be, in addition, proliferation of endothelial cells lining the lymphatic channel (Fig. 188).

The presence of wuchererial worm in the lymph node calls forth a response from the reticulo-endothelial system only when the worm dies or undergoes degenerative changes, but as long as the worm is living or growing, no reaction occurs. The tissue surrounding the degenerated worm undergoes necrosis. The dead worm becomes fragmented or even calcified. Such an area is quickly invaded by the fixed macrophage cells and giant cells appear in order to engulf and absorb the fragments of the dead worm (Figs. 189 & 190). The eosinophilic infiltration which was seen in the earlier stages (while the worm was growing or during parturition) gradually disappears. After the monocytes and the giant cells have done their scavenging work, the fibroblasts begin to appear and are laid down in concentric layers round the nucleus of the dead parasite whose presence however may not be recognised with the maturation of the scar tissue. The end-result therefore is the development of a hyalinised scar tissue (Fig. 191) representing, as it were, the tombstone of the dead wuchererial worm.

Besides the lymph nodes, other organs of the reticulo-endothelial system, such as the liver and spleen, do not take any active part in wuchererial infection. They may however be called upon to deal with the disposal of microfilariae which were circulating in the blood.

HISTOPATHOLOGICAL CHANGES IN THE LYMPH NODE IN WUCHERERIAL INFECTION

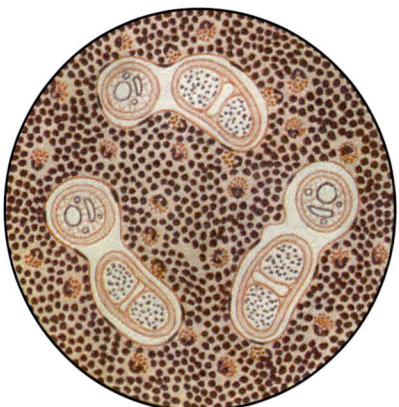

Fig. 186–Males & females of *W. bancrofti* **lodged in a lymph node.**
Showing sections of adult worms within the lumina of lymph vessels (note the double uterus of the female worm). Infiltration of a large number of eosinophil cells can also be seen.

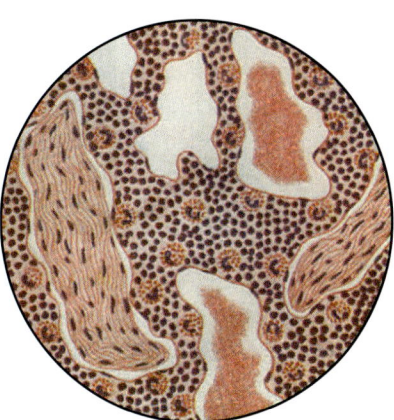

Fig. 187–Lymphoedema or lymph varices.
Resulting from an establishment of collateral circulation due to the partial obstruction of the afferent lymph channels. Two of the lymph vessels are shown to contain recent lymph clots; in two vessels organised clots (later effect of thrombosis) can be seen. The surrounding stroma is infiltrated with a large number of eosinophil cells.

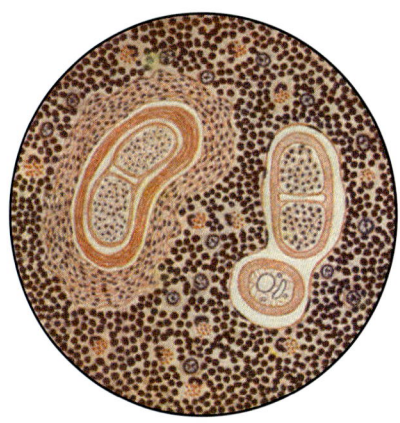

Fig. 188–Obliterative endolymphangitis.
The endothelium lining the lymph vessel occupied by the parasite shows proliferation and the lymph surrounding the parasite has also been thrombosed. The stroma is infiltrated with eosinophil cells and monocytes (macrophages).

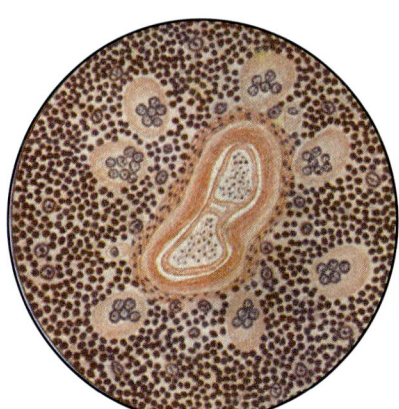

Fig. 189–The occlusion of a lymph vessel.
Strangulating the parasite and causing its degeneration. Macrophages and giant cells have appeared and the eosinophil cells have disappeared; a few plasma cells can also be seen.

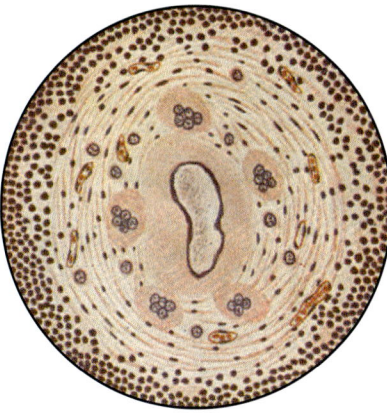

Fig. 190–A "parasitic onion" developing around a degenerated parasite.
The central zone shows a dead calcified worm and surrounding it is a hyaline necrosed mass. In the intermediate zone lie giant cells and macrophage cells. At the periphery, concentric layers of fibro-cellular connective tissue with new capillary blood vessels are to be seen.

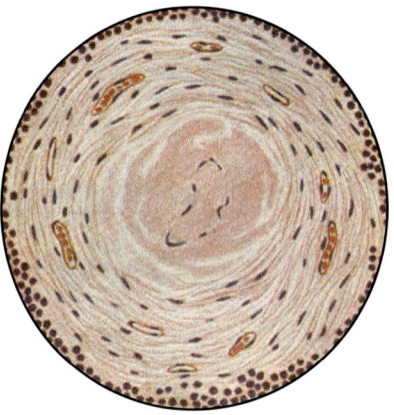

Fig. 191–Formation of a hyaline scar.
The end-result of wuchererial granulation tissue in which the worm has been practically absorbed, leaving only traces of calcified remnants of the worms.

Occult Filariasis (*Meyers-Kouwenaar syndrome*). This is a condition in which there is massive eosinophilia (30 to 80%; absolute count above 3000 per mm^3), generalised lymph node enlargement, hepatosplenomegaly, pulmonary symptoms and absence of microfilaraemia. The adult worm produces the microfilariae continuously, but they do not reach the peripheral blood, because they are destroyed in the tissues. It is an unusual host-reaction to filarial antigen (human or animal), resulting in the development of an eosinophil granuloma in which a large number of eosinophils aggregate around a microfilaria or its remnants. The evidences that this condition is of filarial origin, are as follows: (i) Filarial complement-fixing antibody is present in high titre, (ii) Clinical, haematological and serological manifestations respond readily to microfilaricidal drug, diethylcarbamazine. The species of filarial parasite varies in different localities and it may be either a Wuchereria or a Brugia (human or animal). The syndrome has been reported mostly from India, Sri Lanka, South-East Asia, China, Philippines, Brazil and Africa, i.e., from places wherever filarial infection occurs.

TROPICAL PULMONARY EOSINOPHILIA (*Eosinophilic lung; Weingarten's syndrome*). This is a manifestation of occult filariasis and is characterised by low fever, loss of weight, paroxysmal cough with scanty sputum (may be blood-tinged), dyspnoea (not expiratory) and splenomegaly. Chest radiography shows increased bronchovascular markings or diffuse miliary "mottling" in the lung fields. Microfilaria may be demonstrated in tissues obtained by lung biopsy, although it is difficult to identify the species in tissue sections.

Pathogenic Lesions in Classical Filariasis Caused by *W. bancrofti* (Fig. 192)

1. *Inflammation*—Periodic attacks of fever with lymphadenitis and lymphangitis which are not necessarily due to the presence of parasites but may be the result of sensitisation to the metabolites of the worm located elsewhere.

2. *Dilatation of Lymphatics*—Lymphangiovarix.

3. *Rupture of Lymphangiovarix* (small blood vessels may rupture into the dilated lymphatics): Lymphorrhagia—Lymph scrotum, lymphocele, lymphuria.

   Chylorrhagia (obstruction in the chyle-bearing vessels, thoracic duct)—Chylocele, chyluria or haematochyluria, chylous diarrhoea, chylous ascites and chylothorax.

4. *Hyperplasia of Skin and Connective Tissues*—Elephantiasis (solid oedema) of various parts.

5. *Secondary Bacterial Infection* (with *Streptococcus pyogenes* or *Staphylococcus aureus*)—Septic lymphangitis, abscesses and septicaemia.

Lymphangitis. The parts usually involved are the lymphatics of the testicle and epididymis (epididymo-orchitis), the lymphatics of the spermatic cord (funiculitis), abdominal lymphatics (retroperitoneal lymphangitis) and the lymphatics of the upper and lower extremities; the favourite site for the adults of *W. bancrofti* however is the globus major of the epididymis. The visible lymphatic trunks appear as red congested streaks in the superjacent skin. On palpation, they are found to be painful and appear as cord-like swellings. An acute abdominal symptom may arise as a result of involvement of the retroperitoneal lymphatics. The attack of wuchererial lymphangitis tends to recur periodically once in every month and in some individuals it is related to some particular phase of the moon. It is rather difficult to establish the relationship of attacks of wuchererial lymphangitis to the lunar cycle.

Lymphadenitis. Inflammation of the regional lymph nodes (lymphadenitis) is a frequent accompaniment or may precede an attack of lymphangitis. These are usually found in the groin and sometimes in the axilla. They appear as soft, more or less lobulated masses and are often associated with other wuchererial manifestations. The skin over the swelling is not adherent and unless acutely inflamed, the swelling is not painful and tender.

"Filarial Fever". Filarial lymphangitis is usually accompanied by a rise of temperature ranging from 103° to 104°F which may continue for several days (usually 3 to 5 days). The temperature comes down by crisis with profuse sweating. The fever is associated with a localising sign of inflammation of the lymphatic vessel where the adult worm lies. Examination of blood often shows a transient leucocytosis with an increase of neutrophils; in may also reveal the presence of microfilariae.

Hydrocele. Recurrent attacks of wuchererial orchitis and epididymitis predispose to the occurrence of hydrocele and this condition may exist with or without elephantiasis of the scrotum. The fluid visually contains the microfilariae but the medium being not favourable to their prolonged existence, they die in the hydrocele fluid. The wall of the sac

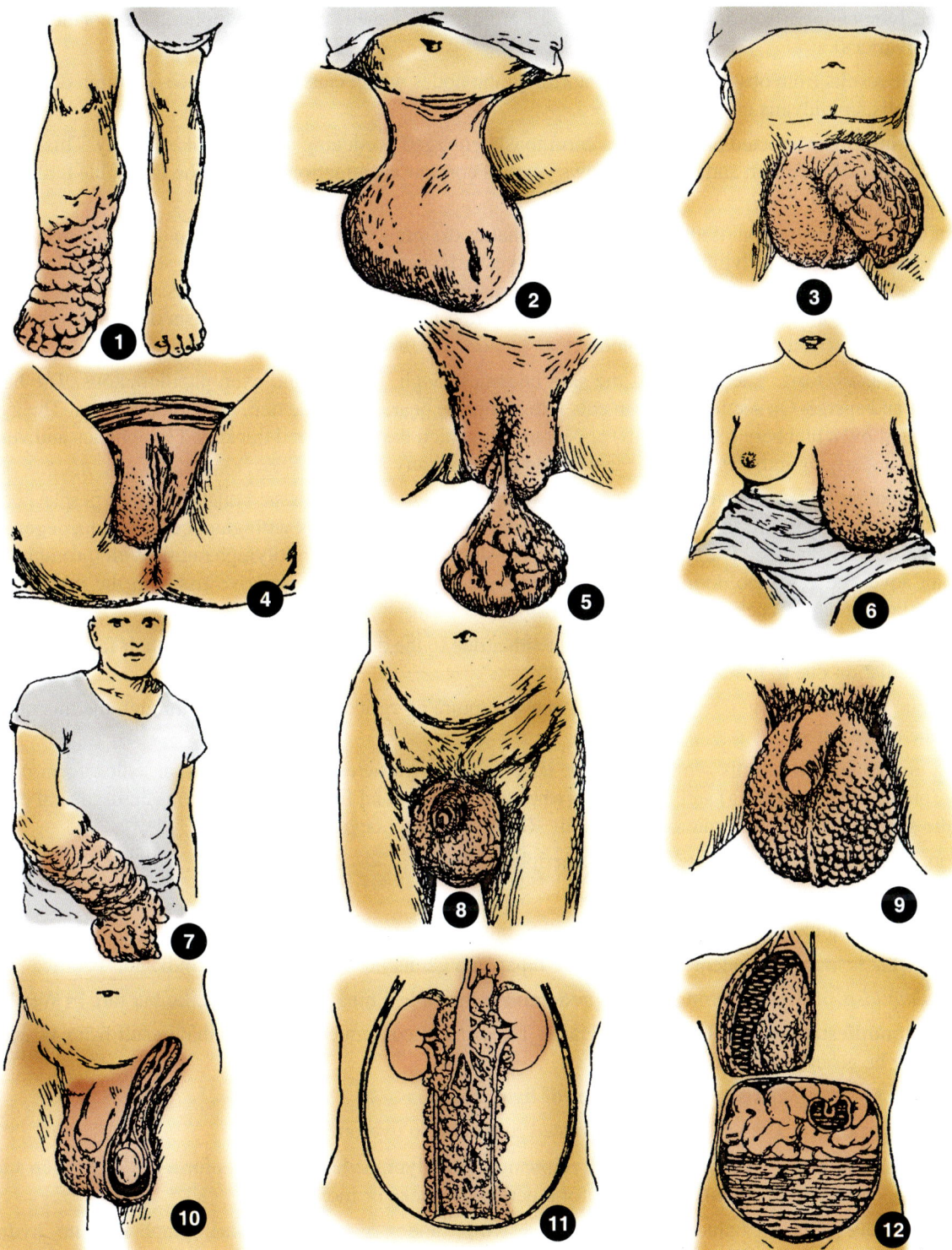

Fig. 192—Pathogenic lesions in classical filariasis caused by *W. bancrofti.*
Elephantiasis of (1) leg, (2) scrotum, (3) penis, (4) labia, (5) clitoris and vulva, (6) breast and (7) forearm; (8) varicose lymph nodes of the inguinal region with lymph scrotum and lymphoedema of the penis; (9) scrotal lymphangiovarices showing vesicles; (10) chylocele and lymph varix of the spermatic cord; (11) chyle varices of the posterior abdominal wall (rupture of these vessels in the urinary tract causes chyluria); (12) chylothorax, chylous ascites and chylous diarrhoea.

is thickened and adult Wuchereriae (living, dead or calcified) may be demonstrated in the wuchererial granulation tissue. The lymphatic vessels in the spermatic cord are also thickened, causing lymphatic varicoceles (funicular lymphangiovariccs).

Hydrocele results from obstruction of para-aortic lymph nodes which causes interference of lymph drainage from tunica vaginalis, epididymis and spermatic cord.

Elephantiasis. The affected part becomes enormously enlarged producing a tumour-like solidity. This is the end-result of wuchererial infection and usually follows years of continuous infection. It is not the inevitable termination of every filarial infection.

CAUSE. Fibrotic constriction of all the afferent lymphatics draining the part. Such a pathological change is brought about by recurrent attacks of lymphangitis over many years. Hypertrophy and hyperplasia, seen in elephantiasis, are the result of excessive protein in the lymph exudate stimulating the connective tissue to excessive growth. Elephantiasis of legs results from obstruction of inguinal or iliac lymph nodes, whereas elephantiasis of scrotum results from obstruction of superficial inguinal lymph nodes.

PATHOLOGICAL ANATOMY. The surface of the skin becomes rough, fissured and even papillomatous. The hairs become rough and sparse. On section, the skin cuts like an unripe pear; it is thickened, dense and fibrous. The subcutaneous tissues show a blubbery (oedematous) appearance in which the dilated and thickened lymphatics and veins can be seen. The underlying muscles and bone usually do not show any alteration.

HISTOLOGICAL EXAMINATION reveals the picture of wuchererial granulation tissue consisting of hyperplasia of connective tissue cells and infiltration of eosinophils, plasma cells and monocytes with giant cells round a degenerating, dead or calcified Wuchereria. The lymphatic vessel also shows obliterative endolymphangitis with thrombus formation. In an advanced case, the dominant lesion consists of hyperplasia of connective tissue in the midst of which remains of defunct adult Wuchereria can be demonstrated.

BLOOD MICROFILARIAE. These are generally absent either due to the death of adult worms or their failure to reach the systemic circulation due to lymphatic obstruction.

Chyluria. Escape of chyle through the urine, due to rupture of varicose chyle vessels through the mucous membrane of the urinary tract.

URINE IN CHYLURIA. It is milk-white in colour. It contains fat particles (dissolves in ether, chloroform or xylol), albumin (precipitates on boiling) and fibrinogen (when allowed to stand forms a coagulum). Microscopical examination of the sediment may reveal microfilaria, a few RBCs and lymphocytes.

BLOOD. Microfilariae may be detected in the peripheral blood.

Geographical variation of Filarial Lesions.

1. *Chyluria* is mainly found in China, Japan and South India but rare in Africa and Pacific.

2. *Hydrocele* is highly prevalent in East Africa, Japan and China but less common in India and Pacific.

3. *Elephantiasis* of leg and scrotum is the predominant lesion in China, India and Pacific but rare in West Africa.

Clinical manifestations of Classical Filariasis. The clinical consequences which may result from *W. bancrofti* infection may be grouped as follows:

A. ASYMPTOMATIC FILARIASIS—These are cases of light infections.

B. SYMPTOMATIC FILARIASIS—These can be divided roughly into two phases:

(a) *Inflammatory phase*—Characterised by lymphangitis and lymphadenitis. It lasts for a few days, then subsides spontaneously and recurs at irregular intervals for a period of weeks or months.

(b) *Obstructive phase*—Characterised by varicose lymph nodes (groin and axilla), lymph scrotum, hydrocele, chyluria and elephantiasis of various parts. These arc found in sites where inflammatory reactions have occurred previously. The lesion results from progressive lymphatic obstruction causing interference of lymph drainage. The obstructive lesions take a long time to develop—may be 20 years. The obstructive phase is punctuated by acute inflammatory reaction.

Diagnosis. The procedures adopted are classified as follows:

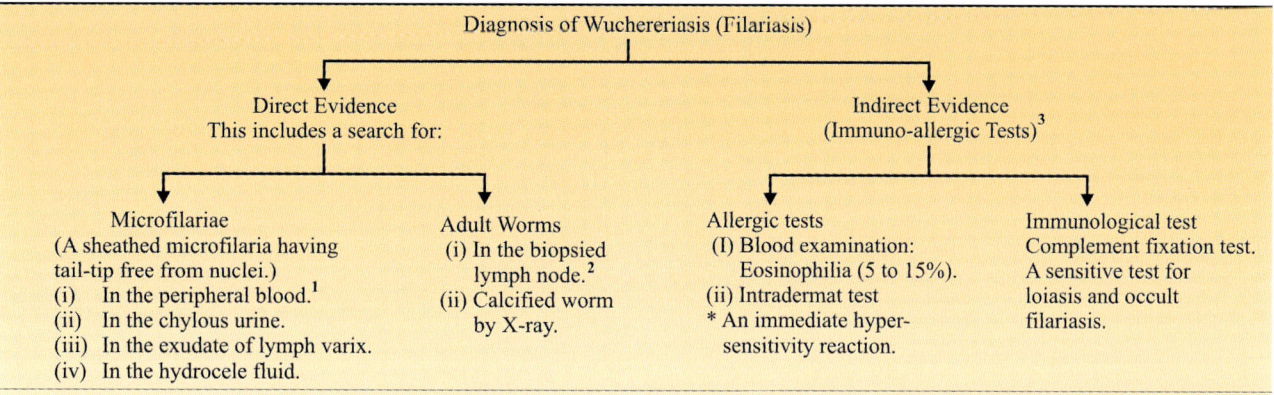

Diagnosis of Wuchereriasis (Filariasis)

Direct Evidence
This includes a search for:

Microfilariae
(A sheathed microfilaria having tail-tip free from nuclei.)
(i) In the peripheral blood.[1]
(ii) In the chylous urine.
(iii) In the exudate of lymph varix.
(iv) In the hydrocele fluid.

Adult Worms
(i) In the biopsied lymph node.[2]
(ii) Calcified worm by X-ray.

Indirect Evidence
(Immuno-allergic Tests)[3]

Allergic tests
(I) Blood examination: Eosinophilia (5 to 15%).
(ii) Intradermat test
* An immediate hyper-sensitivity reaction.

Immunological test
Complement fixation test. A sensitive test for loiasis and occult filariasis.

*Wheal over 2 cm after 30 minutes.

[1]Either in a thin film or a thick film or by concentration methods. The techniques used for the examination of blood for microfilaria are described in Appendix I.

Microfilariae are not found in the peripheral blood in the following conditions: (i) In cases of elephantiasis, due to lymphatic obstruction. (ii) After an attack of lymphangitis, due to the death of the adult worm. (iii) During early allergic manifestations. (iv) In occult filariasis.

Xenodiagnosis. Demonstration of microfilariae in the stomach-blood of the specific mosquito vector which was allowed to bite an infected individual. Compared to concentration methods xenodiagnosis is not very helpful (mosquito abstracts blood to the extent of 1 mm^3).

[2]Tissue change characteristic of wuchererial infection may also be noticed. For purely diagnostic purposes, the lymph node biopsy is not recommended.

[3]Both the complement fixation test and skin test represent group reactions, because antigens used are prepared from any one of these filarial worms: *Dirofilaria immitis* of dog, *Setaria equina* of horse or *Litomosoides carinii* of cotton rat. These are often helpful in the diagnosis of early allergic manifestations.

A fluorescent antibody test has been used for the serological diagnosis of filariasis but found to be not so satisfactory (Sadun, 1963). Serological tests like ELISA test and IHA test can be used for detection of antibodies to larval antigen.

Trop Bio test [ELISA test for detection of CFA (circulating filarial antigens) in serum or plasma] and ICT (immunochromatographic card test) are now available for the detection of adult worm infection and not dependant on the microfilariae periodicity. The specificity of these tests is about 99%.

PCR assay for the detection of microfilaria infection of both *W. bancrofti* and *B. malayi* has been developed but not so much sensitive than microscopic blood examination.

X-ray examination shows calcified adult worm. USG can detect adult *W. bancrofti* in lymphatic vessels of scrotum in infected male and of breast in infected female.

Note: In early allergic manifestations microfilariae do not appear in the circulating blood, hence diagnosis depends on the biopsy of the lymph node adjacent to an area of lymphangitis and occasionally by immuno-allergic tests.

Treatment. The drug having filaricidal action is Diethylcarbamazine. The doses schedule are as follows:

Diethylcarbamazine: 1st day – 50 mg after food. 2nd day – 50 mg three times daily. 3rd day – 100 mg three times daily. 4th day-21st day – 5 mg/kg/day in three divided doses.

Other drugs: Ivermectin—Single oral dose of the drug 150 µg/kg body wt. is used to destroy microfilariae, but there is no macrofilaricidal effect.

Prophylaxis. This consists of the following: (i) destruction of mosquitoes, (ii) reducing the rate of infection amongst insect vectors, (iii) treatment of carriers by using hetrazan and (iv) protection against mosquito bites.

Global elimination programme of lymphatic filariasis. Whole population at risk should be treated with single annual dose of two drugs: Ivermectin 150 µg/kg and albendazole 400 mg in countries of Africa (co-endemic for onchocerciasis) and DEC 6 mg/kg with albendazole 400 mg in other parts of the world. This schedule should be continued for 5-6 years for interruption of transmission. Treatment with DEC-medicated salt daily for 6 to 12 months is an alternative method of treatment. Improved hygienic measures, proper treatment of secondary infection of affected persons and proper care of limb are recommended for morbidity control.

Brugia malayi (Brug, 1927) Buckley, 1960

Common Name: Malayan filaria.

Geographical Distribution. Indonesia, Borneo, Thailand, Vietnam, Malaysia, Burma, Southern China, Korea, Koshima island (Japan), Sri Lanka (now free, WHO 1974), India (either occurring alone or overlapping with bancroftian filaria). In India, it has been chiefly reported from Kerala, Orissa, Madhya Pradesh and Assam.

Habitat. The adult worm is found in the lymphatic system.

Morphology. Morphologically, the adults resemble to those of *W. bancrofti,* being delicate whitish thread like. The mature females vary in length from 4.3 to 5.5 cm and in breadth from 0.13 – 0.17 mm. Mature males measure 1.3 – 2.3 cm. In length and 0.07 to 0.08 mm in breadth. Microfilariae are found at night in the peripheral blood (sometimes sub-periodic and appear in the peripheral blood during the daytime).

Mf. malayi is enveloped in a sheath and shows the following peculiarities as compared to *Mf. bancrofti*:
  (i)   Smaller in size (230 μm by 6 μm); lies folded with head close to tail.
  (ii) Possesses secondary kinks, instead of smooth curves (Fig. 193A).
  (iii) Double stylets at the anterior end.
  (iv) The cephalic space is longer.
  (v)   The nuclei are blurred, hence counting is difficult.
  (vi) Tail-tip is not free from nuclei (Fig. 193B). There are two discrete nuclei—one at the extreme tip of the tail, and the other midway between the tip and the posterior column of nuclei.

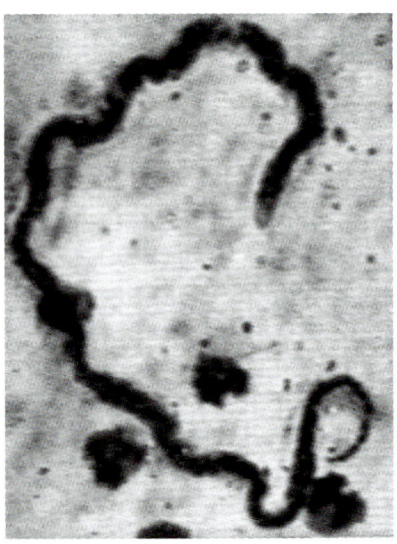

Fig. 193A—*Microfilaria malayi.*
Note the secondary kinks.

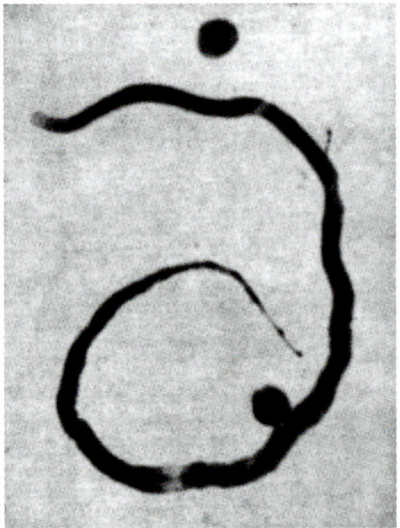

Fig. 193B—*Microfilaria malayi.*
Note the two discrete nuclei at the tail-end: one at the tip which is slightly bulbous and the other at a distance of 10 micrometres (μm).

Life Cycle. Same as that of *W. bancrofti*. The intermediate hosts in India are various species of *Mansonia* (*M. annulifera, M. indiana, M. uniformis*) and one species of *Anopheles (A. barbirostris)* not Culex. Larval development is completed in 6-8 days.

Domestic animals, cats and dogs, may serve as reservoirs of infection (sheathed microfilariae resembling those of *B. malayi* have been found in the blood of these animals in Malaysia, Kenya and India). Monkeys, specially the "leaf monkey" (*Presbytis* sp.) also are important reservoir hosts.

Pathogenicity. Like *W. bancrofti* it causes lymphangitis and elephantiasis (primarily of the lower extremities). Malayan filariasis is characterised by absence of chyluria and rarity of scrotal swellings (recent survey has shown that it is not so rare).

Note: The periodic strain of *B. malayi* is found in man, whereas the subperiodic strain is found in man and a variety of animals in certain areas of Malaysia. *B. pahangi** and other species are found as natural infections in animals alone. The subperiodic strains of *B. malayi* and *B. pahangi* have been incriminated as a cause of "tropical pulmonary eosinophilia" (microfilariae have been demonstrated in the lung biopsy).

Diagnosis. By finding the characteristic microfilariae in the peripheral blood. PCR and DNA probes have also been developed for the diagnosis of the disease.

Treatment. Same as that of wuchereriasis (Bancroftian filariasis).

Prophylaxis. Control measures are directed to protect the individuals from being bitten by infected insect host and the destruction of transmitters. Certain water plants (pistia, water hyacinth and swamp grass) are necessary for the growth of Mansonioides and the removal of these water vegetation often reduces the incidence of infection.

Brugia timori (Partono, Purnomo, Dennis, Atmosoedjono, Oemijati, and Cross, 1977)

(The Timor Filaria)

Human infection with *Brugia timori* is found in Timor Island at the eastern end of the Indonesian archipelago.

No animal reservoir host has yet been discovered. The natural vector mosquito is *Anopheles barbirostris* (*Aedes togoi*) could be infected experimentally by feeding people in eastern part of Flores Island. Adults are found in lymphatic system (but in experimentally infected birds, they have been recovered from lungs, heart and associated large vessels).

Clinical manifestations are milder than other lymphatic filariasis. Lymphangitis, lymphadenitis, lymphoedema (confined below knee) and abscess along the lymph trunk or nodes are common clinical features. Draining abscess may lead to scar formation. Definite diagnosis depends upon the detection of characteristic microfilaria from peripheral blood, collected during night.

In microfilaria, the differences from that of *Mf. malayi* are noted in overall length (310 μm), length : width ratio of cephalic space is 3 : 1 (*Mf. malayi* 2 : 1), 5 to 7 terminal nuclei, sheath not stained with giemsa stain (Fig. 194A).

The laboratory diagnosis, treatment and prophylaxis are similar to those of *B. malayi*.

Onchocerca volvulus (Leuckart, 1893) Railliet and Henry, 1910

Common Name: The convoluted filaria.

SYNONYM: *Onchocerca caecutiens* Brümpt, 1919. Popularly known in America as "blinding filaria".

The generic name Onchocerca means "hooked tail" (from G. *onkos*, hook; *cercos*, tail).

Geographical Distribution. In various parts of Africa and Central America (Guatemala, Venezuela and Mexico); also reported from South Arabia.

Habitat. Adult worm in the subcutaneous connective tissues of man.

Morphology. ADULT WORM. Microscopically the cuticula is seen to be raised in well-marked annular and oblique thickenings; these are more prominent in females than in males. The male measures 3 cm in length by about 0.13 mm in breadth; it has a coiled tail. The female is very long, measuring up to 50 cm in length by 0.4 mm in its greatest diameter. The gravid females may live as long as 15 years.

MICROFILARIAE. These are found in the skin. They are unsheathed and non-periodic. The column of nuclei does not extend to the tail-tip. They measure 300 μm in length by 6 to 8 μm in breadth (Fig. 194B).

Life Cycle. Man is the only definitive host and the intermediate host is a species of a day-biting female "black fly" of the genus *Simulium*. The developmental course of *Mf. volvulus* in Simulium is the same as that of *Mf. bancrofti* in mosquitoes but is completed in 6 days.

Insect vectors. In Africa, they are *S. damnosum* and *S. naevei*. In Central and South America, they are *S. ochraceum* (Mexico and Guatemala) and *S. metallicum* (Venezuela). These are day-biting small flies (1-5 mm long) and the

---

*Other species: *B. pahangi* found in dogs and cats, Malaysia; *B. palei* found in dogs and genet cats, Pate Island, Kenya; *B. ceylonensis* in dogs, Sri Lanka; *B. buckleyi* in hare, Sri Lanka; *B. guyanensis* in the coatimindi, British Guiana; *B. beaveri* in the raccoon, North America; *B. tupaiae* in tree shrew, Thailand.

females suck blood. In Africa two prototypes of *O. volvulus*/*S. damnosum* complex exist—the rain-forest and savannah (Sudan) type. The latter live longer, are in frequent contact with man and have a 30 times higher "transmission potential", hence they cause a very high parasitic load in man.

Pathogenicity. The *infection* is transmitted by the bite of an infected female Simulium. The infective larvae remain localised in the skin and grow into adult worms. The gravid females release actively motile unsheathed microfilariae which migrate in the skin, subcutaneous tissue and eyes until they die (may live as long as 30 months) or ingested by a Simulium. The pathological changes in the skin and eyes result from a hypersensitivity reaction to the dead or dying microfilaria.

The *incubation* period in man is about one year.

O. volvulus causes the disease onchocerciasis in man. The adult worms live in the subcutaneous connective tissues; they do not invade the muscle or viscera. The pathological lesions in onchocerciasis may be divided into two groups as follows:

1. Formation of subcutaneous fibrous nodules (onchocercomas) caused by the adult worms.
2. Ocular lesions caused by microfilariae (metabolites of adult worms may also be responsible).

Subcutaneous Nodules. The sizes vary from a few millimeters to several centimeters (measuring up to 6 cm). They are slow growing tumours and take several years to reach full size. The nodules may be single or multiple, the average number is 3 to 6 but they may be 15 more. They show an uneven distribution. In Africa they are found more on the trunk and limbs than on the head; whereas in America, they are mainly found over the head particularly over the scalp. The explanation is not very clear. It has been said that they occur in the regions where the lymphatics converge or where there is traumatic lymphatic obstruction on pressure points, e.g., strapped head loads or lying on the hips. Simulium habits may also explain the distribution. In Africa, the vector tends to bite on the lower parts of the body, whereas in America, the vector tends to bite about the head and neck. The nodules represent the graveyards of adult worms.

The nodules are raised above the skin surface; they are painless and non-suppurating. On section, they appear as a concentric mass of fibrous tissue with a honeycombed central area containing the adult worms of both sexes remaining intertwined. Dead worms become calcified and initiate foreign body giant cell reaction.

Actively motile microfilariae are found in subepithelial and deeper connective tissue in many areas of the body without any tissue reaction. Only exceptionally the embryos are found in the blood.

Skin lesion such as dermatitis associated with pruritus may be caused by a "toxin" from larva or adult worm. A high eosinophilia is observed in such cases.

Other *complications* which may be observed are:

(1) Development of hydrocele or even lymph scrotum.
(2) Elephantiasis of scrotum and legs.
(3) "Hanging groin" (seen in Africa). The atrophied, inelastic skin of the groin hangs down in a fold containing enlarged, sclerosed femoral or inguinal lymph nodes. The skin shows lichenification and a mottled depigmentation (leopard skin).

Ocular lesions (Ocular onchocerciasis). These are particularly seen in persons with nodules on head or face. They result from the presence of microfilaria which may be found moving about in the substantia propria of the cornea and also in the anterior chamber. The clinical manifestations consist of simple conjunctivitis, small round opacities and pannus in the anterior quadrant of the cornea. Later there may be iridocyclitis, secondary glaucoma and papillitis (optic atrophy), eventually leading to blindness.

Diagnosis. This is based on demonstrating the microfilariae in the shaved pieces of skin and the adult worms inside the excised nodule. Puncturing of the nodule often produces a severe allergic reaction. In cases of ocular lesions, microfilariae may be detected by means of a slit lamp. Blood examination shows a high eosinophilia and immunological tests are also positive.

Skin Test (Mazzotti's test). The appearance of a pruritic papular rash within 24 hours after an oral dose of 50 or 100 mg of diethylcarbamazine suggests the presence of cutaneous microfilaria. The reaction is caused by dead microfilaria of *O. volvulus* killed by the drug.

A fluorescent antibody technique has been employed for the serological diagnosis of onchocerciasis, using microfilariae of *O. volvulus* as antigens. Sera from patients known to have active onchocerciasis reacted positively (Lucasse, 1962).

ELISA (using *O. volvulus* antigen) and CFT have been developed. PCR technique with high specificity for *O. volvulus* and DNA probes are available.

USG is helpful in the detection of deep, non-palpable nodule in patient suffering from this disease.

Treatment. Drugs having specific action include hetrazan (microfilaricidal) and suramin (macrofilaricidal; a toxic drug, to be used with great care). Ivermectin (150 μg/kg once) is drug of choice. It can be repeated after every 6 months up to one year. Mazzotti-type reaction is seen as occational adverse effect of the drug. Fever headache joint pain, pruritus and tender lymph nodes are other adverse effects. Enucleation of nodules is also advised; it helps to reduce not only the danger of ocular complication but also the infection in endemic areas.

Prophylaxis. Control measures should be directed against the insect host.

Mansonella perstans (Manson, 1891) Railliet, Henry and Langeron, 1912

Geographical Distribution. Africa and South America.

Habitat. Adult worms are found in the mesenteric tissues; also in the pleural and pericardial cavities.

Morphology. ADULT WORMS. The male measures 4 cm in length by 0.06 mm in breadth; the female measures 7 cm in length by 0.12 mm in breadth. The distinguishing features are:

 (i) Microscopically, cuticula appears smooth.

 (ii) The anterior end (head) is provided with short cuticular shields, called epaulettes.

 (iii) The tail-end is split and presents a cuticular thickening forming two triangular appendages.

EMBRYOS. *Mf. perstans* are found in the peripheral blood by day as well as by night (non-periodic). The distinguishing features are: (i) smaller in size, (ii) without any sheath, (iii) the tail-end is blunt, and (iv) the nuclei extend to the tail-tip (Fig. 194B).

Life Cycle. The worm passes its life cycle in two hosts:

 (i) In man. Also in chimpanzee and gorilla.

 (ii) In insect. *Culicoides austeni* and *C. grahami*.

Like other microfilariae, *Mf. perstans* follows the same developmental changes in culicoides.

Pathogenicity. Generally considered to be non-pathogenic and usually asymptomatic. Sometimes the infection causes transient swelling like "calabar swelling", fever, headache, pruritus, pain abdomen, articular pain and eosinophilia. Swelling of eyelid, proptosis, nodule in the conjunctiva are also found. These are an immunological response.

Diagnosis. By finding the characteristic unsheathed microfilariae in blood.

Treatment. Hetrazan and ivermectin has no effect on *Mf. perstans*. Specific chemotherapy includes mebendazole (100 mg twice daily for 30 days) or albendazole (400 mg twice daily for 10 days).

Prophylaxis. Protection from insect bite.

Mansonella streptocerca (Macfie and Corson, 1922)

The parasite is found in Central and West Africa. Adult worms have been discovered in the subcutaneous connective tissues of the chimpanzee and in man. The microfilariae have however been found in the skin of the natives of the Gold Coast of West Africa. They are not found in the blood. They measure 180 μm to 240 μm in length and 3 μm breadth. The tail-end is bent in a crook-like curve and the column of nuclei extends to the tail-tip (Fig. 194B). The life cycle has not yet been worked out. The insect vector is *Culicoides grahami* and *C. austeni*. It may produce a purpuric rash similar to onchocerciasis. Microfilariae cause *Streptocerciasis* which is manifested by hypopigmented macule and papule, oedema of the skin, rash and pruritus. Diagnosis is made by demonstration of microfilariae in skin snips. Diethylcarbamazine (2-6 mg/kg for 21 days) eliminates both adult worm and microfilaria of *Mansonella streptocerca*. A single dose of 150 μg/kg body weight of the drug ivermectin also helps in sustained suppression of microfilariaemia in the skin.

Mansonella ozzardi (Manson, 1897) Faust, 1929
Common Name: Ozzard's filaria.

Geographical Distribution. West Indies and parts of Central and South America.

Habitat. Adult worms in the mesentery of man.

Morphology. ADULT WORMS. The *female* measures 7 cm in length by 0.25 mm in breadth. The cuticula is smooth. The tail-end possesses a pair of flap-like papillae. The male is inadequately known and only a single incomplete *male* worm has ever been found.

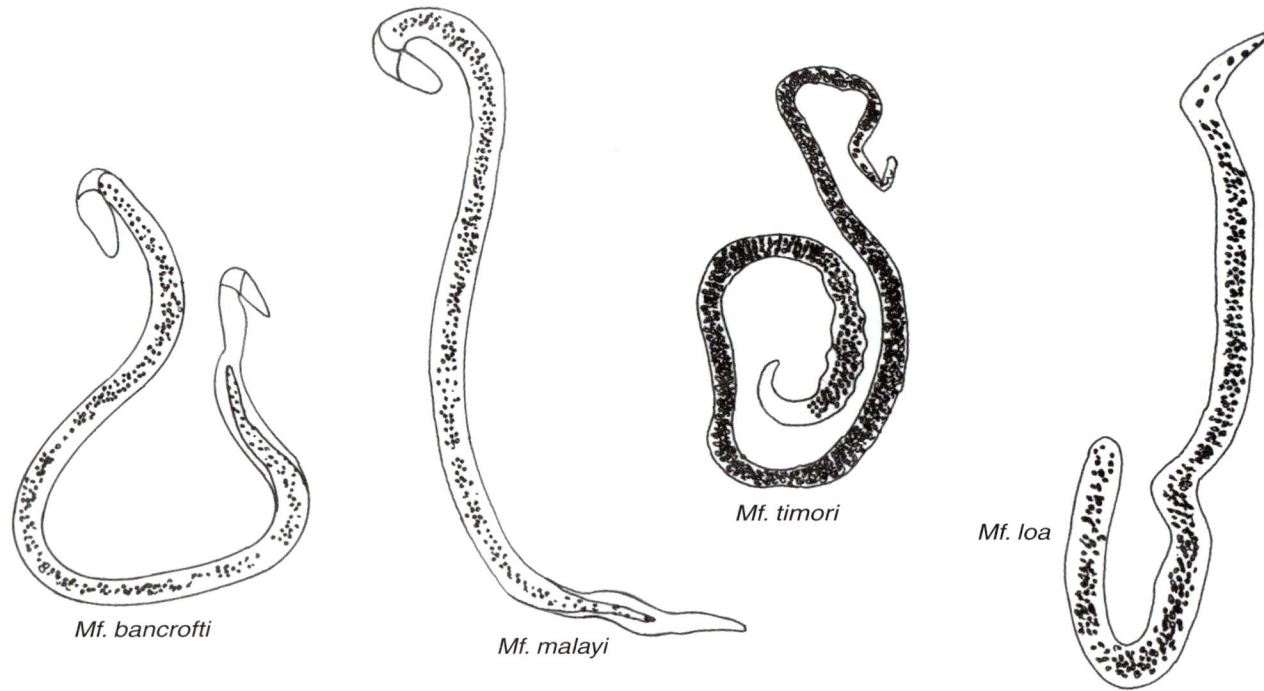

Fig. 194A—Differentiating characteristics of *Mf. bancrofti, Mf. malayi, Mf. timori* **and** *Mf. loa.*

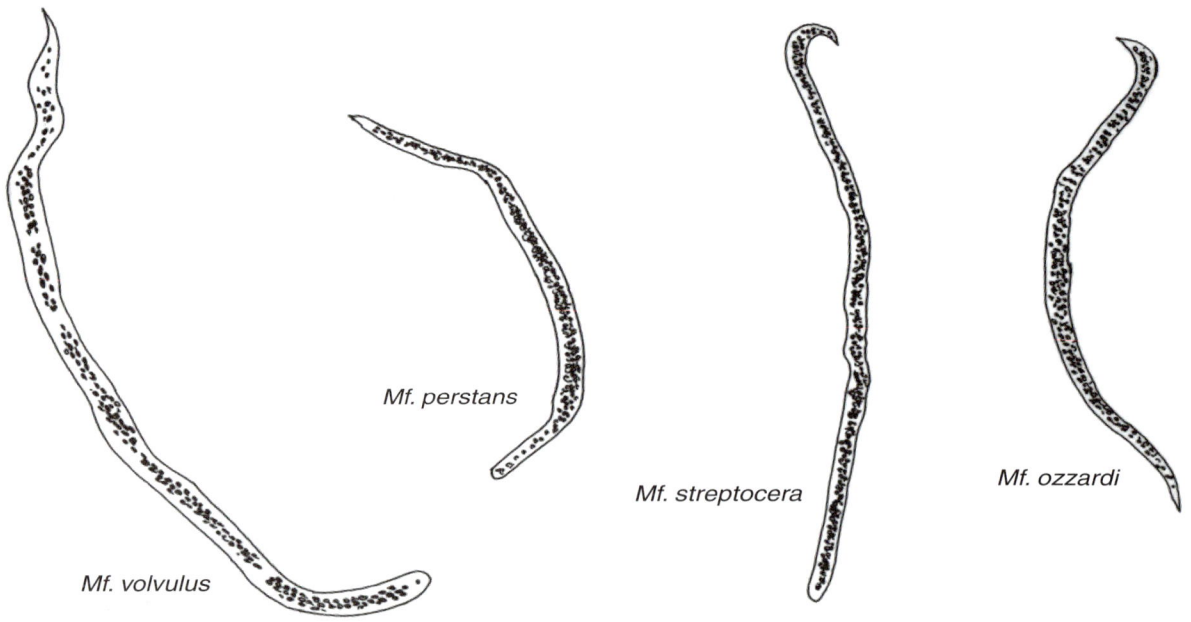

Fig. 194B—Differentiating characteristics of *Mf. perstans, Mf. volvulus, Mf. streptocerca* **and** *Mf. ozzardi.*

EMBRYOS. The microfilariae are found both in the blood and skin. They are small (175-240 μm in length by 4.5 μm in breadth), unsheathed and non-periodic. The tail-end is sharply pointed and the column of nuclei does not extend to the tail-tip (Fig. 194B).

Life Cycle. The insect host of *Mf. ozzardi* is *Culicoides furens* where further development occurs.

Pathogenicity. The worm does not usually produce any pathogenic effect and usually symptomless. Sometimes the infection can produce fever, articular pain, itching and eosinophilia.

Diagnosis. By finding the characteristic unsheathed microfilaria in blood and also in skin snips.

Treatment. Ivermectin (6 mg/kg as a single dose) is used effectively. Mebendazole in the dose of 100 mg twice daily for 10 days or albendazole in the dose of 400 mg twice daily for 10 days is the most effective therapy.

Loa loa (Cobbold, 1864) Castellani and Chalmers, 1913
Common Name: The African eye worm.

"Loa" is the native West African name of the worm.

Geographical Distribution. Central and West Africa.

Habitat. Adult worms in the subcutaneous connective tissues of man; often in the sub-conjunctival tissue of the eye.

Morphology. ADULT WORM. Microscopically, the cuticula is found to have numerous rounded protuberances ("cuticular bosses") which vary in number and arrangement in the two sexes. The *male* measures 3 cm in length by 0.35 mm in breadth. The *female* measures 6 cm in length by 0.5 mm in breadth. The *life span* of adult worms may be 15 years or more.

EMBRYOS. They are found in the peripheral blood by daytime. *Mf. loa* is enveloped in a sheath and measures 300 μm by 7 μm; the column of nuclei extends to the tail-tip (Fig. 194A).

Life Cycle. The worm passes its life cycle in two hosts: man and chrysops (mango or deer flies). Larval development follows the same course as in other microfilariae. The closely related forms found in apes and monkeys appear to be ecologically separate and simian hosts probably do not serve as reservoirs of infection. *Loa loa* is maintained in nature by interhuman transmission. The infection is transmitted by a day-biting female chrysops, *C. silacea* and *C. dimidiata*, both are canopy dwellers; only females suck blood.

Pathogenicity. The worm produces the disease in man called loiasis. Man is infected by the bites of chrysops. The incubation period, i.e., when the worm shows itself, is on an average 3 to 4 years. On entering the human host, the worm migrates rapidly to the various parts of the body through the subdermal connective tissues and shows a special predilection for creeping in and around the eyes. During migration, it causes oedema of subcutaneous tissues, known as "Calabar swellings" or "fugitive swellings". They disappear in course of 2 to 3 days and are regarded as allergic reaction of the tissues to filarial "toxins". Microfilariae can seldom be found during the period of "Calabar swellings", i.e., during the first 4 years of the infection and the diagnosis is based upon history of such "fugitive swellings" associated with intense eosinophilia (30-40%).

Diagnosis. The methods are the same as those for *W. bancrofti*.

Microfilaria can be detected in blood drawn at night. Blood examination reveals high eosiniphilia. Immunodiagnostic tests, like CFT, IFAT and ELISA tests are of limited value. PCR assay has been developed.

Treatment. Hetrazan is an effective remedy for loiasis, causing a quick disappearance of microfilariae from the peripheral blood and even death of adult worm in some cases. Violent allergic reactions which appear in the course of hetrazan therapy may be alleviated by antihistaminics or corticosteroids.

There is often a great risk of development of meningoencephalitis and nephrotic syndrome when cases harbouring a large number of *Mf. loa* (in excess of about 30 per mm^3) are treated with diethylcarbamazine in the dose of 5-10 mg/kg/day. This has been attributed to toxic products liberated from the death of the worm. Hence patients with high microfilaria count are to be treated very cautiously under corticosteroid cover. Ivermectin (200-400 μg/kg in three divided doses for 2 to 4 weeks) is also used effectively. Mebendazole in low doses and albendazole are also effective drugs.

Prophylaxis. This consists of personal protection from the bites of infected flies in the endemic area and destructive campaigns against chrysops.

Filarial Zoonoses

Filarial Zoonoses. Infective larvae of filarial worms which are normally confined to animals are often found in insects biting man. Although they fail to develop into adult worms, these abortive filarial zoonoses have occasionally produced pathological lesions, such as subcutaneous tumours, eye lesions, lymphadenopathy, pulmonary eosinophilia and "coin lesion" in lung simulating neoplasm. There are also records of worms being found in the heart and large blood vessels. Dicrofilariae spp., a common parasite of dogs and cats can cause zoonotic filariasis in man.

In Malaysia *Brugia pahangi*, a parasite of dogs and cats infect man producing lymphangitis and lymphadenitis.

Human Dirofilariasis

Dirofilaria of animals may become adults in man without producing microfilariae. They include;

(1) *Dirofilaria immitis*. A parasite of dog found in the chamber of the right ventricle (dog heart worm). It is prevalent USA, Japan, Australia, Brazil and New Zealand and dog is the definitive host whereas mosquitoes are the intermediate host. By the bite of infected mosquitoes, the man gets infected. The larvae settle in the right heart or in branches of pulmonary artery, because they are not capable of completing their life cycle, in men who are not their natural host. They produce local granulomatous lesion which is seen as "coin shadow" on radiological examination. Diagnosis is confirmed by histological examination of parasite within pulmonary nodule.

(2) *Dirofilaria conjunctivae*. A natural parasite of animals. In U.S.A. it is *D. tennis*, a parasite of raccoons while in Europe, U.S.S.R., Sri Lanka, India, South-East Asia, Italy and East Africa it is *D. repens*, a parasite of dogs and cats.

A few zoonotic human cases (zoonotic filariasis) from where adult Dirofilaria (mostly immature) has been reported are as follows: *D. immitis* from subcutaneous nodules and "coin lesions" in lungs resembling neoplasm; *D. tenuis* and *D. repens* from subcutaneous nodules and abscesses and also from subcutaneous tissue of eyelids and palpebral conjunctiva. *D. immitis* can cause an eosinophilic meningitis in man (Dobson, C. & Welch, J. S. *Trans. Roy. Soc. Trop. Med. & Hyg.*, **68**, 223, 1974).

IHA and bentonite flocculation tests (with anitigen from *D. immitis*) give positive reaction but cross reaction is frequent.

Superfamily DRACUNCULOIDEA

These are long cord-like worms, the mouth being a simple pore and surrounded by circumoral papillae. The oesophagus and intestine are rudimentary. The vulva is in the middle of the body but atrophies before maturity. Females are viviparous and are much longer than males. Larvae are typically "rhabditoid". The worms pass their life cycle in two hosts; cyclops being the intermediate host.

Dracunculus medinensis (Linnaeus, 1758) Gallandant, 1773

Common names: Guinea worm, serpent worm or dragon worm, Medina worm.

The worm has been known from ancient times. Galen (130 to 200 A.D.) gave the name of the disease "dracontiasis". Avicenna (980 to 1037 A.D.), the Arabian physician, named the parasite *Vena medina* as it was common in Medina. In the Bible, it is called the "fiery serpent".

Geographical Distribution. India, Pakistan (Sind and Lahore), Burma, Saudi Arabia, Iraq, Iran, eastern regions of U.S.S.R. (Turkestan), Africa (East, West and Central), West Indies and South America. In India, the parasite is almost eradicated from Punjab, Rajasthan, Madhya Pradesh, Gujarat, Maharashtra and South India. It has not yet been found in Bengal, Assam, Bihar and Orissa.

Habitat. The adult females are usually found in the subcutaneous tissues, especially of the legs, arms and back.

Morphology. ADULT WORMS. *Male.* Although the male worm has not yet been recovered from man (except for one case from India), it has been recovered from experimental animals. The male is much smaller than the female and measures 12 to 30 mm in length by 0.4 mm in breadth.

Female. It is a slender long worm, measuring 60 cm to 1 metre in length with a diameter of 1.5 to 1.7 mm, resembling a piece of long twine thread (Fig. 195). The body is cylindrical, smooth and milk-white in colour. The posterior extremity is tapering and is bent to form a hook. The worm is viviparous and discharges embryos in successive batches for a period of about 3 weeks until the gravid female completely empties its uterine contents. The body fluid is toxic and causes a blister if it escapes into the tissues.

The *life span* of the female is about one year and that of the male is not more than 6 months.

EMBRYOS. These are coiled bodies with rounded heads and long slender tapering tails. They measure 650 to 750 μm in length by 17 to 20 μm in breadth, at the widest part. These embryos are only set free at the time of parturition when the affected part is submerged in water. Further development proceeds in the body of a minute fresh-water crustacean of the genus Cyclops. Unless taken up by cyclops, they can live only for a short period (4 to 7 days).

Life Cycle. The worm passes its life cycle in two hosts: man and cyclops.

   1. *Definitive Host.* Man. Harbours the adult parasite in the subcutaneous tissues.
   2. *Intermediate Host.* Cyclops, in which the embryos undergo certain developmental changes before they become infective to man. *Mesocyclops leuekarti* acts as a host in many regions of the world including India. Other vectors may be *Mesocyclops hyalinus, Thermocyclops vermifer* (the Deccan), *Encyclops serrulatus, Tropocyclops multivolor.*

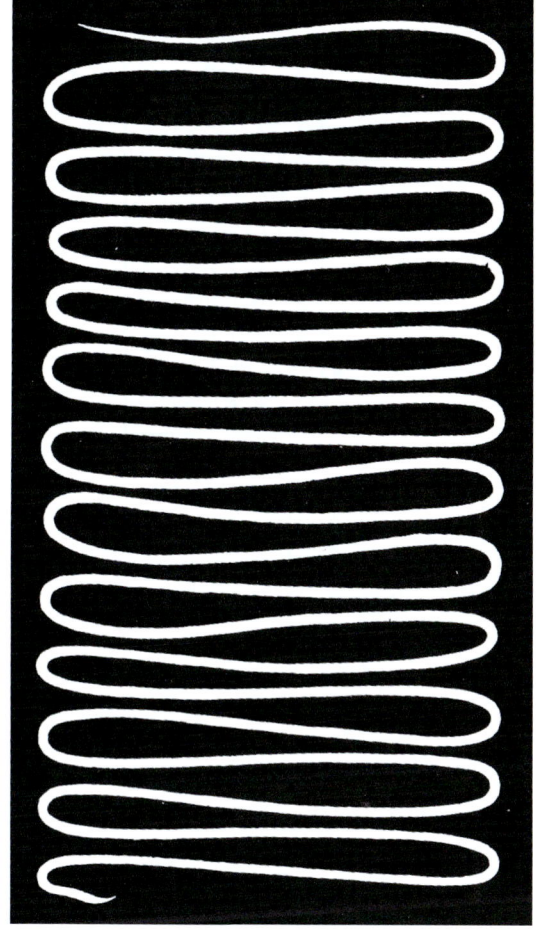

Fig. 195–Female of *Dracunculus medinensis.*
(Natural size)

DEVELOPMENT OF EMBRYOS IN CYCLOPS. Each cyclops can ingest as many as 15 to 20 guinea worm embryos without being inconvenienced in any way. The infected cyclopses usually die at the end of 42 days but with a heavy infection they do not live for more than 15 days (normal span of life of cyclops is about 3 months).

The embryos penetrate the gut-wall within 1 to 6 hours after ingestion and enter the body cavity of the cyclops where they undergo metamorphosis and increase in size (becoming about 1 mm in length). Under favourable conditions it takes about 2 weeks for the development to be completed.

ENTRANCE INTO MAN AND DEVELOPMENT OF ADULT WORMS. The cyclopses containing the infective larvae are swallowed by man with raw drinking water. On reaching the stomach, the cyclopses are digested by the gastric juice and the larvae are liberated. They then penetrate through the gut-wall and enter the retroperitoneal connective tissues where they grow to sexual maturity. The larvae in man become adult males and females. The males die after fertilising the females and disappear within 6 months after infection. The union between males and females occurs early in the deeper connective tissues and not in the intestine. It takes about another 6 months for the gravid female to select its site for discharging the embryos in water. The gravid female migrates and selects only those parts of the skin liable to come in contact with water, such as the backs of water-carriers ("Bhistis"), arms and legs of washermen, and legs of those who fill water in containers in "step wells" and ponds. On reaching the skin surface, it secretes a "toxin", producing a blister which later ruptures and forms an ulcer. Contact with water stimulates the worm to protrude its head through the centre of the ulcer and causes a reflex discharge of a milky fluid containing a large number of coiled embryos ejected from the prolapsed uterus. Thus, the embryos are back again in water and the cycle is repeated (Fig. 196).

Pathogenicity and Clinical Features. Infection with *D. medinensis* in man is known as guinea worm disease or dracunculosis (dracunculiasis or dracontiasis).

Source of Infection—Infected cyclops.

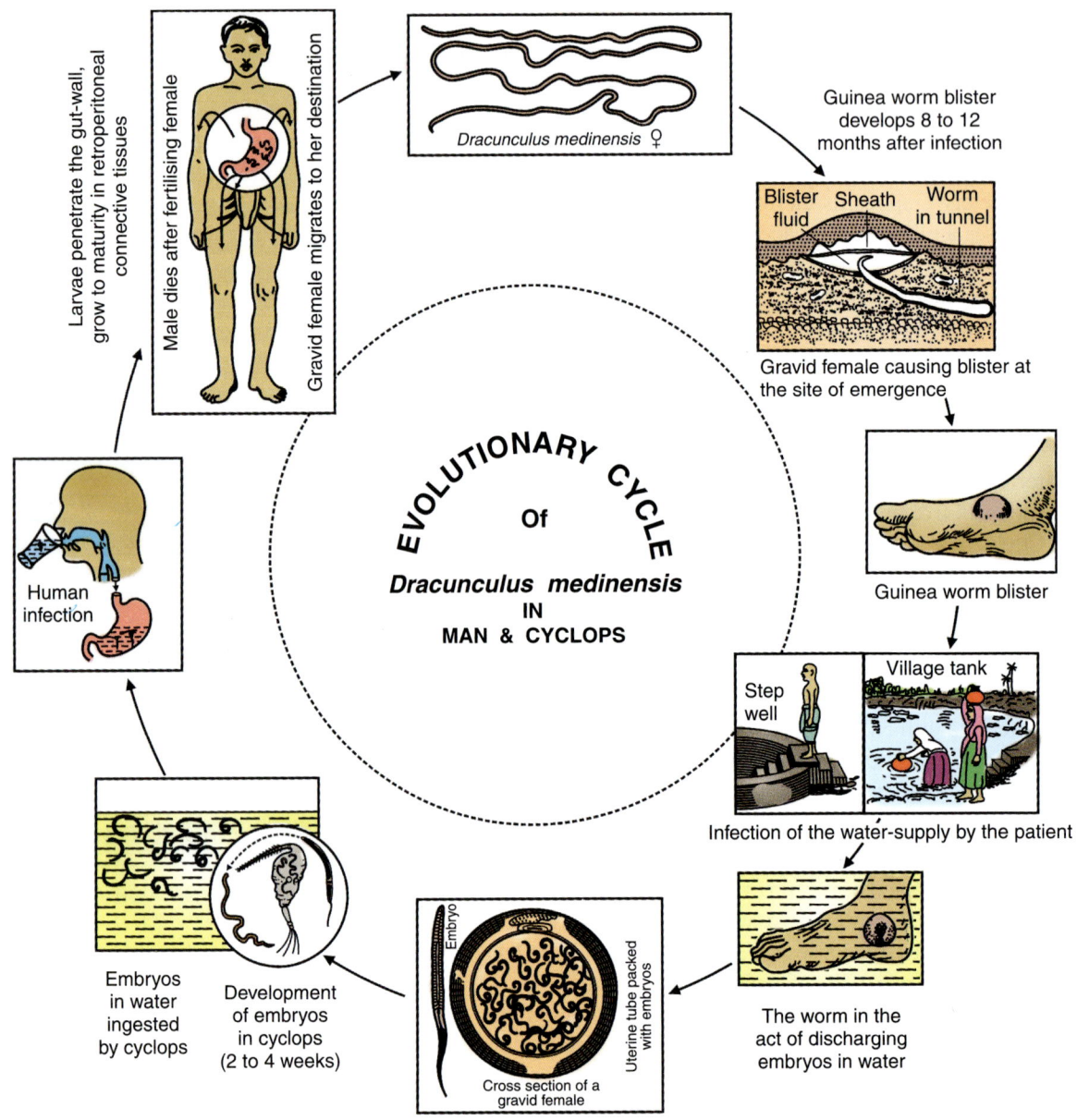

Larvae penetrate the gut-wall, grow to maturity in retroperitoneal connective tissues

Male dies after fertilising female

Gravid female migrates to her destination

Dracunculus medinensis ♀

Guinea worm blister develops 8 to 12 months after infection

Blister fluid — Sheath — Worm in tunnel

Gravid female causing blister at the site of emergence

Guinea worm blister

EVOLUTIONARY CYCLE
Of
Dracunculus medinensis
IN
MAN & CYCLOPS

Human infection

Step well — Village tank

Infection of the water-supply by the patient

Embryos in water ingested by cyclops

Development of embryos in cyclops (2 to 4 weeks)

Embryo — Uterine tube packed with embryos

Cross section of a gravid female

The worm in the act of discharging embryos in water

Fig. 196.
(Morphology after Looss, Leuckart, Fairley & Liston)

Infecting Agent—Larva.

Portal of Entry—Digestive tract, gaining entrance along with drinking water which is neither boiled nor filtered.

Site of Location—Subcutaneous tissues, generally of leg.

Incubation Period—Varies from 8 to 12 months.

PATHOGENIC EFFECTS. The symptoms are manifested during parturition of the female and are due to the liberation of a "toxic" substance causing *allergic manifestation* and *blister formation*. There might also be septic infection as a result of contamination by secondary organisms drawn in by the worm at the time of retraction.

Blister formation (Fig. 197). This lesion appears whenever the female worm makes an attempt to come to the surface of the body where it can readily discharge its embryos. In majority of cases, the female worm chooses some part of the lower extremities but it may be found in lesser degree in arms, trunk, buttock, scrotum, head, neck and female breast. Prompted by instinct, the gravid female proceeds to her destination where it pierces the skin. The head

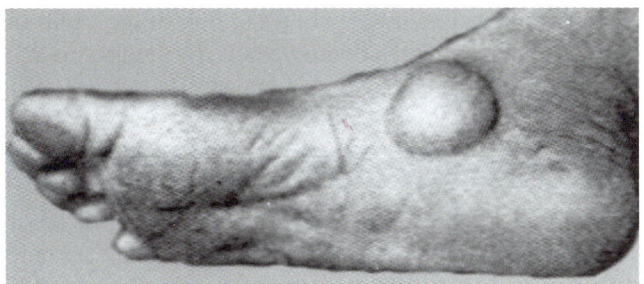

Fig. 197—A guinea worm blister over the medial side of the right foot.

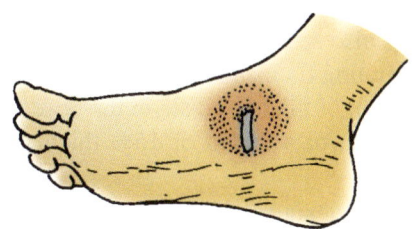

Fig. 198A—The female guinea worm is protruding through the centre of the erosion.

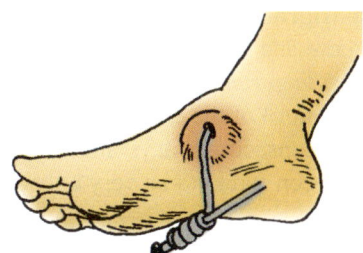

Fig. 198B—An attempt is made to extract the female guinea worm by rolling it round a stick.

of the worm tries to come to the surface resulting in an itching or burning sensation at the area. An irritant secreted by the worm produces a small red spot which is gradually converted into a small bleb or blister. The fluid in the blister is sterile and yellow in colour; it contains many monocytes, eosinophils and neutrophil granulocytes. There are numerous embryos in the fluid. Finally, the blister ruptures, either by itself or by manipulation, revealing a small superficial erosion of ½ to ¼ inch in diameter. A small round hole (large enough to admit a small probe) may be seen at the centre of the erosion, through which the head of the worm is seen to protrude (Fig. 198A), whenever the part comes in contact with water. The central hole leads to a tunnel in the subcutaneous tissue where, the female worm lies.

Laboratory Diagnosis. This consists of the following:

(i)   *Detection of the Adult Worm.* This is possible when the female worm appears at the surface of the skin.

(ii) *Detection of Embryos.* The affected part through which the head of the worm is protruding may be bathed with water to encourage the discharge of embryos from the uterus. The milky fluid containing numerous embryos escapes which can be pipetted off and examined under the microscope.

(iii) *Intradermal Test.* Injection of dracunculus antigen intradermally causes a wheal to appear in the course of 24 hours in positive cases.

(iv) *X-ray Examination.* Worms in deeper tissues after death either become calcified or absorbed. The position of calcified worm may be located by skiagraphy.

(v)   *Blood examination* reveals eosinophilia.

(vi) *Serological Test.* ELISA test and IFA test can detect antibodies to *D. medinensis.*

Treatment. Lambert (1966) obtained good results with a new nitrothiazole compound "ambilhar". In 70 out of 71 patients with dracunculosis the parasites were killed by treatment with this drug. Niridazole (12.5-25 mg/kg orally for 5-7 days) is also effective.

A rational method of extracting the worm is to encourage the parasite to discharge its embryos by careful douching with cold water. It is a common practice in some parts of India that as soon as the female worm shows herself, the end is tied with a fine silk to a match stick or a similar object (Fig. 198B). Then an endeavour is made to roll it inch by inch daily with gentle traction until the whole parasite comes out and this takes about 15 to 20 days. In the hands of a skilled person, extraction of a live worm is much easier than a dead worm. Thiabendazole (50 mg/kg in two divided doses for 3 days) and metronidazole (250 mg 3 times daily for 10 days orally) are used in the treatment.

Prophylaxis. This infection can be prevented by breaking the link of the chain (man-cyclops-man) as follows: (i) prevention of pollution of drinking water by infected individual, (ii) chemical treatment of water-supply for eradication of cyclops, and (iii) drinking of water which is either strained, filtered or boiled.

LARVA MIGRANS

Certain nematode larvae on entering into an unnatural host, man, may not be able to complete their journey through the host's tissues for localisation in their normal abode. Thus, their onward progress is arrested and according to the mode of entrance, two different types of conditions are produced:

1. Entering by skin penetration: *Cutaneous larva migrans or Creeping eruption.*
2. Entering via oral route: *Visceral larva migrans* (Toxocariasis).

Cutaneous Larva Migrans. This is most commonly met with in infection with non-human species of hookworm larvae, e.g., *A. braziliense* and *A. caninum* (see page 215). It is also seen in cases of infection with a spiruroid larva (larva of *Gnathostoma spinigerum*), *Strongyloide* larva and migrating fly maggot, *Gasterophilus* (a form of cutaneous myiasis). For effective control of the condition oral administration of thiabendazole in the dose of 25 mg/kg of body wt. twice daily for two consecutive days and topical application of a cream of 15% thiabendazole powder in a hydrosoluble base have been found to be very encouraging.

Visceral Larva Migrans. Here, after the ingestion of infective stage of the eggs, the second stage larvae are hatched out in the intestine, which invade the intestinal wall and are carried to the extra-intestinal viscera, such as liver, lungs and other organs. In any one of these sites, the progress is arrested by the formation of a granulomatous lesion. The larvae are attacked by phagocytic cells, consisting mainly of eosinophils and histiocytes and occasionally giant cells. The condition, often found in young children, is characterised by high leucocytosis (15,000 to 80,000) and persistent hypereosinophilia (15 to 80 per cent) with or without any constitutional symptom. There may be fever, enlargement of spleen and liver, patchy pneumonitis and hypergammaglobulinaemia. The lesion may occasionally be located in the brain or eye (retina). The common etiological agent for the development of such lesion is infection with a dog ascarid (*Toxocara canis*) or a cat ascarid (*T. cati*). Preventive measures should be directed to the deforming of dogs and cats so that young children are not exposed to the infection. The diagnosis is established by studying the histological characters of the larvae in the granulomatous tissues obtained by biopsy or at autopsy. In the eye, it causes endophthalmitis with a space-occupying granuloma containing the Toxocara larva at or near macula. Ophthalmoscopic examination of the fundus oculi reveals distortion of retina simulating retinoblastoma. Convulsion resulting from lesion in the brain has also been observed. For treatment diethyl-carbamazine (3 mg/kg three times daily for 21 days) and thiabendazole (50 mg/kg three times daily for 7-30 days) have been used with some success.

Accessory aids to diagnosis include the following:

(i) *Haemagglutination test.* Tanned sheep erythrocytes and antigens made from *T. canis* and *A. lumbricoides* when mixed with sera of patients suspected to having visceral larva migrans gave a high titre (above 1 in 80). Strongyloidiasis also gave a high titre.

(ii) *Bentonite flocculation test.* This may also be helpful.

(iii) *ELISA test.* An ELISA test is used now-a-days effectively to detect antibodies against the excretory-secretory antigens of *Toxocara* larvae.

APPENDIX

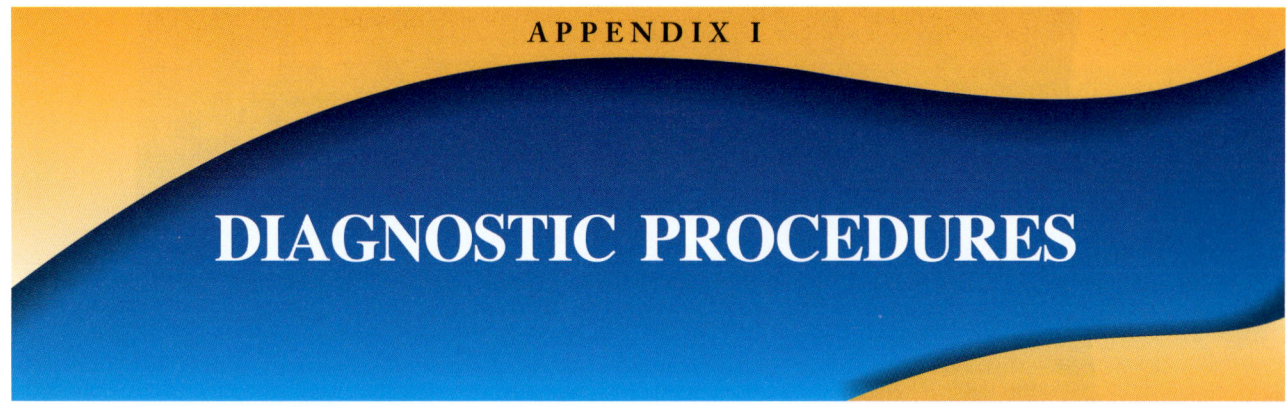

APPENDIX I

DIAGNOSTIC PROCEDURES

A. EXAMINATION OF STOOL FOR PARASITES

FOR PROTOZOAL INFECTIONS

A simple microscopic examination of stool is carried out for the diagnosis of intestinal protozoa. For the demonstration of the trophozoites, an unstained preparation of a fresh material should first be examined when the characteristic movement of the parasite, if any, may be noted. The nuclear character is better studied in stained preparations. A simple method of detecting the cystic forms of the parasite is to examine an iodine-stained preparation of the sample, when the nuclear character can easily be distinguished. The glycogen mass, if present, is stained with iodine but not the chromatoid bars which are seen better in an unstained preparation. Hence, for routine examination both unstained and iodine-stained preparations are made of the same material.

General Rules for Microscopical Examination of the Stool

Preparation:

(i) A minute portion of the faeces is diluted with normal saline (0.9 per cent) and a drop of it is taken on a clean microscopic glass slide. A coverslip No. 1 or No. 0 is then gently put over it, so as to spread out the emulsion into a thin, fairly uniform and transparent layer. This will be used as an unstained preparation.

(ii) Another preparation is made in which a drop of iodine is first added to the drop of saline emulsion and then the coverslip is put on (there must not be so much fluid as to make the coverslip float or move about).

Two such preparations are made either on the same slide or on two different slides.

Note: Addition of iodine kills the organism and therefore, the motility of the parasite is lost but it stains the nuclei and glycogen mass, which are more or less invisible in saline preparation and which now become discernible. Owing to the cessation of movements and also due to the staining, the flagella become recognisable.

Examination:

Both the preparations are first examined under low power objective 2/3rd inch of the microscope and No. 4 Ocular. Starting from one end of the coverslip, the whole slide is examined. Any suspicious object is centred and focussed under high power objective 1/6th inch for a detailed diagnosis.

For the demonstration of flagella in protozoal organisms a *dark ground illumination* may be used for bringing the individual flagellum in sharp relief.

To study the movement of the parasite, a *warm stage* may be fitted with the microscope or the whole microscope may be encased in a wooden chamber inside which an electric bulb is fitted to provide the necessary light and warmth. While examining such preparation precaution should be taken so that the films do not get dried up and for this purpose, the coverslip may be ringed with paraffin or vaseline. It is particularly necessary in cold countries to keep the specimen warm both before and during examination.

Microscopical Examination of Stool for *E. histolytica*

COLLECTION OF STOOL. Essentials to be fulfilled are:

  (i) Stool must be fresh.

 (ii) Receptacle must be clean and dry; no antiseptics should be used to wash it.

(iii) Urine should not be allowed to mix with the stool.

(iv) Oil, oily emulsion, barium or bismuth salts should not be given to the patient before examination.

TO OBTAIN A FRESH SAMPLE:

  (a) The patient is advised to go to the laboratory and to pass a specimen there.

  (b) In the alternative, a soft rubber catheter should be inserted well into the rectum and twisted round several times; when withdrawn, this will contain sufficient material (a fleck of mucus which may be blood-stained) in its "eye" for microscopical examination.

  (c) A proctoscope or a sigmoidoscope should be used for obtaining directly scrapings of the ulcers in the rectum or the sigmoid colon.

PREPARATION OF THE MATERIAL. The microscopical examination of the stool may be carried out unstained in a saline preparation and also in a smear preparation stained with iodine, iron-haematoxylin or any other permanent stains used for the purpose.

(i) *Unstained Preparation.* This is specially useful for the demonstration of the actively motile forms of *E. histolytica*, generally present in symptomatic amoebiasis. A portion of the stool, preferably some mucus, is picked up with a match stick or a wooden tooth-pick or a platinum loop and emulsified with freshly prepared normal saline on a clean glass slide. The resulting mixture should not be too thick and its consistency should be such as to allow a newsprint to be read through it. A clean coverslip No. 1 or No. 0 is placed over it and the excess of fluid, if there be any, may be removed with the help of a filter paper, by slightly tilting the whole slide. If the examination requires a longer time, a ring of vaseline may be applied around the margin in order to avoid drying. Cystic forms can also be detected in a saline preparation of the material. While examining an unstained preparation, the light should be carefully adjusted to get a clear view. For this purpose, the condenser is to be racked down and the iris diaphragm is to be partially closed in order to cut down the illumination. It is convenient to use a mechanical stage so that by moving the stage back and forth, the entire field may be examined in the space of a short time. After the examination is over, the used slides should be placed in a vessel containing 5 per cent lysol.

(ii) *Stained Preparation.* For cysts or dead specimens of trophozoites, stained preparation may be required for the study of the nuclear character for the identification of the species. The iodine-stained preparation is commonly employed for this purpose. But, if a permanent preparation is desired, the film is first fixed and then stained with iron-haematoxylin.

CONCENTRATION METHOD. Chances of finding the cysts of intestinal amoebae and flagellates are greatly increased when a concentrated material is used. When a negative result is obtained from the examination of iodine-stained preparations of a direct smear, the use of a concentration method has often given a positive result. This method is applicable to formed stool and only the cystic forms are detected as the trophozoites are destroyed during the process. The method of Faust *et al* (zinc sulphate centrifugal floatation technique) is recommended.

STAINING METHODS

Iodine Solution. This simple stain is used by the protozoologists in the laboratory to identify cysts of amoebic and flagellated protozoa (Fig. 199) and is usually sufficient for diagnostic purposes.

Lugol's iodine solution is too strong and it must be diluted about five times with distilled water. Such weaker solution may then be used for the staining. The only disadvantage is that the stain deteriorates quickly, hence it should be prepared every two weeks.

Lugol's iodine solution is prepared as follows:

Iodine crystals (powdered)	...	5 g
Potassium iodide	...	10 g
Distilled water	...	100 ml

Potassium iodide is dissolved in distilled water and iodine crystals are slowly added. The solution is then filtered and kept in a stoppered bottle of amber colour.

Dobell and O'Conoor (1921) recommended the use of 1 per cent iodine in 2 per cent potassium iodide solution. Weigert's iodine solution is of the same strength.

Staining for Permanent Preparation

PREPARATION. Smears should be made on a glass slide or on a coverglass which should be uniform.

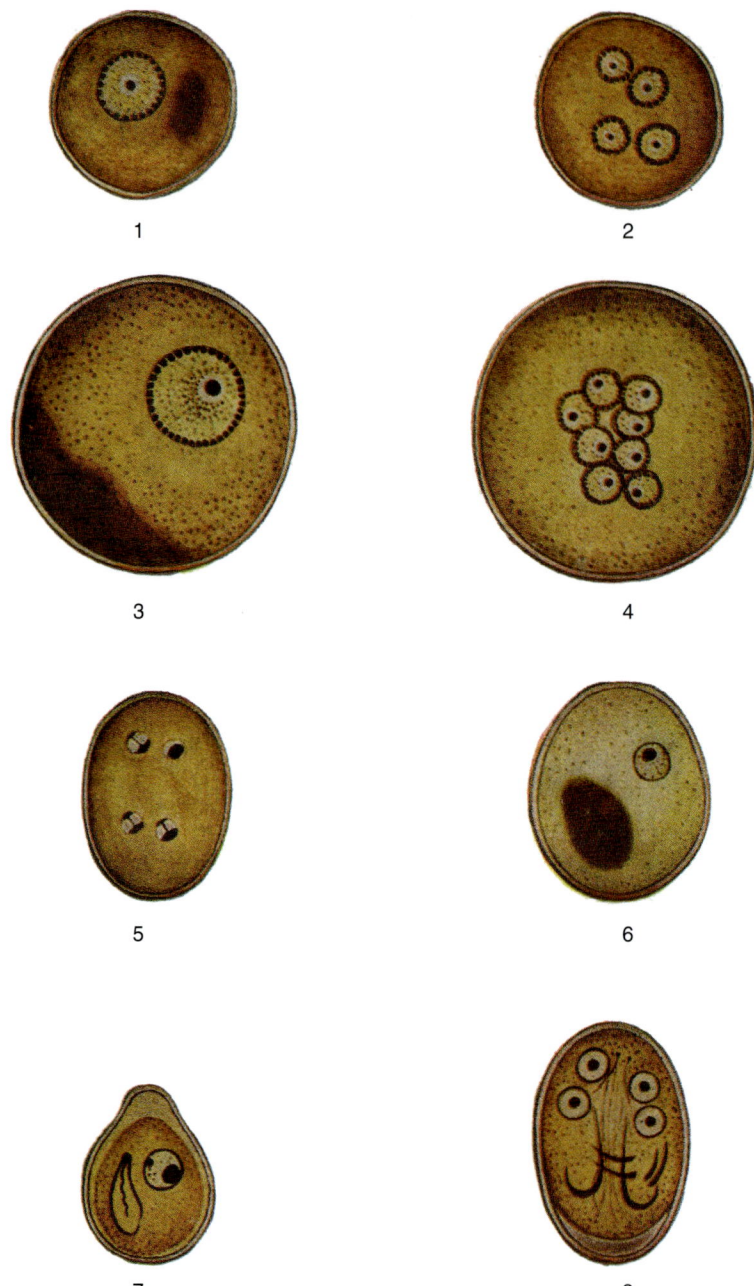

Fig. 199—Cysts of intestinal protozoa of man.
(Stained with iodine.)
1 and 2, *Entamoeba histolytica* (uni- and quadri-nucleate forms); 3 and 4, *Entamoeba coli*
(uni- and octo-nucleate forms); 5, *Endolimax nana*; 6, *Iodamoeba bütschlii*;
7, *Chilomastix mesnili*; 8, *Giardia intestinalis*.

FIXATION: In *Schaudinn's fluid*. The composition is as follows:

Saturated solution of mercuric chloride in distilled water	...	200 ml
95 per cent or absolute alcohol	...	100 ml
Glacial acetic acid	...	15 ml

The smear is kept in this fluid for 5 to 10 minutes. Later to remove the sublimate of mercury, the smear is washed in 50 per cent alcohol and iodised 70 per cent alcohol from 10 to 30 minutes.

STAINED BY HEIDENHAIN'S HAEMATOXYLIN METHOD. Two solutions are employed:

(i) *Staining Solution:*

Haematoxylin crystals (Grübler)	...	1 g
Alcohol, 90 per cent	...	10 ml
Distilled water	...	90 ml

The mixture should be ripened in the sun for a period of ten days when it becomes sherry brown in colour.

(ii) *Mordant Solution :*

Iron alum (Sulphate of iron and ammonium)	...	2 g
Distilled water	...	50 ml

After fixation, the slide is placed in distilled water for 10 minutes. It is then placed in mordant solution for 6 hours. After washing with distilled water, the slide is now put into the staining solution for six hours and if necessary overnight. At this stage, the smear becomes jet black in colour.

DIFFERENTIATION. The mordant solution is diluted with three parts of distilled water. The slide is placed in this solution when some of the black colour gradually comes off. The slide is washed in distilled water and it is examined under the microscope, from time to time, till the nuclear structure is clearly visible.

DEHYDRATION. After washing in distilled water or running tap water, the slide is passed through graded alcohols of 70, 80 and 90 per cent strengths and absolute alcohol, keeping the slide in each solution for 5 minutes. The smear is cleared with xylol and mounted in xylol-balsam.

Note: It is absolutely necessary that the slides should not be allowed to dry at any stage of fixation staining, differentiation, dehydration or cleaning.

FOR HELMINTHIC INFECTIONS

Examination of stool may be carried out by a naked eye examination when the whole of the parasite (adult worm of *Ascaris lumbricoides*, *Ancylostoma duodenale*, *Trichuris trichiura*, *Enterobius vermicularis* and various intestinal flukes) or a part of it (segments of *Taenia saginata* and *T. solium*) may be detected. To search for tapeworm segments, enterobius and ancylostomes, the specimen for examination is diluted with water and poured on to a sieve (meshes 30 to an inch). The faecal matter will be washed away and the worms left may easily be picked out by holding the sieve against a dark background. It is to be remembered that these worms may be passed out in the faeces spontaneously by the host or following the administration of a specific anthelmintic.

In positive cases, detection of adult worms may be difficult at times, but the eggs are generally present in all specimens submitted for microscopical examination. The character of the individual helminthic eggs is sufficiently specific to warrant a correct diagnosis. During identification of eggs, attention should be paid to shape, size, colour and marking on the surface of the egg-shell, the presence of yolk granules, ovum or a differentiated embryo, the existence of an operculum and in specific cases, as in cestodes, the three pairs of embryonic hooklets (Figs. 200 and 201). It may be pointed out that for the detection of helminthic eggs only an unstained preparation is necessary.

Direct Smear. *A simple microscopical examination* of a smear made directly from the sample and viewed under low power will enable one to find the eggs or larvae (as in Strongyloides) when they are present in overwhelming numbers. Enterobius, unless mechanically washed, does not eject any egg in the stool. So washing out stools, preferably after a saline purge, is a sure method of diagnosis. For the purpose of microscopical examination, a thin smear as large as 1½″ × 1″ is made on 3″ × 1″ glass slide and the whole of the smear covered with a coverslip is examined under the microscope.

Concentration Method. Recently various means of concentrating the helminthic eggs have been devised so that they may easily be found. The procedures adopted for the concentration of the eggs may be carried out either by floatation or sedimentation technique. Concentration method used for helminthic eggs may also be employed for protozoal cysts.

FLOATATION TECHNIQUE. The faecal material is dissolved in solution of a higher density than that of the eggs. In this case, the eggs float in the superficial portion of the fluid. It has been observed that all the helminthic eggs float in such a solution except the following: (i) Unfertilised eggs of *A. lumbricoides*, (ii) eggs of *T. saginata* and *T. solium*, and (iii) eggs of all intestinal flukes.

The Strongyloides larvae do not float in salt solution.

(a) *Simple Floatation Technique* (Maplestone, 1940). Willis' technique is of the same principle.

MATERIALS REQUIRED:

1. Glass or metal (tin) "container" of 15 or 20 ml capacity, having a flat bottom, vertical edges and a diameter of not more than 1½ inches.

2. Glass slides 3″ × 2″ instead of 3″ × 1″.

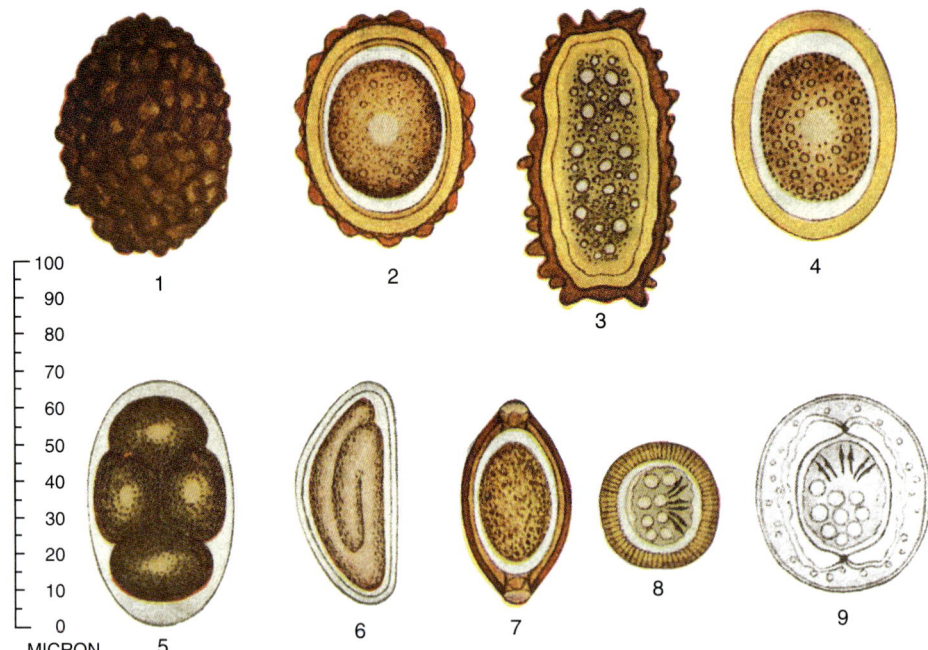

Fig. 200—Helminthic eggs in the stool of man.
1, 2 & 4, Fertilised eggs of *A. lumbricoides*; surface focus; 2, median focus; 4, decorticated
(without the outer envelope); 3, unfertilised egg of *A. lumbricoides*; 5, *N. americanus* or
A. duodenale; 6, *E. vermicularis*; 7, *T. trichiura*; 8, *T. saginata* or *T. solium*; 9, *H. nana*.

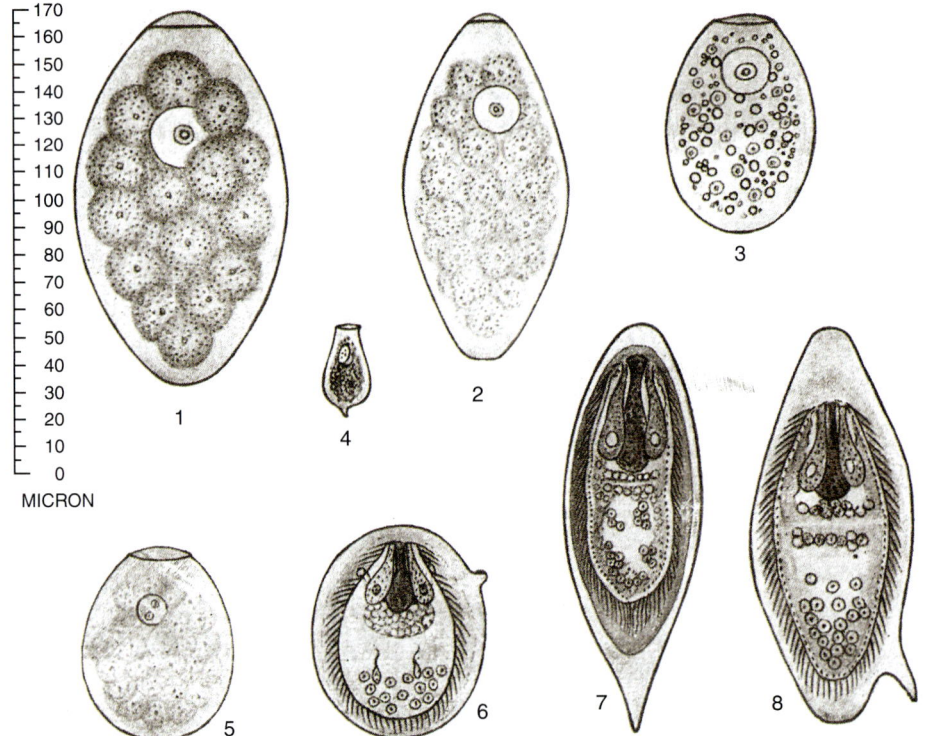

Fig. 201—Helminthic eggs in the stool of man.
1, *F. buski*; 2, *G. hominis*; 3, *P. westermani*; 4, *C. sinensis*; 5, *D. latum*;
6, *S. japonicum*; 7, *S. haematobium*; 8, *S. mansoni*.

3. Saturated salt solution of specific gravity 1.200. This is prepared by allowing an excess of common salt to boil in a basin until a scum forms on the surface. When cooled, it is stored in a bottle, leaving an excess of undissolved salt at the bottom.

4. A sheet of glass on which the "container" is to be placed.

TECHNIQUE. One millilitre of faeces is taken in the "container" and a few drops of salt solution are added. It is then stirred with a glass rod (may be used again after thorough washing) or a small stiff piece of stick (should be discarded after use) so as to make an even emulsion. After this more salt solution (15 or 20 ml according to the capacity of the "container" used) is added till the "container" is nearly full, stirring being continued throughout the process. Any coarse matter, which floats up, may be removed without fear of removing any egg, as the egg takes a long time (20 to 30 minutes) to come to the surface of the fluid. At this stage, the "container" is placed on a level surface (a glass sheet is placed on the laboratory bench). The final filling of "container" is carried out by means of a dropper, until a convex meniscus is formed. A glass slide (3″ × 2″ size) is carefully laid on the top of the "container", so that its centre is in contact with the fluid. The preparation is allowed to stand for 20 to 30 minutes, after which the glass slide is quickly lifted, turned over smoothly so as to avoid spilling of the liquid, and examined under the microscope. A coverslip need not be placed over the fluid, but the surface of the film is to be focussed with 2/3rd in objective, for the detection of eggs.

(b) *Lane's Direct Centrifugal Floatation or D.C.F. Technique*

APPARATUS REQUIRED:

1. Special bucket (for containing the centrifuge tube) with flat bottom and ground-off top, having special carriers with guards to keep the coverslip from slipping out of position.

2. Special coverslip 19 mm square by 0.5 mm thickness.

3. Lane's centrifugal machine.

METHOD. About one to two grammes of faeces is thoroughly mixed with water in a Clayton Lane's centrifuge tube (a small metal hollow tube may be used for thoroughly disintegrating the faecal matter). The faecal emulsion is then centrifuged at a speed of 1,000 revolutions per minute for two minutes. The supernatant fluid is poured off and a saturated solution of common salt having a specific gravity of 1.200 is added to fill ¾ of the tube. After the whole mixture has been vigorously shaken, the tube is filled up to the brim with saturated salt solution so as to expel all air and the thick coverslip is put on. This is then centrifuged at 1,000 r.p.m. for 2 minutes. The coverslip is quickly lifted off and the drop of saline adhering to its undersurface is examined as a hanging-drop preparation.

(c) *Zinc Sulphate Centrifugal Floatation* (Faust *et al*, 1939). A fine faecal suspension is made by taking 1 g of a freshly passed stool and 10 ml of lukewarm distilled water. The coarse particles are removed by straining through a wire gauge (40 meshes to an inch). The filtrate is collected into a Wassermann tube and centrifuged for 1 minute at the rate of 2,500 revolutions per minute. The supernatant fluid is poured off and distilled water is added to the sediment. It is shaken well, centrifuged and the process is repeated 2 or 3 times till the supernatant fluid is clear, which is then poured off. To the sediment is added 3 to 4 ml of a 33% zinc sulphate solution having a sp. gr. 1.80. The sediment is stirred and further zinc sulphate solution is added to fill the tube up to the top and centrifuged again for at least 1 minute at 2,500 r.p.m. The surface film is then removed by a platinum wire loop of 5 mm diameter, on to a clean glass slide, a coverslip is put on and the specimen is examined. For protozoal cysts one drop of iodine solution is added before the coverslip is put on.

SEDIMENTATION TECHNIQUE. The faecal material is dissolved in water or solutions of a density below that of the eggs. In this case, the eggs are concentrated at the bottom.

(a) *Simple Sedimentation*. A sufficient amount of faeces is thoroughly shaken with ten to twenty times its volume of tap water and allowed to settle in a cone-shaped flask (urinalysis flask) for an hour or two. The process is repeated several times till the supernatant fluid is clear. Finally, the sediment at the bottom is examined for the eggs. It is not suitable for protozoal cysts.

(b) *Formol-ether Concentration*. Ritchief's method modified (Ridley and Hagwood, 1956). One gramme of faeces is emulsified in 7 ml of 10% formol-saline and kept for 10 mins. for fixation. It is then strained through an wire gauge (40 meshes to an inch) and the filtrate is collected in a centrifuge tube. To it 3 ml ether is added and the mixture is shaken vigorously for 1 minute. It is centrifuged at 2,000 r.p.m. for 2 minutes and then allowed to settle. The debris are loosened with a stick, the upper part of the test tube is cleared of fatty debris and the supernatant fluid is decanted, leaving 1 or 2 drops. The deposit after shaking is poured on to glass slide, a coverslip is placed over it and the specimen is examined. It does not cause any distortion of protozoal cysts or helminthic eggs and takes only 5 minutes.

Egg Counting Technique. For quantitative estimation of ova or estimating the worm burden. This is employed to determine the egg-laying capacity of a female worm per unit of formed faecal output. These figures are then utilised to estimate the number of worms infecting the patient. On a rough estimate, it is calculated that each female worm produces about 100 eggs per gramme of faeces per day. In hermaphrodite species, such as *Clonorchis* and *Fasciolopsis* the total number of worms is calculated on this basis. In *Nematodes*, however, assuming that the sexes are equally divided, 50 eggs per gramme of faeces represent one worm. Of the various methods of egg-counting, that of Stoll (1923) has gained a wide popularity.

STOLL'S METHOD OF EGG-COUNTING. Four grammes of faeces are mixed with 56 ml of N/10 NaOH in a thick glass tube and thoroughly mixed to make a uniform suspension. This is facilitated by adding a few glass beads and closing the mouth with a rubber stopper and then shaking vigorously. Exactly 0.15 ml of the emulsion is removed by a measuring pipette and placed on a large slide 3″ × 2″ size; a coverslip measuring 22/40 mm is then put over it. With the help of a mechanical stage, all the eggs in the preparation are counted. The number of eggs per gramme of faeces is obtained by mltiplying the count of two such preparations by 100. The average daily output of faeces being known the total egg-production *per diem* can easily be obtained. Considering the consistency of faecal specimen a correction factor (C.F.) is employed to convert the estimate to a formed stool basis as follows (Stoll and Hausheer, 1926):

For mushy-formed stool C.F. is 1.5, for mushy stool C.F. is 2, for mushy diarrhoeic stool C.F. is 3, for frankly diarrhoeic stool C.F. is 4 and for watery stool C.F. is 5.

Note: The quantitative estimation of worm burden calculated from the daily output of eggs in faeces does not provide a correct estimate, because the egg-output of a particular species of worm shows a great variation.

Kato's Cellophane-covered Thick Smear. Kato and Miura (1954) introduced a method which has been found useful in survey work for detecting helminthic eggs and providing a semiquantitative assessment. They employed wettable cellophane strips 22 × 30 mm of 40-50 mm thickness soaked in glycerine-malachite green solution for 24 hours or more to clarify a measured amount of faeces (50-60 mg) spread in an even layer on a glass slide. The strips were placed over the faecal smear, allowed to dry at room temperature for an hour and then examined.

Preservation of Faeces. About 1 to 2 grammes of faeces treated with 8 to 10 ml of 10% formalin is put in a suitable screw-cap vial. Before use the container is to be thoroughly shaken to get a uniform emulsion. Formol-ether concentration technique may be used.

Anal Swab for Enterobiasis. Heller (1876) first recommended anal swabs for the diagnosis of *enterobiasis* and since that time materials have been obtained by scraping with spatulas, curettes, glass slides, rods and other convenient measures. The following have been found to give satisfactory results.

NIH SWAB. Hall (1937) devised a cellophane anal swab commonly referred to as NIH swab (from U.S. National Institute of Health) which has been used with great success by a large number of workers. The constituent parts of NIH swab are as follows: One end of a glass rod (8 to 10 cm long by 4 mm wide) is covered with a piece of transparent cellophane of about one inch square and is held in place by a rubber band. This end of the rod is used for swabbing the anal region. The other end of the rod passes through the rubber cork with which the test tube is closed. After swabbing, the cellophane with the rod may be replaced inside the test-tube and sent to a distant laboratory for examination. A drop of saline is taken on a glass slide and the cellophane end of rod is held over it. The rubber band is then pushed up by a pair of forceps until the cellophane is released. With the rod still held in position, the cellophane is spread out and smoothened in such a way that the material adhering to the cellophane comes to lie in direct contact with the glass slide. A drop of saline is placed over it and a coverslip applied. The eggs thus lie between the glass slide and the cellophane.

SCOTCH CELLULOSE TAPE METHOD. It consists of a length of Scotch cellulose tape (3 to 4 inches long × ¾ inch wide) held with adhesive-side-out at the end of the blade of a wooden tongue depressor by the thumb and index finger. This applicator is then placed first on one side and then on the other side of the anal orifice. After swabbing, the tape is removed and placed with the adhesive-side-down on a drop of toluene on a glass slide.

Faecal Culture. TEST-TUBE FILTER PAPER METHOD—A simple method devised by Haroda and Mori (1955) and modified by other workers (Hsieh 1962) can be utilised for differential diagnosis of hookworm species (and possibly Trichostrongylus or Ternidens in some areas).

About half a gram of fresh specimen of faecal sample is smeared (1-2 mm thick) on strip of sterile filter-paper (15 × 1.5 cm) longitudinally leaving clear spaces at both the ends which is put into sterile test-tube along the side (unsmeared surface being in contact with the wall). The lower end touching the column of sterile water (about 5 to 7 ml) already placed into the tube. Top of the tube is tightly plugged with cotton. The tube thus prepared is incubated at 24°C to 28°C for 7 to 10 days. The filariform larvae will be collected at the bottom of the tube which can be pipetted off to microscope slide for identification. The larvae can be killed by either placing the culture tubes at 50°C water bath for 15 minutes before their removal or by treating the larvae with iodine solution (filtered saturated solution of iodine in 1% KI).

B. EXAMINATION OF BLOOD FOR PARASITES

Examination of Thin Blood Film

PREPARATION (Fig. 202 a, b, c, d, & b_1, b_2):

    (i) Prick the pulp of any finger or lobe of the ear with surgical cutting needle under aseptic condition (area to be pricked is wiped with alcohol and allowed to dry).

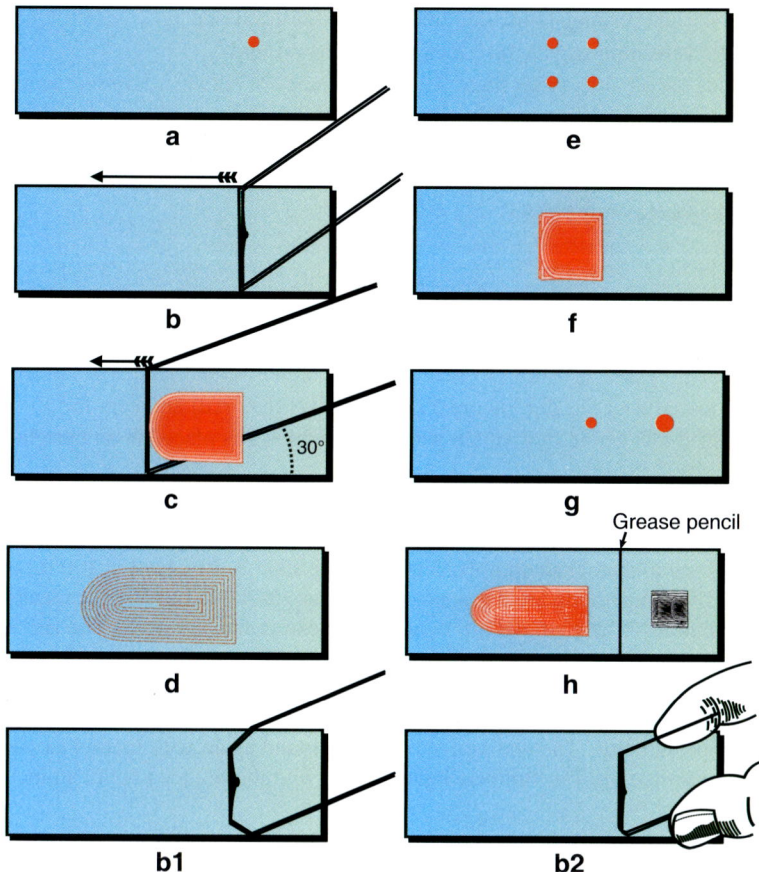

Fig. 202—Preparation of thin and thick films of blood.

a to d, thin film. a, drop of blood at one end of the slide; b, spreader (another glass slide) held at an angle of 45° and pushed in the direction of the arrow; c, making a smear; d, thin blood film completed. b1 and b2, a glass slide with corners cut at one end and a coverslip of haemocytometer used as spreaders. e and f, thick film after James; e, four drops of blood at the corners of a half inch square; f, four drops of blood joined to form a thick film. g and h, thick and thin films on the same slide after Sinton.

(ii) Take a drop of blood not larger than a pin's head on a grease-free clean slide, at a distance of about half an inch from the right end.

(iii) Hold a spreader at an angle of 45 degrees in contact with the drop of blood then lower it to an angle of 30 degrees and push gently to the left, till the blood is exhausted. As the blood is exhausted, the film begins to form"tails"which should end near about the centre of the slide. The spreader may be the smooth edge of a glass slide, with the corners cut off at one end, or a coverslip, preferably the coverslip of a haemocytometer (Fig. 198 b1, b2).

(iv) The film is allowed to dry and labelled by writing across the dried film with a sharp-pointed pencil or a needle.

CHARACTERISTICS OF A GOOD THIN FILM:

(i) The surface of the film is even and uniform.

(ii) The margins of the film do not extend to the sides of the slide.

(iii) The "tails" end near about the centre of the slide.

(iv) It consists of a single layer of red blood cells.

STAINS: *With Leishman's Stain*

(i) Pour Leishman's stain from a drop bottle or by means of a pipette over the dried film and allow it to remain for 30 seconds.

(ii) Dilute the stain with twice its volume of distilled water which should be neutral or slightly alkaline (pH 7-7.2). Cover it to prevent drying.

(iii) Allow the diluted stain to remain on the slide for 10 to 15 minutes.

(iv) Hold the slide under an open tap and flush the stain in a gentle flow of water. The reverse side of the slide may be cleaned by rubbing it well with wet and squeezed cotton wool.

(v) Keep the slide in an upright position (film-side inwards) to drain and dry.

(vi) The dried stained film is examined with 1/12 inch oil-immersion lens.

Note: A properly stained slide has a bluish violet tinge. The correct range of colour is however assured when ionic dissociation of staining radicles occur round about neutral or slightly alkaline pH (7.0 to 7.2).

Alkaline buffer solution is particularly necessary to bring out the Schüffner's dots and is prepared as follows:

Sodium phosphate	…	2 g
Potassium dihydrogen phosphate	…	1 mg
Thymol	…	1 mg
Distilled water	…	1,000 ml

With Giemsa's Stain. The stain can be purchased as a ready-made solution. The method of staining is as follows:

1. The film is first fixed with pure methyl alcohol or ethyl alcohol for 3 to 5 minutes and allowed to dry.

2. Giemsa's stain is diluted by adding 1 drop to each 1 ml of distilled water, neutral or faintly alkaline (*p*H 7-7.2).

3. The diluted stain is poured over the film (about 5 ml per film is required) and kept for 30 to 45 minutes.

4. The slide is then flushed in a gentle flow of tap water, after which it is placed in an upright position with the film-side inwards to drain and dry.

5. The stained film is examined under 1/12 inch oil-immersion lens.

Preparation of Leishman's Stain. The stain is available in the form of powder or tablet. The strength of the solution used for staining is 0.15 per cent of the stain in methyl alcohol (0.15 gram of the stain is dissolved in 100 ml of acetone-free pure methyl alcohol). The materials required for preparation are a ground-glass stoppered bottle of 150 ml capacity, a 100 ml graduated glass cylinder and a glass pestle and mortar. All the articles are thoroughly cleaned and before use, are rinsed with methyl alcohol. The amount of methyl alcohol (100 ml) is first measured in the graduated cylinder. The weighed amount of Leishman's powder (0.15 g) or the requisite number of tablets (each tablet contains 0.15 g of the stain) is placed in the glass mortar and is ground into a paste by adding methyl alcohol in small quantities (about 2 ml each time). The dissolved stain is carefully decanted off, from time to time, into the glass-stoppered bottle. The undissolved stain is ground again with methyl alcohol till no residue is left and the whole methyl alcohol has been used up. The stoppered glass-bottle with the stain is kept in an incubator at 37°C for 24 hours after which it is ready for use.

Examination of Thick Blood Film

Preparation. A big drop of blood is taken on a slide and spread with a needle or with the corner of another slide to form an area of a half-inch square; it may also be prepared by taking 4 small drops of blood (Fig. 202 e & f) and joining the corners of the drops with a needle (James, 1920). The thickness of the film should be such as to allow a newsprint to be read or the hands of a wrist-watch to be seen through the dry preparation. The film is dried in a horizontal position and kept covered by a Petri dish. It is to be noted that in moist climates it takes at least half an hour for the thick films to dry at room temperature. Drying may be accelerated by putting the slide inside an incubator.

Staining. This may be carried out with Leishman's, Giemsa's or Field's stain; if it is desired to use the former two stains, the slide should be dehaemoglobinised before staining.

Dehaemoglobinisation may be carried out:

(i) *With glacial acetic acid and tartaric acid mixture.* The film is flooded with the mixture and as soon as dehaemoglobinisation is complete (indicated by the greyish-white colour of the film), the fluid is drained off by tilting. It is then fixed with methyl alcohol for 3 to 5 minutes. The slide is then washed thoroughly with neutral or slightly alkaline distilled water so that every trace of acid is removed.

(ii) In distilled water by placing the film in a vertical position in a glass cylinder for 5 to 10 minutes. When the film becomes white, it is taken out and allowed to dry in an upright position.

After dehaemoglobinisation the film is stained with Leishman's or Giemsa's stain in the same way as the thin film.

Glacial acetic acid and tartaric acid mixture is prepared as follows: 2 per cent glacial acetic acid, 4 parts and 2 per cent crystalline tartaric acid, 1 part.

Field's Stain (1941). This is a quick method of staining of malarial parasite in thick films (without fixation). The stain consists of two solutions: solution A and solution B. The stains are kept in staining jars with necks wide enough to permit the insertion of a glass slide. The depth of the solution should be about 3 inches, the level being maintained by the addition of fresh solution from time to time.

Technique:

(i) The thick film is placed in solution A for a few seconds (1 to 2 seconds), or till the haemoglobin is removed and no trace of green colouring left.

(ii) It is then removed and immediately rinsed by waving gently in clean water for a few seconds until the stain ceases to flow from the film and the glass slide is free from stain.

(iii) It is then placed in solution B for 1 second.

(iv) It is removed and rinsed gently in clean water for 2 to 3 seconds.

(v) It is then allowed to dry in a vertical position.

Solution A		*Solution B*	
Methylene blue	0.8 g	Eosin (yellow eosin, water soluble)	1 g
Azure I (or Azure B)	0.5 g	Disodium hydrogen phosphate (anhydrous)	5 g
Disodium hydrogen phosphate (anhydrous)	5 g	Potassium dihydrogen phosphate (anhydrous)	6.25 g
Potassium dihydrogen phosphate (anhydrous)	6.25 g	Distilled water	500 ml
Distilled water	500 ml		

The phosphate salts are first dissolved, then the stain is added. Solution of granules of azure I (or azure B) may be facilitated by grinding in a mortar with the phosphate solvent. Each of the prepared solution is set aside for 24 hours and after filtration, it is ready for use. Refiltration may be necessary if there is a scum or a precipitate.

Eosin solution should be renewed as soon as it becomes greenish.

Combined Thick and Thin Films on the Same Slide. This method has been recommended by Sinton(1925) and has been found to be of special value in survey work. Two drops of blood are taken; one, half an inch and another, one inch from the right end of the slide. The former is made into a thick film and the latter into a thin film (Fig. 202 g & h.)

The thick film is first dehaemoglobinised and then stained along with the thin film. The simplest way is as follows: A line with a grease pencil is drawn between the films. The undiluted Leishman's stain is poured over the thin film and after dilution the stain is flooded over the thick film.

Or the thin part of the film is first fixed with methyl alcohol and after drying, the whole slide is flooded with dilute Giemsa's stain and allowed to remain from half to two hours.

J.S.B. Stain. Singh and Bhattacharji (1944) devised a rapid Romanowsky's method of staining malarial parasites by a water soluble stain, which consists of two solutions.

Solution I is made with the following ingredients: methylene blue 0.5 g, potassium dichromate 0.5 g. sulphuric acid (1 per cent by volume) 3 ml, potassium hydroxide (1 per cent) 10 ml and water 500 ml.

Solution II is prepared by dissolving 1 g of eosin (water soluble) in 500 ml of tap water.

The solutions are kept in wide-mouthed stoppered jars 1½ inches diameter by 3½ inches in height; these keep well for several months.

Procedure for Preparing Solution I. The methylene blue is dissolved in 500 ml of water in a narrow-mouth flask; sulphuric acid and potassium dichromate are added one after another, with the formation of a heavy deposit of amorphous purple coloured precipitate of methylene blue chromate. The solution is heated in a water-bath at boiling point for a period of 2 to 3 hours. At the end of this period, the solution turns blue which indicates almost complete polychroming. The solution is allowed to cool at room temperature and the precipitate appears as steel-blue needle-like branched crystals. At this stage, 10 ml of 1 per cent potassium hydroxide is added, drop by drop, with the flask being shaken continuously. A greater portion of the precipitate is dissolved and the liquid is filtered several times till the dye remaining on the filter paper is completely dissolved. The filtrate is blue having a violet iridescence and is a mixture of the azures with only a trace of methylene blue. The solution is left to mature at room temperature for forty-eight hours; the staining qualities of the solution improve with ageing.

Method of Staining Thick Blood Films	*Method of Staining Thick and Thin Films on Same Slide*
1. Immerse the slide in solution I for 10 seconds.	1. Fix the thin smear in methyl alcohol for a second or two and dry.
2. Wash for 2 seconds in a jar containing acidulated tap water adjusted to pH 6.2–6.6 by the addition of 5 per cent acetic or citric acid.	2. Immerse the whole slide in solution I for 30 seconds.
3. Stain with solution II for 1 second.	3. Wash in a jar containing acidulated tap water (pH 6.2 to 6.6).
4. Wash in the same jar (2) for 5 seconds.	4. Stain with solution II for 1 second.
5. Immerse in solution I again for 10 seconds.	5. Wash again in the same jar (3) for 4 seconds.
6. Wash as above for 10 seconds or till the smear gives a pink background.	6. Immerse in solution I again for 30 seconds, or till the smear gives a pink background.
7. Dry and examine.	7. Wash again in acidulated water for 10 seconds
	8. Dry and examine.

Examination of Blood for Malarial Parasites

Time for Taking Blood. The parasites are more easily detected in the film when the blood has been taken several hours after the height of the paroxysm has been reached. Schizogony of *P. vivax*, *P. malariae* and *P. ovale* occurs in the peripheral blood, hence the parasites can readily be demonstrated both during the febrile and afebrile periods in these cases. The parasites in cases of *P. falciparum* infections, however, disappear from the peripheral blood during the afebrile period, hence the best time for demonstrating the falciparum parasites is a few hours after the febrile paroxysm reaches its peak. In general, it may be stated that the blood film should be taken at the time when the patient is seen first and thereafter as occasion arises.

Rules to be Adopted. While drawing blood films for the demonstration of malarial parasites, it will be a convenient and safe procedure to have both thin and thick films either on the same slide or on two different slides, and the examination of stained films should be carried out as follows:

1. A thin film is examined first and if parasites are found, there is no need for examining the thick film.
2. If parasites are not found in the thin film in a few minutes, the thick film should be examined.
3. If parasites are discovered in the thick film but the identity is not clear, the thin film is to be re-examined more thoroughly to determine the nature of the infection.

Remarks on the Examination of Thin Blood Film. In examining a thin film it is desirable to follow certain rules, before a slide can be declared "negative" to malarial parasites, which are as follows:

(i) The area of the film examined should be along the upper and lower margins of the "tail" end of the film, because the parasites are more numerous there.
(ii) A minimum of 100 fields should be examined and the time taken for such examination should be about 8 to 10 minutes. This is based on the observation that in non-immune persons the clinical attack of malaria is associated with the presence of at least one parasite per 100 fields.

Remarks on Thick Blood Film Examination. The red blood cells remain unstained as they are backed by dehaemoglobinisation; the only elements seen in the film are the stained parasites and the leucocytes. In a thick film, the morphology of malarial parasites is distorted, the relationship of red blood cells to parasites or any special change in the red blood cells cannot be observed. Thus, it may be difficult to identify the species of parasite, which is however easier in thin film. Thick films should never be the method of choice nor should it be a substitute for the thin film method; it should be employed only to supplement the latter. A thick blood film may be taken to be actually a concentration method for detecting the parasites as it contains a larger amount of blood in a given area than a thin blood film. Examination of a thick film saves a lot of time as one microscopic field is equivalent to 50 microscopic fields of a thin film. Hence, thick films are often employed in mass surveys for a quick diagnosis and also as a guide to treatment for testing the efficacy of antimalarial drugs.

Appearance of Malarial Parasites in Thick Blood Film (Figs. 203 & 204). Difficulty in identifying the species of malarial parasite in the thick film is due to the fact that owing to the lacking of red blood cells the parasites appear in the unfamiliar setting (absence of the outlines of host-erythrocytes). Further, owing to the lack of fixation, the morphology of the parasite is also altered.

(a) The young trophozoites (ring-forms) of all species appear as streaks of blue cytoplasm with detached nuclear dots and the species cannot be differentiated one from the other. The ring-forms rarely persist but usually appear as broken or irregular rings assuming various patterns. Certain descriptive terms are employed (Field and Fleming, 1938); "comma", where the cytoplasm forms a curved thread with the red nucleus; "swallow" or "gullswing", where a dash of the blue occurs on either side of the red nucleus as two "wings"; "exclamation mark", where the red nucleus occurs below the blue line.

(b) Schizonts and gametocytes (crescents often unmistakable) however retain their normal appearances, although being smaller and less regular in outline; the pigments are seen more clearly. With the disappearance of host-cells, cell-stippling disappears also, such as Schüffner's dots of *P. vivax*, James's dots of *P. ovale*, Maurer's dots of *P. falciparum* and Ziemann's dots of *P. malariae*. Occasionally, *vivax* trophozoites retain the shadowy ("ghost") outlines of the enlarged host-cells with persisting Schüffner's dots.

(c) The nuclei of leucocytes stain a deep purple and are clearly defined, whereas the cytoplasms always appear tattered; the cytoplasmic granules except eosinophils, which have a special resistance, disappear.

(d) The blood platelets stain place purple having a woolly texture and outline.

Examination of Blood for Microfilariae

COLLECTION OF BLOOD. In areas where the microfilaria shows nocturnal periodicity, the blood should be collected between 10 P.M. and 2 A.M. In case of non-periodic microfilaria, the blood may be taken at any time, preferably in the morning.

EXAMINATION OF UNSTAINED PREPARATION. Two or three drops of blood are taken on a clean glass slide and a coverslip is put on. The rim is then smeared with vaseline to prevent drying up of the blood. The slide should be examined next morning under the low

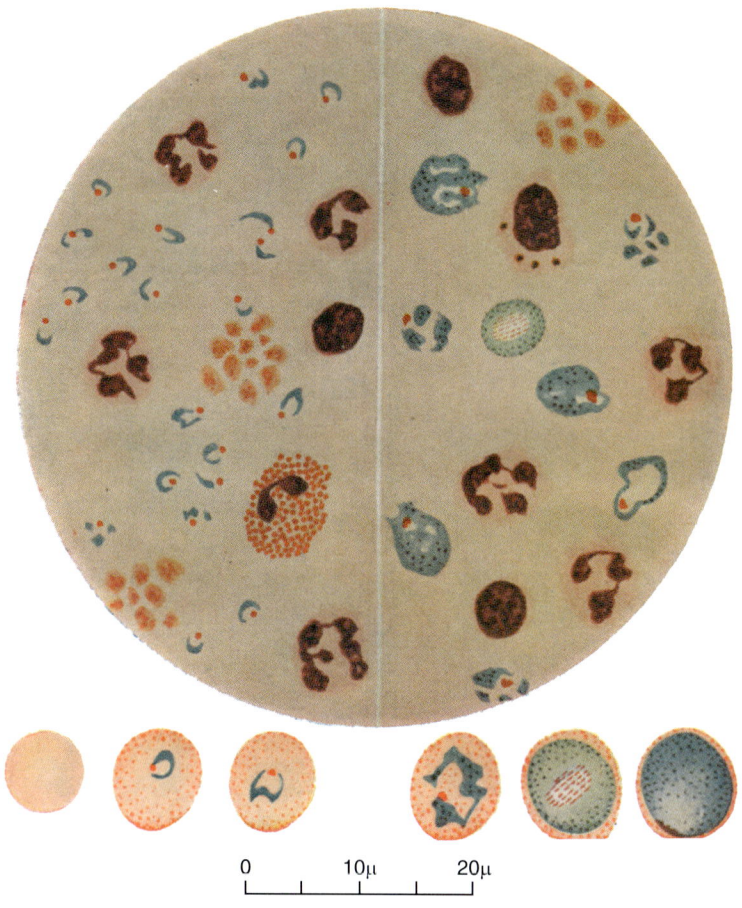

0   10μ   20μ

Fig. 203—*P. vivax* in thick blood film.
(Stained with Leishman's stain after dehaemoglobinisation.)
The left half-field shows the ring-forms (species characters are not distinctive). The right
half-field shows late trophozoite stage and gametocytes. The corresponding appearance
of parasites in thin film is shown below separately under each half.

power objective of the microscope and the microfilaria, if present, may be seen wriggling about in the blood (the microfilaria may remain alive for a period of 24 to 48 hours in such a preparation).

EXAMINATION OF STAINED PREPARATION. For this purpose, a thick film of blood is prepared and kept covered. Next morning, it is dehaemoglobinised by putting the slide in water, dried and fixed in methyl alcohol, and then stained with Lishman's stain, Giemsa's stain or haematoxylin and eosin. Occasionally, the microfilaria may be detected even in a thin film (Figs. 205, 206 & 207).

Haematoxylin and eosin stain. The thick film, after dehaemoglobinisation and fixation, is stained with Delafield's haematoxylin for 5 to 7 minutes (may be steamed over a flame). The stain is washed under tap water and left in the running water for 7 to 10 minutes or till the "blue colour" develops (differentiation may also be done in acid-alcohol). It may be counterstained with dilute Giemsa's stain or 5 per cent aqueous solution of eosin for half a minute. Final differentiation may be made in running tap water.

Vital staining. Either fresh blood or the sediment after dehaemoglobinisation is mixed with methylene blue solution (1 in 5,000 in physiological saline). The living microfilariae of *L. loa*, *O. volvulus* and *D. perstans* take up the stain in 10 minutes, whereas the microfilariae of *W. bancrofti* and *B. malayi* take up the stain much more slowly (Sharp, 1927).

Microfilaria Count. With the help of a haemoglobinometer pipette 20 mm^2 of blood is placed on a clean glass slide, dried as thick film, dehaemoglobinised and stained in the usual manner. The total number of microfilariae in the thick smear multiplied by 50 will give the number per ml of blood.

Concentration Methods. These consist of taking a large quantity of blood (5 to 10 ml) and centrifuging it at a speed of 2,000 revolutions per minute for 2 to 5 minutes. The supernatant fluid is decanted and the sediment is examined for microfilariae. Either the sediment is drawn into a film which is then air-dried, fixed and permanently stained; or the sediment as a whole may be vitally stained. The various concentration methods vary as to the use of dehaemoglobinising agents which may be distilled water, acetic acid (2 per cent), formalin (2 to 5 per cent) or saponin (1 to 10 per cent). The following are some of the methods:

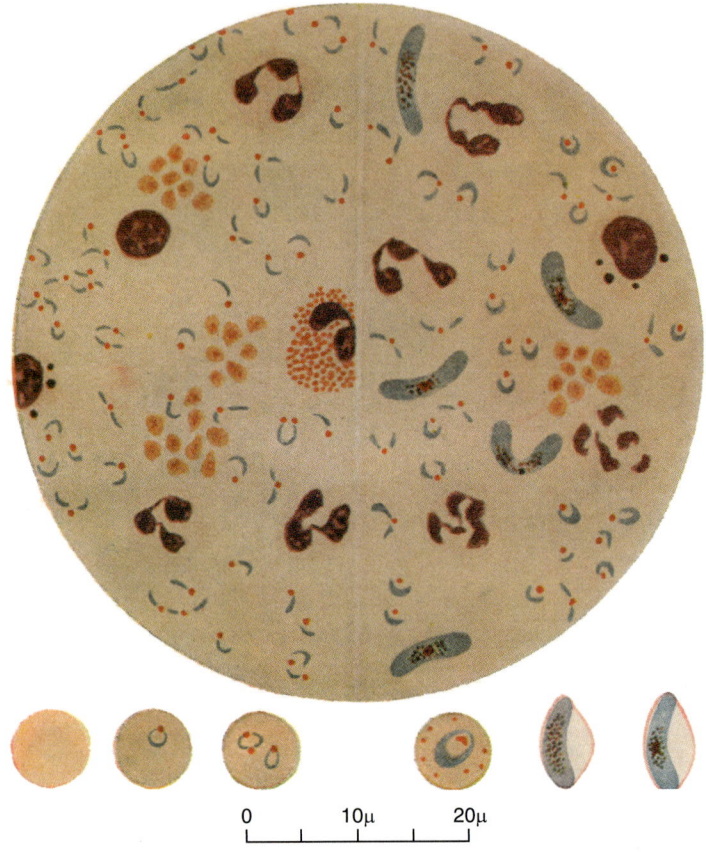

0   10μ   20μ

Fig. 204—*P. falciparum* **in thick blood film.**
(Stained with Leishman's stain after dehaemoglobinisation.)
The left half-field shows the young ring-forms with various cytoplasmic patterns. The
right half-field shows ring-forms of more advanced stage with crescents. The corresponding appearance of parasites in thin film is shown below separately under each half.

(a) One to two ml of blood is taken in a test tube containing 5 to 10 ml of a 2 per cent acetic acid solution. The blood is centrifuged next morning and a smear made from the deposit is stained and examined for microfilariae.

(b) About 5 ml of blood is taken from a vein and is placed in a centrifuge tube containing 10 ml distilled water. The mixture is shaken thoroughly until the blood is lacked. It is then centrifuged and the deposit examined for microfilariae.

(c) About 20 drops of blood are placed in 10 ml normal saline. To this a few drops of 10 per cent saponin solution is added to haemolyse the red blood cells. The specimen is then centrifuged and the living motile larvae may be found in the sediment (Schüffner and Snijders).

(d) About 5 ml of blood is taken in 10 ml of citrated saline (2.5 per cent). Next morning, the blood is dehaemoglobinised by adding 1 per cent saponin solution in normal saline drop by drop, till the haemolysis is completed. A drop of heparin is then added and the mixture is centrifuged. The sediment is examined for microfilariae (Bhaduri, 1948).

(e) One millilitre of blood is mixed with 9 ml of a 2 per cent solution of formalin. The mixture is centrifuged at a speed of 2,000 r.p.m. for 5 minutes; the microfilariae are to be found in the sediment (Knott, 1939).

For Survey Work. Two new techniques for detecting and counting microfilariae are now being used: (i) Counting chamber technique devised by Denham *et al* (1971) in which a measured quantity (20 mm^3) of haemolysed blood is directly examined, and (ii) Membrane filter concentration technique using millipore membrane or nucleopore filter, where the microfilariae liberated from measured quantity (up to 10 ml) of the heparinised blood are examined fresh, or after staining (Bell, 1967; Desowitz & Southgate, 1973).

Hetrazan Provocative Test. Administration of a single dose of diethylcarbamazine (hetrazan) 100 mg orally induces the appearance of nocturnally periodic microfilariae in the peripheral blood in the daytime and is thus useful in carrying out filarial surveys during the daytime. Blood is collected 30-45 minutes after hetrazan administration and is examined by concentration methods.

MICROFILARIA BANCROFTI IN PERIPHERAL BLOOD

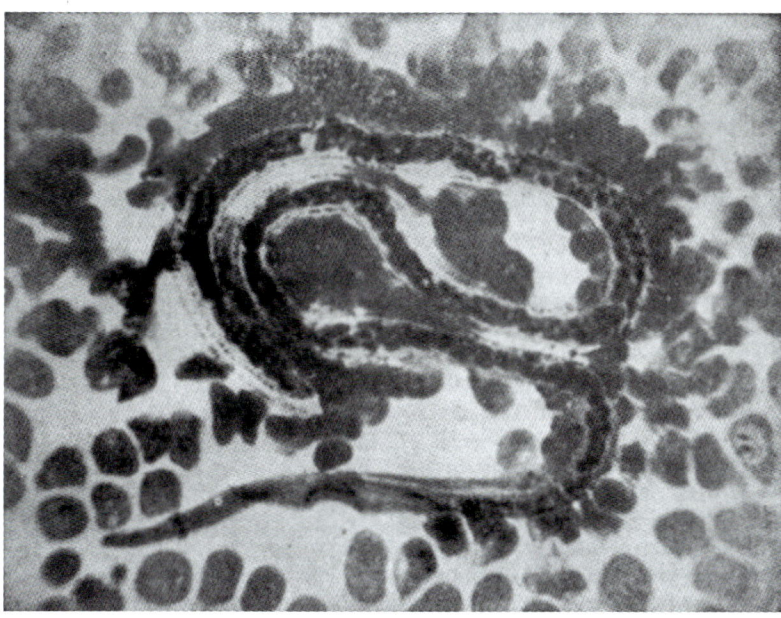

Fig. 205—*Microfilaria bancrofti* **in a thin blood film.**
(Stained with Leishman's stain; seen under oil-immersion lens.)

The subcuticular cells, somatic nuclei and the sheath at the tail-end are well snown:
a trophozoite of *Plasmodium vivax* can be seen on the right marked by arrow.
(From a case of wuchereriasis infected with *P. vivax*.)

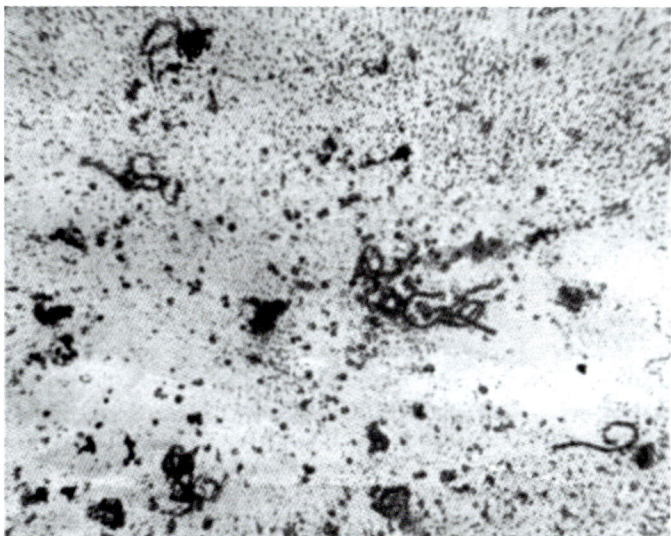

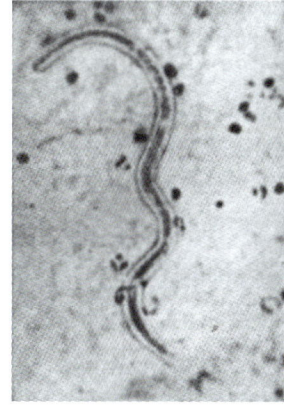

Low power view, showing 9 microfilariae.

Mf. bancrofti, as seen under
higher magnification

Figs. 206 & 207—*Microfilaria bancrofti* **in a thick blood film (concentrated).**
(Stained with Leishman's stain after dehaemoglobinisation.)

C. CULTURAL EXAMINATION

CULTIVATION OF *E. histolytica*

Preparation of the Media. (a) Boeck and Drbohlav's method (modified by Dobell and Laidlaw, 1926). For this purpose, tubes of inspissated blood serum (horse) are first prepared by heating in a serum inspissator as usual. To each of the tubes is added about 3 to 5 ml of a solution of egg albumin so as to cover the solid part of the medium to a depth of 1 ml of the fluid. The medium should be kept in an incubator and taken out immediately before inoculation. Just before inoculation with the material containing Entamoebae, a little sterile rice starch (whole wheat-flour is used by Stone) is added to the medium with a platinum loop. The addition of finely divided starch to the media greatly facilitates the growth.

The *egg albumin solution* is prepared as follows: The surface of the egg-shell is sterilised with alcohol and dried. The shell is perforated with a sterile forceps and the white of the egg is drawn by means of a 5 ml syringe with a stout needle of big bore. The whites of four eggs are dissolved in one litre of sterile Ringer's solution.

The composition of *Ringer's solution* is:

Sodium chloride	...	9 g
Potassium chloride	...	0.2 g
Calcium chloride	...	0.2 g
Distilled water	...	1,000 ml

Rice starch is sterilised by heating it at 180°C for one hour (dry heat).

The cultures are kept at 37°C and subcultures should be made every 2 or 3 days. Trophozoites as well as cystic forms may be used for artificial culture. The amoebae develop best in culture medium having a *p*H of 7.2 to 7.8. It has been shown that the presence of intestinal bacteria introduced along with the inoculating material is necessary for the cultivation of *E. histolytica*.

(b) NIH (National Institute of Health, Bethesda U.S.A.). This common media can be used in place of B.D. media.

Composition:

(i) Fresh egg fluid (albumin)	...	270 ml
Ringer's solution	...	75 ml
(ii) Overlay:		
Locke's solution	...	5 ml
Composition of Locke's solution:		
Sodium chloride	...	8 gm
Calcium chloride	...	0.2 gm
Potassium chloride	...	0.2 gm
Magnesium chloride	...	0.01 gm
Disodium hydrogen phosphate	...	2.0 gm
Sodium bicarbonate	...	0.4 gm
Potassium dihydrogen phosphate	...	0.3 gm
Distilled water	...	1000 ml

The Locke's solution is autoclaved at 15 lbs pressure for 15 mins and final *p*H of fluid is adjusted to 7.1. Egg fluid and Ringer's solution slants are prepared as in Dobell's media. The slants are then overlaid by Locke's solution and autoclaved at 15 lbs pressure for 15 mins. The bottles are incubated overnight to test the sterility.

Antibiotics used in the medium:

(a) Penicilline sodium	...	1000 units/ml of overlay fluid
(b) Streptomycin	...	2.0 mg of streptomycin sulphate per ml of overlay fluid
(c) Acriflavin solution	...	1.0 ml of 0.2 gm acriflavin solution per 5 ml of overlay fluid

Starch—One loopful of freshly prepared rice starch which is autoclaved for 10 mins at 10 lbs pressure is added to the medium just before inoculation.

Technique of Cultivation. Transfers and inoculations are made with a 1 ml sterile capillary glass pipette and not with a platinum loop as required in a bacteriological culture. Ordinary aseptic precautions are to be observed in making inoculation during the cultivation of *E. histolytica* as it has been found that the presence of certain bacteria interferes with the growth of amoeba. Similar precautions are to be taken during transfers, as introduction of any new bacterium will produce a deleterious effect on the parasite. For a successful culture, inoculation should always be made from a fresh stool, preferably passed within fifteen minutes. If in the tropics, the stool is kept covered to avoid contamination, a positive result may still be obtained even from a stool of two hours' standing. When cultures are to be made from formed or semi-formed stool, a little of the fluid (0.5 to 1 ml) taken from the culture tube by means of a sterile capillary pipette is poured on to a small portion of the faecal mass, emulsified and then inoculated. In the case of a fluid or semi-fluid stool, about 0.5 ml of the material is taken up directly and inoculated into the liquid portion of the media.

EXAMINATION. Cultures are to be examined at the end of twenty-four hours. The material is to be collected by 1 ml pipette from the sediment at the bottom of fluid cultures where amoebae are found in large numbers. In slant cultures, the material is to be taken from the surface of the slant at the junction of the fluid by gentle scraping, and the material so loosened is then withdrawn along with the fluid in the capillary pipette. A drop of the fluid so collected is then placed on a clean glass slide, a coverslip preparation made and examined unstained under the microscope. If it is found negative for amoeba, another preparation is examined at the end of forty-eight hours. If it still does not show any amoeba, then a final negative report may be given. It is to be noted that the primary cultures of amoeba do not show many parasites and it seldom exceeds two to four in one microscopic field; in many fields there may be none.

FACTORS HELPING GROWTH OF *E. histolytica*. Yorke and Adams recommended that before implanting the faeces containing the cysts, a preliminary washing is necessary, as normal faeces contain a substance inhibitory to excystation. The cysts obtained after concentration method thus offer a good material for culture, as not only it is rich in cysts but also the inhibitory substance has been removed. Such cysts will readily excyst, provided the media also contain some bacteria. Addition of heat-killed bacteria, introduction of a reducing agent (0.1 per cent cystine hydrochloride or 0.3 per cent neutralised thioglycollic acid) or production of partial anaerobiosis (aeration with nitrogen gas or absorption of oxygen with alkaline pyrogallol) favours excystation in such cases. It is also known that cultivation of bacteria-free excysted amoeba cannot be maintained unless a living bacterium or a flagellate (*T. cruzi*) is present in culture media.

In cultures of intestinal protozoa, *Blastocystis hominis* which is present in nearly every stool, grows readily and thereby prevents the growth of amoebae in such cultures or may even kill the parasites by its overgrowth. It has been suggested that the addition of a small quantity of rice starch or 1 per cent dextrin into the culture media appears to be detrimental to the growth of *Blastocystis hominis*. But the best procedure to overcome this difficulty is to inoculate a kitten *per rectum* with the culture material in which *Blastocystis hominis* is present. The animal develops an acute dysentery and its stool will provide go cultures of *E. histolytica* free from *Blastocystis hominis*.

Morphology in Culture. In cultures, *E. histolytica* shows great avidity for starch granules and feeds on bacteria. All phases of development, both excystation and encystation, are to be seen in culture media. The process of encystment occurs in the course of eighteen to twenty-four hours and excystment starts as soon as the cyst matures. The trophozoites of cultures may be made to encyst under certain circumstances. Cultures inoculated with cysts readily excyst. When trophozoites are inoculated, they multiply rapidly by binary fission.

Trophozoites and cysts do not vary in morphological appearances. The little variation that has been noticed is that the trophozoites are usually larger than the average amoebae and contain numerous bacteria. The motility in cultures is rapid and progressive, exhibiting a marked polarity. The cysts of cultures generally contain one to four nuclei, but sometimes more than four nuclei are observed.

Maintenance of Culture. The medium used for this purpose is either an egg, an agar or a serum slant covered with a fluid medium. A strain of *E. histolytica* can be maintained for more than five years by making subcultures at the end of every forty-eight hours. Special precautions are to be taken that no bacterial contamination takes place during the transfers.

Pure Cultures. Attempts have been made to obtain a culture of *E. histolytica* free from bacteria. The following methods are generally employed:

(a) By cultivating trophozoites obtained from the "pus" of liver abscess free from bacteria.

(b) By employing chemicals such as acriflavine or 1 in 1,000 bichloride of mercury which will injure the bacteria but not the amoebae.

(c) By cultivating cysts washed and free from bacteria.

Pure cultures, however, cannot be maintained for more than one or two generations.

Value of Cultural Examinations:

(i) *In diagnosis*. Compared to a direct microscopic examination and the use of concentration method, cultural examination of the stool for the detection of *E. histolytica* has greatly increased the percentage of positive findings in cases of amoebic infection of the bowel. In making statistical surveys, it is becoming evident that a cultural examination of the stool should be included in the methods employed, as it has been found to be superior to other methods for detection of infective cases.

(ii) It enables one to study the morphological characters of the parasite.

(iii) It may be employed in research work where the efficacy of an amoebicidal drug is being tested.

(iv) It is used to obtain amoebic antigen for specific immunological tests.

CULTIVATION OF LEISHMANIAE

Various culture media such as N.N.N. medium, Solid medium, Semi-defined liquid medium etc. are available for cultivation of leishmania species.

N.N.N. Medium [Novy and McNeal (1904), Nicolle (1908)]*				
N.N.N. medium			Salt agar is prepared as follows:	
This is composed of:			Agar	14 g
Salt agar	2 parts		Sodium chloride	6 g
Rabbit's blood (defibrinated)	1 part		Distilled water	900 ml

The rabbit's blood is added to the liquid agar during cooling. The two are intimately mixed by rotating the tube between the palms of the hands, holding it in a vertical position. The tube is then allowed to set in a sloping position so that the medium may solidify in a slant. When not required, the culture tubes with their mouths covered by sterile rubber caps are kept in an ice chest.

Materials Used: (i) Blood, (ii) Marrow, or (iii) Splenic pulp.

Technique. The material to be cultured is inoculated into the water of condensation of N.N.N. medium; 4 such tubes are inoculated. The tubes are then incubated at 32°C for a period of 1 to 4 weeks. From the tenth day onwards, the tubes are examined for promastigotes. A drop of condensation fluid is taken by means of a capillary pipette or the material is gently scraped from the surface of the medium and is examined in the fresh state. The flagellates, if present, can be seen actively moving in the field. While examining cultures, special care should be taken to avoid contamination. Advantages of seeding into 4 tubes are that one of two tubes can be kept unopened till the end. If there are no flagellates at the end of one mouth, the result may be declared negative.

Solid Medium. This medium (J. C. Ray 1932)** is prepared with agar agar, glucose, beef-heart infusion, peptone, amino acid, glycerin and rabbit's blood in a specially modified test tube. Various addition and alteration has been done to the constituents of this medium afterwards.

The parasite grows in this medium as a thick, grayish-white mucoid spreading lawn. No water of condensation is necessary for the growth of the parasite, but care should be taken so that the medium does not get dry. Usually, the parasite grows within 48 to 72 hours at 24°C which should then be subcultured. The medium is ideal for bulk preparation of antigen. The main disadvantage is that all the strains could not be adopted for the growth on this medium.

Semi-defined Liquid Medium. An easily prepared inexpensive monophasic medium*** which supports continuous culture of Leishmania species promastigotes has been developed. One of them designated as HO-MEM is a modified Eagle's minimal essential medium with Spinner's salts and 10% foetal calf scum. The remarkable increase in parasite number occurs within 5 days of culture. The optimum *p*H for *L. donovani* is 7.2 to 7.4 and optimum temperature is 25° to 26°C. Average doubling time during log growth phase is 10 to 12 hours and this time shortens at mid log phase. HO-MEM is a good medium for transformation of *L. donovani* amistogotes to promastigotes (60 to 80% in 48 hours).

CULTIVATION OF THE MALARIAL PARASITE

It may be pointed out that in actual practice, culture methods are never restored to, for the diagnosis of symptomatic malaria.

Brass and Jone (1912) cultivated malaria parasites in artificial media which could not be maintained more than one cycle. Black (1945) improved the technique of culture.

Trager and Jensen (1976)**** could successfully cultivate human malaria parasite (*P. falciparum*) to observe the erythrocytic schizogony using RPMI1640 medium in in vitro continuous culture technique.

Value of Culture Methods:
1. To obtain erythrocyte stages for the study of antigenic structure.
2. As a source of antigen for sero-epidemiological investigation.
3. To study the sensitivity/resistance of the parasite to various drugs.
4. To observe immuno prophylactic activity.

Trager and Jensen's technique—Malaria parasite is maintained in continuous culture in human erythrocytes, incubated at 38°C, in RPMI 1640 medium with human serum, under an atmosphere with 7% CO_2 and low oxygen (1 or 5%). The parasite

---

* Nicolle, C. (1908). *Compt. Rend. Acad Set.* **146**, 498-499.
** Ray, J. C. (1932). *I.J.M.R.*, **20**, 355.
*** Randy, L. Barens, Rato Brun and Stuart M. Krassner (1976). *Journal of Parasitology*, Vol 62, No. 3, 360-365.
**** Trager, W. and Jensen, J. B. (1976). *Science*, **193**, 673.

material, derived from an infected *Aotus trivirgatus* (Owl monkeys) is diluted more than 100 million times by addition of normal human erythrocytes (Group AB Rh+) at 3 or 4 days intervals. The parasites continued to reproduce their normal asexual cycle of approximately 48 hours but are no longer highly synchronous. They remain infective to *Aotus trivirgatus*.

D. EXAMINATION OF BIOPSY MATERIAL

SPLEEN PUNCTURE

For the Diagnosis of Kala-azar. When the spleen is considerably enlarged, it is one of the most valuable methods for establishing the parasitological diagnosis of kala-azar.

ARTICLES REQUIRED:

1. A 5 ml glass syringe having a sharp needle of 1 to 1¼ inches in length. Sterilisation is done in a hot-air oven. An absolutely dry syringe is essential, as water plasmolyses the parasite.
2. Cotton wool, bandage, Tr. of iodine, alcohol, phenol, Tr. benzoin Co. or collodion.
3. Glass slides and culture tubes (N.N.N. medium).

PREPARATION OF THE PATIENT. Prior to the operation, in order to promote the coagulability of the blood, the patient should be given intravenous or intramuscular injections of calcium gluconate 10% 5 ml for two to three days, the last injection being given on the night before. If, however, the coagulation of blood is normal, the patient need not be prepared in this manner.

PROCEDURE. The patient is made to lie on his back with his left hand underneath the head. The operator stands on the left side and the assistant on the right. The splenic area over which the puncture is to be made is chosen at a spot half to one inch below the costal margin, sterilised by painting with tincture of iodine. The sterilised needle of the syringe is first introduced into the skin and then plunged directly into the spleen by the operator, while the assistant helps in fixing the enlarged spleen by pressing it upwards. During the operation, the patient should be advised to hold his breath to avoid unnecessary movements. Forcible aspiration is now made and some of the splenic pulp or blood is invariably drawn although it may not appear in the barrel of the syringe. The needle is quickly withdrawn. After the splenic puncture, the area is sealed with benzoin or collodion and an abdominal bandage with pressure-pad is applied over the splenic area. The patient should be kept lying down for an hour or two and the pulse rate should be recorded for the detection of any evidence of internal haemorrhage. The patient may be allowed to take food one hour after the puncture. No discomfort is experienced by the patient and only in a small number of cases some tenderness in the splenic area is complained of, for the next 24 hours.

EXAMINATION OF THE MATERIAL. Films are now prepared aseptically by ejecting one or two drops of the fluid on to sterile glass slides which are later drawn in the same manner as ordinary blood films. A little sterile citrated saline is aspirated into the syringe to dilute the splenic juice that is left behind, thereby facilitating the transference of the material into N.N.N. medium. The amastigote forms can be found in stained films and promastigote forms in culture.

CAUTION. The risk of severe haemorrhage can be avoided if the following precautions are taken.

(i) Peripheral blood should be examined to exclude cases of leukaemia.
(ii) Bleeding and coagulation time should be ascertained to exclude any haemorrhagic diathesis.
(iii) Spleen puncture should not be done in cases of kala-azar where jaundice, bleeding from gums and purpura develop in the course of the disease, or where the disease is complicated with severe bronchitis or ascites.

LYMPH NODE PUNCTURE

For the Diagnosis of Kala-azar and African Trypanosomiasis. The skin over the node is sterilised and the node is pressed between the index finger and the thumb. A dry, sterilised hypodermic needle is then inserted into the node. The lymph will enter the needle by capillary attraction and if necessary, a little massage may be applied. The needle is quickly withdrawn and attached to the syringe. The lymph juice is squirted on to a glass slide and a smear preparation made and stained by Leishman's method. Cultures on N.N.N. medium may also be made by taking a little sterile citrated saline and washing the needle with the solution. Cochrane in China, and Kirk and Sati in Sudan, found this method to be useful in the diagnosis of kala-azar. As the lymph nodes are enlarged in certain cases, and the parasites are also demonstrated in such cases of Indian kala-azar, this method is recommended for the diagnosis of kala-azar in India.

For the demonstration of trypomastigote forms of *T. brucei*, the aspirated lymph juice may be examined fresh and unstained. This is a useful procedure in "gambian" sleeping sickness.

LYMPH NODE BIOPSY

Lymph node biopsy, preferably the epitrochlear lymph node, offers an useful aid to the confirmation of *L. donovani* infection. In case of larger lymph node (more than 3 cm in diameter), an attempt may be made to aspirate the gland juice which is then subjected to smear examination and culture in N.N.N. medium, to demonstrate *L. donovani*. In case of failure to demonstrate parasite in affected gland juice, the lymph node may be excised out. The biopsied lymph node is bisected. Scraping from the bisected gland surface before fixation with formal saline may be subjected to culture in N.N.N. medium at 22°C to demonstrate promastigote if any. Smears are stained with Leishman's or Giemsa stain. In lymphatic leishmaniasis, this is the only method to demonstrate parasite.

BONE MARROW BIOPSY

Two methods are generally employed:

1. *Needle or Aspiration Biopsy*. The marrow is aspirated through a wide-bore needle (Salah or Klima type) from the following sites: (i) sternum, (ii) iliac crest (posterior or anterior), and (iii) medial aspect of the upper end of the tibia in children up to 2 years of age. Films are prepared from the aspirated marrow and stained with a Romanowsky stain. Marrow films are examined to study the morphological characters of marrow cells and the presence of parasites.

2. *Trephine Biopsy*. This is particularly useful in the diagnosis of myelosclerosis. Specimens are obtained by means of specially constructed needles for trephining. From the biopsy fragment both films and histological sections can be prepared.

NEEDLE OR ASPIRATION BIOPSY IN CASES OF KALA-AZAR

1. **Sternal Puncture.** (*Note:* The sternal bone is thin and cavity narrow, hence care must be taken when the sternal puncture needle is introduced.)

MATERIALS REQUIRED:

1. *Sternal puncture needle* (Salah type). A short stout needle of the lumbar puncture type, provided with a stylet and a movable guard. The latter is adjusted at a distance of 1.5 to 2 cm from the tip according to the distance required by the needle to reach the marrow and therefore varies with the thickness of the skin and subcutaneous tissues of the thoracic wall. The needle is introduced with the stylet in position.

2. One 2 ml glass syringe for injecting the novocaine and one 10 ml glass syringe for taking the marrow.

3. Two per cent solution of novocaine or one of its substitutes.

4. Cotton wool, alcohol, Tr. of iodine, collodion or Tr. Benzoin Co.

5. Glass slides and culture tubes (N.N.N. medium).

The sternal puncture needle and glass syringes are sterilised in a hot-air steriliser in a test tube.

SITE OF PUNCTURE. Over the mid-sternal region, a little away from the middle line, at the level of second or third intercostal space.

PROCEDURE. The patient is made to lie on his back in the supine position. The area is painted over with Tr. of iodine and alcohol and then anaesthetised up to the periosteum with novocaine solution (1 ml is sufficient). After an interval of 10 to 15 minutes, the puncture is made. The needle is pierced through the skin and subcutaneous tissues up to the periosteum and marrow cavity is reached with a rotary movement, when a loss of resistance will be felt. The style is then taken out and a 10 ml glass syringe (dry and sterilised) is fitted on to the needle and about 0.25 to 0.75 ml of the marrow fluid is aspirated by gentle suction. The patient experiences a dragging pain at this stage. The syringe with the sternal puncture needle is withdrawn and the puncture wound is sealed with collodion or Tr. Benzoin Co.

The material thus obtained is then examined for parasites as described under splenic puncture. Special studies may also be made for the different marrow cells.

2. **Iliac Crest Puncture (Posterior or Anterior).** The technique and procedure of aspiration are the same as for sternal puncture.

(a) For posterior iliac crest puncture, the patient lies on one side with knees drawn up and back flexed as for a lumbar puncture. The needle is inserted perpendicularly 1 cm below the posterior superior iliac spine.

(b) For anterior iliac crest puncture, the patient lies on the back and the needle is inserted into the iliac crest at a point just behind the anterior superior iliac spine.

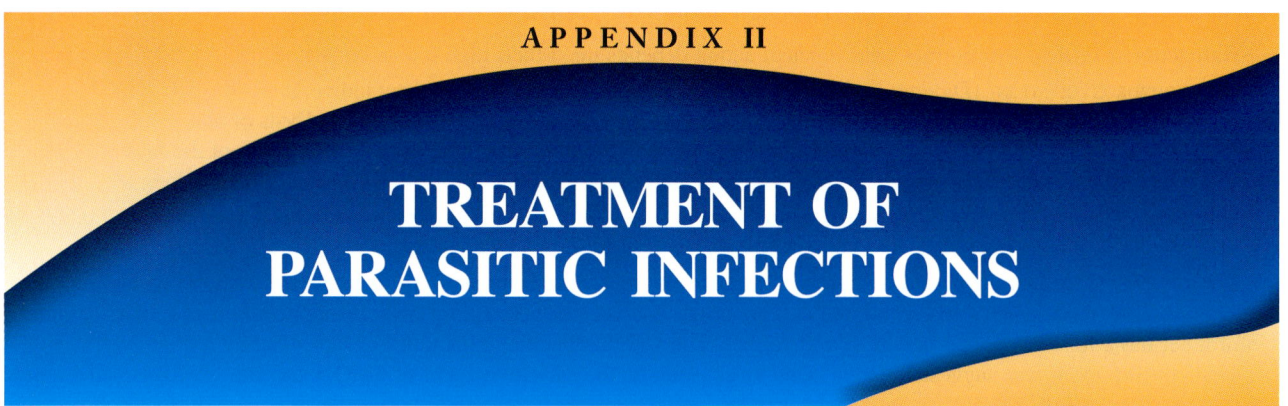

APPENDIX II

TREATMENT OF PARASITIC INFECTIONS

LIST OF DRUGS : DOSAGE AND METHODS OF ADMINISTRATION

AMOEBICIDAL DRUGS

Tissue Amoebicides: (a) Acting on the trophozoites of *E. histolytica* in the intestinal wall, liver and other metastatic areas—Emetine, dehydroemetine (DHE). (b) Acting on the trophozoites of *E. histolytica* in the liver only—4-aminoquinoline (chloroquine).

Emetine. It is the principal alkaloid obtained from the ipecacuanha root (*Cephaelis ipecacuanha*). The salt commonly used for therapeutic action is emetine hydrochloride. When given parenterally, it is a direct-acting tissue amoebicide and not a luminal amoebicide. Hence, it is effective in the treatment of acute amoebic dysentery, amoeboma intestine, hepatic and other forms of metastatic (invasive) amoebiasis. Oral emetine preparations can act as luminal amoebicide. The adult dose is 65 mg dissolved in 1 ml of distilled water, injected daily for 5 to 10 days. Under no circumstances should more than 65 mg be given in 24 hours. One course should not generally exceed more than 650 mg of emetine. The adult dose of 65 mg is not recommended for the treatment of females and weak individuals. The children's dose is proportionately smaller.

Emetine is a very toxic drug, the therapeutic and toxic doses being very close. It is excreted slowly by the kidney, hence there is a risk of cumulative toxicity. For this reason, when a full 650 mg course is required, an interval of 5 to 6 days should be given after the sixth injection.

Route of administration. Intramuscular (I.M.) or deep subcutaneous (S.C.) injections. Intravenous administration of emetine is not recommended in the treatment of amoebiasis.

Side effect. Weakness, muscle pain, nausea, vomiting, diarrhoea and cardiotoxic effect. It is a myocardial poison, leading to a fall of blood pressure (orthostatic hypotension), dyspnoea, precordial pain and tachycardia. ECG changes are flattening or inversion of T waves, widened QRS complexes and arrhythmias.

Caution. During emetine treatment the patient should be on bed rest, the pulse and blood pressure are recorded regularly.

Contraindication. Pregnancy, cardiac, renal and liver disease.

Synthetic Emetine: 2-dehydroemetine (DHE). A less toxic isomer, because it is rapidly eliminated. The adult dose is 60 to 80 mg given I.M. or deep S.C. daily for 5 to 10 days. The various remarks mentioned for emetine also apply to dehydroemetine.

An oral preparation of DHE, containing 20 mg of the compound with a resinate to retard its liberation has been found satisfactory for clinical uses in intestinal amoebiasis. Adult dose is 2 tablets thrice daily for 10 days (Rungs, 1966).

Note: The dose of emetine and dehydroemetine is calculated as 1 mg/kg body weight.

4 -aminoquinoline (*Chloroquine*). It is an antimalarial drug.

CHLOROQUINE. It is effective against hepatic and pulmonary amoebiasis. The doses employed are far in excess of those required for antimalarial activity and are administered to adults as follows: Priming or *loading dose* comprises of 0.3 g of the base (0.5 g of the phosphate) orally twice daily for 2 days. This is necessary to saturate the tissues. *Sustaining or maintenance dose* comprises of 0.3 g of the base (0.5 g of the phosphate) orally once a day for 2 or 3 weeks. *Total dose* varies from 9 to 13 g of chloroquine phosphate (5.4 to 7.8 g of the base). The regimen may lead to some minor toxic manifestations such as, nausea, vomiting, pruritus, headache and disturbed visual accommodation. Higher relapse rates are associated with chloroquine therapy in liver abscess.

Luminal Amoebicides. Acting on *E. histolytica* (trophozoites and cysts) intraluminally.

Direct-acting Luminal or Contact Amoebicides

Halogenated Hydroxyquinolines. Amoebicidal action depends upon their high iodine content.

DI-IODOHYDROXYQUINOLINE (*Diodoquin, Iodoquinol, Embequin*). It contains 63.9 per cent iodine. It is not a satisfactory drug for acute amoebic dysentery. It is effective in the treatment of symptomless carriers and cyst-passers. Cysts of non-pathogenic amoebae if present also disappear after taking the drug. Tablets of 0.65 g administered orally to adults in doses of 2-3 tablets a day for 21 days. The drug may cause *pruritus ari*, thyroid enlargement in some cases and myelo-optic neuropathy after long term therapy.

IODOCHLOR-HYDROXYQUINOLINE : *Clioquinol* (present in entero-vioform). The dosage recommended for adult is 2 to 3 tablets of 0.25 g each, for 10 days. Effective in cases of amoebic dysentery (mild) and cyst-passers.

Kono (1971) from Japan reported a large number of cases of subacute myelo-optic neuropathy (SMON) developing after taking clioquinol (iodochlorhydroxyquinoline) in large doses, a dosage of 1.5 to 3.5 g daily (equivalent to 6-14 tablets of entero-vioform per day), for a prolonged period. It was further observed that banning clioquinol in Japan caused a dramatic fall in the incidence of SMON. It was suggested that a "slow virus" may be the causative agent of SMON and Ota (1970) isolated a new virus from a patient with SMON.

Dichloracetamide Group

DILOXANIDE FUROATE (*Furamide*, Boots, *Entamide*). Issued in tablets, each containing 0.5 g of entamide. Adult dose is one tablet administered orally 3 times a day for 10 days. Effective against intestinal amoebiasis (cyst-passers). The drug is completely non-toxic and causes no serious side-effects (occasional flatulence). Children's dose: 20 mg/kg body weight daily in three divided doses for ten days.

Antibiotics. PAROMOMYCIN (*Humatin*, P. D. & Co.). A direct-acting luminal amoebicide, effective against intestinal amoebiasis. Available in kapseals, each containing the sulphate equivalent to 250 mg paromomycin base. Adult dose is 5 capsules daily for 5 days, totalling 6,250 mg. Dose is calculated as 20 mg/kg body weight. It is administered orally in three divided doses for seven days. Frequent adverse effect is gastrointestinal disturbances and rare adverse effects are renal and auditory damage.

Indirect-acting Luminal Amoebicide. Destroying the intestinal bacteria upon which the *Entamoeba histolytica* is dependent for its growth.

Tetracycline (Oxytetracycline or *terramycin* and chlortetracycline or *aureomycin*). Adult dose 250 mg given orally at 6-hourly intervals for 7 to 10 days. It is often prescribed in acute amoebic dysentery with contact amoebicides (diloxanide furoate).

Both Luminal and Tissue Amoebicides

Metronidazole and its derivative Tinidazole. Metronidazole (*Flagyl*). Both a luminal and tissue amoebicide. Given orally to adults in doses of 800 mg thrice daily for 5 days (dose is higher than that used for giardiasis). It is claimed to be highly effective when used alone. It is relatively non-toxic and can be given to children and patients with heart disease in whom emetine is contraindicated. In mild cases, tinidazole is used in a dose of 2 gm per day in three divided doses for two days and in severe cases, it is used in a dose of 800 mg three times daily for five days. These drugs have little effect on cyst of the parasite.

Imidazole. Imidazole compound such as ornidazole is now used in amoebiasis effectively. The dose is 500 mg twice daily, orally for 5-10 days.

Treatment of Amoebiasis

1. INTESTINAL AMOEBIASIS: (a) For *cyst-passers* (symptomatic or asymptomatic). An attempt is made to keep the incidence of infection down in non-endemic areas. One of the contact amoebicides is used, such as entamide furoate, paromomycin, diodoquin, milibis, metronidazole or oral emetine preparations.

(b) For *acute amoebic dysentery*. The aim will be to cure the disease and minimise the chances of relapse, hence 2 or more drugs are often used in combination or successively. Symptoms are rarely controlled by emetine or DHE I.M. for 3-4 days. Contact amoebicides (oral or iv metronidazole, oral entamide and diodaoquin) are used to eradicate intestinal organisms (*vide supra*).

(c) For *mild dysenteric attack*. Contact amoebicides (entamide furoate or diodoquin) or metronidazole are used with tetracycline. In addition, chloroquine may be given to protect the liver or eradicate subclinical hepatic infection.

2. HEPATIC AMOEBIASIS (Amoebic liver abscess). Emetine or DHE for 10 days or chloroquine for 21 days. Followed by a contact amoebicide, entamide furoate or diodoquine to eradicate the intestinal trophozoites and cysts. Alternatively metronidazole or tinidazole may be given which acts both as a luminal and tissue amoebicide.

Test of cure. One month after completion of treatment stool is to be examined for cysts of *E. histolytica* for 6 consecutive days. Ideally it should be repeated at 3-monthly intervals for a year.

DRUGS FOR GIARDIASIS

Mepacrine (*Atebrin*). For adults, one tablet (0.1 g) thrice daily for 3 to 5 days and for children half a tablet twice daily for 3 days.

Metronidazole (*Flagyl*). A derivative of imidazole. Schneider (1961) reported good results with this drug. The standard dose for adult is 200 mg, given orally, thrice daily for 5 days. Side-effects include mild digestive disturbances. Flagyl is also useful in *T. vaginalis* infection and in all types of amoebiasis.

Tinidazole. It is used in a dose of 2 gm once orally.

Furazolidine. It is an effective drug (100 mg 4 times daily × 7 to 10 days). It is preferred to children inspite of its slow action in control of the disease.

DRUGS FOR TRICHOMONIASIS

Metronidazole. One tablet (0.2 gm) 3 times daily for 7 days or 2 gm (10 tabs) in a single dose. The sexual partner should be treated similarly over the same day period. Sexual partner should abstain from coitus or condom protection against re-infection during coitus should be insisted untill both partners are made free of *Trichomonas vaginalis*. In stubborn infection where repeated courses of drug are required, it is recommended that intervals of 4 to 6 weeks should be allowed between courses. Uncoated Metronidazole vaginal inserts may be used concurrently with oral medication. One insert should be used daily for 7 days.

Metronidazole crosses the placental barrier and enters the foetal circulation rapidly. It is contraindicated during first trimester of pregnancy by FDA, U.S.A. as its effects on foetal development are not definitely known. During second and third trimesters of pregnancy, metronidazole probably should be restricted to those patients in whom topical measures have proved inadequate.

Tinidazole. It is closely related in structure and activity to metronidazole. It may be given orally in the dose of 150 mg twice a day for 7 days or 150 mg three times daily for 5 days.

Furazolidine. Nifuroxime (Tricofuron) vaginal suppositories—One suppository twice daily for 2 to 3 weeks.

TRYPANOCIDAL DRUGS

For the Treatment of African Trypanosomiasis

Suramin (*Antrypol, Naphuride sodium, Bayer "205"* or *Germanin*).

A urea-substitution compound. It is most effective in early stages in clearing the blood infection. Dosage for adult is 1 g, dissolved in 10 ml of distilled water, given intravenously (rarely intramuscularly) every week for 10 weeks. To avoid idiosyncrasy, the initial dose should be 0.2 to 0.5 g, thereafter 1 g.

Toxic symptoms include damage to renal parenchyma (appearance of albumin and granular casts in the urine), polyneuritis and dermatitis.

For prophylaxis in adults, 1 gm intravenously every two to three months.

Pentamidine isethionate. An aromatic diamidine. Issued in ampoules of 200 mg in powder form. Solution to be freshly prepared. Adult dose is 4 mg per kilogramme of body weight. Initial adult dose is 100 to 200 mg. A course of treatment consists of 10 intramuscular injections, given daily or on alternate days. It is effective in clearing trypanosomes from the blood.

For prophylaxis in adults a single dose of 175 to 200 mg intravenously for every 6 months.

Melarsoprol (Mel. B.). A compound of melarsen oxide and BAL (dimercaprol); contains trivalent arsenic. It is very effective both in "gambian" and "rhodesian" sleeping sickness when the central nervous system is involved. Adult dose is 3.6 mg per kilogramme of body weight, given intravenously on each of 4 consecutive days, then rest period for one week and later a second course (one or two series are required). It has given good results in cases refractory to other forms of treatment, but its toxicity is high and should be given under close supervision. The main toxic effect is an arsenical encephalopathy.

Mel. W. It belongs to melaminyl series of trivalent arsenicals. It is a water soluble form of Mel. B. It has the advantage of being given intramuscularly. It is given in the same doses as Mel. B. A series of 3 to 4-days course is given, each daily dose is at a level of 3.6 mg per kg body weight (Nodenot *et al* 1960). If necessary, it may be repeated after a couple of weeks.

Eflornithine. It is an irreversible inhibitor of ornithine decarboxylase. It is used I.V. in *T. brucei* gambiense in haemolymphatic stage and with C.N.S. involvement stage in a dose of 400mg/kg/day in four divided doses for 15 days. Adverse drug reactions are similar to those of other cytotoxic drugs, such as bone marrow depression, gastorintestinal disturbances, alopecia, convulsion. The adverse drug reactions are reversible.

For the Treatment of South American Trypanosomiasis

Benznidazole. It is used orally in acute cases of *T. cruzi* infection in dose of 5-10 mg/kg/day in 2 divided doses for 30-90 days. Allergic rash, dose depended polyneuropathy, g.i. disturbences, psychological disturbances are frequent adverse effects of the drug. The drug metabolites may act on parasite by interaction with DNA.

Nifurtimox. The drug shows promising result in the treatment of acute and early chronic cases of *T. cruzi* infection. It is given orally 8-10 mg/kg/day in four divided doses for 90-120 days. The mechanism of action of the drug is not completely known. Frequent adverse effects are anorexia, vomiting, weight loss, loss of memory, insomnia, tremors, paresthesia, polyneuritis, weakness, convulsion.

LEISHMANICIDAL DRUGS

For the Treatment of Kala-azar

Antimonials. Trivalent antimonials—No longer used. Pentavalent antimonials—Drug of choice.

Sodium Antimony Gluconate. Strengths of 20 mg, 40 mg and 100 mg of antimony per ml are available. This salt is the least toxic and is quickly eliminated, hence higher daily doses can be administered without any ill effects. On an average, about 6 to 8 g of antimony are required to sterilise an adult patient. It is administered intramuscularly.

Megulamine antimonoate is an alternative drug and is recommended iv/im in a dose of 20 mg stibamine/kg/day for 20-28 days.

Non-metallic Compound (Aromatic diamidine) Pentamidine Isethionate. The drug can be given as a 10 per cent solution by intramuscular injection and as a 1 per cent solution by intravenous injection, but the former method is to be preferred as compared to the latter. The average individual dose (both for adult and children) is 4 mg per kilogramme body weight. A course consists of 12 to 15 injections given daily or on alternate days. A second course after an interval of 10 to 15 days, may be required in areas where the disease is known to be resistant. The drug is supplied in the form of a powder in dose of 200 mg in sealed ampoules.

Useful in antimony resistant cases and cases of kala-azar complicated with pulmonary tuberculosis.

Amphotericin B (*Fungizone*), an antifungal agent, is also used in severe visceral leismaniasis, muco-cutaneous leishmaniasis and resistant cases of Kala-azar; but for its nephrotoxicity, it should not be the first choice and requires great care in administration. In drug-resistant cases, splenectomy followed by specific chemotherapy may be helpful (Morton and Cooke, 1948). It is administered in the dose of 0.1 mg/kg of body wt. daily by slow i.v. infusion, well diluted in 0.5 litre 5% dextrose, (given over 6 hours). It may be increased to 0.25 mg/kg of body wt. Total dose should not be more than 2 gm.

Liposomal Amphotericin B. It is less toxic drug and now used in treatment of visceral leismaniasis in several countries in a dose of 3.4 mg/kg/day, i.v. for 5 days and another injection of the drug in the same dose on 10th day. In immunicompromise patient upto 10 injections are given. In combination with lipid, amphotericin B is delivered at the site of intracellular infection and facilates rapid cure of the disease.

Paromocycin (aminosidine). It is an aminoglycoside antibiotic and is effective in a dose of 15 mg/kg/day i.v. or i.m. for three weeks. The drug can be used in treatment of visceral leismaniasis either alone or in combination with antimonial drugs.

Miltefosine. It is an alkyl-phospholipid and oral antineoplastic agent. It is an effective oral drug approved for visceral leishmaniasis. A daily dose of 100 mg/kg of body weight for 28 days cures the disease dramatically. It can not be used in pregnancy due to its teratogenic effect. Nephrotoxicity g. i. disturbances and rarely skin rash are usual side effects.

Note : Interferon Y, imidazole, allopurinol show antileishmanial activity, but their use has limited value.

Treatment of resistant cases of Kala-azar: Certain cases are encountered in which ordinary treatment fails to cure the visceral infections which are referred to as resistant and mostly reported from Mediterranean areas, South America, Sudan and recently from India. These cases require prolonged treatment with higher doses of antimony; two or three courses may be repeated at fortnightly intervals. Sometime, a change to another antimony compound produces the desired result. Aromatic diamidine appears to be the drug of choice and promises a higher rate of cure. There is an increase incidence of visceral lismeniasis in immunocompromised patients and rise of acquired resistance to antimonial drugs is also noted.

For the treatment of Oriental sore (large and multiple) and Espundia. Pentavalent preparations of antimony are the drugs of choice. In resistant cases of espundia pyrimethamine and amphotericin B may be tried. Pyrimethamine is given in 3 courses with a rest period of 8 days during the courses. For the first 2 courses 50 mg by mouth daily for 10 days and for the third course 25 mg daily for 10 days are given. Folic acid should be given concurrently. In purely cutaneous lesion, a single intramuscular injection of cycloguanil pamoate in doses 5 mg base/kg has been found to be very effective. Paramomycin ointment 2 gm/day for 20 days is used in cutaneous leishmaniasis. Ketaconazole, fluconazole, itraconazole are alternative drugs.

ANTIMALARIAL DRUGS

Antimalarial drugs are classified as follows:

  (i) Arylaminoalcohols compounds (quinine, quinidine, chloroquine, amodiaquine, mefloquine, halofantrine, lumefantrine, piperaquine, primaquine, tafenoquine).

 (ii) Antifols (pyrimethamine, proguanil, chlorproguanil, trimethotrim).

(iii) Artemisinine compounds (artemisinin, di-hydroartemisinin, artemether, artesunate, arte-ether).

Many antibacterial drugs (sulphonamides, sulphones, macrolides, chloramphenicol, tetracycline, lincosamides) also have slow antimalarial action and are used in combination with other antimalarial drugs. Resistance has been reported only in sulphonamides.

Drugs active against sensitive *P. falciparum* are also active against others species of plasmodium. Most of the antimalarial drugs act predominantly in the middle third of the life cycle of the parasite, when synthetic and metabolic activities are increased to a great extent. No antimalarial drug is able to prevent rupture and reinvasion once the schizont is formed.

Quinine. Main use at present is for the treatment of drug-resistant *P. falciparum* malaria. Salts used are quinine hydrochloride, bihydrochloride, sulphate or bisulphate.

Modes of Issue. As powders (for mixtures), tablets of 325 mg (5 grs) each (for oral administration) and ampoules of quinine bihydrochloride 325 mg/ml (for parenteral administration).

Dosage and Methods of Administration: (a) *Per-oral.* The standard method recommended for an adult is as follows: 650 mg of the salt three times a day for 10 to 14 days.

The drug is either prescribed in acid mixture or in the form of tablets. An alkaline mixture should be given about half an hour before the administration of the drug.

Children's dose is about one-twentieth of the adult dose for each year.

Side-effect. Cinchonism (buzzing in the ears, deafness, fullness in the head and dizziness); hypersensitive reaction (thrombocytopenic purpura and drug fever), mild haemolysis in G-6-PD deficient individuals.

Effect on Parasite. A drug acts on early ring forms (trophozoites), kills gametocyte of *P. vivax*, *P. ovale* and *P. malariae*. For effective action, the plasma concentration of quinine is to be maintained at the level of 5 mg per litre for 4 to 6 days. No action on mature gametocytcs of *P. falciparum*.

For suppressive therapy. A daily dose of 650 mg is required; hence not recommended.

(b) *Parenteral.* Intramuscular injections: In adults, about 325 to 650 mg of quinine bihydrochloride dissolved in 5 ml of re-distilled water, having a *p*H of 3.5, is injected into the gluteal muscles (buttock) about 3 inches below the highest point of the iliac crest, deep into the muscles and well massaged. Not more than three injections on successive days are required and oral therapy should be quickly resumed as soon as the condition of the patient permits such a procedure. Intramuscular injection is specially indicated in pernicious malaria and cases where nausea and vomiting prevent absorption of the drug from the gastrointestinal tract.

Intravenous quinine is required in cases of pernicious malaria to obtain a quick action on the parasite in the shortest possible time, as delay under the circumstances may cause death. The dose recommended for adults is 650 mg of quinine bihydrochloride dissolved in 20 ml of sterile normal saline with 5% glucose. The injection should be given slowly at the rate of 2 ml per minute and the solution should be freshly prepared and warmed to the body temperature. The dose should never exceed 650 mg. Usually, one dose will be required and a second injection, if necessary, may be repeated after 8 to 12 hours. As the effect of intravenous quinine passes off quickly, an intramuscular injection of 650 mg of quinine should be given to supplement it. In a case of complicated falciparum malaria along with specific drug therapy, general treatment should also be carried out, such as measures to combat medical shock or dehydration (fluid and electrolytes), to treat severe anaemia (blood transfusion), to prevent intravascular coagulation (heparin) and to lessen cerebral oedema (dexamethasone or prednisolone, frusemide).

Quinidine. Although it is an active antimalarial drug but has cardiotoxic effect. So, it is usually not used in malaria.

Mepacrine (*Atebrin*, *Quinacrine*), **9-aminoacridine derivative.** Now rarely used as it is less effective than chloroquine and more toxic drug. It is a yellow crystalline powder, bitter to taste and sparingly soluble. Tablets of mepacrine hydrochloride, each 0.1 g (100 mg), containing 0.78 g of the base or active substance, are used for oral administration. They are given after meals in doses of 0.1 g three times a day for 5 days, totalling 1.5 g. For an effective schizonticidal action an initial "loading" dose of 0.2 to 0.3 g three times a day may be necessary. The patient is advised to take water freely and also sodium bicarbonate in doses of 15 grains (1 g), dissolved in a glass of water along with each dose of the drug.

Mepacrine may be used in combination with quinine or paludrine but it has no distinct advantage. Mepacrine and primaquine when given concurrently produce toxicity and should not be used.

For Suppressive therapy. In adult, a single dose of 0.1 g daily and in semi-immune subjects 0.3 g once weekly. To be taken about 15 days before possible exposure.

Side-effects. Yellow discolouration of the skin; occasionally psychotic disturbances and some gastro-intestinal discomfort. Prolonged use may lead to skin lesions resembling *lichen planus*.

Note: Some physicians do not recommend mepacrine to children.

Chloroquine, a 4-aminoquinoline derivative. The drug of choice for acute attack.

Two salts are used: Chloroquine phosphate (Aralen, Avlochlor, Resochin) and Chloroquine sulphate (Nivaquine). Chloroquine phosphate is issued as white tablets, each weighing 0.5 g (contains 0.3 g of the base) and 0.25 g (contains 0.15 g of the base) and used commonly. The drug should not be taken continuously as a prophylactic major, for more than 5 years, without regular ophthalmic checkup as it may cause irreversible retinopathy.

Effect on Parasitic Cycle. One of the potent drugs which has yet been discovered (Fairly, 1949). The drug acts on the early ring forms (trophozoites). It probably causes lysosome damage or inhibition of nucleic acid synthesis of parasite. It has no action on mature gametocytes of *P. falciparum* and does not affect the tissue stage of the parasite.

For Overt malaria. Tablets of 0.5 g are administered orally in the following doses to an adult:

First day 2 tablets *stat* and 1 tablet 6 hours later. Second day 1 tablet and third day 1 tablet, totalling 5 tablets of 0.5 g (2.5 g). Children's dose is proportionately smaller. To prevent recrudescence of *P. falciparum* chloroquine base 300-600 mg orally once a week should be continued for 4 to 8 weeks. If parasitaemia persists after 72 hours, chloroquine-resistant strains are suspected and indicates the administration of quinine.

For Suppressive therapy. One tablet of 0.5 g (0.3 g base) is given to an adult once a week. For children weekly dose is as follows: 0.2 years 37.5 mg base, 3 to 5 years 75 mg base and 6-12 years 150 mg base.

Note: Strains of *P. falciparum* in certain countries of the Far East (Thailand) and South America do not respond to normal therapeutic dosage with chloroquine. Such resistant strains may be introduced in an area that has already reached the maintenance phase of eradication. Chloroquine-resistant strains are also resistant to other drugs but not to quinine.

For *Parenteral injection* (intramuscular and intravenous) ampoules of chloroquine in aqueous solution are available in strength of 40 mg base per ml (5 ml contain 20 mg chloroquine base). Intravenous injection should be given slowly in very dilute solution (the same precaution being taken as in intravenous quinine). Parenteral injection of chloroquine is not recommended to children.

Amodiaquine (*Camoquin, Cam-aqi*), **a 4-aminoquinoline derivative.** Issued as 0.2 g base tablet. For treatment it is administered orally to adults in doses of 0.6 g base *stat*, then 0.4 g base daily for 2 days. For mass treatment in rural areas a single dose of 0.6 g base is used. *For suppressive therapy*, 0.4 g base orally once a week to adults is given. Reliance is however now placed more on chloroquine than on amodiaquine. It is toxic drug and cross resistance can occur.

8-aminoquinoline derivatives

(a) **Pamaquine** (*Plasmoquine, Plasmochin*). This was the first to be synthesised in 1927. Two salts were used: Pamaquine hydrochloride and pamaquine naphthoate; the latter for oral administration. As the margin of safety between the effective therapeutic dose and the toxic dose is very small, it is no longer recommended.

(b) **Primaquine phosphate.** Tablets containing 7.5 mg or 15.0 mg of the base are available. The adult dose is 15 mg of the base daily and administered orally in single or divided doses for 10 to 14 days. In case of 14 days' treatment, two courses of 7 days with a 7-day interval may be given. The patient receiving primaquine should be kept in bed and plenty of fluid should be given. Should not be given to children. The dose 22.5 to 30 mg base/day is required for relatively resistant strains which is found in East Asia and Oceania.

Effect on Parasitic Cycle. It is a polyvalent gametocytocidal, having a marked action on the crescents of *P. falciparum*. It exercises some inhibitory effect on hypnozoite forms. It can destroy the pre-erythrocytic forms. Thus, this group appears to fulfil the criteria of an efficient (ideal) antimalarial drug having observable effect on pre-erythrocytic, erythrocytic, latent hepatic stage and gametocyte stages. Unfortunately, the drug is too toxic to be of any use as a prophylactic.

It may be prescribed to an adult for radical cure (eradicating latent hepatic stage either concurrently or after the clinical cure with a powerful drug (chloroquine or quinine)).

Side-effects. Mild degrees of cyanosis may result from methaemoglobinaemia and there may be colicky abdominal pain. In glucose-6-phosphate dehydrogenase-deficient individual, it causes haemolysis and haemoglobinuria. In mild form of G-6PD deficiency, primaquine in a dose of 0.75 mg/kg (45 mg) once weekly for six weeks is recommended.

(c) **Tafenoquine** formally known as etaquine and belongs to 8-aminoquinolone group. It is 13 times more active than primaquine as hypnozoitocidal drugs. It also has schizontocidal activity and useful in both vivax and falciparum. It is effective and less toxic than primaquine. The drug causes oxidant haemolysis in G-6PD deficient patient.

Halofantrine (*Halfan*). It is 9-phenathrene methanol. In spite of its potent action over parasite fatal ventricular tachycardia have resticted its use. It is used in a dose of 500 mg three times daily for three days follwed by repetition of same dose after seven days. The mode of action is similar to that of quinine.

Lumefantrine. The fixed combination with artemether produces more effective action and cures the patient rapidly. This combination is now used for prophylaxis and treatment of malaria in many countries. The mode of action is similar to that of quinine.

Mefloquine hydrochloride, quinoline-methanol (WR 142, 490). It is found to be extreamly effective both in treatment and suppression of falciparum malaria and vivax malaria. It is available as a tablet and dose is 15 mg to 25 mg/kg/day. The mode of action is similar to that of quinine. Unlike quinine, the mefloquine does not bind to DNA. No action is on gametocytes and hypnozoites. It has very long half-life and resistant strains are selected more quickly than any other anti-malarial. The drug is used for treatment of multidrug resistant strains of *P. falciparum* in a dose ranging from 0.1 to 1.5 gm and in drug resistant *P. vivax* malaria. Side effects such as abdominal cramps, vomiting etc. are not uncommon. Mefloquine is safe for at least 2 years and contraindicated in first trimester of pregnancy, during lactation period, cardiac conduction disorders, neuropsychiatric disorders, epilepsy. Use of artesunate with mefloquine improves the tolerance and absorption of the drug mefloquine and helps to cure the disease rapidly and effectively. Mefloquine should not be used to people receiving quinine, to avoid cardiovascular effects but no interaction has been demonstrated.

Note: Quinidine, quinine, mefloquine and halofantrine are structurally similar and they can compete for blood and tissue binding sites.

Dihydrofolate Reductase Inhibitors (DHFR inhibitors)

An enzyme complex (DHFR) which helps in the synthesis of folic acid in the malarial parasite is present. Antifols (proguanil, pyrimethamine, chlorproguanil, trimethoprim) inhibit the enzyme complex causing interference in folic acid synthesis and parasite dies.

(a) **Proguanil (Chloroguanide).** A biguanide derivative. It is a colourless, bitter crystalline substance. It is rapidly excreted and free from toxic effect. It has no antifolate activity in man. Issued as tablets of 0.1 g (100 mg) or 0.3 g (300 mg) of proguanil hydrochloride (paludrine).

Effect on Parasitic Cycle. It destroys the erythrocytic stages (asexual blood forms) of the parasite, acting on the dividing schizonts (not the drug of choice for the treatment of non-immunes). It is mainly used for suppressive therapy and for continuous prophylaxis, it is the drug of choice. It has also some action on pre-erythrocytic stages of *P. falciparum* and may be regarded as a true causal prophylactic. It also prevents the sporogony cycle inside the mosquito. The parasite readily acquires resistance which is even transmitted to the mosquito vector.

For Suppressive therapy. Proguanil is given as a weekly dose of 0.3 g (300 mg) or a biweekly dose of 0.1 g to adults and a daily dose of 0.1 g, to non-immune adults. For children a daily dose is as follows: 0-1 year 25 mg, 2.5 years 50 mg.

Proguanil (chloroguanide) and the dichlorobiguanide (chlorproguanil) are considered as the safest antimalarial drugs.

(b) **Pyrimethamine (Daraprim).** It is chemically related to proguanil. It is an antifolate agent and daily dose may cause megaloblastic anaemia. It is a slow-acting drug and acts mainly on mature forms. It is not the drug of choice for the treatment of acute malaria in non-immune subjects. It inactivates gametocytes and prevents their development in the mosquito. *For suppressive therapy* 50 mg (2 tablets) orally once a week or 25 mg (1 tablet) twice a week to adults is given. Resistance to the drug develops readily. For children 0.5 years 12.5 mg and 6-12 years 25 mg once a week, thereafter adult doses should be given. The tablets have an attractive flavour and children should not have an easy access to them, because overdosage may cause fatality.

(c) **Trimethoprim** (pyrimidine derivative). Structure similar to folate. It exhibits synergism with long-acting sulphonamide. A single administration of trimethoprime 500 mg with sulfalene 750 mg has been found to be very effective in malaria, particularly in chloroquine-resistant *P. falciparum* infections.

Antagonist of p-aminobenzoic acid (PABA)

Sulphonamides and Sulphones. Long-acting sulphonamide like sulphodoxin, sulphomethoxins, sulphodimethoxine etc. are used in combination with pyrimethamine, particularly in chloroquine-resistant *P. falciparum* infections. Sulphodoxin with trimethoprim or pyrimethamine are also effective drugs against multi-resistant strain of *P. falciparum* infections.

Sulphones such as DDS and DADDS have also been used in combination with other drug (pyrime-thamine) for the treatment of resistant strains of *P. falciparum*.

Fansidar (each tablet contains sulphodoxin 500 mg combined with 25 mg pyrimethamine) in a dose of 3 tablets at once, is used in chloroquine-resistant *P. falciparum*.

Artemisinin and its derivatives (Artemether, Artesunete, Arteether): These are rapidly acting sesquiterpenes isolated from the Chinese wood plant *Artemisia annua* (*quinghaosu*).These compounds get concentrated in erythrocytes where they liberate peroxide radicals which kill the parasite. They have wide spectrum of action on asexual malarial parasite, from medium sized ring forms to early schizonts form but not active against intra-hepatic forms. They reduce gametocyte carriage and thus transmission. No significant resistance to this drug is yet noticed. Side-effect is serious neurotoxicity. Quinine intravenously is co-administered with artemisinin compounds to ensure that no recrudescence can occur. For treatment of acute falciparum malaria combination containing artesunate (4 mg/kg/day for three days), chloroquine, amodiaquine and sulphodoxine – pyrimethamine combination are sometimes preferred.

Artemisinin and its derivatives are used for mefloquine resistant and multidrug resistant case of *P. falciparum* malaria. In falciparum malaria, artemisinin derivatives prevent progression to severe form of the disease effectively. The dose of artemisinin is 25 mg/kg thrice daily on first day, 25 mg/kg once daily on second and third day. Mafloquine in a dose of 15 mg/kg may be added to second and third dose in resistant cases. Artimisinin is less active than the derivatives. It is not metabolized to di-hydroartemisinin. DHA is two to ten times more potent in comparison with artemisinin. The three derivatives, artemether, arte-ether and artesunate are synthesized from di-hydroartemisinin and converted back to it within the body.

(a) **Artemether:** It is used in a dose of 80 mg i.m. twice daily on first day followed by 80 mg i.m. once daily for next 4 days has been recommended. Oral form is also available.

(b) **Arte-ether:** The drug is more lipophilic than Artemether. It has an extensive cerebral distribution and thereby delays recrudescence in cerebral malaria caused by *P. falciparum*. I.V quinine is co-administered with artemisinin compounds so that no recrudescence occurs. Arte-ether also exhibits gametocytocidal action on *P. falciparum*. The dose of arte-ether in adult is 15 mg once daily by i.m. or i.v. route for 3 consecutive days. The dose for children is 3 mg/kg per day for 3 days. Adverse effects on CNS are more with arte-ether.

(c) **Artesunate:** It is used orally in a dose of 120 mg once daily on first day followed by 60 mg daily for 4 days and can be used i.m or i.v route in a dose of 50 mg twice daily for 4 days. In severe cerebral malaria, a second dose of 60 mg may be added on first day, 6 hours after first dose. The dose in children is 2 mg/kg/day for five days.

New drugs:

Atovaquone. It is hydroxynaphthoquinone (inhibitor of electron transport chain in mitochondria of the parasite). Its long half life (70 hours) may lead to selection of resistant organisms. Recrudescence (30%) occurs. Dose is 200 mg twice daily for three days and can be combined with proguanil or tetracycline. It acts mainly during trophozoite blood stage.

Atovaquone-proguanil (*Malarone*). This new broad-spectrum anti-malarial drug is highly active against multi-drug resistant *P. falciparum* malaria. The combination contains atovaquone 250 mg and proguanil 100 mg.

Pyronaridine. It is structurally, closely similar to amadiaquine and now used in fixed combination with artesunate in many countries against multi drug-resistant *P. falciparum*. It has been developed in China and used in China and in other countries.

Piperaquine. It is a bisquinoline compound and its hydroxy derivative is active against multidrug resistant *P. falciparum*. The fixed combination with de-hydroartemisinin or primaquine or trimethoprim is used in China, Vietnam and Cambodia.

Note: Antibacterial drugs with antimalarial activities include tetracycline, doxycycline, clindamycin, azithromycin, chloramphenicol and fluoroquinolones. Doxycycline and azithromycin are more active and most widely used both for prophylaxis and treatment. Tetracycline is active against all species of malaria. Clindamycin is effective like tetracycline and can be used safely in pregnant mother and children.

Drug-resistant Plasmodia

The term "resistance" is applied to signify when a parasite strain is able to survive or to multiply, or both even after the administration and absorption of adequate recommended therapeutic dose or a higher dose of an active schizonticidal drug but within the limits of tolerance of that subject (WHO, 1967). Resistance may be of various grades and denned as follows (WHO, 1968):

Grade 1 (R_1 level)—Asexual parasites in blood are cleared, but recrudescence follows.

Grade 2 (R_2 level)—Asexual parasites in blood are not cleared, but markedly reduced.

Grade 3 (R_3 level)—Asexual parasites in blood are not markedly reduced.

Strains of *P. vivax* and *P. malariae* may vary in their responses to antimalarial drugs, but drug-resistance is applied to *P. falciparum* and *P. vivax* also. Reports from Asia and Africa showed that the use of proguanil and cycloguanil pamoate caused the appearance of resistant strain and this character is also transmitted through the anopheline vectors. The use of pyrimethamine in Asia, Pacific, South America and Africa also caused the appearance of drug-resistant parasite. Chloroquine resistant strain is also reported from South-east, Asia, South America and from Africa. Hence, neither of these drugs should be used alone for mass chemotherapy or chemoprophylaxis where resistance to that particular drug exists. It is in these groups of cases multiple drug regimen is advocated. Cross-resistance is another potential source of drug-resistance.

The prevention of resistance is achieved by the use of combination of antimalarial drugs with different mechanisms of actions and with different drugs targets. The two drugs which do not have common mode of action are prefered

Multiple drug regimen. The following preparations (dose for non-immune adults) are used :

Chloroquine-resistant *P. vivax* (following drugs are used)

Quinine sulphate 650 mg 3 times daily for 3-7 days with Doxycycline 100 mg twice daily for 7 days

Or Mefloquine 750 mg stat followed by 500 mg, 12 hours later.

Chloroquine-resistant *P. falciparum* (following drugs are used)

Quinine sulphate 650 mg 3 times daily 3-7 days with Doxycycline 100 mg twice daily for 7 days or with Tetracycline 250 mg 4 times daily for 7 days or with Fansider (Pyremethamine and sulphadoxine combination) 3 tablets as a single dose on last day of quinine therapy.

Or Atovaquone Proguanil (Malarone) 2 tablets twice daily for 3 days

Or Mefloquine 750 mg stat followed by 500 mg 12 hours later

Or Artesunate 4 mg/kg/day for 3 days with Mefloquine 750 mg stat followed by 500 mg 12 hours later (25 to 10 mg/kg)

Mefloquine-resistant *P. falciparum* (following drugs are used)

Quinine sulphate 650 mg 3 times daily 3-7 days with Doxycycline 100 mg twice daily for 7 days or with Tetracycline 250 mg 4 times daily for 7 days.

Or Artesunate 4 mg/kg/day for 3 days with Mefloquine 750 mg stat followed by 500 mg 12 hours later.

Note: The drug resistance is mostly encountered with synthetic antimalarials but not with quinine. Proguanil and pyrimethamine resistant strains respond to chloroquine and chloroquine-resistant strains respond to quinine.

Mechanism. Resistance develops by the usage of a metabolic bypass of the pathway blocked by the relevant drug. Resistance develops more easily with those drugs, such as proguanil and pyrimethamine, which inhibit the folic acid-folinic acid cycle but less so with the drugs, such as quinine, mepacrine and 4-aminoquinoline, which act on the glycolytic cycle of the growing parasite before division.

Chemotherapy and Chemoprophylaxis of Malaria

Before chemotherapy the "immunity" status of the individual is to be assessed and the species of Plasmodia infecting the individual is also determined. For the treatment of non-immunes, i.e., those with a recent history of exposure to infection should be given a standard schizonticidal drug for clinical cure (eradication of erythrocytic phase) and the drug of choice is 4-aminoquinoline, chloroquine. For radical cure* of *P. vivax, P. malariae* and *P. ovale* infections an 8-aminoquinoline, primaquine is to be used concurrently or after the clinical cure. *P. falciparum* infection in non-immunes is always dangerous and should be promptly treated. As there is no latent hepatic stage phase, primaquine is not required but to prevent recrudescence the schizonticidal drug should be continued for some time (chloroquine base 300 mg once a week for a month).

For the treatment of immunes, i.e., those exposed to continuous and repeated infections oral schizonticides given on one day only are usually quite adequate. A complete eradication of erythrocytic phase may not be required, because the integrity of the immunity depends upon the E phase of the parasite.

For chemoprophylaxis, the schizonticidal drugs should be started just before entering an endemic area and taken regularly and continuously during the stay (possible exposure) and also for one month after leaving the area. Mefloquine is to be commenced about 15 days before entering a malarious area (possible exposure) to allow an adequate blood level of the drug to be attained, to detect adverse reaction before travel and to switch over to alternative drugs (chloroquine, proguanil, doxycycline) if required.

Doses of antimalarial drugs given are for the non-immuned adults. For immuned and partly immuned, the first few doses are usually enough. For children, the doses must be scaled down and at present, the doses are calculated not from age but on weight basis and body surface area (BSA).

It is to be noted that no drugs are available at present which can destroy sporozoites, hence it is not possible to prevent infection (no true prophylaxis exists). Symptoms of infection can however be suppressed while residing in a malarious area and all the schizonticidal drugs can be used for this purpose. The suppressant drug, chloroquine, may be incorporated into common salt used for normal daily preparation of food. This form of indirect drug distribution is often referred to as Pinotti's method (1960).

As a control measure, chemoprophylaxis is no longer recommended to younger, or to other populations except for temporary use to soldiers, police forces, serving in highly endemic areas and travelers coming from non-endemic areas.

Choice of regimen is decided by length of stay, level of malaria transmission, level of drug resistance, area to be visited, presence of underlying disease in the traveller and concomitant medication advised.

High chloroquine resistance area: Mefloquine 250 mg – 1 tablet weekly **or** Malarone (Atovaquone 250 mg + Proguanil 100 mg) – 1 tablet daily (from two days before travelling to one week after return) **or** Doxycycline 100 mg – 1 tablet daily.

Moderate chloroquine resistance area: Chloroquine 150 mg base – 2 tablets weekly with Proguanil 100 mg – 2 tablets daily.

Chloroquine sensitive area: Chloroquine 150 mg base – 2 tablets weekly **or** Proguanil 100 mg – 2 tablets daily.

---

*Radical cure with primaquine to prevent relapses should be the aim when the patient leaves the endemic area but it is of no use if he remains in the endemic area.

DRUGS FOR BALANTIDIASIS

Oxytetracycline. A course consists of 0.5 g of the drug administered orally to adults at 6-hourly interval for a period of 7 to 10 days.

Diodoquin. This drug is administered orally in the dose of 650 mg three times daily for twenty days.

Metronidazole. It is used in a dose of 750 mg three times daily for 5 days.

DRUG FOR ISOSPORIASIS

Trimethoprim-sulfamethoxazole. These drugs are used as a combination drug (TMP in a dose of 160 mg in combination with SMX 800 mg once in a day).

DRUG FOR CRYPTOSPORIDIOSIS

Nitozoxanide. It is recommended in a dose of 500 mg twice daily for three days.

DRUG FOR CYCLOSPORIASIS

Trimethoprim-sulfamethoxazole. This combination is drug of choice (TMP 160 mg in combination with SMX 800 mg, twice daily for 7-10 days).

DRUGS FOR BABESIOSIS

Clindamycin. It is used in a dose of 1.2 gm twice daily intramuscularly or intravenously for 7-10 days with oral quinine in a dose of 650 mg three times daily after food for 7-10 days. Oral clindamycin in a dose of 600 mg three times daily for 7-10 days can be used in place of its intravenous therapy.

Atovaquone. It is effective in a dose of 750 mg twice daily with azithromycin in a dose 600 mg daily 7-10 days effective.

DRUGS FOR MICROSPORIDIOSIS

Albendazole. It can be used in a dose of 400 mg twice daily for 21 days.

Fumagillin. It is 5-fluorouracil compound and is effective in a dose of 60 mg/kg/day for 14 days. The drug can be used with albendazole also.

DRUGS FOR PNEUMOCYSTOSIS

Co-trimoxazole. High dose of co-trimozole (100 mg/kg/day of suphamethoxole and 20 mg/kg/day of trimethoprim) is given in two to four divided doses orally or intravenously in all stages of severity of *P. carinii* infection. In HIV infected person treatment is continued intravenuously for 21 days, whereas in other cases of immunosuppression states, the treatment is continued for shorter period of 14 to 17 days. In cases of mild infection, oral co-trimozole is recommended.

Clindamycin. It is used in a dose of 450 to 600 mg orally, four times daily with primaquine in a dose of 15 mg/kg orally daily. This treatment may be continued for 21 days in all severe stages of PCP infection. I.V. clindamycin can be given for first 7 to 10 days and then can be switched over to oral therapy. It is also administered to those patients who do not responed to co-trimozole and pentamidine

Dapsone. It is used in a dose of 100 mg/day with trimethoprim in a dose of 20 mg/kg/day.

Atovaquone. The drug is used in a dose of 750 mg twice daily for 21 days and is less effective.

Trimetrexate with follinic acid. Trimetrexate in a dose of 45 mg/m^2 daily i.v. is used with folinic acid 20 mg/m^2 four times daily. Trimetrexate is a methotrexate analogue and is given with follinic acid to protect the cells of the human body from methotrexate induced toxicity.

Pentamidine. In patient with severe pneumonia, it is given in a dose of 4 mg/kg/day i.v. is used for 21 days. It has high efficacy, but greater toxicity like nephrotoxicity. Hypoglycaemia, hypotension, nausea, vomiting are other side-effects.

INTESTINAL ANTHELMINTICS

Anthelmintic drug (G. *anti*, against; *helmins*, worm) may either destroy the worms (vermicide) or help the expulsion of the worms without killing them (vermifuge). It may be pointed out that any drug which produces active catharsis can expel a large number of helminths which have not anchored to the intestinal wall and hence, may be regarded as a vermifuge (L. *vermis*, worm; *fugare*, to chase away).

General Rules to be Followed in the Treatment of Intestinal Helminthiasis

1. A specific diagnosis should be made first. It is to be noted that a multiple helminthic infection is common in tropical countries. Even helminthiasis may be associated with protozoal infection. In all such cases, the specific therapy should be first directed to the one causing greater pathogenic effects.

2. The general condition of the patient should be assessed, such as the presence of anaemia, cirrhosis of liver, nephritis and pregnancy. Most of the anthelmintic drugs are not well tolerated by alcoholics and therefore, in mass therapy, taking of alcohol should be forbidden.

3. A light diet in the evening and sometimes a saline purgation at night before the anthelmintic treatment may be given with a view to freeing the bowel and thus exposing the worms to the direct action of the drugs.

4. Administration of anthelmintic in the morning on an empty stomach. The drug may be administered orally as tablet, in gelatin capsules or as an emulsion.

5. No food upto 2 hours after the specific medication. Sometimes, a post-purgative is necessary in order (i) to eliminate the injured parasites which might recover, if left in the intestine or might be disintegrated and absorbed giving rise to toxic manifestation and also (ii) to prevent any absorption of the drug, thereby reducing the toxicity.

6. No food is advised till the bowels move.

7. All stools after specific medication should be collected and examined for the expelled worms.

8. A follow-up examination of the stool is necessary to assess the success of the treatment and a second course of treatment may be repeated, if the helminthological evidence of infection reappears.

Anthelmintics for Intestinal Nematodes

Tetrachlorethylene ($C_2 Cl_4$), B.P. It is a heavy liquid insoluble in water. It is not used now a days.

Bephenium hydroxynaphthoate (*Alcopar*, B.W. & Co.). It is now used rarely.

Piperazine Salts (citrate, adipate or phosphate). Available in the form of syrup (citrate), wafers, tablets and granules (phosphate). Effective against enterobiasis and ascariasis; also have some effects on Trichuris and Heterophyes. No preliminary treatment and no "follow-up" measures are necessary.

For *ascariasis*, a single dose of 3 to 4 g is given to adults and children over 6 years and 2 to 3 g to I children under 6 years. It is preferable to give the drug at bed time and the affected worm may be evacuated next day by a saline purge (worms are intact and in the living state but not actively motile). For a single dose, 150 mg per kg of body weight with a maximum of 4 g a day.

For *enterobiasis*, a single or divided daily dose for 7 successive days. Dosage for such a course varies 1 in different age groups according to body weight and the daily dose is calculated as 50 to 75 mg per kg body weight up to a maximum of 2 g.

Piperazine is one of the most satisfactory drugs for enterobiasis but repeated doses are required and vomiting may occur. Relapses are frequent unless every member of the infected group is treated at the same time and hygienic measures are taken to avoid reinfection.

Recently the standard 7-day course of piperazine treatment of enterobiasis has been replaced by a single dose method, using a combination of piperazine phosphate and standardised senna ("senokot") in the form of flavoured granules (pripsen); 40 grains of these granules (about 1 teaspoonful) contain 1 g of piperazine phosphate and 7 mg of sennosides A and B. It is given in the following doses: For a child over 6 years and to an adult, 4 teaspoonfuls (160 grs) of the granular preparation containing 4 g of piperazine and for a child under 6 years, 3 teaspoonfuls (120 grs) of the granular preparation containing 3 g of the piperazine. It may conveniently be given along with milk. Side-effects are practically nil except some griping and loose motions in some cases. This single dose treatment has been found to be more effective than the usual 7-day course and favourable results have already been reported by various authors. The aim of the treatment is to maintain an adequate concentration of piperazine within the intestine long enough to ensure complete evacuation of all the paralysed worms by normal peristalsis. Senna has been found to be more useful than saline, because it produces a normal peristalsis by stimulating Auerbach's plexus (White and Scopes, 1960; Kagan, 1961).

Thiabendazole. A broad-spectrum anthelmintic. Effective against strongyloidiasis, ascariasis, enterobiasis and hookworm infections; weakly effective against trichuriasis, and ineffective against tape-worm infections. It is also useful in creeping eruption and trichinelliasis (Botero, 1965).

Dosage. 25 mg/kg body weight twice a day for 2 days. Given after evening meals in a suspension or as tablets (base or pamoate). A 20 per cent solution of thiabendazole, 2 g a day orally for 5 days has been found to be satisfactory remedy for cutaneous larva migrans caused by A. braziliense (Baranski and Carnerio, 1966).

Side-effects. Anorexia, nausea, vomiting, abdominal cramps, urticaria and rash; evidence of some degree of toxicity of nervous system, such as disorientation and other mental disturbances, are seen. All these side-effects resolve with the stoppage of the drug.

Pyrantel pamoate or embonate (*Combantrin*, Pfizer). A useful broad spectrum anthelmintic.

Adult dose is 10 mg (base)/kg body weight, given as a single dose (or for 2 consecutive days) after break-fast in a suspension or chewable tablets. Others have recommended 20 mg base/kg body weight. A purge is given 3 hours after the drug and stools examined for expelled worms up to 48 hours. Tolerance is excellent and side-effects are absent. It is claimed to be the drug of choice in enterobiasis and ascariasis. It is also effective in hookworm infection. It has no significant effect in trichuriasis.

Mebendazole (R-17,635). A yellowish powder almost insoluble in water. Chemically, it is methyl-N-[5(6)-benzoyl-1-2-benzimidazolyl]carbamate. It acts directly on the nematode, probably by blocking the glucose uptake. None of the drug is absorbed from the gut.

Adult dose is 200 mg by mouth twice daily for 4 days. Issued as 100 mg tablet. The drug is taken preferably with water after breakfast. It has no side-effects. No prior or post-treatment is necessary. The efficacy of this drug is not increased by the higher or repeated doses and the therapeutic effect is not related to the age and weight of the persons treated. It has polyvalent therapeutic action and is considered to be one of the best drugs so far available for the treatment of helminths.

Chaia and Cunha* administered the drug to Brazilian school children (from 7-17 years) in doses of 200 mg twice daily for 4 consecutive days (total dose 1600 mg). They observed the cure rate as follows: For ascariasis 100%, trichuriasis 96-100%, enterobiasis 100% and hookworm infection 84.2–100%. It is effective against Strongyloides of rat but not of man.

Albendazole. It is broad-spectrum anthelmantic which is effective against common nematodes. In nematode infection usual dose for adult and children above two years of age is 400 mg as a single oral therapy. For strongyloidiasis 400-800 mg per day is recommended for three days.

DRUGS FOR TRICHINELLIASIS

Mebendazole. It is used in a dose of 200 – 400 mg/kg/day three times daily for 3 days and then 400 – 500 mg three times daily for 10 days.

Albendazole. It is effective in a dose of 400 mg. twice daily for 7 – 14 days.

Steroids are co-administered with mebendazole or albendazole to control serious effects of acute inflamation.

DRUGS FOR TRICHURIASIS

Mebendazole. It is recommended in a dose of 100 mg twice daily for three days or 500 mg once in a day.

Albendazole. It is given in a dose of 400 mg daily for 3 days.

Ivermectin. It is used in a dose of 200 μg/kg/day in combination with albendazole in a dose of 400 mg.

DRUGS FOR STRONGYLOIDIASIS

Ivermectin. It is recommended in a dose of 200 μg/kg daily for three days and should be repeated after seven days. For strongyloides hyperinfection the drug is given on first day, second day, fifteenth day and sixteenth day.

Albendazole. It is administered in a dose of 400 mg daily.

Mebendazole and Thiabendazole. They can be used effectively in treatment of the disease. The dose of thiabendazole is 50 mg/kg/day in two divided doses for two days. Maximum dose is 3 gm/day.

DRUG FOR TRICHOSTRONGYLIASIS

Levamisole. It is used as single oral dose of 2.5 mg/kg. It causes spastic paralysis of the parasite and eliminates it from the intestine. It is rapidly absorbed to attain high plasma concentration within two hours and also eliminated within three hours. Adverse effects are nausea, vomiting, abdominal pain, headache and dizziness.

FILARICIDAL DRUGS

Drugs for Filariasis (*W. bancrofti, B. malayi, B. timori, Loa loa, O. volvulus, M. streptocerca*)

Diethylcarbamazine (*Hetrazan, Banocide*). This is a synthetic piperazine derivative, issued in the form of 50 mg tablets for oral administration. It is generally given in doses of 2 mg per kg body weight, three times a day after meals, for a period of 3 weeks; if necessary the period may be extended. Thus, an individual weighing 75 kilogrammes will require 2 × 75 = 150 mg of

---

*Chaia, G. and Cunha, A. S. (1971). Therapeutic action of mebendazole (R-17, 635) against human helminthiasis. Reprinted from *Folia Med.*, 63, 834-52. (Abstracted in *Trop. Dis. Bull.*, Sept. 1972, p. 922).

hetrazan or three 50 mg tablets thrice daily (450 mg a day).

The drug is effective against microfilariae of *W. bancrofti*, *B. malayi*, *B. timori*, *O. volvulus*, *Loa loa* and *M. streptocerca*. It has a specific action in occult filariasis. It has no direct lethal action, but sensitises microfilariae so that they are readily phagocytosed by macrophages. Its macrofilaricidal effect is seen against the adult worms of *L. loa*, *W. bancrofti*, *B. malayi*, *B. timori* and *M. streptocerca*.

In some cases, allergic reaction due to release of foreign protein from dead worms have been observed. It may appear a few hours after start of treatment. It may be systemic and local. Systemic reactions are fever, headache, joint pain, dizziness, anorexia, vomiting, malaise, shortness of breath but they pass off soon. On the other hand, local reactions include lymphadenitis, lymphoedema, formation of abscess. Local reactions occur later and last long period. Severe reaction to diethylcarbamazine is found in persons affected with *O. volvulus* or *Loa loa*.

Ivermectin. It is used as oral drug in the dose of 150 μg/kg. It eliminates microfilaria of *W. bancrofti*, *B. malayi*, *B. timori*, *Loa loa*, *M. streptocerca*, *M. ozzardi*, *O. volvulus*. Side-effects are similar to that of diethylcarbamazine. It should not be used during pregnancy, lactation period and to children below 5 years of age. As it has no effect over adult worm, repetition of treatment at half yearly or yearly interval is recommended. Drug causes intrauterine degeneration and temporary sequestration of unborn microfilaria. Side-effects are itching, rash, muscle and joint pain, dizziness, tender lymphadenopathy and conjunctivitis. Sometimes, hypotension and bronchoconstriction are observed as side-effects.

DRUGS FOR FILARIASIS (*Mansonella perstans*)

Mebandazole. It is administered in a dose of 100 mg twice daily for 30 days and gives good result in treatment.

Albendazole. It is given in a dose of 400 mg twice daily for 10 days and is also effective drug.

DRUG FOR FILARIASIS (*Mansonella ozzardi*)

Ivermectin. It is administered as a single dose of 6 mg and produces long-term reduction in microfilaraemia.

DRUG FOR FILARIASIS (*Mansonella streptocerca*)

Diethylcarbamazine (DEC) and **ivermectin** are useful for treatment of the disease.

DRUGS FOR DRACUNCULOSIS

Thiabendazole. It is given orally for 3 days in the dose of 50-100 mg/kg of body wt.

Metronidazole. It is effective in the dose of 25 mg/kg of body wt., orally, daily for 10 to 20 days **or** 250 mg three times daily for 10 days.

Niridazole ("ambilhar"). It is a nitrothiazole compound and used in a dose of 12.5-15 mg/kg daily, orally for 7-10 days. It should be used carefully in elderly people, patients whose transminase level is unusually high and those with coronary defects. Side-effects are retro-orbital headaches, nausea, vomiting and abdominal colic. Urine is coloured red. Neuropsychological symptoms (anxiety, psychomotor agitation and mental disorientation) are seen but resolve with the stoppage of the drug. A temporary aspermatogenesis has been observed in experimental animals but there is no evidence of this in man (Acta Tropica, 1966).

DRUGS FOR ONCHOCERCIASIS

Diethylcarbamazine. It is administered in a dose of 25 mg on first day, 50 mg on second day and then increase to 100 mg twice daily, for 5 to 7 days. Total dose is 1.3 gm.

Ivermectin. It is administered as single oral dose of 15 μg/kg and should be repeated 6 to 12 months after initial treatment. It causes rapid elimination of microfilaria from skin.

DRUGS FOR LOIASIS

Diethylcarbamizine. It is recommended in a dose of 9 to 12 mg/kg/day in three divided doses for two weeks and repetition with this drug regimen is necessary. In case of severe infection, very small doses of DEC combined with steroid should be started initially and care must be taken about development of mazzoti reaction in case of treatment of patient having loiasis with onchocerciasis.

Ivermectin. It is given in a dose of 200 to 400 μg/kg and has been reported to be a safe and effective drug.

Mebendazole and albendazole. The drugs are used to cure the disease.

Anthelmintics for Intestinal Cestodes

Niclosamide (Yomesan). It is a salicylamide derivative and has been found to be an effective cestodicidal. It is a white, odourless powder, insoluble in water and dispensed in 0.5 g tablets. The drug is well tolerated. In *Taenia* and *H. diminuta* infections, a single dose of 2 gm in persons above 6 yrs of age, 1 gm between 2 yrs and 6 yrs of age, and 0.5 gm below 2 yrs of age are administered. A saline purgative 2 hours after administration of anthelmintic may be recommended for effective worm expulsion.

It is drug of choice against *H. nana*. It is also an effective drug against *D. caninum*, *Diphyllobothurium latum*, *T. solium* and *T. saginata*. It should be given orally, daily after breakfast, for 7 days in the following dosage schedules:

In person above 6 years of age : 2 gm on first day then 1 gm. daily for remaining 6 days.

In children from 2 years to 6 years of age: half the above mentioned dose.

In children below 2 years of age: One fourth of adult dose.

Niclosamide is not recommended in cysticercosis where albendazole or praziquantel are used.

Bethional. It is dichlorophenol derivative and is given in taeniasis (*T. saginata* and *T. solium* infection) orally, in a single dose of 2 gm followed by a saline purgative 2 hours later.

Albendazole. It is benzimidazole derivative having a broad-spectrum anthelmintic property being effective against common nematodes and cestodes. It is available in tablet and suspension form having 400 mg of the base per tablet and per teaspoonful of suspension. The drug is well tolerated with negligible side reactions.

In tapeworm infection, for adult and children above two years of age the dose is 400 mg/day for 3 days. Occasional adverse effects are diarrhoea, abdominal distress. In cysticercosis, it is used in a dose of 400 mg twice daily for 30 days and can be repeated, if necessary.

Praziquantel. The drug is a pyrazinoisoquinoline derivative, which is effective against a wide range of cestode infections in animals and human. It is a colourless crystalline powder, bitter to taste. At the lowest effective concentration, it causes increased muscular activity followed by constriction and spastic paralysis of worms and at the higher therapeutic concentration, vacuolization and vesculation of the tegument of the parasites and death of worms. It causes increased membrane permiability to certain monovalent and divalent cations, especially, calcium. Maximum concentration in plasma occurs by 1 to 2 hours, half-life of praziquantal in plasma is 1-5 hours due to its rapid metabolism. There is yet no evidence of mutogenic, carcinogenic and teratogenic effects from various studies done so far.

In taeniasis (*T. solium* and *T. saginata*) the drug in the dose of 10 mg/kg and in *D.caninum* and *D. latum* infection, the drug in the dose of 25 mg/kg as a single dose gives promising result. For larval cestodes (e.g. cysticercus in human) prolonged dose of 50-100 mg/kg/day in three doses for one month is recommended.

For *hymolepsis nana* – single dose of 20 mg/kg is recommended.

Anthelmintics for Intestinal Trematodes

Oxamiquine. This highly effective drug is used for the treatment in all stages of *S. mansoni* infection only (orally in a dose of 15 mg/kg twice daily for two days). It is an accepted cheap schistosomicide drug both for the treatment of individual patient and in mass treatment programme.

Hexyresorcinol B.P. ("Caprokol" or "hexylresorcinol crystoids").

Chemically it is 1,3-dihydroxy-4-hexylbenzene. It is a white crystalline substance, insoluble in water but soluble in alcohol, ether, chloroform and oils. It has an objectionable taste and has an irritant action on the mucous membrane. It is administered orally in the form of a pill, having a specially processed hard gelatin coating, available in doses of 0.1 - 0.2 g. The adult dose is 1g and the children's dose is 0.1g per year up to the age of 10 years. The drug is given on an empty stomach as a single dose (swallowed as a whole and not to be chewed). Although post-purgation is not essential, it may sometimes be necessary to expel the dead worms. Hexylresorcinol is used in infection by *F. buski* and *E. ilocanum*. It is a true vermicide and is also effective against *Ascaris lumbricoides* and hookworms (more effective against *N. americanus* than *A. duodenale*) but now superseded by other drugs.

Praziquantel. It is effective against wide range of trematode infection. For *Clonorchis sinensis* and *Opisthorchis viverrini*— three oral doses of 25 mg/kg of body weight on the same day are required. The oral dose of 75 mg/kg of body weight daily in three doses for two consecutive is required for *Paragonimus westermani*.

SCHISTOSOMICIDAL DRUGS

Oxamniquine. It is a synthetic derivative of lucanthone used for treatment of *S. mansoni* infection. The dose of the drug is decided by age of the patient and geographical distribution of the infection. The dose varies from 15 mg to 60 mg/kg for two to three days and the dose can be given as single dose or two divided doses, always after food. The treatment should not be given during first trimester of pregnancy, in patient with epilepsy. Side-effects are vomiting, diarrhoea, abodominal distension, dizziness, drowsiness, headache, hallucination and state of exitement convulsion, mild eosinophilia (due to host reaction to dead worms). Orange to red discoloration of the urine may follow the therapy.

Praziquantel. It is a pyrazinoisoquinoline derivative which is effective against schistosomiasis in man.

For *S. haematobium*, *S. mansoni* and *S. intercalatum*—a single oral dose of 40 mg/kg of body weight and for *S. japonicum*—two doses of 30 mg/kg of body weight orally at twelve hours interval are quite effective. In some areas, for *S. mansoni* and mixed infection higher dose upto 60 mg/kg of body weight (in three divided) may be required.

In *S. mekongi*, one day oral treatment by praziquantal in a dose of 60 mg/kg of body weight (in three divided doses) has been found to be effective.

Frequent adverse effects are abdominal discomfort nausea, sweating, fever, sedetion and blood eosinophilia. Occasional adverse effects are headach and dizziness.

DRUGS FOR FASCIOLIASIS

Bithionol (*Actamer*, *Eitin*). It is a dichlorophenol derivative. Yokogawa *et al* (1961) found it to be an effective and safe remedy. They gave it in doses of 30-50 mg per kg body weight per day in 3 subdivisions, every other day by mouth, for 10 to 15 days. Side-effects were mild and transient and include nausea, vomiting, abdominal pain and diarrhoea. Also effective in paragonimiasis.

Triclabendazole. It is effective in a dose of 10 mg/kg once in a day.

Nitazoxanide (Cryptaz). It is found to be an effective drug against fascioliasis, ascariasis, trichouriasis and hookworm. Nitazoxanide includes both nitazoxanide and its derivative tizoxanide. The dose is 100-400 mg twice daily for three days. Prednisolone in a dose of 5-10 mg/day may control toxaemia and antibiotics are used to treat acute cholangitis due to secondary bacterial infection.

DRUG FOR FASCIOLOPSIASIS

Praziquantel. It is given in a dose of 70 - 75 mg./kg./day in three divided doses for one day.

DRUGS FOR CLONORCHIASIS AND OPISTHORCHIASIS

Praziquantel. It may be used in a single dose of 40 mg/kg. Higher doses 75-120 mg/kg/day in three divided doses for one to two days are required to cure heavy infection.

Albendazole. It is recommended in a dose of 10 mg/kg/day for seven days.

DRUGS FOR PARAGONIMIASIS

Bithionol. The dosage schedule should be followed as mentioned against fascioliasis (30-50 mg/kg in alternate day for 10-15 days).

Praziquantel. It is effective in a dose of 70-75 mg/kg/day in three divided doses for two days.

Triclabendazole. It is administered in a dose of 5 mg/kg once daily for three days or 10 mg/kg in a single dose.

Niclofan. It is used in a single dose of 2 mg/kg.

DRUG FOR OPISTHORCHIASIS

Praziquantel. It may be given in a single dose of 40 mg/kg.

DRUGS FOR ECHINOSTOMIASIS

Mebendazole, albendazole, praziquantel, bithionol, hexylresorcinol crystoids and niclosomide are used.

Praziquantel in a dose of 15 mg/kg is recommended.

DRUG FOR HETEROPHYIASIS

Praziquantel. It is administered in a single dose of 10-20 mg/kg.

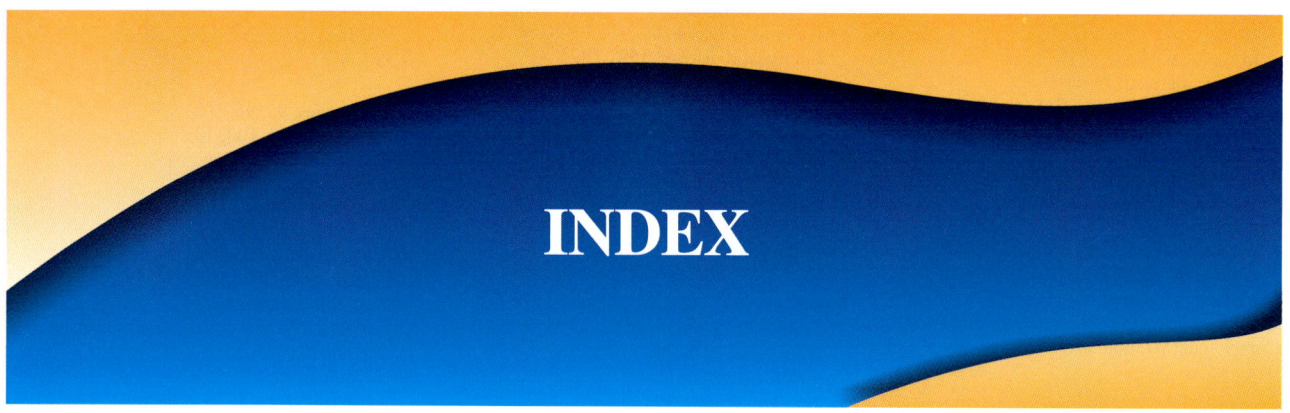

INDEX